Interpretation of Equine
Laboratory Diagnostics

Interpretation of Equine Laboratory Diagnostics

Edited by

Nicola Pusterla

University of California-Davis
California, USA

Jill Higgins

Equine Consulting Services-Penryn
California, USA

WILEY Blackwell

Registered Office(s)
John Wiley & Sons, Inc., 111 River Street, Hoboken, NJ 07030, USA

Editorial Office
111 River Street, Hoboken, NJ 07030, USA

For details of our global editorial offices, customer services, and more information about Wiley products visit us at www.wiley.com.

Wiley also publishes its books in a variety of electronic formats and by print-on-demand. Some content that appears in standard print versions of this book may not be available in other formats.

Library of Congress Cataloging-in-Publication Data

Names: Pusterla, Nicola, 1967– editor. | Higgins, Jill, 1977– editor.
Title: Interpretation of equine laboratory diagnostics / edited by Nicola Pusterla, Jill Higgins.
Description: Hoboken, NJ : Wiley, 2017. | Includes bibliographical references and index. |
Identifiers: LCCN 2017026727 (print) | LCCN 2017027883 (ebook) | ISBN 9781118922811 (pdf) |
    ISBN 9781118922804 (epub) | ISBN 9781118739792 (cloth)
Subjects: | MESH: Horse Diseases–physiopathology | Horse Diseases–diagnosis |
    Diagnostic Techniques and Procedures–veterinary | Clinical Laboratory Techniques–methods
Classification: LCC SF951 (ebook) | LCC SF951 .I58 2017 (print) | NLM SF 951 |
    DDC 636.10896075–dc23
LC record available at https://lccn.loc.gov/2017026727

Cover Design and Images: Courtesy of Nicola Pusterla

Set in 10/12pt Warnock by SPi Global, Pondicherry, India
Printed and bound by CPI Group (UK) Ltd, Croydon, CR0 4YY

C9781118739792_040124

Contents

Contributors

Monica Aleman
Department of Medicine and Epidemiology
School of Veterinary Medicine
University of California
California
USA

Barry Ball
Gluck Equine Research Center
Department of Veterinary Science
University of Kentucky
Kentucky
USA

Barbara A. Byrne
Department of Pathology, Microbiology and
Immunology
School of Veterinary Medicine
University of California
California
USA

Kelli L. Barr
Department of Infectious Diseases and Pathology
College of Veterinary Medicine
University of Florida
Florida
USA

Ashley G. Boyle
Department of Clinical Studies
New Bolton Center
School of Veterinary Medicine
University of Pennsylvania
Pennsylvania
USA

Marjory B. Brooks
The Comparative Coagulation Laboratory
Animal Health Diagnostic Center

College of Veterinary Medicine
Cornell University
New York
USA

Alan Conley
Department of Population Health and Reproduction
School of Veterinary Medicine
University of California
California
USA

Beate Crossley
California Animal Health and Food Safety Laboratory
Department of Medicine and Epidemiology
School of Veterinary Medicine
University of California
California
USA

Joshua B. Daniels
Department of Microbiology, Immunology and
Pathology
College of Veterinary Medicine & Biomedical Sciences
Colorado State University
Colorado
USA

Ghislaine A. Dujovne
Department of Population Health and Reproduction
School of Veterinary Medicine
University of California
California
USA

Krista E. Estell
Department of Medicine and Epidemiology
School of Veterinary Medicine
University of California
California
USA

Julia B. Felippe
Cornell University
College of Veterinary Medicine
New York
USA

C. Langdon Fielding
Loomis Basin Equine Medical Center
California
USA

Carrie J. Finno
Department of Population Health and Reproduction
School of Veterinary Medicine
University of California
California
USA

Janet Foley
Department of Medicine and Epidemiology
School of Veterinary Medicine
University of California
California
USA

Nicholas Frank
Department of Clinical Sciences
Cummings School of Veterinary Medicine
Tufts University
Massachusetts
USA

Connie J. Gebhart
Veterinary and Biomedical Sciences
University of Minnesota
Minnesota
USA

Alonso Guedes
University of Minnesota
Minnesota
USA

Jill Higgins
Equine Consulting Services-Penryn
California
USA

Ashley Hill
California Animal Health and Food Safety Laboratory
Department of Medicine and Epidemiology
School of Veterinary Medicine
University of California
California
USA

Emir Hodzic
Department of Medicine and Epidemiology
School of Veterinary Medicine
University of California
California
USA

Robin Houston
William R. Pritchard Veterinary Medical Teaching Hospital
School of Veterinary Medicine
University of California
California
USA

Amy L. Johnson
Department of Clinical Studies – New Bolton Center
University of Pennsylvania School of Veterinary Medicine
Pennsylvania
USA

Jennifer Jeske
Department of Medicine and Epidemiology
School of Veterinary Medicine
University of California
California
USA

Christian M. Leutenegger
IDEXX Laboratories, Inc.
California
USA

Maureen T. Long
Department of Infectious Diseases and Pathology
College of Veterinary Medicine
University of Florida
Florida
USA

K. Gary Magdesian
Department of Medicine and Epidemiology
School of Veterinary Medicine
University of California
California
USA

Melissa Mazan
Cummings School of Veterinary Medicine
Tufts University
Massachusetts
USA

Linda Mittel
Department of Population Medicine and Diagnostic
Sciences
College of Veterinary Medicine
Cornell University
New York
USA

SallyAnne L. Ness
Hospital for Animals
College of Veterinary Medicine
Cornell University
New York
USA

Jorge Nieto
Department of Surgical and Radiological Sciences
School of Veterinary Medicine
University of California
California
USA

Jed Overmann
Veterinary Clinical Sciences Department
College of Veterinary Medicine
University of Minnesota
Minnesota
USA

Angela Pelzel-McCluskey
United States Department of Agriculture
Animal and Plant Health Inspection Service
Veterinary Services
Colorado
USA

M. Cecilia T. Penedo
Veterinary Genetics Laboratory
School of Veterinary Medicine
University of California
California
USA

Robert H. Poppenga
California Animal Health and Food Safety Laboratory
System and
Department of Molecular Biosciences
School of Veterinary Medicine
University of California at Davis
California
USA

Nicola Pusterla
Department of Medicine and Epidemiology
School of Veterinary Medicine

University of California
California
USA

M. Judith Radin
Department of Veterinary Biosciences
The Ohio State University College of Veterinary
Medicine
Ohio
USA

Camilla J. Scott
William R. Pritchard Veterinary Medical Teaching
Hospital
School of Veterinary Medicine
University of California
California
USA

Leslie Sharkey
Department of Veterinary Clinical Sciences
College of Veterinary Medicine
University of Minnesota
Minnesota
USA

Sharon J. Spier
Department of Medicine and Epidemiology
School of Veterinary Medicine
University of California
California
USA

Nicole Stephenson
Department of Medicine and Epidemiology
School of Veterinary Medicine
University of California
California
USA

Mary H. Straub
Department of Medicine and Epidemiology
School of Veterinary Medicine
University of California
California
USA

Sandra D. Taylor
Department of Veterinary Clinical Sciences
College of Veterinary Medicine
Purdue University
Indiana
USA

Josie Traub-Dargatz
Colorado State University
College of Veterinary Medicine and
Biomedical Sciences
Department of Clinical Sciences
Colorado
USA

Jan Trela
Department of Surgical and Radiological Sciences
School of Veterinary Medicine
University of California
California
USA

Wendy Vaala
Merck Animal Health
New York
USA

Anita Varga
Gold Coast Veterinary Service and Consulting
California
USA

Bettina Wagner
Department of Population Medicine and
Diagnostic Science
College of Veterinary Medicine
Cornell University
New York
USA

W. David Wilson
Department of Medicine and Epidemiology
School of Veterinary Medicine
University of California
California
USA

Preface

As equine practitioners, we are blessed to be in a field that is constantly and rapidly advancing. With the discovery of emerging or re-emerging diseases, equine practitioners, like ourselves, are challenged to not only understand these new entities, but also be able to use appropriate diagnostic tests and adequately interpret their results. The objectives of this book are to help equine veterinarians with the interpretation of equine laboratory diagnostics as they apply to hematology, clinical chemistry, serology and molecular diagnostics. There are currently incredible equine medical texts that address the laboratory diagnostic approach of certain diseases. However, much of their focus is devoted to the clinical presentation, pathophysiology of the disease, and treatment options. This book represents a unique compilation of both established and new diagnostics that are routinely offered by diagnostic laboratories across North America in an easy-to-use manual written by leading experts in the various fields. Our goal was to link the principles of clinical pathology in hematology, clinical chemistry, serology, molecular diagnostics, and genetics with clinical understanding and then translate the results of such investigation into a format that is readily usable by the busy equine veterinarian. This book is a quick reference guide for veterinary students, veterinary technicians and equine veterinarians, who have a need for laboratory diagnostics in their daily equine practice and studies. One of the main challenges in the veterinary profession we've experienced is locating accurate information on the meaning of certain diagnostic laboratory results taking into account their potential advantages and pitfalls. Who has the time to stay up-to-the-minute current with the newly-developed assays and to develop a level of comfort with their use without having any specific experience in interpretation of their results? This book offers an easy and practical introduction to currently available tests, helps with understanding of the results by providing examples, presents comparative data on test performance, and makes reference to the laboratories that offer such testing.

It is our personal goal to make professional life a little bit easier for our fellow hardworking equine veterinarians who are also doing double time being great moms and dads, husbands and wives, and all of the other roles that we play. Our hope is that this manual will become your go-to, quick reference guide that frees up your time to do the things that really matter... caring for horses, training the next generation of equine veterinarians, and making a difference in this world. Thank you to everyone who believed in the idea behind this book and to our families for allowing us the time and opportunity to work on it together. It has been a fun adventure!

Nic and Jill

Veterinary Diagnostic Testing

Linda Mittel

Department of Population Medicine and Diagnostic Sciences, College of Veterinary Medicine, Cornell University, New York, USA

1.1 Introduction

Most veterinary diagnostic laboratories have websites or booklets describing requirements for diagnostic sampling. These resources have descriptions of the sample needed, volume, temperature requirements for shipping, and other valuable information to assist the referring veterinarian.

Obtaining diagnostic samples from animals may present zoonotic disease exposure to the veterinarian. The veterinarian should always be aware of zoonotic diseases, transboundary diseases and even potential bioterrorism acts when collecting diagnostic samples. One of the most recognized potential zoonotic exposures for veterinarians is rabies and this should be on the differential in any neurological case. Any neurological case should be carefully handled when obtaining brain or any samples from the horses.

Additionally, foreign animal diseases (FAD)/transboundary diseases should be on the differential when clinical signs suggest such. International movement of horses legally and illegally may introduce FADs into the United States and consultation with the USDA and state veterinarians should be done prior to any sampling should veterinarians have any concerns about these possibilities.

Veterinary diagnostic testing utilizes many of the rapidly developing testing platforms including PCR, sequencing, multi-array, and MALDI-TOF to assist in diagnosis. Testing procedures are changing frequently and veterinarians must familiarize themselves with their referral laboratories' website or contact the lab to stay abreast of new sampling requirements, and tests.

Many large state veterinary diagnostic laboratories are full-service laboratories and provide assistance to veterinarians in diagnostic plans, choosing tests and samples for suspected illnesses. State veterinary laboratories may be accredited by the American Association of Veterinary Laboratory Diagnosticians (AAVLD), which is an organization that promotes the improvement of veterinary diagnostics and standards for testing (see www.aavld.org/mission-vision-core-values). Veterinarians should work closely with their laboratory to be assured that they are familiar with the most current and correct sample collection and handling required by the laboratory.

Most laboratories have specialized sections for testing which include: clinical pathology, anatomical pathology, endocrinology, coagulation, bacteriology, virology, molecular diagnostics, and toxicology. Referral to other laboratories is routinely done by large laboratories due to the extensive testing requirements and recognized expertise of other laboratories.

1.2 Diagnostic Sampling

1.2.1 Whole Blood

One of the most frequently tested body fluids in the equine is blood.

- Most veterinary blood tests are done on whole blood, plasma or serum.
- A number of different blood tubes, transport vials, and so on, should be available to veterinarians at all times to obtain diagnostic samples such as CBCs and blood chemistries.
- Some blood tests require specialized collection tubes or containers that are not routinely stocked at veterinary practices and may be purchased from the laboratory.
- Consultation with your laboratory or review of their website should be done prior to blood sample collections to ensure quality and diagnostic samples.
- Special attention should be made to the specimen, the manner of collection, appropriate transport container, temperature requirements, correct test requests, and

complete paperwork. Most laboratories welcome assisting veterinarians to help ensure the correct samples are collected.

1.2.2 Order of Draw

The order in which blood samples are drawn when multiple blood collection tubes are being collected from the animal is called "order of draw." Although this is not routinely practiced in veterinary medicine, it is suggested to follow the order of draw. Advanced techniques and the improved detection levels in diagnostic tests may cause inaccurate results from carry over between tubes with additives. It has been determined which additives affects test results and drawing the blood in the correct order is necessary, but some researchers feel the difference is minimum. The order of draw for most veterinary applications is: sterile tubes (blood cultures), light blue, red top, or SST, dark green, and purple (Box 1.1). If additional tubes are going to be drawn consultation with the lab should be done.

1.3 Collection, Preparation, and Handling

1.3.1 Blood Collection Tubes

Various types of evacuated blood-drawing supplies should be kept on hand in a clinic or in an ambulatory vehicle for equine diagnostic testing. Additional blood collecting supplies may include specialized blood-drawing needles, needle holders, and butterfly collection device needles.

There are numerous specialized blood collection tubes that are used in human medicine that can be used in veterinary diagnostic testing for special and routine tests (Figure 1.1). These tubes include: (1) trace element tube (royal blue cap), (2) thrombin based clot tube with activator gel for serum separation (orange cap), (3) glucose determinations (gray cap), (4) lead determination (tan caps), purple/lavender caps, and (5) blood culture collection tubes and DNA testing tubes (yellow capped with sodium polyanethol sulfonate (SPS) and others for specified tests.

Important facts about evacuated blood collection tubes:

- Expiration date
  - Blood collection tubes expiration dates are stamped on the tubes.
  - Out of date tubes may lose vacuum because of dried out stoppers and cause incomplete seals, incomplete filling of tube, and additives may become inactive over time.
  - Plastic collection tubes may not maintain the same shelf life as glass.
- Tube size and complete fill
  - Evacuated tubes are designed to auto-fill to a designated amount and should be allowed to fill until blood stops flowing automatically.
  - Under-filling tubes with additives will adversely affect results.
  - If there is a likelihood that a tube will not be filled to the correct volume, smaller tube sizes should be used to ensure the correct dilution of blood to the additive. Blood collection tubes/containers come in various sizes.

Box 1.1 Key points of blood sampling.

- Review the referral laboratory website or contact the lab to obtain information.
- Required sample type: plasma, serum, whole blood, etc.
- Animal preparation: fasting, at rest, after exercise, after medications, etc.
- Volume of required sample. The minimum volume allows one single analysis including instrument dead volume.
- Collection tube type and size: EDTA, heparin, citrate, glass, plastic tube, microtube, etc.
- Sample handling after collection: clotting time, centrifugation, temperature requirements.
- Shipping and handling requirements: receipt at the laboratory within stated time, chilled, frozen, room temperature, and so on.
- Do not freeze sera in glass tubes.
- Storage temperature is specified as room temperature (15–30 °C), refrigerated (2–10 °C), or frozen (−20 °C or colder).

- Samples after collection should immediately be placed in appropriate temperature holding areas until testing is begun or until prepared for shipping to referral lab.
- An air-dried blood smear should accompany EDTA samples for hemogram if testing not performed within 3–5 h post collection.
- Slides should be labeled with a pencil or diamond point pen.
- Cells in collection tubes with anticoagulants/additives may develop artifactual changes; therefore, air-dried slides should be made to prevent these changes.
- Slides should be placed in slide mailers away from moisture and formalized tissues/samples. Formalin fumes affect air dried slides and may render cytology smear nondiagnostic.

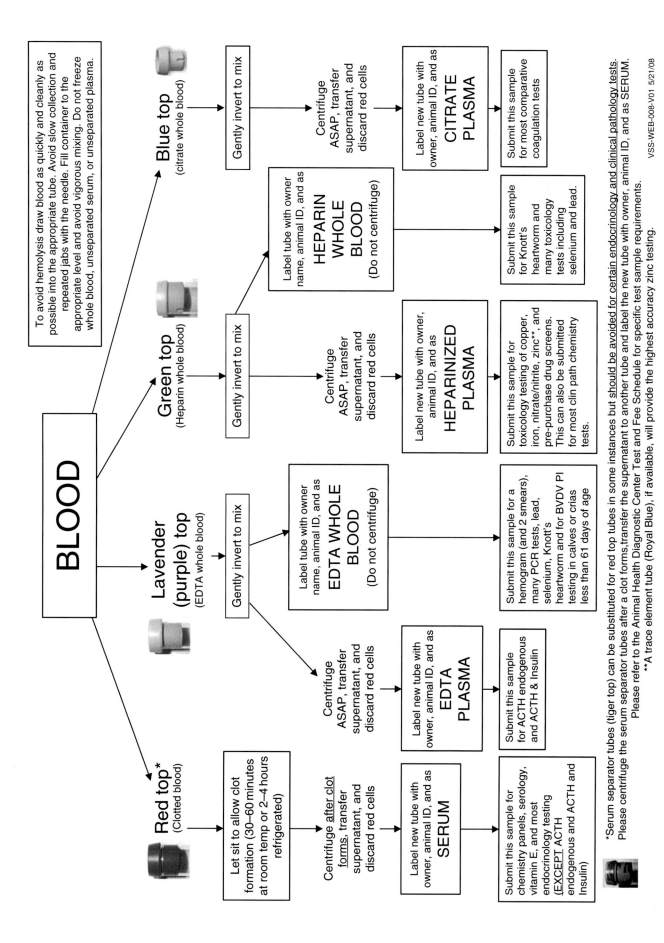

BLOOD

To avoid hemolysis draw blood as quickly and cleanly as possible into the appropriate tube. Avoid slow collection and repeated jabs with the needle. Fill container to the appropriate level and avoid vigorous mixing. Do not freeze whole blood, unseparated serum, or unseparated plasma.

Red top* (Clotted blood)

Let sit to allow clot formation (30–60 minutes at room temp or 2–4 hours refrigerated)

Centrifuge after clot forms, transfer supernatant, and discard red cells

Label new tube with owner, animal ID, and as SERUM

Submit this sample for chemistry panels, serology, vitamin E, and most endocrinology testing (EXCEPT ACTH endogenous and ACTH and Insulin)

Lavender (purple) top (EDTA whole blood)

Gently invert to mix

Label tube with owner name, animal ID, and as EDTA WHOLE BLOOD (Do not centrifuge)

Submit this sample for a hemogram (and 2 smears), many PCR tests, lead, selenium, Knott's heartworm and for BVDV PI testing in calves or crias less than 61 days of age

Centrifuge ASAP, transfer supernatant, and discard red cells

Label new tube with owner, animal ID, and as EDTA PLASMA

Submit this sample for ACTH endogenous and ACTH & Insulin

Green top (Heparin whole blood)

Gently invert to mix

Label tube with owner name, animal ID, and as HEPARIN WHOLE BLOOD (Do not centrifuge)

Submit this sample for Knott's heartworm and many toxicology tests including selenium and lead.

Centrifuge ASAP, transfer supernatant, and discard red cells

Label new tube with owner, animal ID, and as HEPARINIZED PLASMA

Submit this sample for toxicology testing of copper, iron, nitrate/nitrite, zinc**, and pre-purchase drug screens. This can also be submitted for most clin path chemistry tests.

Blue top (citrate whole blood)

Gently invert to mix

Centrifuge ASAP, transfer supernatant, and discard red cells

Label new tube with owner, animal ID, and as CITRATE PLASMA

Submit this sample for most comparative coagulation tests

*Serum separator tubes (tiger top) can be substituted for red top tubes in some instances but should be avoided for certain endocrinology and clinical pathology tests. Please centrifuge the serum separator tubes after a clot forms, transfer the supernatant to another tube and label the new tube with owner, animal ID, and as SERUM. Please refer to the Animal Health Diagnostic Center Test and Fee Schedule for specific test sample requirements.

**A trace element tube (Royal Blue), if available, will provide the highest accuracy zinc testing.

VSS-WEB-008-V01 5/21/08

Figure 1.1 Blood flow chart. *Source:* Courtesy of Linda Mittel.

- Adhere to volume requested by laboratory because requested volume is used for verification of results, add-on tests, and parallel (acute and convalescent serology) testing.
- Necessary volume should be calculated prior to collecting samples.
- Mature normal sized horses should yield 4 ml of serum from each 10 cc blood drawn: 5 ml of plasma should be obtained from 10 ml of whole blood.
- These volumes may vary with hydration, health status (anemia) and other conditions.
- Foals or seriously anemic animals may require that smaller volumes of blood be taken.
- Microtubes ranging from 200 to 600 microliters and other blood collection tubes are readily available ranging in sizes from 2 to 10 ml.
- Butterfly collection lines/winged infusion sets may be used to obtain blood samples in the case of inaccessibility to the jugular veins, small vessel size, fractious animals, or difficult approaches.
- Butterfly collection lines/winged infusion sets can be placed directly into the blood collection tube, but a syringe should be attached to butterfly lines to obtain the blood to prevent vessels collapse from undue pressures. Note that butterfly collection needles/winged infusion sets have been recognized to be one cause of a large number of needle sticks to technicians and staff. Appropriate care should be done to prevent this.
- Blood may be drawn directly into syringes and transferred to appropriate tubes. Special transfer devices are available to transfer blood from syringe to collection device/tube.
- Special handling of these samples drawn by syringes must be done to prevent hemolysis, damage to the cells, and under/over filling of the tubes. The needle should be removed from syringe carefully (do not recap) and push the plunger steadily, but gently to prevent hemolysis and run the blood down the side of the opened tube. The correct volume should be placed in the tube and immediately stoppered and inverted as required.

1.4 Blood Sample Handling after Collection

All blood samples should be collected and gently mixed by inverting the tubes immediately after collection. The inside of certain tubes is sprayed with additives and sample must be inverted multiple times to allow contact with the additive and mixing of the blood.

- EDTA, heparin and other additive invert 8–10 ×
- SST, red top and plastic serum tubes invert 5 ×
- Sodium citrate tubes invert 3–4 ×
- Blood culture vials invert 8–10 ×

Plasma and serum are obtained from different types of tubes. Plasma is obtained from whole blood with an additive/anticoagulant. Serum is obtained from clotted blood.

1.5 Centrifugation of Blood Samples

Blood samples and other diagnostic samples may need to be centrifuged to separate components.

- The normal waiting time for blood to clot is ~30 min.
- Centrifugation of clotted blood to obtain serum or anticoagulated blood to obtain plasma is typically done at 1000–1200 g for 10–15 min. Some blood collection tube manufacturers have specific centrifuge speed requirements and review of these requirements may be necessary prior to sample handling.
- Temperatures during centrifugation should be between 20–22 °C. If analytes are temperature-labile, centrifugation should be done at 4 °C or refrigerated.
- Serum collection
  - Serum collection tubes should be handled as suggested by tube manufacturer and as required by the laboratory.
  - Blood collected in a plain red top tube, serum separator tube (SST), or a tube to obtain serum should be allowed to clot at room temperature for a minimum of 30 min and no longer than 2 h before centrifugation and removal of the clot.
  - Special serum collection tubes are available to expedite clotting within 30 min. Orange capped SST tube with thrombin manufactured by Becton Dickson allows for clotting in 5 min and is commonly used in emergency situations.
  - The premature spinning of samples prior to full clotting will cause difficulty in separating the clot from the sera and may cause hemolysis, change in electrolytes, and analytes that may adversely affect results.
  - Refrigeration prior to the clot formation may affect results and cause spurious values particularly potassium levels.
  - Hemolyzed blood can adversely affect blood chemistry analytes.
  - Blood potassium, and total bilirubin can be affected by hemolysis.
  - Tubes should be spun in a centrifuge after clotting and serum should be promptly removed with a disposable pipette and placed into another plain red top tube or transport vial and stored at designated temperature.

- Vitamin E and bilirubin are light sensitive and should be wrapped in aluminum foil or stored in dark container as should all light sensitive samples.
- Ammonia, certain blood coagulation testing, and ACTH are temperature sensitive. These analytes must be collected and chilled/frozen immediately.
- Some serum samples for serological testing may be kept at room temperature, but it is best to refrigerate or freeze sera after collection and during shipment.
- Sera should be frozen to prevent protein breakdown and bacterial contamination,
- particularly when samples will be held longer periods of time (2–3 weeks) for parallel testing of acute and convalescent serum samples.
- Serum separator tubes (SST) or "tiger tops" (ref) have a special gel that allows for easier separation of the sera from the clot after centrifugation. This gel does not make a complete seal between the cells and serum (or plasma) and the tube should be centrifuged and serum removed from the cells to prevent changes in analyte values.
- SST tubes should not be re-centrifuged because potassium values will be spuriously elevated.
- Plasma collection
  - Plasma is obtained from whole blood tubes with additives or anticoagulants such as EDTA, heparin, and citrate.
  - Whole blood is spun in a centrifuge and the supernatant, plasma, is removed with a disposable pipette. There are plasma collection tubes with gel to aid in the separation of the plasma from the cells. Plasma is collected and placed in a transport vial or plain red top tube. It is imperative to identify the plasma source (EDTA plasma, citrated plasma, etc.) because the additives/anticoagulant may affect the test and some tests are validated with a specific plasma type and it required for testing.

1.6 Blood Culture Sampling

- Blood cultures are used in veterinary medicine in cases of sepsis, fevers of unknown origins, and other potential bacteremia/fungemic conditions. Use of blood cultures will assist in identification of the infectious agent associated with the illness and decrease the overuse of antibiotics.
- Specialized blood culture vials/tubes are required.
- A set of both anaerobic and aerobic blood culture samples should be drawn at the same time.
- Three sets (aerobic and anaerobic) should be drawn over a 24-h period. Sampling should occur prior to initiating therapy. In critically ill animals in need of antimicrobial therapy, two sets of blood cultures can be drawn within 15 min of each other and antimicrobials administered afterward.
- Samples should be drawn as a fever is rising to optimize isolating of bacterial organisms.
- Aseptic collection techniques are critical to prevent sample contamination and subsequent confusion on the interpretation and validity of results.
- Blood culture vials are available with resins to remove antimicrobials from blood for culture.
- Inoculated blood culture vials should be protected from temperature extremes, bright light and never be chilled.
- Blood culture vials should be taken to the laboratory as soon as possible (within 3 h) after collection, but if shipped to a referral lab, vials should be maintained at room temperature prior to and during shipping. Samples must be shipped overnight.
- Ship the blood culture vials in an insulated container to prevent temperature extremes.
- Patient identification should be noted on vial, time, and location of draw (which vein used, etc.) to prevent future resampling blood cultures in the same area.

1.7 Laboratory Validation of Blood Samples

Blood tests are validated on specific types of blood samples or products (plasma or serum) and reference values are established using these validated samples. Certain tests are required to be done on specific specimens; that is, CBCs must be done on whole blood from EDTA tubes or capillary tubes with EDTA anticoagulant in the tube.

- Heparinized whole blood causes distortion of the RBCs and is not acceptable for a hemogram.
- The specific type of plasma should be identified, that is, heparinized plasma, citrated plasma or EDTA plasma and noted on transport tube along with other animal identification, date, and initials of the person who drew the sample.
- Heparinized plasma is used for some toxicology testing.
- EDTA plasma is used for testing ACTH.
- Citrated plasma is used in coagulation studies.

Each laboratory may have their own specific requirements and this should be reviewed prior to sampling. Every veterinary laboratory does not have the same requirements.

1.8 Specimens, Transport Containers, and Media for Various Disciplines

1.8.1 Clinical Pathology

Emergency testing and routine tests are the norm for this section and turnaround times are usually quick. There are many routine tests that are performed in this section, but sophisticated testing is also done such as flow cytometry, immunophenotyping, and body fluid analysis (synovial fluid, pulmonary fluid, abdominal fluid, cerebrospinal fluid). Clinical pathology testing compliments most other laboratory sections and is often one of the first tests requested in diagnostic workups.

The section on blood collection and testing in this manual applies to most of the blood sample submissions to clinical pathology. Other equine samples that are processed in clinical pathology require special handling/collection include:

- Tracheal wash fluid, joint/synovial fluid, cerebrospinal fluid, bronchoalveolar lavage fluid, bone marrow, urine, and various needle aspirates submitted for cytological evaluation and analysis require submission in a sterile red top/EDTA tube.
- If cytological evaluation is requested, air dried smears of the fluid from either the red top tube or the EDTA tube should be sent with the sample in order to preserve the cellular components from breakdown and facilitate interpretation. These slides should be sent in slide mailers and kept dry.
- If culture will be requested on body fluid samples, a sterile red top tube or vial should be sent in addition to the EDTA sample. EDTA is bactericidal and not acceptable for aerobic or anaerobic bacterial culture or fungal culture. A sterile red top tube or sterile transport vial is required for aerobic fluid culture.
- Anaerobic culture on fluid samples requires the use of an anaerobic transport media. Anaerobic vials, large mouth screw top lids, vials with septum for needle injections or bottles are available for fluids, and tissues. Saturated swabs are not the preferred sample.
- Synovial fluid should be placed in a sterile red top and EDTA tube. Air dried slides should be made and submitted. Samples with small number of cells may require that the sample be cytospinned and slides made from the pellet on arrival at the lab to obtain a good representation of the cellular components.
- Bronchoalveolar lavage (BAL) samples should be sent in an EDTA blood collection tube and a plain red top tube chilled for overnight delivery. Air dried smears made direct from the EDTA tube should be submitted

with the fluids (cells in a low protein fluid such as the saline lavage fluid may breakdown and become difficult to identify).
- Tracheal wash samples should be placed in both, a sterile red top tube for culture and an EDTA tube for cytological evaluation. Air dried smears should be made from the EDTA sample tube.

1.8.2 Microbiology

This lab section is responsible for the growth, identification, and antibiogram of bacteria, yeasts, and fungal agents. The advent of new technology has allowed for quick and novel bacterial identification. The MALDI-TOF™ machine has revolutionized the identification time of bacteria to minutes versus days. PCR and sequencing are other testing platforms that are used for bacterial and fungal identification. Collaboration with the molecular section of the laboratory is done many times to assist in identifications.

- Bacterial sampling and transport media
  - Sampling for isolation of bacteria and fungi may require specialized transport media (TM) to allow shipping/transfer to a referral laboratory.
  - Anaerobic and aerobic blood culture has specialized collection media. Amies transport media with or without charcoal and modified Stuart's medium are three of the commonly used aerobic bacterial TM. Amies TM with charcoal is used in veterinary medicine for the isolation of fastidious organisms such as *Taylorella* sp. and is required in contagious equine metritis regulatory testing.
  - Specialized enteric TM are available for assisting in the recovery of enteric organisms such as Para Pak™ transport media. This TM does not need refrigeration after inoculation for shipment.
  - Anaerobic vials, jars with large mouth lids, and tubes are available for fluids, tissue samples, and swabs, respectively. Some manufacturers sell anaerobic culture tubes with screw top tubes with special injection septum for liquid sample introduction or for swab introduction. Anaerobic transport media is required for swabs, body fluids, small pieces of tissue for anaerobic bacterial isolation. Anaerobic culture can be performed on fresh tissue that is > 2–3 cm in diameter (where the center of the tissue has maintained anaerobic conditions). The samples should arrive to the laboratory within 24 h of collection.
  - Tied off loops of bowel can be submitted for anaerobic enteric culture where laboratory will culture contents/tissue for anaerobes.
  - Fresh tissues samples must arrive chilled or frozen within 24 h after animal's death whereas inoculated

anaerobic transport media must be kept at room temperature for shipping and handling and arrive within 24 h.

- *Clostridium* toxin tests can be done on fresh feces, but toxin proteins are extremely heat-labile and samples should be frozen as soon as obtained and shipped frozen within 24 h of collection.
- Proper inoculation and handling of the anaerobic TM before inoculation and during is required to maintain anaerobic conditions. Tubes should be stored upright and when inoculating so to prevent loss of gas cap (see https://ahdc.vet.cornell.edu/docs/Anaerobic_Culture-Inoculation_of_Anaerobic_Transport_Media.pdf).
- Inoculated anaerobic transport media must be maintained at room temperature.
- Botulism PCR testing is done for the presence of *Clostridium botulinum* genes in feed, intestinal tissue and feces. This testing is done at the National Botulism Reference laboratory at the University of Pennsylvania, School of Veterinary medicine (www.vet.upenn.edu/veterinary-hospitals/NBC-hospital/diagnostic-laboratories/national-botulism-reference-laboratory).

- Fungal sampling and transport media
  - Transport media used for suspect systemic fungal infections is the same as for bacterial cultures. Consultation with the lab prior to suspect fungal submission is suggested. The use of molecular testing (PCR) for fungal identification directly from the clinical sample requires special handling and bacterial transport media cannot be used.
  - Dermatophytes do not require specialized TM.
  - Skin scrapings, hair, and horn/hoof samples should be sent in dry containers/paper envelopes to prevent moisture condensation and overgrowth with contaminants.
  - Skin, corneal fluid, tissue samples/biopsies should be placed into sterile screw top transport vials with a drop of sterile saline, chilled, and shipped for arrival to lab within 24 h.
  - Systemic fungal infection swab samples can be transported in aerobic and anaerobic bacterial media (Port a cul™) or the previously discussed anaerobic containers.
  - Inoculated bacterial transport media with fungal samples should be shipped and handled as discussed in the bacterial section.
  - Swabs obtained from the cornea, uterus/endometrium, and other locations should be inoculated into aerobic or anaerobic transport media and shipped chilled or room temperature, respectively. Actual tissue sample is preferred for culture.

- All samples must be shipped overnight and arrive chilled to the laboratory to prevent overgrowth by contaminants.
- If both fungal and bacterial testing is to be done, two swabs should be obtained to assure adequate sample volume.

1.8.3 Molecular Testing

The development of molecular assays has increased the breadth of testing for infectious pathogens. Molecular diagnostic laboratories utilize various molecular diagnostic modalities, including nucleic acid amplification techniques, and sequencing technologies.

- Universal viral transport medium (liquid) is available from various manufacturers and is room temperature stable for viral transport, maintenance, and long-term freeze storage.
- All body fluids including whole blood, serum, CSF, respiratory fluid samples, urine, and feces are acceptable samples for viral testing.
- Viral isolation is still very important even with the advent of PCR. Isolation allows for vaccine development, anti-viral treatments, and identification of novel agents. However, viral isolation requires that the sample contains at least a moderate viral load in order to successfully grow virus.
- Bacterial transport media cannot be used for viral PCR testing.
- Dacron- or rayon-tipped swabs are preferred for PCR and viral testing.
- Freezing tissues and samples can preserve samples for later viral testing, however, repeated freeze thaw is not recommended.

1.8.4 Parasitology

The parasitology section provides identification of parasites by various methods. These include direct fecal smear examinations, fecal flotations, fresh and fixed tissue samples for parasite identification, whole parasite identification, serological, and molecular testing.

- Fecal floatation testing requires 1–2 normally formed fecal balls (approximately 10 g of feces) from an average horse for quantification. Samples should be sent in a clean anaerobic leak-proof containers/plastic bag. Samples should not be submitted in an exam glove or rectal sleeve.
- Fresh feces submitted for fecal floatation must not be exposed to temperature extremes. Eggs may rupture/hatch in sample and the sample may become nondiagnostic.

- The McMaster, Wisconsin, and other modified methods may be used to obtain approximate numbers of strongyle egg counts and are frequently performed in private veterinary clinics.
- Testing fecal samples for tapeworms, *Anaplocephala perfoliata*, by floatation is not a reliable test due to the intermittent shedding of eggs by the adult tapeworms. Serological testing has been developed but has not gained favor due to the inability to interpret positive results in horses that have been successfully treated for tapeworms, but still remain seropositive.
- Fecal sampling for floatation to assist in determining resistance patterns using fecal egg count reduction test (FECRT) should be obtained 10–14 days post administration of an anthelmintic.
- Fecal samples that cannot be tested soon after collection (within 7 days or less) may be placed into TM such as 10% formalin or polyvinyl alcohol to assist in preserving the ova and the delicate trophozoites forms seen with enteric protozoal infections.
- Fecal samples for larval parasite and identification (strongyle family) should be fresh, kept at room temperature, and contain large numbers of ova on fecal floatation (>100 epg) to insure adequate numbers of larval hatching for identification.
- Lungworms, *Dictyocaulus arnfieldi* can be diagnosed in fresh fecal samples, but requires active floatation techniques and special sugar solutions. Clinical signs or suspect disease should be provided to parasitology lab to allow proper techniques to be performed. Baermann testing is used for diagnosis of lungworms if eggs are not found in fecal samples that have been tested by active floatation methods.
- Pinworms are not routinely found in fecal floatations and the "cellophane tape test" can be used to assist with diagnosis of pinworms ova (cellophane tape is stuck to a clear glass side and examined microscopically).
- Enteric protozoal infections are not thought to be pathological in apparently normal equine adults and foals, but antigen (fecal) ELISA detection tests are readily available for *Giardia*, and cryptosporidium.
- EPM causative agents, *Neospora hughesi* and *Sarcocystis neurona* antibody levels can be detected in serum and CSF by IFAT and ELISA. IHC and PCR are available for detection of the organisms in neurological tissue, but may not be rewarding due to the focal localized areas of infection.
- Skin scrapings and entire/partial parasites submitted for identification must be submitted in a clean escape-proof container such as plain red top blood collection tube or transport vial with screw top lid. Isopropyl alcohol in a red top tube/leak-proof vial can be used to transport and preserve ticks, mites, and other parasites.
- Skin scrapings should be obtained after lightly scraping the affected area until small drops of fresh blood are seen.
- Tissue samples or fresh tissue biopsies for parasite evaluations such as *Oncochera* sp. can be submitted in clean leak-proof containers with a few drops of sterile saline to keep samples moist and prevent dessication of parasite.
- Skin parasites maybe "washed out" during histological sample processing; therefore, a fresh biopsy in addition to the fixed sample should be submitted in a transport vial that prevents desiccation for parasite evaluation.

1.8.5 Toxicology

Toxicology laboratories utilize various types of analytical equipment and instruments, techniques for the detection, identification, and quantification of organic, inorganic, and toxic compounds. Vitamins and mineral testing are often performed in these laboratories. The accurate diagnosis of a toxicosis like many other diseases is made by utilizing information made from criteria. Forensic and legal cases tested in toxicology have stringent requirements for sampling, identification, shipping, and handling. These should be reviewed prior to obtaining samples to prevent serious errors in sampling. Chain of custody may be necessary particularly in forensic cases and possible legal cases. This should be discussed with the laboratory and client that is requesting testing so that the samples are not compromised for use in legal cases.

Drug screens for regulatory, and pre-purchase drug screens have specific requirements such as (1) sample type (i.e., whole blood, urine), (2) blood tube collection types, including EDTA, heparin or serum, and (3) testing volumes. It is critical to follow the laboratory guidelines for testing and sampling since many of these drug screens are associated with legal repercussions and cannot be redrawn.

Ante-mortem samples may include whole blood (blood tube additives may vary on testing and should be discussed with toxicologist), serum, urine, hair, body fluid, reflux, and feces. If unable to contact toxicologist prior to testing whole blood, tubes with EDTA or heparin are generally acceptable. Certain drugs are protein-bound and necessary sampling tubes may vary with each compound; therefore, using both tubes would prevent errors on the part of the submitter.

Samples should be placed in individually identified containers such as plastic sealable bags, sterile urine sample cups or wrapped in aluminum foil for testing lipophilic toxins. Excess air should be removed from plastic bags. Samples should be frozen as soon as possible and kept frozen in a deep freezer (not frost free) until analyzed. Serum should be removed from the clot and frozen.

SST tubes are not appropriate for drug monitoring or toxicological analysis. The gel in SST extracts lipophilic substances which is most drugs; therefore, causing falsely low drug concentrations.

Testing plant materials and forage for possible toxicities should include part of the leaves, stems, flowers and roots. Forage samples should be kept cool and dry or even frozen. Photographs of suspect plants showing stems, roots, flowers, seeds, should be submitted along with plants if available.

Post mortem/necropsy cases should always include a complete "tox set" and be held frozen until needed for testing. This link describes the information and suggested samples for toxicological workups and drug screens (https:// ahdc.vet.cornell.edu/docs/Toxicology_Submissions_and_ Analytica_Screens.pdf). The "tox set" can be used if necessary after histopathology results are obtained or for use in ancillary testing. Tissue material from a necropsy should include brain, liver, kidney, fat, urine, aqueous humor or intact eyeball, skin (site of exposure), heart blood collected in lithium heparinized blood collection tubes, stomach, reflux, intestinal contents, and feces. Collect stomach, intestine, and feces last to prevent contamination of entire carcass. Each sample or tissue should be placed in individually identified container similar to the ante-mortem testing. Most toxicological samples should be frozen and stored in a non-frost proof freezer. Other samples to collect may include paint chips, soil, supplements, and feed, forages, water, and cohort blood and urine samples.

1.8.6 Virology

The virology diagnostic section provides testing for viral agent detection and monitoring in multiple species using viral isolation and serology as the mainstay of testing. The development of PCR and molecular testing has increased the breadth of testing, and this section now utilizes various diagnostic modalities including, nucleic acid amplification techniques, and sequencing technologies.

Fresh tissue samples, and body fluids and products in viral transport media are acceptable samples. Some viruses are unable to be cultured easily or even at all and PCR techniques are being used successfully with these viruses. Viral transport media may optimize viral isolation and can be used in PCR techniques.

- Viral isolation requires that sample has a high viral load in to grow virus. Low numbers of viruses in sample may cause false negatives.
- Multiple species tissue cell lines may be necessary to isolate viruses from various animal species.
- Viral isolation is still very important even with the advent of PCR. Isolation allows for vaccine development, anti-viral treatments, and identification of novel agents.
- Turnaround time with viral isolation may range from 3–30 days.
- Bacterial transport media cannot be used for PCR testing.
- Dacron or rayon flocked swabs are preferred for PCR and viral isolation.
- Acceptable samples for viral isolation or PCR includes nasal swabs, body fluids/discharges, and target tissue samples.
- Universal Transport Medium, is a room temperature stable viral transport media for collection, transport, maintenance, and freezer storage.

1.8.7 Immunology/Serology

This laboratory section is responsible for testing areas that include allergies, autoimmune diseases and presence of antibodies in serum or other body fluids such as CSF, peritoneal fluid, and aqueous humor. Testing includes various platforms such as serum neutralization (SN), hemagglutination inhibition (HI), complement fixation (CF), Western Blot, ELISA, flow cytometry, multiplex, indirect fluorescent antibody (IFA), agar gel immunodiffusion (AGID), microscopic agglutination, serum hemagglutination inhibition (SHI), and cytokines. Most serology tests use an antigen as a reagent to capture antibodies.

- Serum is the most common sample tested, but other body fluids that are validated can also be used such as peritoneal fluid, CSF, and so on.
- Serum should be obtained in a clot tube (SST or red top) and allowed to clot at room temperature and centrifuged. Serum should be removed and placed in a transport tube.
- Acute samples and convalescent sera should be submitted together for parallel testing. Convalescent sera should be drawn 10–21 days after illness depending on agent to be tested for.
- Leptospirosis MAT serum samples should be drawn approximately 10 days post beginning of suspected illness. Further, antimicrobial treatment may blunt leptospirosis antibody response.
- *Anaplasma phagocytophilum* IFA titers develop 5–7 days after infection with agent.
- Titers associated with *Borrelia burgdorferi*, EHV-1/-4, *S. neurona*, *N. hughesi* may produce lifelong antibodies and positive titers are not always associated with active illness.
- Vaccine titers do not correspond to disease-protective levels in animals.
- IgM is the first isotype to elevate after infection followed by IgG.

1.8.8 Anatomical Pathology

Surgical biopsies, post mortem gross examinations, and histology are the most frequently submitted cases. Histology is the most frequently requested test and supporting stains and tests assist in diagnosis.

- Formalin preservation of tissues or biopsy samples should be done as soon as possible to prevent autolysis. The minimum dilution of formalin to tissue should be 10:1.
- Small pieces of tissue are required to allow for fixation. Large pieces of solid tissue should be cut into pieces that are 0.5 cm thick to allow fixation of tissues.
- Formalin preserved tissue should not be allowed to freeze.
- Bouin's solution may be used for fixation of delicate tissues such as with ophthalmic, intestinal tissues and reproductive histological evaluation.

1.8.9 Endocrinology

This laboratory section tests reproductive and metabolic hormones, and vitamins in the horse. This includes progesterone, PMSG, testosterone, granulosa cell tumor testing, metabolic testing including ACTH, leptin, and thyroid tests.

- Serum is the preferred sample for the majority of equine tests except for ACTH testing.
- Serum should be removed after centrifugation from the blood collection tube after clot formation and placed into a plain red top tube or transport vial.
- Hemolyzed samples may adversely affect results.
- Blood collection tubes with activators, SST tubes and activators, or any additives are not acceptable for serum collection.
- Sera should be chilled/frozen after removal from clot and shipped to laboratory to arrive chilled.
- EDTA whole blood testing for Cushing's disease should be chilled immediately after collection and prior to centrifugation. Equine ACTH testing requires EDTA plasma that has been collected after gravitational separation should not be frozen, but chilled. Proteolytic enzymes that may be still in plasma may affect results and cause ACTH values to be inaccurate. Do not place EDTA whole blood too close to ice packs prior to plasma separation for the same reason. EDTA plasma must be frozen as soon as possible after removal from cells and placed in a plain plastic red top tube or plastic transport vial. EDTA plasma should not be placed back into EDTA tubes for transport to laboratory.

If liquid additives have been used as the tube additive sample dilution may occur.

1.8.10 Coagulation

Vascular injury is the most common cause of hemorrhage in the horse, but there are various conditions in the horse that may cause hemostatic failure. Diagnostic testing can aide in this determination, but careful sampling techniques, proper collection and handling are necessary to obtain accurate meaningful results. If the animal is excited splenic contraction may occur and cause elevated blood cell counts and increased platelet counts, alcohol from the skin preparation, sedatives, and analgesics may also affect the results.

There are primary hemostatic (platelet plug tests) and secondary hemostatic and fibrinolysis assays (fibrin clot formation/coagulation) available to assist in the diagnosis.

- Primary hemostatic tests include platelet counts that can be obtained from a stained blood smear by examination of the feathered edge of a smear to detect platelet clumping. This can be done in a clinical pathology laboratory when a CBC is done.
- Routine EDTA tubes used for hemograms are acceptable for making blood smear for platelet evaluation. This requires a careful venipuncture (atraumatic and away from recent venipuncture sites) directly into an evacuated EDTA (purple cap tube), heparin (light green cap) or citrate (light blue cap) collection tube. Complete fill of the tube for the proper ratio for testing is required. After collection mix by inverting 8–10 times. The sample should remain at room temperature, and the smear prepared as soon as possible after collection.
- Secondary hemostatic and fibrinolytic assays are often done with POC units. Automated POC units are available in clinical settings for stall-side testing and require the same correct careful sampling handling as in primary testing. Sample must be collected into a citrate blood collection tube (light blue tube), allow complete autofill, and mix by inversion 8–10 times. Sample may be drawn through intravenous catheter, but sample must be obtained after the catheter has been flushed with 20 cc of sterile calcium free saline. Maintain citrate blood collection tube at room temperature until it is centrifuged. Following centrifugation, place the plasma into a plastic tube. Ship sample chilled or frozen to the laboratory. Hemolyzed samples are not acceptable.

Further Reading

AHDC. https://ahdc.vet.cornell.edu/docs/Blood_Tubes_ and_Labeling_Guidelines.pdf. [Online] 2016. https:// ahdc.vet.cornell.edu/docs/Blood_Tubes_and_Labeling_ Guidelines.pdf.

Arronson DM. 1987. Bor. Annals of Internal Medicine. 106(2): 246–253.

Asirvatham JR, Moses V, and Bjoransen L. 4, April 2013. Errors in potassium measurement: A laboratory perspective for the clinician. North American Journal of Medical Sciences, 5: 255–259.

Baron EJ, Miller JM, Weinstein MP, Richter SS, Gilligan PH, Thomson RB Jr, et al. 2013. A guide to utilization of the microbiology laboratory for diagnosis of infectious diseases: 2013 recommendations by the Infectious Diseases Society of America (IDSA) and the American Society for Microbiology (ASM)(a). Clin Infect Dis. 57(4): e22–e121.

BD Vacutainer Venous Blood Collection Tube Guide. 07 2010.

BD. BD Vacutainer Venous Blood Collection. [Online] 2010. [Cited: October 20, 2015.] https://www.bd.com/ vacutainer/pdfs/plus_plastic_tubes_wallchart_ tubeguide_VS5229.pdf.

Bowen Raffick AR and Remaley AT. 2014. Interferences from blood collection tube components on clinical chemistry. Biochemia Medica, 24: 31–44.

Brooks MB. 2008. Equine coagulopathies. In BW Parry (ed.), Veterinary Clinics of North America. Philadelphia: Elsevier Saunders, Vol. 24, p. 335–355.

Center or Phlebomtony. [Online] https://www.phlebotomy. com/pt-stat/stat0510.html.

Dow SW, Jones RL, and Rosychuk RAW. 1989. Bacteriologic specimens: Selection, collection, and transport for optimum results. The Compendium Small Animal, 11: 686–701.

Frank C, Madden DJ, and Duncan C. 2015. Field necropsy of the horse. Veterinary Clinics of North America Equine Practice 31: 233–245.

Guder WG, Narayanan S, Wisser H, and Zawta B. 2009. Diagnostic Samples: From the Patient to the Laboratory: The Impact of Preanalytical Variables on the Quality of Laboratory Results, 4th Updated Edn. John Wiley & Sons, Ltd, p. 124.

Henry JB and Kurec AS. 1996. The clinical laboratory: Organization, purposes and practices. In JB Henry (ed.), Clinical Diagnosis and Management by Laboratory Methods. Vol. 19. Philadelphia: WB Saunders,

LabCorp. Microbiology Specimen Collection and Transport Guide. [Online] 2015. www.LabCorp.com.

Lappin VS and Michael R. 2012. Enteric protozoal infections. In CE Greene (ed.) Greene's Infectious Disease of Dog and Cat, 4th Edn. Elsevier, pp. 785–792.

Marjani A. 2006. Effect of storage time and temperature on some serum analytes. The Internet Journal of Laboratory Medicine. 2(2): 1–6.

McPherson RA and Pincus MR. 2011. Henry's Clinical Diagnosis and Management. Philadelphia: Elsevier/ Saunders.

Meridian Biosciences, Inc. Meridian Bioscience, Inc. [Online] www.meridianbioscience.com/.

Sanger. Sample Collection for Microbiological Samples. 2008.

Tuck MK, Chan DW, Chia D, Godwin AK, Grizzle WE, Krueger KE, et al., 2009, Standard Operating Procedures for Serum and Plasma Collection: Early Detection Research Network Consensus Statement Standard Operating Procedure Integration Working Group. Journal of Proteome Research, 8: 113–117.

Willard MD and Tvedten H. 2012. Small Animal Clinical Diagnosis by Laboratory Methods. St. Louis: Saunders, an imprint of Elsevier Inc.

Young A. 1990. Blood culture: Indications and technique. Equine Veterinary Education, 2: 38–40.

2

Basic Techniques and Procedures

Emir Hodzic

Department of Medicine and Epidemiology, School of Veterinary Medicine, University of California, California, USA

2.1 Introduction

A small fraction of microorganisms can be categorized as pathogens, or having the ability to incite infectious disease processes in a host. It has been shown that the term "pathogen" can be applied to very few microorganisms, even fewer if pathogenicity is defined as causing infectious disease at all times (Goldmann and Pier, 1993). Traditionally, accurate and prompt identification of pathogenic microorganisms in clinical samples has been a responsibility of microbiologists in a laboratory setting. The effectiveness of the microbiology laboratory depends on appropriate sample selection, collection, and transportation. So, the significance of microorganism detection in clinical samples needs to be discussed between microbiologists and clinicians with regard to maintaining sample quality as well as taking into consideration the roles of the host and environment.

Rapid, sensitive, and specific detection of pathogenic microorganisms is essential for the effective treatment of an infected host. Diagnostic methods in microbiology have a task to make microorganisms "visible" and "measurable," so the methods are either qualitative (presence/absence) or quantitative (absolute number of pathogens, colonies, plaques, or genes).

Until very recently, efforts to detect and identify microorganisms have depended on *in vitro* analysis, where bacteria are grown in culture. Based on Koch's postulates, a bacterium must be shown to grow outside the body in culture in order to prove that it causes disease. In the past, this criterion has posed a problem, as many bacteria are particular in their growth requirements. However, since at least a fraction of microorganisms is not so particular, these efforts have yielded an array of diverse microbial cultivation techniques. Microbial cultivation methods opened up an unsuspected world of microscopic life and presumed causative agents of infectious diseases (Relman, 1998). Over the

years, researchers have pointed out two reasons why the majority of bacteria do not culture: (1) some bacteria only grow in specific conditions offered by the host including a very narrow pH, the right nutrient availability, and so on; and (2) certain bacteria only grow in the presence of certain other species of bacteria (Lamoth and Greub, 2010).

Current testing methods of detecting pathogenic microorganisms have to answer these three basic questions: (1) Is something there (qualitative testing)? (2) If there, how much is present (quantitative testing)? (3) If there, what is it (identification testing) (Moldenhauer, 2008)? Issues in detecting pathogenic microorganisms are as follow: *sensitivity* – detection volume and presence of interfering substances that reduce assay sensitivity; *specificity* – detection of the right organism, or group of organisms; *quantification* – precision and accuracy.

Commonly used methods of pathogen detection include: microscopy, cultivation, biochemical methods, bio-testing, immunological methods, and molecular methods (Murray et al., 1995a, Gracias and McKillip, 2004, Petti, 2007, Lazcka et al., 2007, Nayak et al., 2009). None of these methods are 100% efficient, so it is highly recommended to utilize more than one method, which depends on sample type, clinical symptoms, and suspected pathogen (Pickup, 1991). For bacterial detection, traditional microbiology has proved a time-consuming procedure. Organisms have to be isolated and grown, and usually a series of biochemical tests must be completed for identification (Kaspar and Tartera, 1990). Molecular methods are necessary if the traditional methods provide poor results. Techniques such as the polymerase chain reaction (PCR) used for the amplification of pathogen-specific DNA sequences have proved to be sensitive. However, when using environmental samples, a degree of sample preparation is required since impurities contained within the sample may inhibit the PCR. Furthermore, the

Interpretation of Equine Laboratory Diagnostics, First Edition. Edited by Nicola Pusterla and Jill Higgins.
© 2018 John Wiley & Sons, Inc. Published 2018 by John Wiley & Sons, Inc.

use of small sample volumes means that the cells often has to be concentrated to obtain the desired sensitivity (Radstrom et al., 2004).

2.2 Essential Prerequisites for High-Quality Bacteria Detection

The effectiveness of the laboratory diagnostics depends on the appropriate sample selection, collection, and transportation. If sample collection and handling are not priorities for clinicians, the laboratory can do very little to advance patient care. It is the laboratory's responsibility to provide the necessary information, which should include specific criteria for safety, selection, collection, transportation, sample acceptability, and labeling.

During sample collection, the clinicians should abide by the *safety procedures* in order to protect themselves, the personnel handling the samples, and the sample integrity. All sample collection procedures must be performed while wearing gloves, laboratory coat, and, where appropriate, masks. All sample containers must be leak-proof within a sealable, leak-proof plastic bag. Leaking containers or syringes with needles must never be transported to the laboratory (OSHA, 2011, Gimenez-Marin et al., 2014, CLSI, 2011).

Sample(s) selection should be on the basis of signs and symptoms that represent the disease process, and should be collected before administration of antimicrobial agents. Some infectious diseases are distinctive enough to be identified clinically. Most pathogens, however, can cause a wide spectrum of overlapping clinical syndromes in animals. Conversely, a single clinical syndrome may result from infection with any one of many pathogens. The manifestations of an infection depend on many factors, including the site of acquisition or entry of the microorganism; organ or system tropisms of the microorganism; microbial virulence; the age, sex, and immunologic status of the patient; underlying diseases or conditions. The signs and symptoms of infection may be localized, or they may be systemic. Samples selected for microbiologic examination should reflect the disease process and be collected in sufficient quantity to allow complete microbiologic examination. For example, the number of microorganisms per milliliter of a body fluid or per gram of tissue is highly variable, ranging from less than 1 to 10^8 or 10^{10} colony-forming units (CFU). Swabs, although popular for sample collection, frequently yield too few cells for accurate microbiologic examination and should be used only to collect material from the skin and mucous membranes. Because skin and mucous membranes have a large and diverse indigenous flora, every effort must be made to minimize sample contamination

during collection (Washington, 1996, Rabenau et al., 2010, Panel et al., 2010). If possible, samples should be collected before the administration of antibiotics. Above all, close communication between the clinician and the microbiologist is essential to ensure that appropriate samples are selected and collected and that they are appropriately examined.

Although sample processing is usually well standardized in the diagnostic laboratory, *preanalytic procedures* outside the laboratory usually follow with considerable variability. It has been shown that preanalytic errors make up to 85% of all laboratory errors, with 95% of them occurring outside the laboratory. For example, false negative results may occur due to sample degradation during inadequate transport. Additionally, contamination in the field/during sample collection may cause false-positive results, which could have severe consequences. The main issues of concern during sample transport and storage include sample integrity, contamination, sample identity, and the risk of environmental hazards due to infectious material (Endler and Slavka, 2010, Gimenez-Marin et al., 2014). Samples collected from potentially infected animals are considered hazardous, so the transport outside of the laboratory is subject to national and international regulations. All samples must be *promptly* transported to the diagnostic laboratory, preferably within 2 h. In general, samples for detection of bacterial agents should not be stored for more than 24 h, and no more than 2–3 days at 4 °C for viruses (Miller and Holmes, 1995).

Detection methods depend more and more on the quality of the *sample preparation*. Samples are very heterogeneous (stool, plasma, CSF), so preparation must be a factor to consider in order to achieve results within a reasonable amount of time. Thus, the increasing need for speed and precision in new detection methods illustrates the importance of sophisticated methods for sampling and sample preparation within the overall process. The proper development and adaptation of sample preparation toward the endpoint detection method applied is essential for exploiting the whole potential of the complete workflow of any diagnostic method. The overall goals of sample preparation are: (1) to concentrate the target bacteria, as bacteria may be at low concentrations and detection methods commonly use only small sample volumes; (2) to remove or reduce the effects of inhibitory substances, as sample matrices may be incompatible with the analytical methods; and (3) to reduce the heterogeneity of samples in order to ensure negligible variations between repeated sampling. If homogenized thoroughly, the pooling of samples will facilitate a high throughput analysis.

Quality assurance and *quality control* in the routine diagnostic laboratory must be taken into consideration. Unfortunately, quality assurance and quality control guidelines are not always properly developed or they are highly diverse between laboratories as only a limited number of standards and reference materials are available. Components that are required for validation of used microbiological diagnostic tests or test systems should include: (1) internal and external run control; (2) participation in inter-laboratory test results comparison; (3) validation of employee competence; (4) calibration and maintenance of instruments, and (5) correlation with clinical findings (Raggam et al., 2010, Madej et al., 2010).

2.3 Microbiological Methods for Pathogen Detection

When a new and promising microbiological diagnostic technique is developed, microbiologists quickly incorporate it into pathogen detection methods. For example, the advent of PCR as a DNA amplification technique led to the emergence of methods that rely on PCR for the detection of various pathogens. Although these methods are PCR-based, they normally incorporate other familiar techniques such as culturing and microscopic examination. Microscopy, culture, biochemical, biosensors, immunological, and molecular techniques are used in various pathogen detection methods. Most pathogen detection methods include enrichment (a culture technique) and enzyme-linked immunoassay (an immunological technique) or polymerase chain reaction (a genetic technique) (Yousef, 2008).

2.3.1 Microscopy

The first step in processing clinical material is microscopic examination of the specimen. Direct examination is a rapid, cost-effective aid to identify microorganisms and enumerate cells. Visible microorganisms may denote the presumptive etiological agent, guiding the laboratory in selecting appropriate isolation media and the clinician in selecting empirical antibiotic therapy.

Modern microscope instruments are designed to produce magnified visual or photographic images of objects too small to be seen with the naked eye. The microscope must accomplish three tasks: (1) produce a magnified image of the sample, (2) separate the details in the image, and (3) render the details visible to the human eye or camera. For microscopic examination, it is sufficient to have a compound binocular microscope equipped with achromatic objectives, wide-field oculars, a mechanical stage, a sub stage condenser, and a good light source. For examination of wet-mount preparations, a dark field condenser, or condenser and objectives for phase contrast, increases image contrast. An exciter barrier filter, dark field condenser, and ultraviolet light source are required for fluorescence microscopy. Microscope objectives are the most important components of an optical microscope because they determine the quality of the images that the microscope is capable of producing. There is a wide range of objective designs available that feature excellent optical performance and provide for the elimination of most optical aberrations. Standard bright-field objectives, corrected for varying degrees of optical aberration, are the most common and are useful for examining samples with traditional illumination techniques. Other, more complex, methods require specific objective configurations, which often include placement of a detector on or near the rear focal plane (Chapin, 1995, Drent, 2005, Abramowitz et al., 2002).

Microscopes can be separated into several different classes. One grouping is based on what interacts with the sample to generate the image, light or photons (optical microscopes), electrons (electron microscopes), or a probe (scanning probe microscopes). Alternatively, microscopes can be classed on whether they analyze the sample via a scanning point (confocal optical microscopes, scanning electron microscopes and scanning probe microscopes) or analyze the sample all at once (wide-field optical microscope and transmission electron microscopes). The most commonly used are *compound microscopes* that are light illuminated. The image seen with this type of microscope is two-dimensional (2D) enabling views of individual cells, even living ones. It has high magnification but low resolution (Conchello and Lichtman, 2005, Centonze Frohlich, 2008). *Fluorescence microscopy* is the most rapidly expanding microscopy technique employed today, both in the medical and biological sciences, a fact which has spurred the development of more sophisticated microscopes and numerous fluorescence accessories. Epifluorescence, or incident light fluorescence, has now become the method of choice in many applications (Michalet et al., 2003). A *dissection microscope* is light illuminated and the image appears in 3D. It is used for dissection utilizing a laser light. Laser light scans across the sample with the aid of scanning mirrors and then the image is placed on a computer screen (Foldes-Papp et al., 2003). The *digital microscope* uses the power of the computer to view objects not visible to the naked eye. The computer software allows the monitor to display the magnified sample. An advantage of digital microscopes is the ability to email images, as well as comfortably watch moving images for long periods. A *scanning electron microscope* uses electron illumination.

The image is seen in 3D and has high magnification and high resolution. The sample is coated in gold and the electrons bounce off to give the exterior view of the sample. The pictures are in black and white. A *transmission electron microscope* is electron illuminated and gives a 2D view. The electron beams pass through the thin slices of sample and have high magnification and high resolution (Grogger et al., 2000).

Microorganisms present in collected clinical or pathological samples are transparent and the best approach to distinguish them is to use dyes or biological stains. Differentially stained samples are the most helpful for presumptive identification of the majority of pathogens. The Gram stain and acid-fast stain are examples of differential stains. There are other miscellaneous stains such as periodic acid-Schiff, toluidine blue O, Giemsa, and Wright stains. In addition, the fluorescence stains aid in identification of microorganisms because of the specific attachment of the fluorochromes in the dyes to microorganism components.

2.3.2   Culture Techniques

Culturing in microbiology refers to the transfer of an organism from its ecological niche (e.g., organ, tissue, body fluid, exudate), transient vehicle (e.g., food), or storage medium (as in case of stock culture), into a growth-permitting laboratory medium. In many instances, isolating and culturing microorganisms either in artificial media or in a living host confirms the cause of an infection. Bacteria (including mycobacteria and mycoplasmas) and fungi are cultured in either liquid (broth) or on solid (agar) artificial media. The inoculated medium is then incubated at an optimum growth conditions and for a suitable length of time to allow cell multiplication, resulting in a culture of the organism.

Liquid media provide greater sensitivity for the isolation of small numbers of microorganisms; however, identification of mixed cultures growing in liquid media requires subculture onto solid media so that isolated colonies can be processed separately for identification. Growth in liquid media also cannot ordinarily be quantitated. Solid media, although somewhat less sensitive than liquid media, provide isolated colonies that can be quantified if necessary and identified. Some genera and species can be recognized on the basis of their colony morphologies. The laboratory medium could be non-selective, selective, or differential, depending on the goal of the culture technique.

Non-selective culturing relies on using growth-permitting non-selective media. "Enrichment," which is used extensively in pathogen detection methods, is a non-selective culture technique. Buffered peptone water, for example, is used to enrich environmental samples in *Salmonella* spp. (Thomason et al., 1977).

Selective media allow the growth of target bacteria, while inhibiting the growth of other microbial populations. For example, organisms that have the ability to utilize a given sugar are screened easily by making that particular sugar the only carbon source in the medium, allowing for the growth of the target microorganism only. Likewise, the selective inhibition of some types of microorganisms can be studied by adding certain dyes, antimicrobials, salts, or specific inhibitors that will affect the metabolism or enzymatic systems of the organisms. For example, media containing potassium tellurite, sodium azide or thallium acetate at different concentrations will inhibit the growth of all Gram-negative bacteria. Media supplemented with the antimicrobial penicillin or crystal violet inhibits the growth of Gram-positive bacteria. Tellurite agar is used to select for Gram-positive organisms, and nutrient agar supplemented with the antimicrobial penicillin can be used to select for the growth of Gram-negative organisms (Holt et al., 1994).

Screening is a culture technique used to distinguish target from non-target microorganisms. Laboratory media supplemented with differential agents are used in screening. These agents allow analysts to visually detect the target microorganisms in a microbial population. Acid producing bacteria, for example, are distinguished from non-acid producers when suitable pH indicators are included in carbohydrate-containing agar media (Holt et al., 1994, Zhou et al., 2011).

Selection and screening are executed simultaneously using selective-differential media. For example, xylose lysine desoxycholate agar is a selective-differential medium often used in culture-based methods for detection of *Salmonella* spp. This medium contains sodium desoxycholate that selects for *Enterobacteriaceae*, and phenol red, a pH indicator that reveals acid production by non-*Salmonella* isolates. When executed properly, selection and screening, done sequentially or simultaneously, enable analysts to isolate target microorganisms as pure cultures (Holt et al., 1994).

Cultures are generally incubated at 35–37 °C in an atmosphere consisting of air, air supplemented with carbon dioxide (3–10%), reduced oxygen (microaerophilic conditions), or no oxygen (anaerobic conditions), depending upon requirements of the microorganism. Since clinical samples from bacterial infections often contain aerobic, facultative anaerobic, and anaerobic bacteria, such samples are usually inoculated into a variety of general-purpose, differential, and selective media, which are then incubated under aerobic and anaerobic conditions. The duration of incubation of cultures also varies with the growth characteristics of the microorganism. Most aerobic and anaerobic bacteria will grow overnight, whereas some mycobacteria require as many as 6–8 weeks.

2.3.3 Biochemical Methods

Although classification based on genetic divergence highlights the evolutionary relationships of bacteria, classification based on the morphological and biochemical features of bacteria remains the most practical way to identify these organisms. A definitive identification scheme for bacteria was presented in *Bergey's Manual of Determinative Bacteriology* (Holt et al., 1994). Bacteria are classified on the basis of many characteristics: cell shape, nature of multicellular aggregates, motility, formation of spores, and reaction to the Gram stain. Important in the identification of a genus and species of bacteria are biochemical tests, including the determination of the kinds of nutrients a cell can use, the products of its metabolism, the response to specific chemicals, and the presence of particular characteristic enzymes.

The methods available use a combination of tests to establish the enzymatic capabilities of a given bacterial isolate as well as the ability of the isolates to grow or survive the presence of certain inhibitors. Enzyme based test are designed to measure the presence of a single enzyme as well as a complete metabolic pathway. Examples of single enzyme tests are as follows: catalase test, coagulase test, pyrase test, hippurate hydrolysis test, oxidase test, indole test, Dnase test, *ortho*-Nitrophenyl-β-galactoside test, urease test, methylene red test, and Voges Proskauer test. In addition, establishing inhibitor profiles are useful in identification of isolated microorganisms (Holt et al., 1994, Murray et al., 1995b, Lennox and Ackerman, 1984).

The classification systems frequently used for alternative methods are based on how the technology works; for example, growth of microorganisms, viability of microorganisms, presence/absence of cellular components or artifacts, nucleic acid methods, traditional methods combined with computer-aided imaging (which might also be considered automation of an existing method), and combination methods. *Growth-based technologies* are based upon the measurement of biochemical or physiological parameters that reflect the growth of the microorganisms. Examples of these types of methods include: ATP bioluminescence, colorimetric detection of carbon dioxide production, and measurement of change in headspace pressure, impedance, and biochemical assays. *Viability-based technologies* do not require growth of microorganisms for detection. Differing methods are used to determine if the cell is viable, and if viable cells are detected, they can be enumerated. Examples of this type of technology include solid phase cytometry, flow fluorescence cytometry, and optical imaging with NADH detection (Moldenhauer, 2008).

2.3.4 Biosensors

Conventional methods are used despite their long turnover times because of their high selectivity and sensitivity. Biosensors are particularly attractive as a means to detect and identify pathogenic microorganisms due to their specificity and sensitivity, the potential to shorten the time span between sample uptake and results, and the competitive cost. Biosensors also allow the analysis of complex sample matrices (Lazcka et al., 2007, Love and Jones, 2008). To provide protection, that is, timely warning of the presence of a pathogen, environmental samples are often analyzed using biosensors. This presents an additional problem, in that other microorganisms will also be present within the sample. The detector needs to be able to discriminate the pathogen of interest from the background, and this can be achieved in a number of ways. These include: (1) detection of an increase in the number of particles, (2) detection of an increase in biological particles, (3) detection of pathogenic biological agents, or (4) the specific identification of a biological agent. The use of biosensors for sensitive specific detection of a pathogenic microorganism still remains a significant challenge, and success is often dictated by the nature of the detection element (the specific ligand) and the choice of target analyte (Ivnitski et al., 1999).

The basic biosensor framework includes a substrate such as silicon, glass or polymers such as polymethyl methacrylate, polydimethyl siloxane, and so on, coated with a conductive layer like polysilicon, silicon dioxide, silicon nitrite, metal like gold, and metal oxides. A suitable detection system includes specific capture molecules like antibodies, enzymes, DNA/RNA probes, and phage-derived biomolecular recognition probes. Highly sensitive sensors (e.g., thickness shear mode and immunosensor) can be fabricated using piezoelectric materials such as quartz crystal, potassium sodium tartrate, lithium niobate, and so on as a substrate, coupled with electromechanical detectors (Nayak et al., 2009). High sensitivity, ease of operation, high accuracy and wide detection capacity can be achieved with optical biosensors that utilize fiberoptics, optoelectronic components, complementary metal oxide semiconductors, and fluorescence/phosphorescence, reflectance, chemiluminescence, light scattering, or refractive index for the detection purpose (Lazcka et al., 2007, Velasco-Garcia, 2009).

The expeditious growth in the development of biosensors and the involvement of multidisciplinary research activities in this field has led to the immense application of this technology. Biosensors, as a method for detection of pathogenic microorganisms, have been applied in healthcare, detection of food and water-borne pathogens, in agriculture, and in defense.

2.3.5 Immunology-Based Methods

The field of immunology-based methods for bacteria detection provides very powerful analytical tools for a wide range of targets. Immunoassay technique is based on the interaction between an antigen and antibody, and the technology required for detecting or quantifying this interaction. There is a large variety of immunoassays, and these techniques are used broadly in many fields including toxicology and pathogen detection. Enzyme-linked immunosorbent assay (ELISA) (Herrmann, 1995) test is the most established technique nowadays as well as the source of inspiration for many biosensor applications. Another detection method based on immunological techniques is the fluorescent immunoassay. Both assays can be adapted to detect antigens that originate specifically from the targeted bacterial pathogen. Hence, these techniques are useful screening or identification tools in pathogen detection methods. Immunology-based methods require specific antibodies, which are among the most important molecules, with limitless applications in the field of biology, microbiology, medicine, and agriculture. For example, the most rapid diagnostic tests used in food or clinical laboratories are based on antigen-antibody reactions (Banada and Bhunia, 2008).

The antibody's ability to recognize and bind with high affinity to specific antigenic sites (epitopes), even in a complex mixture, is exploited for qualitative and quantitative measurement of the antigens. Thus, antibody application is broad – it is not only used for detection and classification of the antigens, but also for understanding the microheterogeneity among proteins resulting from recombinant or somatic mutations. The production and selection of a suitable antibody is imperative for the successful design of an immunoassay, which depends on the assay parameters: the choice of a polyclonal or monoclonal antibody; of purified or native sera; of fragmented, bispecific, or fusion proteins; and the relative cost (Herrmann, 1995).

Additionally, immunoassays can utilize immunomagnetic separation (Perez et al., 1998), a pre-treatment and/or pre-concentration step, that can be used to capture and extract the targeted pathogen from the bacterial suspension by introduction of antibody coated magnetic beads (Gu et al., 2006). Immunomagnetic separation can then be combined with almost any detection method; for example, optical, magnetic force microscopy, magnetoresistance (Baselt et al., 1998) and hall effect (Lazcka et al., 2007). Custom derivative magnetic beads are available from a number of companies. Beads of widely ranging sizes (from a few nanometers up to a few tens of microns) may be chosen depending on the application. While large beads may be used for the measurement of intermolecular forces, smaller particles are best for the detection of small analytes where high sensitivity is critical. In the case of whole bacteria, the use of beads in the low micrometer range may provide the right balance between time and sensitivity.

2.3.6 Molecular Detection and Identification of Microorganisms

The ultimate goal in microbial testing is to accurately and sensitively detect pathogens in real-time or as quickly as possible. Molecular diagnostics offer many advantages over traditional microbiological and immunological methods for the detection of pathogenic microorganisms. These include faster processing time as well as greater potential for intra-species identification and identification of antibiotic susceptibility and strain typing. Molecular diagnostics is revolutionizing the clinical management of infectious disease in a wide range of areas, including pathogen detection, evaluation of emerging novel infections, surveillance, early detection of bio threatening agents, and antimicrobial resistance profiling (Yang and Rothman, 2004).

Polymerase chain reaction is a molecular technique for in vitro amplification of a DNA fragment via enzymatic replication. Products of PCR amplification (amplicons) are separated on agarose gel, stained, and the resulting fluorescent DNA bands are detected. The original techniques of PCR are being superseded by real-time PCR technique that allows detection of PCR amplification products while they are formed (Heid et al., 1996). PCR is an extremely powerful, rapid method for diagnosis of microbial infections and genetic diseases, as well as for detecting microorganisms in environmental and food samples (Radstrom et al., 2004). PCR has advantages over conventional laboratory practices as it offers rapid and accurate detection of infectious agents, which is a crucial for the timely administration of appropriate treatments. PCR is particularly useful for the identification of organisms that cannot be cultured, or where culturing conditions are insensitive or require prolonged incubation times. Thus, PCR has opened up new possibilities for the detection of slow-growing pathogens, intracellular bacteria as well as viable, but non-cultivable, pathogens (Tenover et al., 1999, Traore et al., 2006, Glynn, 2008).

Real-time PCR monitors the accumulation of PCR product in a reaction while it is taking place, compared to endpoint detection of the PCR product in conventional PCR. These technologies provide quick, sensitive, quantitative detection of PCR products in a closed-tube format, thereby significantly reducing the risk of contamination (Csordas et al., 2004, Raoult et al., 2004).

Fluorescent technologies employed are either nonspecific, using dyes such as SYBR Green I or SYBR Gold, which are minor groove-binding dyes and intercalate into the PCR product during amplification; or specific, using probes to detect specific sequence amplification in the PCR. A number of different fluorescent probe chemistries have been employed in real-time PCR assays, including hydrolysis probes (TaqMan, Beacons) and hybridization probes (FRET). While the mechanism of fluorescent signal generation is different for each of the probe chemistries, the fluorescent signal generated by the probes or minor groove-binding dyes is directly proportional to the amount of PCR product generated (Bustin, 2002, McKillip and Drake, 2004). Real-time PCR is quantitative, with a broader dynamic range than conventional PCR.

Clearly the method with the least risks of variability for genotypic identification would be *sequencing* the entire chromosome or a gene of the unknown organism and comparing the sequence to others in an identification database. The sequences are generated by a modification of the polymerase chain reaction, and the relatedness of the derived sequence to others in the proprietary database is determined as the basis for the identification. This technology has several advantages. It can be used to identify filamentous fungi, bacteria, and yeast. It can also be used to identify slow-growing organisms, or even those that cannot be cultured. The major disadvantage of the system is the high costs associated with it in terms of dedicated facilities, personnel training, time, and consumables.

2.4 Challenges to Current Detection Methods

Results of conventional detection methods are not very amenable to quantitative interpretations. Even the most practiced culture methods are not as quantitative as some analysts may have anticipated. Therefore, the accuracy required for microbiological criteria or specifications are not attainable by conventional detection methods. Real-time PCR is highly reproducible and allows for the *quantification* of microorganisms or physiological changes in gene expression. The dynamic range of the performed calibration curve can be up to nine orders of magnitude from $<10^1$ to $>10^{10}$ starting molecules, depending on the applied standard material.

Bacterial cell density differs from sample to sample, and from animal to animal, so the reliability of the used method depends on its *detection limit* in a quantitative sense.

This means a method with a detection limit of a single bacterium per certain amount of heterogeneous organic matter is likely acceptable. Some methods have smaller detection limits, which results in inability of detecting or quantifying small bacterial populations without cell propagation steps. Amplification of the bacterial cell population, or any cellular components targeted by the analysis, is a prerequisite for successful detection. Enrichment has been used reliably to augment the pathogen's population, but this technique is the most time-consuming step in the analysis (Pusterla et al., 2010).

Important questions when choosing a microbiologic detection method are: *which traits to analyze* and *how many tests are needed for identifying a bacterial pathogen?* Being prokaryotic single-celled organisms, bacteria have a simple morphology, which cannot be used as a basis for their classification or identification. However, microbiologists should carefully consider these morphological characteristics before they develop a battery of identification tests. Sometimes it is impossible to identify a bacterium reliably on the basis of a single test (Murray et al., 1995b, Holt et al., 1994). Serological tests are used extensively in pathogen identification, and some immunoassay techniques have been automated. It is difficult, however, to correlate serological properties of an isolate with its genotypic or other phenotypic traits. Therefore, it is unreliable to use only serological techniques to identify a causative agent or track diseases. Genetic techniques were introduced in pathogen detection methods by targeting characteristic sequences in bacterial genomes. There is no doubt that molecular techniques are valuable in modern detection methods, but several problems remain, such as inhibition of PCR or determination of viable and nonviable targets. It is generally agreed that the most acceptable approach for identifying an isolate is to integrate all available phenotypic and genotypic traits. Assembling and assimilating all data on an isolate's diverse traits should aid the analyst in making a sound judgment about its identity.

References

Abramowitz M, Spring, KR, Keller, HE, et al. 2002. Basic principles of microscope objectives. Biotechniques, 33: 772–774, 776–778, 780–781.

Banada PP and Bhunia AK. 2008. Antibodies and immunoassays for detection of bacterial pathogens. In: M Zourob, S Elwary, and A Turner (eds), Principles of Bacterial Detection: Biosensors, Recognition Receptors and Microsystems. New York, NY: Springer.

Baselt DR, Lee GU, Natesan M, et al. 1998. A biosensor based on magnetoresistance technology. Biosens Bioelectron, 13: 731–739.

Bustin SA. 2002. Quantification of mRNA using real-time reverse transcription PCR (RT-PCR): trends and problems. J Mol Endocrinol, 29: 23–39.

Centonze Frohlich V. 2008. Phase contrast and differential interference contrast (DIC) microscopy. J Vis Exp 6(17): pii: 84.

Chapin K. 1995. Clinical microscopy. In: PR Murray (ed.) Manual of Clinical Microbiology. 6th edn. Washington, D.C.: ASM Press.

CLSI 2011. Laboratory Quality Control Based on Risk Management; Approved Guideline. Wayne, PA: Clinical and Laboratory Standards Institute. In: Document, C. EP23-A.

Conchello JA and Lichtman JW. 2005. Optical sectioning microscopy. Nat Methods, 2: 920–931.

Csordas AT, Barak JD and Delwiche MJ. 2004. Comparison of primers for the detection of Salmonella enterica serovars using real-time PCR. Lett Appl Microbiol, 39: 187–193.

Drent P. 2005. Properties and selection of objective lenses for light microscopy applications. Microscopy and Analysis, 19: 5–7.

Endler G and Slavka G. 2010. Stability of the specimen during preanalytic. In: HH Kessler (ed.) Molecular Diagnostics of Infectious Diseases. Graz, Austria: Deutsche National Bibliothek.

Foldes-Papp Z, Demel U, and Tilz GP. 2003. Laser scanning confocal fluorescence microscopy: an overview. Int Immunopharmacol, 3: 1715–1729.

Gimenez-Marin A, Rivas-Ruiz F, Perez-Hidalgo Mdel M, et al. 2014. Pre-analytical errors management in the clinical laboratory: a five-year study. Biochem Med (Zagreb), 24: 248–257.

Glynn B. 2008. Rapid nucleic acid-based diagnostics methods for the detection of bacterial pathogens. In: M Zourob, S Elwary, and A Turner (eds.) Principles of Bacterial Detection: Biosensors, Recognition Receptors and Microsystems. New York, NY: Springer.

Goldmann DA and Pier GB. 1993. Pathogenesis of infections related to intravascular catheterization. Clin Microbiol Rev, 6: 176–192.

Gracias KS and Mckillip JL. 2004. A review of conventional detection and enumeration methods for pathogenic bacteria in food. Can J Microbiol, 50: 883–890.

Grogger W, Hofer F, Warbichler P, et al. 2000. Quantitative energy-filtering transmission electron microscopy in materials science. Microsc Microanal, 6: 161–172.

Gu HW, Xu KM, Xu CJ, et al. 2006. Biofunctional magnetic nanoparticles for protein separation and pathogen detection. Chem. Commun.: 941–949.

Heid CA, Stevens J, Livak KJ, et al. 1996. Real time quantitative PCR. Genome Res, 6: 986–994.

Herrmann JE. 1995. Immunoassays for the diagnosis of infectious diseases. In: PR Murray, EJ Baron, MA Pfaller, et al. (eds.) Manual of Clinical Microbiology. Washington, D.C.: ASM Press.

Holt JG, Krieg NR, Sneath PHA, et al. 1994. Bergey's Manual of Determinative Bacteriology, Baltimore, Maryland, Williams & Wilkins.

Ivnitski D, Abdel-Hamid I, Atanasov P, et al. 1999. Biosensors for detection of pathogenic bacteria. Biosensors & Bioelectronics, 14: 599–624.

Kaspar CW and Tartera C. 1990. Methods for detecting pathogens in food and water. Methods in Microbiology, 22: 497–534.

Lamoth F and Greub G. 2010. Fastidious intracellular bacteria as causal agents of community-acquired pneumonia. Expert Rev Anti Infect Ther, 8: 775–790.

Lazcka O, Del Campo FJ, and Munoz FX. 2007. Pathogen detection: a perspective of traditional methods and biosensors. Biosens Bioelectron, 22: 1205–1217.

Lennox VA and Ackerman VP. 1984. Biochemical identification of bacteria by replicator methods on agar plates. Pathology, 16: 434–440.

Love TE and Jones B. 2008. Introduction to pathogenic bacteria. In: M Zourob, S Elwary, and A Turner (eds.) Principles of Bacterial Detection: Biosensors, Recognition Receptors and Microsystems. New York, NY: Springer.

Madej RM, Davis J, Holden MJ, et al. 2010. International standards and reference materials for quantitative molecular infectious disease testing. J Mol Diagn, 12: 133–143.

Mckillip JL and Drake M. 2004. Real-time nucleic acid-based detection methods for pathogenic bacteria in food. J Food Prot, 67: 823–832.

Michalet X, Kapanidis AN, Laurence T, et al. 2003. The power and prospects of fluorescence microscopies and spectroscopies. Annu Rev Biophys Biomol Struct, 32: 161–182.

Miller JM and Holmes HT. 1995. Specimen collection, transport, and storage. In: PR Murray (ed.) Manual of Clinical Microbiology. 6th Edn. Washington, D.C.: ASM Press.

Moldenhauer J. 2008. Overview of rapid microbiological methods. In: M Zourob, S Elwary, and A Turner (eds), Principles of Bacteria Detection, Biosensors, Recognition Receptors and Microsystems. 1st Edn. Montreal Canada: Springer.

Murray PR, Baron EJ, Pfaller MA, et al. 1995a. Manual of Clinical Microbiology, Washington, DC, American Society for Microbiology.

Murray PR, Baron EJ, Pfaller MA, et al. 1995b. Manual of Clinical Microbiology, Washington, D.C., ASM Press.

Nayak M, Kotian A, Marathe S, et al. 2009. Detection of microorganisms using biosensors-a smarter way towards detection techniques. Biosens Bioelectron, 25: 661–667.

OSHA 2011. Laboratory safety guidance. In: Occulational Safety and Health Administration, USDOL (ed.). Available online at (https://www.osha.gov/Publications/laboratory/OSHA3404laboratory-safety-guidance.pdf) accessed June 2017.

Panel TDRDEE, Banoo S, Bell D, et al. 2010. Evaluation of diagnostic tests for infectious diseases: general principles. Nat Rev Microbiol, 8: S17–29.

Perez FG, Mascini M, Tothill IE, et al. 1998. Immunomagnetic separation with mediated flow injection analysis amperometric detection of viable *Escherichia coli* O157. Anal Chem, 70: 2380–2386.

Petti CA. 2007. Detection and identification of microorganisms by gene amplification and sequencing. Clin Infect Dis, 44: 1108–1014.

Pickup RW. 1991. Development of molecular methods for the detection of specific bacteria in the environment. Journal of General Microbiology, 137: 1009–1019.

Pusterla N, Byrne BA, Hodzic E, et al. 2010. Use of quantitative real-time PCR for the detection of *Salmonella* spp. in fecal samples from horses at a veterinary teaching hospital. Vet J, 186: 252–255.

Rabenau HF, Raggam RB, and Salzer HJF. 2010. Choice of adequate sample material. In: HH Kessler (ed.), Molecular Diagnostics of Infectious Diseases. Graz, Austria: Deutsche National Bibliothek.

Radstrom P, Knutsson R, Wolffs P, et al. 2004. Pre-PCR processing: strategies to generate PCR-compatible samples. Mol Biotechnol, 26: 133–146.

Raggam RB, Kessler HH, and Rabenau HF. 2010. Qality assurance and quality control in the routine molecular diagnostic laboratory. In: HH Kessler (ed.), Molecular Diagnostics of Infectious Diseases. Gratz, Austria: Bibliographic Nationalbibliothek.

Raoult D, Fournier PE, and Drancourt M. 2004. What does the future hold for clinical microbiology? Nat Rev Microbiol, 2: 151–159.

Relman DA. 1998. Detection and identification of previously unrecognized microbial pathogens. Emerg Infect Dis, 4: 382–389.

Tenover FC, Jones RN, Swenson JM, et al. 1999. Methods for improved detection of oxacillin resistance in coagulase-negative staphylococci: results of a multicenter study. J Clin Microbiol, 37: 4051–4058.

Thomason BM, Dodd DJ, and Cherry WB. 1977. Increased recovery of salmonellae from environmental samples enriched with buffered peptone water. Appl Environ Microbiol, 34: 270–273.

Traore H, Van Deun A, Shamputa IC, et al. 2006. Direct detection of Mycobacterium tuberculosis complex DNA and rifampin resistance in clinical specimens from tuberculosis patients by line probe assay. J Clin Microbiol, 44: 4384–4388.

Velasco-Garcia MN. 2009. Optical biosensors for probing at the cellular level: a review of recent progress and future prospects. Semin Cell Dev Biol, 20: 27–33.

Washington JA. 1996. Principles of diagnosis. In: S Baron (ed.) Medical Microbiology. 4th Edn. Galveston (TX): University of Texas Medical Branch at Galveston.

Yang S and Rothman RE. 2004. PCR-based diagnostics for infectious diseases: uses, limitations, and future applications in acute-care settings. Lancet Infect Dis, 4: 337–348.

Yousef AE. 2008. Detection of bacterial pathogens in different matrices: Current practices and challenges. In: M Zourob, S Elwary, and A Turner (eds), Principles of Bacterial Detection: Biosensors, Recognition Receptors and Microsystems. New York, NY: Springer.

Zhou P, Hussain SK, Liles MR, et al. 2011. A simplified and cost-effective enrichment protocol for the isolation of *Campylobacter* spp. from retail broiler meat without microaerobic incubation. BMC Microbiol, 11: 175.

3

Point-of-Care Testing

C. Langdon Fielding

Loomis Basin Equine Medical Center, California, USA

3.1   Introduction

Point-of-care (POC) testing is the analysis of clinical specimens as close to the patient as possible. The testing may be stall-side or in the immediate vicinity at a nursing station. As computers and machines become smaller and more portable, nearly all testing could potentially be considered point-of-care. The readily available "hand-held" tests that equine veterinarians can perform stall-side are included next.

3.2   Advantages of POC Testing

Equine veterinarians with POC testing capabilities will have a unique advantage in rapid diagnosis, prognosis and treatment. It is important to determine which testing is cost effective for a given practice setting. POC analyzers can be separated into multi-test analyzers (MTA) versus single-test analyzers (STA). MTAs are a single machine that can be used to measure a variety of parameters, but are typically more expensive than STAs. STAs tend to be inexpensive and often easy to use. Ambulatory practitioners may find it more practical to own one MTA as opposed to multiple STAs.

3.3   Considerations for POC Testing

- Cost of the analyzer
- Cost per test
- Number of anticipated tests per year
- Ease of testing
  - If a given test is very challenging to perform, this will limit the use and increase the testing time.
  - If failure rate is high, then the additional costs associated with the extra time or supplies must be included.

3.4   Specific POC Tests to Consider

3.4.1   Blood Ammonia

Ammonia measured in the blood comes primarily from the gastrointestinal tract, however, it can also be produced in muscle and kidney. Ammonia is produced during exercise both from deamination of AMP, as well as catabolism of branched-chain amino acids. The deamination of AMP rises rapidly with increasingly intense exercise and is the primary route of ammonia production during high intensity work. Ammonia can be cleared by a variety of organs but liver and muscle are the major routes.

The measurement of ammonia is relevant in the fields of emergency and critical care, internal medicine, and sports medicine. Critical patients with gastrointestinal ileus, equine coronavirus infection, and hepatic failure can all experience life-threatening hyperammonemia (Hasel et al., 1999, McGorum et al., 1999). Sports medicine clinicians measure blood ammonia levels to help determine level of fitness and response to training (Lindner et al., 2006).

POC testing of ammonia allows immediate measurement after sample collection which negates the need for sample processing and freezing if measurement will be delayed. STA machine can measure blood ammonia concentration within minutes (PocketChem BA, Woodley Equipment Company, UK).

3.4.2   Creatinine

Creatinine is produced from the breakdown of creatine and creatine phosphate. Creatinine is freely filtered in the glomerulus but may undergo active secretion in horses (Bickhardt et al., 1996). The creatinine concentration is inversely related to GFR and is often used as an indirect measure of renal function. Even small increases

Interpretation of Equine Laboratory Diagnostics, First Edition. Edited by Nicola Pusterla and Jill Higgins.
© 2018 John Wiley & Sons, Inc. Published 2018 by John Wiley & Sons, Inc.

(as little as 0.3 mg/dl) in creatinine in a normally hydrated person may indicate the presence of acute kidney injury (AKI) and similar changes in horses should be monitored carefully (Kellum and Lameire, 2013). Increased creatinine concentration can also be seen with post-renal problems including rupture of the urinary system (ureters, bladder, and urethra) or obstruction of the urinary system. In foals, creatinine can be significantly elevated at birth but may be related to placental dysfunction. In newborn foals with normal renal function, increased creatinine values typically return to normal within 48–72 h (Chaney et al., 2010). Creatinine is most commonly measured along with other parameters on a variety of MTAs.

Uses in equine practice: The measurement of creatinine is relevant in the fields of general equine practice, emergency and critical care, internal medicine and anesthesia. The POC measurement of creatinine is useful for field practitioners as many medications used in equine practice have some degree of nephrotoxic potential (NSAIDs, aminoglycosides, tetracycline, etc.). Ideally renal function should be tested before starting treatment with nephrotoxic medications, and during the course of therapy.

3.4.3 Electrolytes

Sodium (Na^+), potassium (K^+), and chloride (Cl^-) are the most commonly measured electrolytes. The measurement of the ionized forms of calcium (Ca^{++}) and magnesium (Mg^{++}) has applications in equine practice as well.

Sodium is the predominant extracellular cation. The sodium concentration represents the balance between the total amount of sodium in the body (and indirectly potassium as well) and the total amount of water. Determination of the sodium concentration is important for evaluating fluid balance and managing renal failure cases.

Potassium is the predominant intracellular cation. Increased extracellular concentrations of potassium can be life-threatening. Hyperkalemia is frequently seen with renal failure and hyperkalemic periodic paralysis (HYPP). Hypokalemia is commonly encountered in anorexic horses receiving large volumes of intravenous fluids containing dextrose.

Chloride is the predominant extracellular anion. The chloride concentration frequently changes in conjunction with the sodium concentration. Chloride has a significant role in acid-base balance particularly when the difference between the sodium and chloride concentration changes dramatically. Treatment of acid-base disturbances without knowledge of the chloride concentration can be challenging.

Most analyzers determine a group of electrolyte concentrations which typically include a minimum of sodium, potassium, and chloride. Calcium, blood gases, and other acid-base variables are often included in combination with the basic electrolytes.

The measurement of electrolytes is relevant in the fields of general equine practice, emergency and critical care, internal medicine, and anesthesia.

3.4.4 Blood Gases/Acid-Base Parameters

Arterial blood gases are used to evaluate the respiratory system, as well as acid-base balance. The arterial partial pressure of oxygen (PaO_2) generally represents lung function and more specifically the ability of the lungs to transfer oxygen from inhaled air into the arterial blood. The arterial partial pressure of carbon dioxide ($PaCO_2$) generally represents the adequacy of ventilation. The measurement of pH and bicarbonate (HCO_3^-) concentration is important for understanding and treating acid-base disorders.

Analyzers that measure blood gas or acid/base variables will commonly measure these parameters as a group and are often combined with electrolytes and measured on MTAs. The measurement of blood gases/acid-base parameters is relevant in the fields of anesthesia, critical care, and internal medicine. Blood gas measurement is not typically performed in a field situation in general equine practice.

3.4.5 Lactate

L-Lactate is produced during anaerobic metabolism and primarily cleared by the liver and kidneys. Increased concentrations of lactate are commonly associated with increased production or decreased clearance. Lactate has been shown to have prognostic value in a variety of equine conditions and is commonly measured in emergency situations on admission, as well as for serial monitoring during treatment (Hashimoto-Hill et al., 2011, Tennent Brown et al., 2010).

The measurement of L-lactate is relevant in the fields of emergency and critical care, internal medicine, and sports medicine. Lactate determination can be performed on both STAs and MTAs. The low analyzer cost for lactate testing combined with a low per test cost makes it ideal even for ambulatory practitioners that have a moderate emergency caseload.

3.4.6 Cardiac Troponin I

Cardiac troponin I (cTnI) is a specific marker of myocardial damage. It can be increased in a variety of circumstances including heart failure, toxic injury to the myocardium, or myocardial injury secondary to systemic inflammation/disease (Díaz et al., 2014, Davis et al., 2013). Uses in equine practice are generally restricted to emergency and critical care or internal medicine cases. Testing for cTnI is currently available for POC testing on an MTA (i-STAT Handheld analyzer, Abaxis, Union City, CA).

3.4.7 Glucose

Blood glucose monitoring has many applications in equine practice, including in the management of sick neonatal foals and horses with insulin resistance. It also has prognostic value in critically ill horses (Johnson et al., 2012, Hassel et al., 2009, Hollis et al., 2008). The measurement of glucose is relevant in the fields of emergency and critical care, internal medicine, anesthesia, and general equine practice. There are numerous analyzers (both STA and MTA) that are available, but many STAs are inexpensive. The cost per test is extremely low making this another ideal entry level POC diagnostic test.

3.4.8 Clotting Times (PT and PTT)

The coagulation system is complex and closely linked to the inflammatory cascade. PT, or prothrombin time, was originally considered to evaluate extrinsic clotting cascade. PTT, or partial thromboplastin time, was originally considered to evaluate intrinsic clotting cascade. PT and PTT are typically measured in critically ill horses, cases of unexplained bleeding, or prior to a surgical/invasive procedure. Uses in equine practice are generally restricted in the fields of emergency and critical care, internal medicine, and surgery. The rapid determination of PT and PTT are an essential test for most equine ICUs

3.4.9 Serum Amyloid A

Serum Amyloid A (SAA) is a positive major acute phase protein that increases with inflammatory diseases. In equine practice, SAA testing is often used as a screening tool to identify occult or early infection that may not be otherwise evident from the physical examination or other blood testing. SAA can also be used to monitor the response to treatment (i.e., antimicrobials, post-surgery) (Daniel et al., 2015, Belgrave et al., 2013). The testing of SAA has only recently become available for POC testing and is measured on an STA. The measurement of SAA is relevant in the fields of internal medicine, emergency and critical care, and general equine practice.

3.4.10 Triglycerides

Triglycerides are a type of lipid that circulates in the blood. Measurement is particularly important in ponies and miniature horses that are in a negative energy balance, especially during lactation and pregnancy (McKenzie, 2011). If these animals become anorexic, they can develop hyperlipidemia or hyperlipemia with significant morbidity and mortality in severe cases. Even in full-sized breeds of horses, triglyceride concentrations can increase with anorexia and disease. Hypertriglyceridemia may be present with pars pituitary intermedia dysfunction (PPID) or equine metabolic syndrome. The measurement of triglycerides is relevant in the fields of internal medicine, emergency and critical care, and general equine practice.

3.5 Conclusion

The addition of POC testing is likely to raise the level of care that an equine veterinarian can provide. It is important to evaluate the costs and benefits of this type of investment. In the author's experience, many veterinarians enthusiastically enter the world of equine POC testing only to be plagued by expired cartridges and a poor return on investment.

References

Bickhardt K, Deegen E, and Espelage W. 1996. Kidney function tests in horses – methods and reference values in healthy animals. *Dtsch Tierarztl Wochenschr.* 103: 117–122.

Belgrave RL, Dickey MM, Arheart KL, and Cray C. 2013. Assessment of serum amyloid A testing of horses and its clinical application in a specialized equine practice. *J Am Vet Med Assoc.* 243: 113–119.

Chaney KP, Holcombe SJ, Schott HC 2nd, and Barr BS. 2010. Spurious hypercreatininemia: 28 neonatal foals (2000–2008). *J Vet Emerg Crit Care (San Antonio).* 20: 244–249.

Daniel AJ, Leise BS, Burgess BA, Morley PS, Cloninger M, and Hassel DM. 2015. Concentrations of serum amyloid A and plasma fibrinogen in horses undergoing emergency abdominal surgery. *J Vet Emerg Crit Care (San Antonio).* doi: 10.1111/vec.12365.

Davis TZ, Stegelmeier BL, Lee ST, Green BT, and Hall JO. 2013. Experimental rayless goldenrod (Isocoma pluriflora) toxicosis in horses. *Toxicon.* 73: 88–95.

Díaz OM, Durando MM, Birks EK, and Reef VB. (2014) Cardiac troponin I concentrations in horses with colic. *J Am Vet Med Assoc.* 245: 118–125.

Hasel KM, Summers BA, and De Lahunta A. 1999. Encephalopathy with idiopathic hyperammonaemia and Alzheimer type II astrocytes in equidae. *Equine Vet J.* 31: 478–482.

Hassel DM, Hill AE, and Rorabeck RA. 2009. Association between hyperglycemia and survival in 228 horses with acute gastrointestinal disease. *J Vet Intern Med.* 23: 1261–1265.

Hashimoto-Hill S, Magdesian KG, and Kass PH. 2011. Serial measurement of lactate concentration in horses with acute colitis. *J Vet Intern Med.* 25: 1414–1419.

Hollis AR, Furr MO, Magdesian KG, Axon JE, Ludlow V, Boston RC, and Corley KT. 2008. Blood glucose concentrations in critically ill neonatal foals. *J Vet Intern Med.* 22: 1223–1227.

Johnson PJ, Wiedmeyer CE, LaCarrubba A, Ganjam VK, and Messer NT 4th. 2012. Diabetes, insulin resistance, and metabolic syndrome in horses. *J Diabetes Sci Technol* 6: 534–540.

Kellum JA and Lameire N; for the KDIGO AKI Guideline Work Group. 2013. Diagnosis, evaluation, and management of acute kidney injury: a KDIGO summary (Part 1). *Crit Care* 17: 204.

Lindner A, Signorini R, Brero L, Arn E, Mancini R, and Enrique A. 2006. Effect of conditioning horses with short intervals at high speed on biochemical variables in blood. *Equine Vet J Suppl.* 36: 88–92.

McGorum BC, Murphy D, Love S, and Milne EM. 1999. Clinicopathological features of equine primary hepatic disease: a review of 50 cases. *Vet Rec.* 145: 134–139.

McKenzie HC 3rd. 2011. Equine hyperlipidemias. *Vet Clin North Am Equine Pract.* 27: 59–72.

Tennent-Brown BS, Wilkins PA, Lindborg S, Russell G, and Boston RC. 2010. Sequential plasma lactate concentrations as prognostic indicators in adult equine emergencies. *J Vet Intern Med.* 24: 198–205.

4

Test Performance
Christian M. Leutenegger

IDEXX Laboratories, Inc., California, USA

4.1 Introduction

Diagnostic test performance is characterized by its diagnostic accuracy, which relates to the ability of a test to discriminate between the anticipated target condition and health. Measures of diagnostic accuracy are determined in validation experiments and are quantitatively described by a test's sensitivity and specificity, predictive values, area under a receiver-operating-characteristic (ROC) curve, Youden's index, and diagnostic odds and likelihood ratios.

The validation phase itself can be split into an analytical and clinical part; the analytical validation determines particular test characteristics such as precision, reproducibility, spiking, recovery and linearity checks, and analytical limit of detection (Box 4.1). The clinical validation is run with defined samples from clinically affected or healthy individuals and aims to fully answer the discriminative power of the test between the target condition and health by defining diagnostic sensitivity and specificity, predictive values, ROC curves, likelihood ratios, and Youden's index (Box 4.2).

4.2 Analytical Validation

Analytical performance of a diagnostic test requires the use of the target analyte in a stable sample matrix environment in order to determine the quality of the diagnostic test itself. The stability of the target analyte by itself and mixed into the sample matrix are important variables to determine and are somewhat different depending on the diagnostic test use.

4.3 Minimum Information for Diagnostic Tests

Every new diagnostic entering a validation protocol should be accompanied by a diagnostic test manual that includes some basic information: intended use of the test (disease diagnostics, monitoring, screening, wellness testing); description of the analytical test principle; specification of instrumentation and equipment; reagent and disposable list; standard operating procedure (SOP); sample type requirements; description and definition of calibrators and control material; safety procedures; waste management; time to result calculations; and approximate costs.

4.4 Precision

Precision of a test measures the closeness of a series of repeat measurements of the same material and expressed as a coefficient of variation (CV) in percent. CV is calculated using the standard deviation (SD) and mean (X_{mean}) of all measurements in the formula $CV = (SD \times 100\%)/X_{mean}$. Precision should be analyzed over the intended dynamic range of the diagnostic test using a dilution series of the target analyte in the stable sample matrix. For virtually all diagnostic procedures, precision varies with target analyte concentration: CVs are usually higher at the end of the standard curve with very low target analyte concentrations and have to be defined to determine acceptance of the test.

Interpretation of Equine Laboratory Diagnostics, First Edition. Edited by Nicola Pusterla and Jill Higgins.
© 2018 John Wiley & Sons, Inc. Published 2018 by John Wiley & Sons, Inc.

Box 4.1 Analytical validation.

Minimum Information for diagnostic tests
Precision (within-run and between-run)
Accuracy
Spiking recovery and linearity checks
Control material
Method comparison
Analytical sensitivity and specificity
Additional analytical performance tests

Box 4.2 Clinical validation.

Overlap tests
Sample selection process for clinical validation
Diagnostic sensitivity and specificity
Predictive values
ROC curve
Likelihood ratios

Within-run precision can be assessed in different ways. A practical approach is to use a representative number of patient specimens containing different target analyte concentrations and analyze in duplicate. Then, the determined quantitative target analyte concentrations are grouped into three groups (low, medium, high concentration), SD and CVs calculated for each group, and statistically tested for significant differences using modified F-tests. Results can be graphed as a precision profile by plotting CVs (on the y-axis) versus analyte concentration (x-axis).

4.5 Accuracy

An alternative term for accuracy is bias or systematic error and is defined as agreement between the mean of repeat measurements on the same sample against the true value. Because naturally occurring samples with known concentrations are difficult to obtain, an appropriate sample matrix is normally spiked with known concentrations of the target analyte. Alternatively, accuracy can be determined by comparing a new diagnostic test to an existing test. In that case, additional parameters such as constant systematic error (consistent differences between the two methods indicating method dependent error) and proportional systematic errors (inconsistent differences between the two methods, related to additional variables than the test methods themselves) can be determined.

4.6 Spiking Recovery and Linearity Checks

Spiking recovery experiments can be carried out in different ways. One method requires the existence of the target analyte in pure form and known concentration, to be spiked into the sample matrix with known concentration of the target analyte. The difference between those concentrations gives information about how much of the analyte can be recovered in the spiked sample. Recovery is normally expressed as percentage of recovery compared to the known concentration and should be around 100%, with acceptance criteria to be defined specifically for each diagnostic test.

A different test characteristic is assessed by using spiked sample matrix diluted in sample matrix without presence of measurable target analyte (zero calibrator). It is important to use a sample matrix that is identical or as close as possible to the sample type intended to be used for the diagnostic test as a zero calibrator to prevent a bias resulting in a proportional systemic error. The difference between expected and measured analyte concentration is then investigated in a linear regression analysis. The confidence interval of the slope should be close to 1, indicating 100% recovery. It is also important to test for linearity by using a Runs-test, also called Wald–Wolfowitz test. This is a non-parametric statistical test that checks for randomness in a two-valued data set.

4.7 Control Material

Defined and stable control material is produced in order to test multiple lab locations for accuracy in tests called external quality assurance, ring trials or proficiency testing. The control material, coded with different concentrations of analyte mixed with zero calibrator samples are tested in replicates and analyzed using a Wilcoxon Signed Rank test, depending on sample distribution. Means and or medians are compared to the expected concentrations of the target analyte to determine the bias of the analytical method, expressed in percentages.

4.8 Method Comparison

The systemic error is assessed by analyzing the same sample set with the new diagnostic test and comparing the results to a gold standard test. The goal is to prove that the new diagnostic test compares to the gold standard test within the inherent precision ranges of both methods, based on acceptance criteria.

4.9 Analytical Sensitivity and Specificity

Analytical sensitivity and specificity are distinctly different terms than diagnostic or clinical sensitivity and specificity and produce confusion in the diagnostic use of laboratory test results.

Analytical sensitivity describes the limit of detection of a particular diagnostic test at the molecule level, meaning what the smallest amount of target analyte is which can be measured in the appropriate sample matrix in a reliable fashion. For DNA testing, for example, it is important to determine how many nucleic acid equivalents can be detected within a single PCR reaction. For that purpose, dilution series of known concentrations of target DNA are analyzed in replicates. If very low analytical sensitivity has to be obtained for a particular test, a larger number of replicates are necessary to obtain single digit analytical sensitivity, due to the randomness of molecular distribution within a highly dilute sample.

Specificity at the analytical level refers to the ability of a diagnostic test to measure the particular target analyte and not a closely related analyte. Again, for molecular diagnostic tests, this is confirmed by sequencing the PCR product using outside primers in order to confirm the recovered nucleotide sequence is identical to the targeted nucleic acid sequence of the PCR test.

Diagnostic sensitivity and specificity will be further specified in the next section.

4.10 Additional Analytical Performance Tests

Parameters associated with the sample matrix which influence the test characteristics have to be analyzed before a test enters the clinical validation phase. For example, high contents of lipids, bilirubin, hemoglobin, and glucose in blood samples, mucus on swabs or nasal washes, soil or litter contaminants in fecal material can all influence the analytical behavior of a diagnostic test, and influence diagnostic performance indices. Depending on the target analyte it may be useful to examine the effects of these substances in detail. To that effect, many of these interfering substances can be obtained in pure form, such as unconjugated bilirubin and glucose, hemoglobin, lipids, and so on. For molecular tests, the influence of PCR inhibition is of particular importance. Humic acid for example, a well-known soil substance to cause complete inhibition of the DNA poly-merase enzyme, can be purchased in pure form. It can be used to (1) test the nucleic acid extraction method and its ability to remove humic acid and (2) test the reverse transcription reagents and the PCR mastermix for its susceptibility to humic acid inhibition. In order to test for absence of inhibition, molecular diagnostic laboratories are using specialized and dedicated quality controls such as a spike-in Inhibition Positive Control (IPC), which is analyzed with a specific PCR test: by comparing the known concentration with the recovered concentration of the IPC analyte, the inhibitory component in the nucleic acid eluate can be assessed. Particular acceptance criteria have to be worked out for different sample types and diagnostic tests.

Other than sample matrix components, there are additional variables which have to be assessed separately, such as medication and interfering diseases. The presence of excess amounts of antibodies in the blood stream has the potential to complex out a target antigen and render it undetectable. In such instances, protocols have to be validated to release the target protein from its masking antibody.

Related to sample matrix conditions are considerations of collection protocols, storage containers, handling and shipping conditions, type of anticoagulants, venous site of blood sampling, and so on. These factors can affect test performance significantly and have to be considered when random test result deviations occur.

4.11 Clinical Validation

Once analytical variables of a diagnostic test procedures are defined, clinical sample analysis becomes the focus of the validation. In order to prevent a bias in the determination of the clinical usefulness of a new procedure, a blind, prospective validation adhering to certain criteria should be utilized.

4.12 Study Design in the Clinical Validation Phase

Definition of the appropriate clinical target population is instrumental in the determination of the clinical utility of a diagnostic test. For example, patients with illnesses on the list of differential diagnosis should be included into the test sample set. The total number of test subjects in general should be in the 50–100 range. Patient selection and proper definition of inclusion criteria are essential for this clinical validation phase and depend on the test under investigation and the diagnostic application. The patients selected for the validation phase have to be tested independently of the laboratory test being investigated. All these factors influence study design and the outcome of the validation. Existing definitions given by the Standards for Reporting of Diagnostic Accuracy should be considered.

4.13 Diagnostic Sensitivity and Specificity

The diagnostic or clinical sensitivity (DSE) and specificity (DSP) indices are different from their analytical counterpart. Diagnostic sensitivity is the percentage of patients with a given disorder who are correctly identified by the diagnostic test. High analytical sensitivity does not guarantee high or acceptable diagnostic sensitivity. With other words, DSE is the probability of getting a positive test result in the patient group with the disease.

Diagnostic specificity is the percentage of patients (with a differential disease) or individuals (healthy) who do not have a given condition who are identified by the assay correctly as negative for the condition. Or with other words, DSP represents the probability of a negative test result in a patient group (or healthy individuals) without the disease. Analytical specificity issues of a diagnostic test for example has a direct influence on the perceived diagnostic sensitivity and therefore has to be considered to play a role in the clinical validation process.

Test results are considered positive or negative depending on the upper or lower limit of the reference interval. For molecular tests, presence of absence of the target nucleic acid is considered positive or negative. For select quantitative molecular tests, medically relevant cutoff values have to be determined during the clinical validation, which then are used to calculate performance indices. In order to calculate DSE and DSP, test results are tabulated in a 2×2 table and calculated as follows: $DSE = TP/(TP + FN)$ and $DSP = TN/(FP + TN)$

	Disease Present	Disease Absent
Test Positive	True Positive (TP)	False Positive (FP)
Test Negative	False Negative (FN)	True Negative (TN)

Neither DSE or DSP are influenced by the disease prevalence. For that reason, study results can be transferred in between studies with different disease occurrence. Disease spectrum however does influence sensitivity and specificity.

4.14 Predictive Values

Predictive values describe the probability of having the disease of interest (or absence thereof) in an individual with a positive result (or a negative result, respectively).

The positive predictive value (PPV) describes the probability of having the disease state of interest in an individual with a positive result; therefore, PPV represents the proportion of patients with positive test result in the total group of individuals with positive test results or $(TP/(TP + FP))$.

The negative predictive value (NPV) describes the probability of not having the disease state in a subject with a negative test result; therefore, the NPV represents the proportion of patients/healthy individuals with a negative test result in the total group of individuals with negative test results, or $(TN/(TN + FN))$.

In contrast to DSE and DSP, PPV and NPV are dependent on disease prevalence in the examined population. For that reason, predictive values cannot be transferred from one to another study in which prevalence differences existed. Prevalence affects PPV and NPV differently: PPV is increasing, while NPV decreases with the increase of prevalence of the disease.

4.15 Receiver-Operating-Characteristic (ROC) Curve

ROC curves are used to assess the overall diagnostic accuracy of the test. In order to plot a ROC curve, the values for DSE and DSP are plotted in a x-y graph while changing the cutoff values over the spectrum of test results. The shape of the curve and the area under the curve is an indicator of the discriminative power of the test. The closer the curve bends into the upper left hand corner, which is equivalent with a larger area under the curve, the better is the discriminating power of the test between diseased and non-diseased samples (value of 1.0). In extreme, the value is 1 indicating full discrimination; if the line is straight between the x-y cross point and the upper right corner, there is no discriminating power of the test (value of 0.5; Figure 4.1).

4.16 Likelihood Ratios

Diagnostic accuracy can also be characterized by calculating positive and negative likelihood ratios (LR). LR tells us how many times more likely particular test results are in individuals with the disease than in those

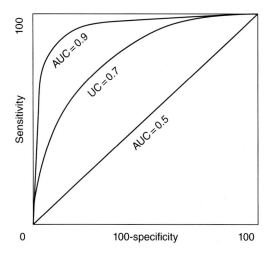

Figure 4.1 A Receiver-Operating-Characteristic (ROC) curve can be plotted by creating the DSE-DSP pairs over the range of selected cutoff values. Tests with poor performance and low discriminative power tend toward the diagonal line. Tests with good performance and discriminative power tend to bend upwards and to the left upper corner. The best performance, characterized by a DSE of 100% and DSP of 100% is located at the top left corner in the ROC graph.

without the disease. When both probabilities are equal, then the test has not discriminative power and is of no value; LR = 1.

Positive LR (LR+) tells us how much more likely a positive test result is to occur in patients with the disease compared to those without the disease: LR+ = DSE/(1-DSP). LR+ are normally above 1 because a diagnostic test does normally correlate with disease. Excellent diagnostic tests have LR+ of 10 or higher. The higher the LR+, the better the diagnostic tests' ability is in ruling-in the diagnosis.

Negative LR (LR−) tells us how much less likely the negative test result is to occur in a patient than in an individual without the disease: LR− = (1-DSE)/DSP. LR− is normally less than 1 because it is less likely that a negative test result occurs in subjects with disease than in subjects without the disease. Excellent diagnostic tests have LR− of <0.1. The lower the LR- value, the better the diagnostic tests' ability is in ruling-out the diagnosis.

Further Reading

STARD: Standards for Reporting Studies of Diagnostic Accuracy: Bossuyt PM, Reitsma JB, Bruns DE, Gatsonis CA, Glasziou PP, Irwig LM, et al. 2003. The STARD statement for reporting studies of diagnostic accuracy: explanation and elaboration. Clin Chem. 49(1): 7–18.

QUADAS: Quality Assessment of Diagnostic Accuracy Studies: Whiting P, Weswood ME, Rutjes AW, Reitsma JB, Bossuyt PN, and Kleijnen J. 2006. Evaluation of QUADAS, a tool for the quality assessment of diagnostic accuracy studies. BMC Med Res Methodol. 6: 9.

CLIA: Clinical Laboratory Improvement Amendments. FDA website www.fda.gov

ACCE framework: Analytical validity, clinical validity, clinical utility and associated ethical, legal and social implications. Mattocks CJ, Morris MA, Matthijs G, Swinnen E, Corveleyn A, et al. 2010. A standardized framework for the validation and verification of clinical molecular genetic tests. Eur J Hum Genet. Dec; 18(12): 1276–1288.

CLSI: Clinical and Laboratory Standards Institute: Wayne PA. Quality management for molecular genetic testing; approved guideline. CLSI document MM20-A. Clinical and Laboratory Standards Institute, 2012.

5

Enzymes
Leslie Sharkey

Department of Veterinary Clinical Sciences, College of Veterinary Medicine, University of Minnesota, Minnesota, USA

5.1   Introduction

The measurement of enzyme activities is a critical component of the routine serum biochemical profile. While low values are rarely diagnostically significant, elevations can be used to determine the spectrum of tissues involved in a pathologic process and to estimate the severity of the condition. Serial assessments can aid in evaluating progression of pathology or response to therapy. The presence of most diagnostic enzymes in the blood is incidental and reflects release due to routine cell turnover in tissues. Because these enzymes rarely serve any biological purpose in the blood, their concentrations are not regulated, thus reference intervals tend to be wide. Therefore, elevations are often expressed in fold elevations above the upper limit of the reference interval. While some enzymes originate from a single tissue, many have multiple potential sources. As a result, most test panels include multiple diagnostic enzymes that are interpreted together in the context of the history, physical examination, and other laboratory data to determine the most likely tissues involved. The tissue content of enzymes varies by species, so it is important to use equine-specific enzyme panels. In some cases, the enzyme data in combination with other clinical data can lead to a diagnosis, but in many cases additional diagnostic investigation may be required to determine a specific pathologic process.

5.2   Sample Collection and Methodologic Considerations

Measurement of enzyme activities in the blood is typically performed using serum. Lipemia, icterus, and hemolysis can all interfere with the analysis depending on the specific assay system, so it is important to avoid these if possible and to be aware of possible artifacts.

Most commercial and academic laboratories will evaluate samples for potential interferences and indicate any concerns about data validity on subsequent reports. Samples should be collected atraumatically and serum should be removed from cells as soon after clotting as possible (optimally <30 min) to avoid leakage of enzymes from blood cells and artifactual elevations in some enzymes. Most analyzers perform functional assays to evaluate serum enzyme activities, evaluating either the consumption of substrate or accumulation of a product; this means that machines and reagents developed for human medical practice can be used, but laboratory and species-specific reference intervals are necessary. Age of the animal can also impact expected values, and specific reference intervals for neonatal foals should be used to avoid diagnostic errors.

5.3   General Principles of Diagnostic Enzymology Data Interpretation

There are three non-mutually exclusive general mechanisms for increased serum enzyme activities: cell damage, enzyme induction, and decreased clearance from circulation (not a significant issue for diagnostically relevant enzymes in equine practice). Cell damage enzymes reflect either reversible or irreversible cell damage associated with cell blebbing or increased cell membrane permeability secondary to cell injury or death. Enzymes in this category include AST, SDH, CK, and sometimes GGT in the horse. Enzyme induction reflects increased cellular production associated with tissue hyperplasia or exposure to drugs, hormones, or other regulatory substances. Enzymes in this category include ALP and GGT.

Evaluation of diagnostic enzymes generally involves using the patterns of enzyme elevations to identify probable tissues involved and evaluating the magnitude to

Table 5.1 Summary of diagnostic enzymes, their tissues sources, mechanisms for increase, and basics of interpretation.

Enzyme	Tissue source	Mechanism of increase	Interpretation
Aspartate aminotransferase (AST)	Hepatocytes, muscle (skeletal and cardiac), erythrocytes	Cell damage	Due to lack of tissue specificity, interpret in conjunction with CK, SDH, and evidence of in *vitro* or *in vivo* hemolysis
Creatine Kinase (CK)	Muscle (skeletal and cardiac, possible a small amount from smooth muscle)	Cell damage	Considered muscle-specific and most often increases due to skeletal muscle damage. Is a very sensitive indicator of damage, so small elevations (<5000–10,000 IU/L) are considered nonspecific and can be associated with transport or injections. Myopathies are often associated with more robust to massive increases (>50,000 IU/L). Because of the short serum half-life of CK, persistent elevations suggest ongoing muscle damage
Sorbitol dehydrogenase or iditol dehydrogenase (SDH)	Hepatocytes	Cell damage	Favored because of tissue specificity for the liver, but may be less sensitive for the detection of damage than AST, possibly related to a shorter half-life in circulation
Gamma glutamyltransferase (GGT)	Wide distribution but most serum activity originates from the biliary epithelial cells, less from hepatocytes	Cell damage, solubilization from bile canalicular membrane by bile acids, and induction	Primarily considered an indicator of post-hepatic cholestasis and biliary hyperplasia, although it is also used as a nonspecific screening test for liver disease and values do increase in association with some gastrointestinal pathology; foals have a higher reference interval for GGT compared with adult horses, cause not specified
Alkaline phosphatase (ALP)	Biliary epithelial cells, hepatocytes, bone, intestine	Solubilization from bile canalicular membrane by bile acids, and induction	Reflects bone growth in foals (100-fold increase in newborns, falling over the first month of life and normalizing by 2–4 years), indicative of cholestatic liver disease. Can be elevated with intestinal pathology (colic), possibly due to increases in intestinal source ALP

estimate the severity of the process. Increasing values over time suggest progression of disease, while decreasing ones tend to suggest resolution; however, enzyme exhaustion due to a paucity of remaining viable tissue is also possible (Table 5.1). Evaluation of trends is likely more prognostically relevant than the magnitude of elevation at an isolated point in time.

5.4 Specific Diagnostic Enzymes and Their Interpretation

- *Age-related changes.* Foals have several unique features in their diagnostic enzyme data, so clinicians should have general awareness of age-related features of equine clinical chemistry data and should consult age-specific reference intervals or submit a serum sample from an unaffected control foal for reference if no reference intervals are available. ALP is elevated due to bone growth and GGT due to unknown endogenous causes, which can lead to the erroneous presumption

of cholestatic liver disease in neonatal foals, especially because serum bilirubin values are also higher in the first two weeks of life (Box 5.1) (Brewer et al., 1991, Hank et al., 1993, Patterson and Brown, 1986, Rumbaugh and Anderson, 1983). Dystocia or other trauma will result in variable increases in AST and CK due to muscle damage, but the responses are not specific to the age of the foal (see next).
- *Muscle damage.* Elevations in CK and AST are sensitive indicators of muscle damage in horses. Mild damage that may occur secondary to transport, exercise, or injections is reflected in smaller elevations, while trauma, surgery, or hypoperfusion can cause intermediate changes, and myopathies result in the most severe elevations. There is overlap between causes depending on the severity and time relative to the injury. For example, a report describing presumed immune-mediated myositis in 37 horses found a mean serum CK activity of 9,746 U/L with a range from 260–139,183 U/L, demonstrating the wide variation of values that can be associated with a single histologically defined disease process (Lewis et al., 2007). Because of differences

---

Box 5.1 Clinical example

A 3-week-old Friesian colt presented for diarrhea, lethargy, and inappetance; adequate passive transfer was confirmed by serum IgG testing. On physical examination, the colt was depressed with normal vital signs, signs of mild dehydration, and perineal staining. His CBC was unremarkable other than the presence of toxic neutrophils indicative of inflammation. The following enzyme values were obtained on his serum biochemical profile (serum bilirubin was within reference intervals):

ALP	H	624 U/L	(48–148)
GGT	H	65 U/L	(3–18)
SDH		6 U/L	(1–7)
AST		190 U/L	(162–316)
CK		237	(82–303)

The increases (H) in ALP and GGT were interpreted to be age related. The foal received fluid therapy, antimicrobials, anti-inflammatory medication, a biosponge, and probiotics. He responded well and was discharged two days later.

Box 5.2 Clinical example

Illustration of variation in enzyme values for horses presenting with muscle damage associated with different clinical presentations. Note the mild elevations with the puncture wound, the slightly greater elevations occurring secondary to a surgical colic (but still attributed primarily to skeletal muscle damage: poor tissue perfusion and iatrogenic causes), and the more dramatic increases associated with post-anesthetic myopathy, with the CK peaking and falling earlier than the AST.

Condition	SDH (1–7 U/L)	AST (162–316 U/L)	CK (82–303 U/L)
Puncture wound	4	443	542
Small intestinal intussusception	1	768	2892
Post-anesthetic myopathy day 1	12	7009	>20,000
Day 2	6	10,400	>20,000
Day 4	2	10,082	9,129

---

in cell release and clearance from the blood, CK tends to increase rapidly and is cleared quickly after an acute episode, while AST increases are slightly delayed and more persistent due to a lag in clearance. See Box 5.2 for some clinical examples. Pre-operative muscle enzyme activities may have prognostic significance in horses with surgical colic, with higher values for CK and AST noted in horses with lesions causing intestinal ischemia and in non-survivors (Krueger et al., 2014). Increases were attributed to endotoxin-mediated damage to muscle, and while statistically significant, the differences between survivors and non-survivors were relatively modest. Interestingly, neither GGT nor SDH levels varied with lesion type or prognosis.

- *Hepatocellular damage.* SDH is the most specific indicator of hepatocellular damage in the horse, with AST and GGT also used as more sensitive but less specific indicators. Thus, when SDH is elevated, there is a high degree of confidence that hepatocellular damage is the cause, while a normal value does not exclude hepatocellular damage, especially if GGT and/or AST are simultaneously elevated. These changes can reflect the magnitude of the damage, but are not specific to the cause. While hepatocellular damage can signal primary liver disease, it is important to remember that systemic hypoperfusion, anemia, and secondary effects from gastrointestinal pathology can also cause hepatocellular damage in the absence of primary hepatic pathology. A study evaluating serum biochemical data

---

Box 5.3 Clinical example

Clinical examples of enzyme elevations in three horses presenting with primary intestinal conditions. Note the increasing magnitude of enzyme elevations associated with the severity of the intestinal pathology and systemic circulatory compromise (H=high).

Condition	ALP (48–148)	GGT (3–18)	SDH (1–7 U/L)	AST (162–316 U/L)	CK (82–303 U/L)
Colonic impaction and torsion	H 288	15	4	H 421	204
Nephrosplenic entrapment	H 162	H 21	H 8	H 439	H 1229
Epiploic foramen entrapment, infarction, and gastric rupture	H 424	H 23	H >50	H 713	H 10,377

---

in horses undergoing liver biopsy concluded that no single test or combination of tests could reliably differentiate the horses with and without histologic evidence of liver disease (Durham et al., 2003).

- *Post-hepatic cholestasis.* GGT and ALP are the primary indicators of post-hepatic cholestasis, along with hyperbilirubinemia. Acute biliary obstructions are uncommon in the horse, but may be associated with cholelithiasis or colonic displacement. More commonly, milder forms of post-hepatic cholestasis may occur secondary to hepatocellular swelling, infiltration of the liver parenchyma by inflammatory or neoplastic cells, or to fibrosis associated with infectious liver disease and toxic insults. In horses, it can be difficult to achieve a definitive interpretation of post-hepatic cholestasis using the serum biochemical profile alone because the combination of anorexia-induced hyperbilirubinemia and colic-associated elevations in ALP and GGT (see the next bullet point) results in a similar pattern on the serum biochemical profile.
- *Intestinal disorders and systemic disease.* Intestinal disorders can result in secondary hepatic pathology via ascending infection of the biliary tract, exposure of the liver to endotoxin and bacteria carried by the portal circulation, and secondary to hypoperfusion associated with shock and sepsis. Hepatocytes are also susceptible to hypoxic injury associated with anemia, generally reflected in increased hepatocellular injury enzymes such as SDH, AST, and GGT. Specifically, proximal enteritis has been shown to cause elevations in ALP, AST, and GGT (SDH was not reported), presumably due to secondary hepatic pathology that was confirmed in a small number of horses that were necropsied; none of the horses had evidence of liver disease prior to the presentation for proximal enteritis (Davis et al., 2003). Likewise, a subset of horses presenting with surgical colic had elevated serum SDH and GGT activities, with high GGT values more likely to persist after surgery, but these values were not strongly prognostic (Underwood, 2010). High liver enzyme activities (GGT and SDH) were common in a study of hospitalized neonatal foals, primarily associated with sepsis, perinatal asphyxia syndrome, and proximal enteritis, but did not appear to be prognostic (Haggett et al., 2011). Approximately half of horses with right dorsal displacement of the colon had elevations in serum GGT activity, while only 2% with left dorsal displacement had increases, suggesting that the right displacements may impinge on bile flow (Gardner et al., 2005). Box 5.3 illustrates clinical examples of extra-hepatic causes of enzyme elevations.

References

Brewer BD, Clement ST, Lotz WS, and Gronwall R. 1991. Renal clearance, urinary excretion of endogeneous substances, and urinary diagnostic indices in healthy neonatal foals. J Vet Intern Med 5: 28–33.

Davis JL, Blikslager AT, Catto K, and Jones SL. 2003. A retrospective analysis of hepatic injury in horses with proximal enteritis (1984–2002). J Vet Intern Med 17: 896–901.

Durham AE, Smith KC, and Newton JR. 2003. An evaluation of diagnostic data in comparison to the results of liver biopsies in mature horses. Eq Vet J 35: 554–559.

Gardner RB, Nydam DV, Mohammed HO, Duscharme NG, and Drivers TJ. 2005. Serum gamma glutamyl transferase activity in horses with right or left dorsal displacements of the large colon. J Vet Intern Med 19: 761–764.

Haggett EF, Magdesian KG, and Kass PH. 2011. Clinical implications of high liver enzyme activities in hospitalized neonatal foals. J Am Vet Med Assoc 239: 661–667.

Hank AM, Hoffman WE, Sanecki RK, Schaeffer DJ, Dorner JL. 1993. Quantitative determination of equine alkaline phosphatase isoenzymes in foal and adult serum. J Vet Intern Med 7: 20–24.

Krueger CR, Ruple-Czerniak A, and Hackett ES. 2014. Evaluation of plasma muscle enzyme activity as an indicator of lesion characteristics and prognosis in horses undergoing celiotomy for acute gastrointestinal pain. BMC Veterinary Research 10 (Suppl 1): 57–64.

Lewis SS, Valberg SJ, and Nielsen IL. 2007. Suspected immune-mediated myositis in horses. J Vet Intern Med 21: 495–503.

Patterson WH and Brown CM. 1986. Increase of serum gamma-glytamyltransferase in neonatal Standardbred foals. Am J Vet Res 47(2): 461–463.

Rumbaugh GE and Adamson PJ. 1983. Automated serum chemical analysis in the foal. J Am Vet Med Assoc 183: 769–772.

Underwood C, Southwood LL, Walton RM, and Johnson AL. 2010. Hepatic and metabolic changes in surgical colic patients: a pilot study. J of Vet Emerg Crit Care 20: 578–586.

6

Kidney Function Tests
Leslie Sharkey

Department of Veterinary Clinical Sciences, College of Veterinary Medicine, University of Minnesota, Minnesota, USA

6.1 Introduction

The kidney plays a central role in fluid, electrolyte, acid-base, and mineral balance. It contributes to the regulation of erythrocyte production via erythropoietin, and glomerular damage can result in serum albumin abnormalities. Therefore, while blood urea nitrogen (BUN) and serum creatinine (Cr) are the most common indicators of kidney function, many other serum biochemical analytes can be influenced by renal disease and should be evaluated in conjunction with the BUN and Cr. Discussion of these analytes in this chapter will be restricted to their interpretation in altered kidney function. Proper diagnostic evaluation of kidney parameters requires a complete urinalysis concurrent with the serum biochemical profile. While loose diagnostic inferences can be made without a urinalysis, these conclusions are speculative without simultaneous chemical and microscopic evaluation of urine. Even with a complete clinicopathologic data set, complete characterization of renal pathology may require biopsy. A large study of 151 renal biopsies in horses revealed a complication rate of 11%, primarily hemorrhage or colic signs, but only a single fatality (Tyner, 2011). Over 90% of biopsies yielded a histologic diagnosis, however, correlation with necropsy findings was reported to be limited at 72%.

6.2 Blood Urea Nitrogen (BUN)

Urea is synthesized in the liver from bicarbonate and ammonia. Urea is the major route of nitrogen excretion, so protein catabolism contributes to BUN concentrations. Elimination is primarily renal, where it is freely filtered by glomeruli and undergoes passive tubular resorption. Thus, reduced tubular flow rates will increase reabsorption, increasing blood concentrations. A proportion of urea is excreted in the intestine, where it can undergo microbial digestion, and this route of elimination may be increased in horses with renal disease. Increases in BUN indicate azotemia, which is classified as pre-renal, renal, or post-renal based when interpreted in the context of the physical examination findings and urinalysis (Table 6.1). There are no unique sample collection and handling requirements for BUN measurement. Dietary protein content and muscle catabolism will have minor positive influences on BUN in horses.

Once dietary and metabolic considerations have been eliminated, the primary cause for increased BUN is decreased glomerular filtration rate (GFR). BUN may become elevated earlier than creatinine, especially in pre-renal azotemia because of increased tubular reabsorption. The greatest elevations in BUN are observed in severe renal or post-renal azotemia, although the degree of elevation at presentation is not strictly predictive of the cause or reversibility of azotemia. The relationship of increased BUN with decreased GFR is non-linear. Significant (>75%) decreases in GFR are required to cause an increased BUN, and relatively large decrements in GFR are associated with minimal increments in BUN early in renal disease, while relatively minor additional decreases in GFR are associated with relatively greater increases in serum urea and Cr concentrations. Decreases in BUN can be associated with increased renal excretion associated with high tubular flow rates. In many species, low BUN can be a feature of hepatic insufficiency, but studies of horses with liver disease suggest this is not a common finding in the equine (Durham et al., 2003).

6.3 Creatinine (Cr)

Cr is derived primarily from muscle, with skeletal muscle contributing >90% of the serum Cr. For this reason, variation in muscle mass may influence serum

Interpretation of Equine Laboratory Diagnostics, First Edition. Edited by Nicola Pusterla and Jill Higgins.
© 2018 John Wiley & Sons, Inc. Published 2018 by John Wiley & Sons, Inc.

Table 6.1 Classification of azotemia. Urine specific gravity (USG).

Type of azotemia	Degree	USG	Clinical signs	Causes
Pre-renal	Mild to moderate	>1.035	Dehydration, poor pulse quality, prolonged capillary refill time, pale or red mucous membranes	Dehydration, cardiac disease, shock (hemorrhagic, anaphylactic, septic, neurogenic)
Renal	Mild to severe	<1.020, often 1.008–1.014	Depend on duration and severity	Congenital, inflammatory/infectious, toxic, neoplastic
Post-renal	Mild to severe	Variable	Dysuria, renal colic, abdominal distention, note that urine volume may be decreased but some animals will continue to pass urine	Urolithiasis, trauma, neoplasia

Cr. Cr is freely filtered in the glomerulus, with minimal to no tubular reabsorption, although small amounts may be secreted in the presence of azotemia. A low level of excretion via the gastrointestinal tract is also possible. Serum Cr has a similar non-linear relationship with GFR as BUN, being a relatively insensitive indicator of renal dysfunction early in disease, while large increases may be seen late in disease with relatively minimal decrements in GFR. There is no unique sample collection or handling requirement for Cr. The most commonly used method for Cr measurement, the Jaffé reaction, does have some analytical considerations. The presence of some compounds, such as proteins, glucose, ketone bodies, and a few drugs, are "non-creatinine chromagens," meaning that they cause a positive interference because the assay recognizes them as Cr. Bilirubin can cause a negative interference. While muscle damage can result in release of Cr, with normal renal function, this is rapidly cleared from the circulation. Cr is generally used as an indicator of decreased GFR. Hypercreatininemia in neonatal foals has been associated with impaired placental function, in which case levels should rapidly decline the first few days after birth. One study of 28 neonatal foals with hypercreatininemia failed to identify significant placental pathology in most cases, although a diagnosis of neonatal encephalopathy was common (Chaney et al., 2010). The authors noted resolution of this "spurious" hypercreatininemia within 72 h with appropriate neonatal therapy and high survival rates, while foals with acute renal failure tended to have more severe azotemia that did not resolve with treatment despite similar presenting serum Cr values (Chaney et al., 2010). Foals with spurious hypercreatininemia were reported to have mean serum Cr of 13.6 mg/d, with a standard deviation of 7.5. (See Box 6.1 for a clinical example.)

6.4 Classification of Azotemia

Azotemia is classified into three non-mutually exclusive types: pre-renal, renal, and post-renal (see Table 6.1). Pre-renal azotemia reflects a decreased GFR that is the result of poor renal perfusion primarily due to systemic causes such as dehydration, low cardiac output, and conditions of inadequate vascular tone, including shock (see Box 6.1 and Box 6.2). The degree of azotemia is generally mild to moderate, there are supportive clinical signs such as prolonged capillary refill time or poor pulse quality, and if renal function is intact, compensatory mechanisms should result in renal concentration of urine to a specific gravity of >1.035 (Geor, 2007). Clinicians must beware that fluid therapy or diuretic use will influence urine specific gravity, evaluated should be performed prior to initiation of treatment. Marked decreases in renal perfusion that initially manifest as pre-renal azotemia can cause ischemic renal injury. This can exacerbate existing renal pathology or act alone or synergistically with renotoxic medications such as non-steroidal anti-inflammatories and some antibiotics to cause renal azotemia. One study of renal parameters in horses presenting with primary gastrointestinal disease and a Cr >3.0 mg/dl observed that the presence of reflux, hypochloridemia, and abnormal rectal examination findings was associated with persistence of azotemia beyond 3 days of treatment for the primary disease (Groover et al., 2006). Horses with persistent azotemia had significantly higher Cr than horses resolving within 3 days of presentation (5.2 vs 3.9 g/dl), with 4 of the 26 horses in the study ultimately treated for a diagnosis of acute renal failure.

The hallmark of renal azotemia is inappropriately concentrated urine (<1.020, but often isosthenuria) in the presence of azotemia and/or dehydration. This is primarily due to renal tubular dysfunction and is indicative

A 9-hour old Percheron/Paint cross colt presents for generalized weakness. He was born during the night and found in the morning cold and unable to stand. Meconium was not passed. He has been treated with 1 pint of colostrum and antibiotics. On presentation, the colt was quiet, recumbent, and depressed. He was estimated to be 8% dehydrated, was hypothermic, had a constant machinery heart murmur consistent with a patent ductus arteriosus and weak peripheral pulses. No suckle reflex could be elicited. CBC revealed a regenerative left shift with toxic change and a relative erythrocytosis.

BUN		22 mg/dl	(13–23)
Cr	H	4.2 mg/dl	(0.7–1.7)
Calcium		12.2 mg/dl	(10.4–12.9)
Phosphorus	H	4.9 mg/dl	(1.7–4.4)
Albumin	L	2.7 g/dl	(2.9–3.9)
Globulin	L	0.7 g/dl	(1.9–3.9)
Sodium		138 mmol/L	(130–140)
Chloride		98 mmol/L	(95–103)
Potassium		4.1 mmol/L	(3.6–5.1)
Bicarbonate		26.6 mmol/L	(25–31)
Anion Gap		16	(10–16)

Although no urine specific gravity was performed, the hypercreatininemia was attributed to either placental dysfunction (organ was not available for evaluation) or spurious hypercreatininemia. A mild pre-renal azotemia could not be excluded; however, the BUN was within reference intervals. Abdominal ultrasound revealed an intact urinary bladder. The increased phosphorus was interpreted to be evidence of bone growth normal for the age of the foal. Mildly low albumin was not considered clinically relevant, and a serum IgG snap test was normal after the colt received 2 units of plasma. He was also treated with fluids and antibiotics, to which he responded well. Two days after presentation, the serum Cr concentration had normalized (1.3 mg/dl), while the hyperphosphatemia was persistent, supporting the initial interpretation.

A 2-year-old Paint stallion presents for a 2-day history of lethargy and mild colic signs transiently responsive to non-steroidal anti-inflammatory medication and nasogastric administration of mineral oil. On presentation, he was quiet and responsive with normal heart and respiratory rates, but a mild fever. His mucous membranes were tacky and he had a prolonged capillary refill time. Gut sounds were present but decreased, and 28 l of reflux was obtained over the following 24 h. Initial rectal examination revealed a distended large colon with a partial left dorsal displacement, however, 24 h later, the left kidney could not be palpated and there was concern for a nephrosplenic entrapment. CBC revealed neutropenia with mild toxic change and a mild relative erythrocytosis.

BUN	H	39 mg/dl	(13–23)
Cr	H	2.4 mg/dl	(0.7–1.7)
Calcium		11.1 mg/dl	(10.4–12.9)
Phosphorus	H	4.7 mg/dl	(1.7–4.4)
Albumin		3.6 g/dl	(2.9–3.9)
Sodium	L	127 mmol/L	(130–140)
Chloride	L	89 mmol/L	(95–103)
Bicarbonate		28.6 mmol/L	(25–31)
Anion Gap		14	(10–16)

The neutropenia was consistent with acute inflammation, while the polycythemia and physical examination findings were consistent with dehydration and decreased perfusion. Although a urine specific gravity was not available for confirmation, the mild azotemia was interpreted to be most likely pre-renal on this basis. Hyperphosphatemia was the result of decreased GFR. Electrolyte losses were presumed to be gastrointestinal, and there were no acid-base abnormalities at presentation despite reflux and poor perfusion. The stallion was taken to surgery for the presumed entrapment, which was confirmed and corrected during an exploratory laparotomy. An enterotomy was also performed to relieve colonic distension by gas, fluid, and food material. The horse recovered well with no additional signs of colic and laboratory data normalized. This is an example of presumed pre-renal azotemia that resolved with correction of underlying gastrointestinal causes.

of renal disease, however, it is important to note some conditions in which other factors may interfere with renal tubular function, such as osmotic diuresis or medullary washout. Renal azotemia can be mild to severe, and pre-renal azotemia may contribute to the degree of severity, so the patient should be re-evaluated after correction of pre-renal factors. Post-renal azotemia is characterized by obstruction of urine flow distal to the kidneys. Variable degrees of decreased urine production, dysuria, abdominal distention, and pain can accompany post-renal azotemia, which can be mild to severe in degree. Urolithiasis is the most common cause, but congenital abnormalities, neoplasia, and trauma can also cause post-renal obstruction. Complete obstruction of urine flow for an extended period can be detrimental to renal tubular cells, causing renal azotemia.

6.5 Other Biochemical Analytes in Conditions of Decreased GFR

6.5.1 Minerals

- Magnesium can be increased due to reduced renal elimination.
- Calcium can be normal in horses with renal failure, although acute renal failure tends to be associated with hypocalcemia, while chronic renal failure tends to be associated with hypercalcemia (LeRoy et al., 2011, Schott, 2007). Hypercalcemia appears to be the result of failure of renal elimination of dietary calcium, and can be ameliorated by dietary modification from high calcium alfalfa to lower calcium grass hay (Schott, 2007). Hypercalcemia associated with equine renal dysfunction does not appear cause clinical signs and does not have prognostic significance (LeRoy et al., 2011, Schott, 2007).
- Hyperphosphatemia can be associated with pre-renal azotemia and with renal azotemia in cases of acute renal failure. In contrast, horses with chronic renal failure characterized by hypercalcemia, there is a compensatory hypophosphatemia.

6.5.2 Electrolytes

- Sodium values may be high, low, or within reference intervals in horses with pre-renal azotemia depending on the underlying cause. Hyponatremia is more common than hypernatremia in horses with both acute and chronic renal failure due to inability of the renal tubules to appropriately reabsorb sodium. Thus, inappropriately high urinary fractional excretion of sodium can be an indicator of renal disease and will be discussed in the urinalysis chapter. Post-renal azotemia can likewise be associated with hyponatremia, in this circumstance due to inability to excrete water with a dilutional effect on remaining extracellular sodium concentrations. While abnormalities in sodium can reflect underlying renal dysfunction, sodium loss via other routes (gastrointestinal, cutaneous) that results in hyponatremia can likewise impair the renal medullary concentration gradient required for optimal urine concentration. Thus, hyponatremia can be the result or the cause of impaired renal function.
- Serum chloride values typically mirror serum sodium concentrations.
- Although serum potassium concentrations can be variable in equine renal disease, they can provide important information. Polyuria often leads to excessive renal losses of potassium, and decreased feed intake can contribute to hypokalemia. In contrast, conditions associated with decreased urine output, such as acute renal failure, acute on chronic renal failure, and post-renal causes of azotemia tend to result in hyperkalemia because of failure of renal elimination of this electrolyte.

6.5.3 Acid-Base

Acid-base balance is often normal until terminal stages of renal dysfunction, at which point a high anion gap acidosis occurs because of failure to eliminate uremic acids. Lactic acidosis can also contribute due to associated dehydration, or when other pre-renal causes of decreased tissue perfusion are present. If there is concurrent reflux with subsequent hypochloremic metabolic alkalosis, a mixed acid-base disorder may be observed.

6.5.4 Albumin

Serum albumin concentrations may be high, low, or normal in pre-renal azotemia. Dehydration due to restricted access to water or loss of protein-poor fluids (i.e., sweating, some types of diarrhea) can lead to hyperalbuminemia, while loss of protein-rich fluids such as blood or exudative effusions can result in hypoalbuminemia. Serum albumin levels are reduced in horses with glomerular damage due to selective loss of this relatively small protein through damaged filtration pores; significant proteinuria will be noted on urinalysis that can be better quantified by measuring the urine protein:creatinine ratio. Tubular damage can cause lower magnitude proteinuria due to failure of renal reabsorption of the normally filtered protein load, but this rarely leads to hypoalbuminemia (see Box 6.3). Anorexia and poor nutrition associated with chronic renal failure can contribute to hypoalbuminemia as well.

Box 6.3 Case example of a horse in renal failure.

A 13-year-old Arab stallion presents with a history of treatment with large doses of non-steroidal anti-inflammatory (NSAID) medication during a horse show earlier in the month, during which he also had mild diarrhea. After the show, the stallion was noted to be lethargic and anorexic, so additional NSAIDs were administered. The horse has lost approximately 150 pounds since the horse show. On presentation, the stallion is bright and alert, appears to be normally hydrated, and had notable dental calculus of his incisors. All CBC data were within reference intervals.

BUN	H	71 mg/dl	(13–23)
Cr	H	6.1 mg/dl	(0.7–1.7)
Calcium	H	17.1 mg/dl	(10.4–12.9)
Phosphorus	L	1.3 mg/dl	(1.7–4.4)
Magnesium	H	3.2 mg/dl	(1.3–2.3)
Albumin	L	2.8 g/dl	(2.9–3.9)
Sodium	L	125 mmol/L	(130–140)
Chloride	L	92 mmol/L	(95–103)
Potassium		4.3 mmol/L	(3.6–5.1)
Bicarbonate		28.8 mmol/L	(25–31)
Anion Gap	L	9	(10–16)

Urine specific gravity: 1.010

Glucose, bilirubin, ketones: negative

3+ proteinuria

Urine sediment: no cells, many calcium carbonate crystals

The moderate to marked azotemia and isosthenuria was indicative of renal azotemia, with little support for a pre-renal component in the physical examination or laboratory data. Note the hypercalcemia and secondary hypophosphatemia most consistent with a chronic process. Hypoalbuminemia with marked proteinuria in a urine with a normal sediment examination indicates that glomerular damage is likely an important component of the renal pathology, although the history of weight loss suggests a nutritional component cannot be excluded. The low anion gap is the result of the hypoalbuminemia. Failure of renal reabsorption of sodium and chloride indicative of tubular dysfunction was confirmed by inappropriate high urinary electrolyte excretion. This horse also had increased urinary GGT concentration (153 U/L, normal <5) supportive of ongoing acute renal tubular damage (see the urinalysis chapter). The horse responded to supportive care for a clinical diagnosis of acute on chronic renal failure, and a biopsy was not performed. The long-term prognosis was considered guarded to poor.

References

Chaney KP, Holcombe SJ, Schott HC, and Barr BS. 2010. Spurious hypercreatininemia: 28 neonatal foals (2000–2008). J Vet Emerg Crit Care 20: 244–249.

Durham AE, Smith KC, and Newton JR. 2003. An evaluation of diagnostic data in comparison to the results of liver biopsies in mature horses. Eq Vet J 35: 554–559.

Geor RJ. 2007. Acute renal failure in horses. Vet Clin Equine 23: 577–591.

Groover ES, Woolums AR, Cole DJ, and LeRoy BE. 2006. Risk factors associated with renal insufficiency in horses with primary gastrointestinal disease: 26 cases. J Am Vet Med Assoc 228: 572–577.

LeRoy B. Woomums A, Wass J, Davis E, Gold J, Foreman JH, et al. 2011. The relationship between serum calcium concentration and outcome in horses with renal failure presented to referral hospitals. J Vet Intern Med 25: 1426–1430.

Schott HC. 2007. Chronic renal failure in horses. Vet Clin Equine 23: 593–612.

Tyner GA, Nolen-Walston RD, Hall T, Palmero JP, Couëtil L, Javscias L, et al. (2011) A multicenter retrospective study of 151 renal biopsies in horses. J Vet Intern Med 25: 532–539.

7

Carbohydrates
Leslie Sharkey

Department of Veterinary Clinical Sciences, College of Veterinary Medicine, University of Minnesota, Minnesota, USA

7.1 Introduction and Physiology

Glucose measurement is an important metabolic indicator that is highly regulated in all species. Food intake, glycolysis, glycogenolysis, and gluconeogenesis all contribute to supporting blood glucose levels in the normal range across a wide range of nutritional conditions. Glucagon, corticosteroids, catecholamines, and growth hormone all increase plasma glucose concentrations, while the primary hormone lowering glucose is insulin. Not surprisingly, clinicians will encounter hyperglycemia far more often than hypoglycemia in their patients, although immaturity of some metabolic pathways in the neonate leads to higher prevalence of hypoglycemia in this cohort.

7.2 Glucose

7.2.1 Methodology

Reference laboratory analyzers utilize robust methods with high accuracy and precision to evaluate serum glucose. All point of care analyzers should be validated against these methods across the full range of diagnostically relevant values. Additional detail on point of care testing can be found in Chapter 3. Attention to optimal sample collection and handling is important for accurate glucose measurement. Most importantly, separate serum from cells within 1 hour of collection in the horse if the sample is kept at room temperature. Storage at 4 °C prevents a statistically significant decline in glucose concentration for at least 8 h (Collicutt et al., 2015). This may be an attractive alternative to collection in sodium fluoride potassium oxalate, which has previously been cited as the anticoagulant of choice to prevent *in vitro* glycolysis, however recent work calls the validity of this practice into question (Collicutt et al., 2015, Rendle et al., 2009).

7.2.2 Hyperglycemia

Stress, excitement, and pain are common causes of hyperglycemia in the horse, and may be accompanied by corticosteroid or epinephrine-mediated changes in the leukogram. The early phases of endotoxemia can also be associated with hyperglycemia (see Box 7.3 and Chapter 11). Diabetes mellitus is uncommon in the horse, but when identified, is typically type II. Equine pituitary pars intermedia dysfunction (PPID) can also be associated with hyperglycemia.

7.2.3 Hypoglycemia

The potential for pre-analytical error to contribute to hypoglycemia should always be evaluated, particularly when clinical signs are absent. While true hypoglycemia is rare in adult horses, even those with liver failure or experiencing starvation, it is relatively common in ill neonatal foals (McGorum et al., 1999, Divers, 2011). Hypoglycemic foals are often septic, starving, or rarely, have liver dysfunction, with <50 mg/dL glucose potentially indicative of a poorer prognosis (Divers, 2011, see Box 7.1). Paraneoplastic hypoglycemia, while also rare, has been reported in horses in association with renal or hepatic neoplasia (Baker et al., 2001, Swain et al., 2005, Wong et al., 2015).

Box 7.1 Case example of a foal with severe hypoglycemia.

An 18-hour-old Thoroughbred colt presented for signs of respiratory distress after an unobserved foaling the previous day. The foal initially stood and nursed, but gradually became weaker and was bottle fed overnight. On presentation, the foal was laterally recumbent, nonresponsive, and shocky. Peripheral pulses were not palpable and extremities were cold. The capillary refill time was >8 s, and severe expiratory wheezes could be ausculted in all lung fields with crackles in the cranioventral fields. The CBC revealed severe neutropenia with lymphopenia and hyperfibrinogenemia.

Glucose	L	15 mg/dl	(75–116)

The severe hypoglycemia is even more dramatic given that foal serum glucose is usually slightly higher than adult (Axon and Palmer, 2008). This foal died shortly after presentation and necropsy revealed severe necro-suppurative bronchopneumonia, with in utero infection suspected based on the extent of lung involvement.

7.2.4 Evaluation of Glycemic Control

It may be helpful to assess glucose and insulin responsiveness if equine metabolic syndrome, insulin resistance, or PPID is suspected in a patient (Frank and Tadros, 2014). These tests should be performed after an overnight fast and samples should be drawn in the morning. Results may be confounded by stress, excitement, pain, or exercise. It is very important to use the individual laboratory reference intervals, as test methodology for hormones like insulin will affect expected results.

- Fasting insulin and glucose
  - Equine metabolic syndrome is suggested by normal glucose or hyperglycemia, hyperinsulinemia, and hypertriglyceridemia. Increased leptin concentration (>4 ng/L) also supports a diagnosis of this condition.
  - Type 2 diabetes mellitus is characterized by hyperglycemia with normal or increased fasting insulin (referred to as non-compensated or compensated insulin resistance, respectively; see Box 7.2).

Box 7.2 Case example of a horse with PPID and secondary type 2 diabetes mellitus.

A 22-year-old Arabian gelding presented for weight loss and elevated liver enzymes. While his appetite varied, he was never completely off feed. On physical examination, moderate hirsutism was noted, and he had a pendulous abdomen. His body condition score was 3/9. His CBC was within normal limits. The following abnormalities were seen on his chemistry panel.

Test	Unit	Patient	Reference intervals
AST	IU/L	1251	170–370
ALP	IU/L	1747	80–187
GGT	IU/L	2164	7–20
SDH	IU/L	263	4–14
Triglyceride	mg/dL	925	10–60
Glucose	mg/dL	384	83–114
Bile acids	μmol/L	103	4–12

Urinalysis

Color/appearance	Yellow, opaque
Specific gravity	1.025
pH	8.0
Protein (mg/dl)	Trace
Blood	+
Glucose	++
Acetone	Negative
Bilirubin	Negative
Sediment	0–1 RBC/hpf
	0–1 squamous epithelial cells/hpf
	Many calcium carbonate crystals

- The marked increases in liver enzymes and bile acids are compatible with impaired liver function, likely due to hepatic lipidosis.
- The hyperglycemia, glucosuria and hypertriglyceridemia indicate metabolic dysregulation, compatible with diabetes mellitus.
- Given the age of the horse and the physical findings of hirsutism and weight loss, PPID with secondary type 2 diabetes mellitus was suspected.

After an overnight fast, blood was drawn for additional testing.

	Unit	Patient	Reference interval
Endogenous ACTH	pg/mL	124	9–35
Fasting Insulin	pmol/L	116	29–179
Fasting glucose	mg/dL	291	83–114

- The increased endogenous ACTH is compatible with PPID.
- Normal fasting insulin in a patient with hyperglycemia is compatible with uncompensated type 2 diabetes mellitus.

Type 1 diabetes mellitus in the horse is rare and characterized by hyperglycemia and hypoinsulinemia. Glycosuria and ketonuria may be detected.

- Glucose tolerance testing
  - There is a variety of testing protocols for assessing glucose tolerance and insulin sensitivity. See Chapter 60 for details on performing these testing procedures.

- The oral sugar test can be used to screen for equine metabolic syndrome by assessing glucose and insulin response to an oral sugar load.
  - After an overnight fast, a baseline blood sample is obtained and Karo Light Corn Syrup (0.15 mL/kg) is given per os. Blood samples are collected at 60 and 90 min.
  - Equine metabolic syndrome is indicated by an insulin concentration >420 pmol/L (>60 µU/mL) and/or glucose >125 mg/dL at either 60 or 90 min following an oral sugar load.
  - Insulin between 315–420 pmol/L (45–60 µU/mL) suggests mild or early equine metabolic syndrome (see Box 7.3).
- Combined glucose insulin test
  - After an overnight fast, a baseline blood sample is collected. Intravenously administer 150 mg/kg glucose as 50% dextrose, immediately followed by 0.10 IU insulin iv.
  - Glucose is measured at 0, 1, 5, 15, 25, 35, 45, 60, 75, 90, 105, 120, 135, and 150 min.
  - Insulin is measured at baseline and 45 min.
  - A horse is insulin resistant if the glucose exceeds the baseline concentration for more than 45 min.
  - Insulin >695 pmol/L (>100 µU/mL) at 45 minutes is consistent with compensated insulin resistance or excessive pancreatic response to a sugar load.

Box 7.3 Case example of a horse with equine metabolic syndrome.

An 11-year-old warm blood mare was noted by her owner to be "an easy keeper lately." On physical examination, she had a body condition score of 8/9 with adiposity of the nuchal crest, between the shoulder blades, and over the croup. The CBC and chemistry profile were with within normal limits. After an overnight fast, an oral sugar test was performed and the following data obtained.

	Glucose (mg/dL)	Insulin (pmol/L)
Fasting	87	194
60 minutes	147	377
90 minutes	154	475
Fasting reference interval	83–114	<300

Plasma endogenous ACTH was 5.9 pmol/L (reference interval 2.0–10.0).

Although fasting glucose and insulin were normal, an insulin >420 pmol/L and glucose >125 mg/dL at 90 min indicate insulin dysregulation and equine metabolic syndrome. The normal endogenous ACTH excludes PPID as a cause of the insulin resistance. Dietary management to decrease obesity was instituted.

7.2.5 Fructosamine

- Fructosamine refers to the irreversible, non-enzymatic glycation of albumin, and its concentration reflects blood glucose concentrations over the previous 2–3 weeks. While it has proven useful in evaluating glycemic control and in distinguishing excitement-induced hyperglycemia in small animals, few studies have evaluated the usefulness of fructosamine in horses. Effects of season, age, or breed on this analyte have not yet been established.
- Fructosamine was increased and correlated with glucose and indicators of insulin resistance in horses with laminitis (Knowles et al., 2012).
- Fructosamine concentrations were found to be increased in horses with PPID but did not distinguish between animals treated with pergolide (Gehlen et al., 2014) or those with laminitis (Knowles et al., 2014).
- Fructosamine may be increased in mares during early lactation (Filipovic et al., 2010).

7.3 Ketones

Production of ketones from long chain fatty acids and their use as an energy source occurs during periods of negative energy balance. Ketones include acetone, acetoacetate, and ß-hydroxybutyrate (ß-HB) with ß-HB most commonly measured in the blood. Transient ketonemia may occur following exercise in horses (Bruss, 2008). ß-HB increases in mares during pregnancy and early lactation (Filipovic et al., 2010, Bazzano et al., 2014). Though less common than in similarly affected small animals, ketones may sometimes be detected in the urine of horses with type 1 and type 2 diabetes mellitus (Tasker, 1966, Ruoff et al., 1986).

References

Axon JE and Palmer JE. 2008. Clinical pathology of the foal. Vet Clin Equine 24: 357–385.

Baker JL, Aleman M, and Madigan J. 2001. Intermittent hypoglycemia in a horse with anaplastic carcinoma of the kidney. J Am Vet Med Assoc 218: 235–237.

Bazzano M, Giannetto C, Fazio F, Arfuso F, Giudice E, and Piccione G. 2014. Metabolic profile of broodmares during late pregnancy and early post-partum. Reproduction in Domestic Animals. 49: 947–953.

Bruss ML. 2008. Lipids and ketones. In: JJ Kaneko, JW Harvey, and ML Bruss (eds). Clinical biochemistry of Domestic Animals, 6th Edn. Burlington MA: Elsevier, pp. 81–115.

Collicutt NB, Garner B, Berghaus RD, Camus MS, and Hart K. 2015. Effect of delayed serum separation and storage temperature on serum glucose concentration in horse, dog, alpaca, and sturgeon. Vet Clin Pathol 44: 120–127.

Divers TJ. 2011. Metabolic causes of encephalopathy in horses. Vet Clin Equine 27: 589–596.

Filipovic N, Stojevic Z, and Prvanovic N. 2010. Serum fructosamine concentrations in relation to metabolic changes during late pregnancy and early lactation in mares. Berliner und Münchener Tierärztliche Wochenschrift. 123: 169–173.

Frank N and Tadros EM. 2014. Insulin dysregulation. Equine Vet J. 46: 103–112.

Gehlen H, May A, and Bradaric Z. 2014. Comparison of insulin and glucose metabolism in horses with pituitary pars intermedia dysfunction treated versus not treated with pergolide. J Equine Vet Sci. 34: 508–513.

Knowles EJ, Menzies-Gow NJ, and Mair TS. 2014. Plasma fructosamine concentrations in horses with pituitary pars intermedia dysfunction with and without laminitis. Equine Vet J. 46:249–251.

Knowles EJ, Withers JM, and Mair TS. 2012. Increased plasma fructosamine concentrations in laminitic horses. Equine Vet J. 44: 226–229.

McGorum BC, Murphy D, Love S, and Milne EM. 1999. Clinicopathologic features of equine primary hepatic disease: a review of 50 cases. Vet Record 145: 134–139.

Rendle DI, Heller J, Hughes KJ, Innocent GT, and Durham AE. 2009. Stability of common biochemistry analytes in equine blood stored at room temperature. Eq Vet J 41: 428–432.

Ruoff WW, Baker DC, Morgan SJ, and Abbitt B. 1986. Type II diabetes mellitus in a horse. Equine Vet J 18: 143–144.

Swain JM, Pirie RS, Hudson NPH, Else RW, Evans H, and McGorum BC. 2005. Insulin-like growth factors and recurrent hypoglycemia associated with renal cell carcinoma in a horse. J Vet Intern Med 19: 613–616.

Tasker JB. 1966. Laboratory aids to diagnosis in equine practice. J Am Vet Med Assoc. 148: 384–390.

Wong D, Hepworth K, Yaeger M, Miles K, and Wilgenbusch C. 2015. Imaging diagnosis-hypoglycemia associated with cholangiocarcinoma and peritoneal carcinomatosis in a horse. Vet Radiol Ultrasound 56: E9–E12.

8

Lipids
M. Judith Radin

Department of Veterinary Biosciences, The Ohio State University College of Veterinary Medicine, Ohio, USA

8.1 Introduction

Triglycerides and cholesterol are measured as indicators of lipid and energy metabolism. These analytes are part of the routine biochemistry panel or may be added by request. Conditions that result in a negative energy balance such as anorexia, pregnancy, or lactation can trigger development of dyslipidemias. In the equine species, this is most often characterized by increased concentrations of triglycerides with variable increases in cholesterol as the balance between fat mobilization and utilization becomes dysregulated. With rising serum triglycerides anorexia often worsens, and the dyslipidemia becomes self-perpetuating. Hyperlipemia may be associated with fatty infiltration of organs such as the liver and kidney, contributing to organ failure and death of the patient. Predisposing factors for development of dyslipidemias include obesity, diet, stress, and breed. Definitions of various terms used in describing altered triglycerides and cholesterol in the horse are given in Box 8.1.

8.2 Normal Metabolism

Serum triglyceride concentration reflects dietary intake and hepatic synthesis. There are several sources of fatty acids that may be used for triglyceride synthesis.

- Pancreatic lipases release fatty acids and glycerol from dietary triglycerides. Fatty acids absorbed from the diet are esterified to triglycerides by intestinal epithelial cells and released via the lacteals into the circulation in the form of chylomicrons.
- Hepatic synthesis is the major source of triglycerides in the blood of horses. Hepatocytes take up nonesterified fatty acids (NEFA) from the blood and synthesize triglycerides. Triglycerides are then incorporated into very low-density lipoproteins (VLDL) and released into the circulation.

- Triglycerides from chylomicrons and VLDL are hydrolyzed to fatty acids and glycerol by lipoprotein lipase (LPL) on endothelial cells in the extrahepatic tissues. The resultant glycerol and fatty acids may be used as energy sources by tissues such as muscle. In adipose tissue, the fatty acids are re-esterified into triglycerides for storage in adipocytes. Insulin increases LPL activity, promoting uptake of fatty acids and storage as triglycerides in adipocytes during times of ample energy intake.
- Volatile fatty acids are produced by bacterial fermentation of dietary carbohydrates in the large intestine of the horse. Acetate and butyrate may be used for fatty acid and subsequent triglyceride synthesis by adipose tissue.
- Mobilization of energy stores from adipocytes is mediated by hormone sensitive lipase (HSL) that hydrolyzes triglycerides to glycerol and NEFA. HSL is the rate limiting enzyme for mobilization of triglyceride stores in adipocytes. HSL activity is inhibited by insulin, thus promoting triglyceride storage when adequate glucose is available. HSL activity is increased by glucagon, corticosteroids, and catecholamines, promoting mobilization of fat stores in times of negative energy balance or stress.

Serum cholesterol concentration is modulated by a variety of mechanisms. Because plants and microbes do not make cholesterol, herbivores such as the horse cannot obtain cholesterol from the diet. In the horse, cholesterol concentrations depend on a balance between synthesis, utilization, and excretion.

- Cholesterol is primarily synthesized in the liver. The rate limiting enzyme in cholesterol synthesis is 3-hydroxy-3-methylglutaryl-CoA (HMG-CoA) reductase. HMG-CoA reductase activity is increased by insulin and thyroid hormones and decreased by glucagon and corticosteroids.
- Cholesterol is incorporated into VLDL or high-density lipoproteins (HDL) by hepatocytes and released into the circulation. HDL may incorporate cholesterol from

Interpretation of Equine Laboratory Diagnostics, First Edition. Edited by Nicola Pusterla and Jill Higgins.

Box 8.1 Definitions

Dyslipidemia

- A disorder of lipid metabolism that is characterized by abnormal (usually increased) concentrations of triglycerides and/or cholesterol. The cause may be genetic or acquired.

Lipemia

- Turbidity or lactescence of the serum or plasma due to increased triglyceride concentrations (increased VLDL and/or chylomicrons).

Hyperlipidemia

- Elevated concentrations of triglycerides and/or cholesterol.
- Some authors define this as triglyceride concentrations of 100–500 mg/dL with no lactescence or hepatic lipidosis.
- Hyperlipidemia may be seen in all breeds of horses.

Hypertriglyceridemia

- Triglyceride concentration exceeding the reference interval
  - >100 mg/dl with no lipemia, organ lipidosis, or clinical disease may be seen in all breeds of horses
  - >500 mg/dL with or without gross lipemia is a severe form that may be seen in large breed horses and may be accompanied by fatty infiltration of organs and disease.

Hyperlipemia

- Triglycerides >500 mg/dL with gross lipemia of the serum
- Accompanied by hepatic and renal lipidosis
- Most commonly seen in ponies, donkeys, and miniature horses; less common in large breeds

---

extrahepatic sources through reverse cholesterol transport. Hypercholesterolemia often accompanies hypertriglyceridemia due to incorporation of cholesterol into VLDL.
- Cholesterol is used for the synthesis of steroids, sex hormones, vitamin D, and cellular membrane components.
- Hepatocytes use cholesterol to produce bile acids. A major route of cholesterol excretion is through the bile.

8.3 Sample Collection and Methods

- Increased triglyceride concentrations may be detected by visual examination of a serum or plasma sample. The sample will have a hazy appearance when triglycerides are >300 mg/dL and become opaque when triglyceride concentrations exceed 600 mg/dL (Figure 8.1). Hypercholesterolemia does not contribute to the lactescence of the sample.
- Triglycerides and cholesterol may be measured in serum, heparinized plasma, or EDTA plasma.
- While not routinely measured in horses, NEFA may be measured as an indicator of fat mobilization. NEFA is measured in serum or EDTA plasma. Heparinized plasma or serum obtained using a serum separator tube are not recommended as baseline NEFA concentrations will be higher and concentrations will rise with storage of the plasma (Stokol and Nydam, 2005).
- A fasting sample is recommended, especially if part of an evaluation for equine metabolic syndrome. The recommended procedure is to leave one flake of hay in

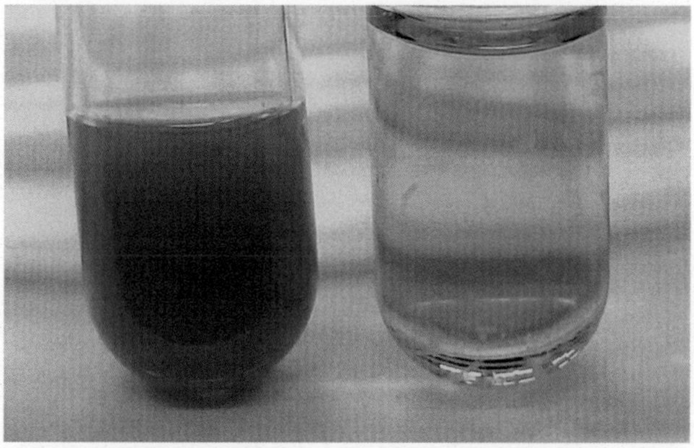

Figure 8.1 The sample on the left is serum from a Quarterhorse with hypertriglyceridemia and hyperbilirubinemia. Notice how the sample is opaque from the hyperlipemia. Anorexic horses often become hyperbilirubinemic, imparting the dark yellow to orange color to the sample. The sample on the right is serum from a normal horse.

the stall after 10:00 pm and draw the sample in the morning (Frank, 2011).
- Serum or plasma should be separated from cells soon after the sample is drawn and refrigerated. Triglycerides and cholesterol are stable for a week at 4°C, for 3 months at −20°C, and for years at −70°C. In samples with marked hyperlipidemia, some precipitation of lipoproteins may occur with freezing and thawing. NEFA are stable for up to 72 h at 4°C and for 1 month at −70°C.
- All three assay methodologies typically involve enzymatic reactions followed by spectrophotometric reading of a color change. Consequently, like other colorimetric assays, these are subject to potential interferences such as icterus, hemolysis, and even severe lipemia.

The reference laboratory should be able to provide guidelines for interpretation of interferences in relation to their specific test methodology.
- Interpretation of results should be relative to laboratory established reference intervals.

8.4 Disorders of Lipid Metabolism

8.4.1 Role of Negative Energy Balance

- Negative energy balance occurs when energy demand exceeds intake and may be seen with anorexia, pregnancy, lactation, food deprivation, or heavy exercise. Increased mobilization of fat stores is a normal response to negative energy balance. As blood glucose and insulin concentrations fall, HSL is no longer inhibited by insulin, resulting in hydrolysis of triglycerides stored in adipocytes. NEFA increase within hours of withholding feed (Frank et al., 2002, 2003). NEFA also rapidly rise during exercise and may remain elevated during recovery from exercise (Yoo et al., 2007, Westermann et al., 2008). Glycerol and NEFA released from the adipocytes are metabolized for energy. NEFA that are not metabolized by ß-oxidation are re-esterified to triglycerides in hepatocytes and released into circulation as VLDL.
- As anorexia progresses, an imbalance between lipolysis, ß-oxidation of NEFA, and hepatic production of VLDL develops. Even in otherwise healthy horses and ponies, increases in triglycerides, VLDL and cholesterol are observed after several days of fasting (Frank et al., 2002, Naylor et al., 1980, Bauer, 1983).
- Hepatic production of VLDL out paces the ability of extrahepatic tissues to clear triglycerides from the circulation (Watson et al., 1992).
- Hepatic lipidosis ensues as triglyceride production exceeds cellular export of VLDL. This results in an accumulation of fat in the hepatocytes.
- Marked elevations in triglycerides have been associated with a poor prognosis as tissue lipidosis ensues, contributing to organ dysfunction; however, mortality may be reduced by aggressive therapy.

8.4.2 Insulin Resistance as a Contributing Factor

- The imbalance between lipolysis and NEFA utilization is exacerbated by predisposing factors such as breed, obesity, pregnancy, equine metabolic syndrome, advancing age, pituitary pars intermedia dysfunction (PPID), endotoxin, or illness. These predisposing conditions have insulin resistance as a common factor.
- Insulin resistance is characterized by impaired insulin signaling. This results in decreased inhibition of HSL and an inappropriate rate of lipolysis.

- Some breeds are predisposed to insulin resistance (Frank, 2011).
- Stress hormones released during illness contribute to insulin resistance by decreasing insulin secretion and insulin actions. Corticosteroids and epinephrine also stimulate activity of HSL, enhancing lipolysis and release of NEFA into the circulation.
- Endotoxemia results in insulin resistance (Vick et al., 2008, Tóth et al., 2009, 2010) and may promote development of dyslipidemias. LPL-mediated clearance of triglycerides is inhibited and hepatic VLDL synthesis is increased with endotoxemia.
- As the availability of NEFA exceed utilization by extrahepatic tissues and storage capacity of adipocytes, triglycerides may accumulate in extrahepatic tissues such as kidney and muscle, resulting in lipotoxicity and organ failure. Azotemia (increased BUN and creatinine) may result from a combination of pre-renal factors such as dehydration and renal failure secondary to lipotoxicity.

8.5 Patterns of Dyslipidemia

8.5.1 Large Breed Horses

- Food deprivation is characterized by increases in triglycerides, cholesterol, total bilirubin and NEFA, while glucose and insulin are decreased. In large breed horses, triglycerides may exceed 100 mg/dL, but would not be expected to exceed 500 mg/dL in the absence of complicating factors. NEFA may increase 16–20-fold (Naylor et al., 1980, Frank et al., 2002). In healthy horses experiencing food deprivation, triglyceride and NEFA concentrations plateaued after several days. Triglyceride, cholesterol, and NEFA levels rapidly normalized after regaining access to food.
- Anorexia complicated with illness such as colic, gastroenteritis, respiratory disease, or other causes of inflammatory disease can result in triglyceride concentrations exceeding 500 mg/dL. Reports vary on the presence or absence of visible lipemia and may depend on the severity of the hypertriglyceridemia (Naylor et al., 1980, Dunkel and McKenzie, 2003). Azotemia (increased BUN and creatinine) was frequently reported in association with hypertriglyceridemia and hyperlipemia (see Box 8.2).

8.5.2 Small Breed Horses and Donkeys

- Ponies and donkeys may develop primary hyperlipemia. Triglycerides often exceed 500 mg/dL and cholesterol levels may double within several days of food deprivation in otherwise healthy ponies (Bauer, 1983). Spontaneous cases are most often associated with

---

Box 8.2 Clinical example

A 28-year-old Grade Gelding in good body condition presented for anorexia, fever and colic of 15 hours duration. On physical exam, he had profuse nasal discharge that contained feed material. He was anesthetized on Day 1 and an esophageal obstruction comprised of impacted grain and hay was relieved. There was marked edema and inflammation of the pharynx and larynx, and a full thickness mucosal tear was present at the site of the obstruction. Auscultation of the lungs was compatible with inhalation pneumonia. The horse was treated with antibiotics and a nasogastric tube was placed.

Test	Unit	Day 1	Day 8	Reference intervals
PCV	%	55	36	27–44
WBC	$\times 10^9$/L	2.1	8.2	4.7–10.6
Neutrophils	$\times 10^9$/L	0.6	5.7	2.4–6.4
Lymphocytes	$\times 10^9$/L	1.4	2.0	1.0–4.9
Monocytes	$\times 10^9$/L	0.1	0.5	0–0.5
Fibrinogen	mg/dL		803	193–422
AST	IU/L	251	314	170–370
ALP	IU/L	195	535	80–187
GGT	IU/L	23	26	7–20
CK	IU/L	445	204	150–360
Cholesterol	mg/dL	113	217	51–97
Triglyceride	mg/dL	115	1123	10–60
Total bilirubin	mg/dL	3.4	6.9	0.6–1.8
Glucose	mg/dL	206	78	83–114

The remainder of his laboratory data was unremarkable.

Day 1

- The increased PCV was likely due to splenic contraction as a result of pain. He had a leukopenia with a marked neutropenia, due to endotoxemia.
- The mild elevation in ALP and GGT was suggestive for cholestasis. The increase in total bilirubin may reflect both cholestasis and anorexia. At this time point, there was a mild increase in triglycerides and cholesterol. These increases were a response to anorexia, endotoxemia, and the stress of illness. The hyperglycemia also reflected stress and pain.

The horse remained off feed as the inflammation in the esophagus and larynx began to heal. Because the choke was considered secondary to dental disease, the gelding was sedated on Day 6 and his teeth were floated. Endoscopic examination of the esophagus showed healing of the mucosal tear but ongoing inflammation of the larynx, pharynx, and esophagus.

Day 8

- The PCV and leukogram were normal; however, the fibrinogen concentration was elevated, compatible with the ongoing inflammation in the lungs and esophagus.
- The gelding had marked hypertriglyceridemia and hypercholesterolemia. The cholestatic enzymes (ALP and GGT) further increased, raising the concern for development of hepatic lipidosis. Bilirubin was also increased, compatible with anorexia and cholestasis. He became hypoglycemic due to a negative energy balance secondary to ongoing anorexia.

Aggressive enteral feeding was instituted on Day 8. A re-check of his triglycerides on Day 10 showed rapid improvement at 189 mg/dL. The horse was discharged to the care of his owner several days later.

This case is a good example of how anorexia combined with complicating conditions can result in hyperlipidemia. While marked hypertriglyceridemia may be associated with a poor outcome, this case illustrates that aggressive therapy to correct the negative energy balance along with treatment of the primary disease may lead to resolution of the dyslipidemia.

Box 8.3 Clinical example

A 20-year-old miniature donkey stallion was presented for lethargy and inappetance. Five days ago, he refused to eat his grain; however, he was on spring pasture so the owner was not initially concerned. He became progressively depressed and ceased eating altogether. On physical examination, the donkey was obese with a body condition score of 8 out of 9. Ventral strabismus was observed in his right eye and he was ataxic. A heavy strongyle burden was found on fecal examination.

Test	Unit	Patient	Reference intervals
AST	IU/L	711	170–370
ALP	IU/L	492	80–187
GGT	IU/L	1011	7–20
SDH	IU/L	32.1	4–14
CK	IU/L	360	150–360
Triglyceride	mg/dL	1284	10–60
Total bilirubin	mg/dL	0.5	0.6–1.8
Glucose	mg/dL	266	83–114

The hypertriglyceridemia and increased liver enzymes were consistent with primary hyperlipemia and hepatic lipidosis. The neurologic signs were attributed to hepatic encephalopathy. The hyperglycemia was due in part to stress. However, there likely was a component of insulin resistance associated with obesity. While the underlying cause of his initial inappetance was not determined, the heavy parasite burden in an obese miniature donkey may have set the stage for development of a negative energy balance and consequent hyperlipemia. Due to a poor response to therapy and worsening neurologic signs, the donkey was humanely euthanized.

---

pregnancy or early lactation and may be exacerbated by obesity or stress (Hughes et al., 2004). A familial predisposition for hyperlipemia has been suggested for Shetland ponies (Jeffcott and Field, 1985, see Box 8.3).

- In miniature horses, hyperlipidemia or hyperlipemia most often develops subsequent to a primary that which results in anorexia and inflammation; although primary hyperlipemia may occur (Mogg and Palmer, 1995).
- The plasma is grossly lactescent and fatty infiltration of the liver and other organs occurs. Insulin concentrations may be increased and blood glucose decreased.

8.5.3 Neonates and Foals

- Triglycerides and cholesterol concentrations are often higher in healthy foals compared to their mares, and these increases may persist for 4–9 months (Bauer et al., 1989, Axon and Palmer, 2008, Aoki and Ishii, 2012). Because laboratory reference intervals are frequently developed by sampling adult horses, this needs to be kept in mind when interpreting biochemical panels from foals.
- In healthy, nursing foals, triglycerides have been reported to be up to 2–4-folds higher than the adult reference intervals by 1 day of age (Bauer et al., 1989, Aoki and Ishii, 2012). Triglycerides peak around 1 week of age and can be as much as 4–6-fold greater than the adult reference interval at that time. Cholesterol concentrations are increased at birth and appear to peak at 1 day of age by up to 2–5-fold over adult reference intervals. Cholesterol concentration remains 2–3-fold increased over adult reference intervals for at least 4 months, gradually decreasing over time. NEFA can be 4–5 times higher at birth in the foal compared to the mare, but drop to levels similar to the mare within a day (Aoki and Ishii, 2012). Post prandial effects of nursing likely contribute to the wide variation reported in normal foals.
- Sick foals that become anorexic and fail to nurse often develop hypertriglyceridemia, which may be associated with a poor outcome (Myers et al., 2009, Barsnick and Toribio, 2011, Armengou et al., 2013, see Box 8.4). NEFA increase in septic and in nonseptic sick foals as a result of lipolysis (Armengou et al., 2013). Hypoglycemia may be seen in sick foals and is usually more severe in foals that are septic. Some foals may respond to parenteral nutrition with hyperglycemia due to insulin resistance or impaired insulin responses.

Box 8.4 Clinical example

This filly was born on Day 1. The delivery was induced due to suspected placentitis in the mare. The filly was depressed, did not nurse well, and was recumbent much of the time. A nasogastric feeding tube was placed on Day 1 and colostrum was administered. After that, the feeding tube was used to administer her mare's milk. The filly also was started on intravenous fluids with 50% dextrose. By Day 2, the filly developed diarrhea. Additional treatments included antibiotics, a nonsteroidal anti-inflammatory drug, gastroprotectants, Lactaid, and an intestinal adsorbent.

Test	Unit	Day 1	Day 2	Day 3	Day 4	Reference intervals (adult)
PCV	%	37	29	31	27	27–44
WBC	$\times 10^9$/L	4.1	1.9	1.1	1.9	4.7–10.6
Neutrophils	$\times 10^9$/L	2.1	1.1	0.7	1.1	2.4–6.4
Lymphocytes	$\times 10^9$/L	1.9	0.7	0.4	0.7	1.0–4.9
Monocytes	$\times 10^9$/L	0.1	0.1	0	0.1	0–0.5
Total protein	gm/dL	3.3	4.3	3.9	3.8	6.4–7.9
BUN	mg/dL	52	51	31	13	13–27
Creatinine	mg/dL	7.1	3.9	2.3	1.3	0.8–1.7
Albumin	gm/dL	2.4	2.5	2.3	2.2	2.8–3.6
Globulin	gm/dL	0.9	1.8	1.5	1.6	3.6–4.3
Total bilirubin	mg/dL	3.2	5.0	6.6	7.1	0.6–1.8
Direct bilirubin	mg/dL	0.2	0.5	0.4	0.5	0.1–0.3
AST	IU/L	90	170	166	164	170–370
ALP	IU/L	1873	1660	1635	1110	80–187
GGT	IU/L	12	16	14	14	7–20
SDH	IU/L	4.8	2.5	2.1	3.4	4–13
CK	IU/L	832	658	670	184	150–360
Triglyceride	mg/dL	68	500	85	47	10–60
Glucose	mg/dL	28	126	184	105	83–114
Foal IgG	mg/dL		423	766		>800

This is a case of a filly with suffering from sepsis and fetal stress due to placentitis and placental insufficiency.

- The foal is leukopenic and neutropenic, compatible with sepsis. The lymphopenia on Days 2–4 indicates stress (response to endogenous steroids).
- The increases in BUN and creatinine are likely due to placental insufficiency and fetal stress and as expected, declined over several days. Dehydration also may have contributed.
- The foal is hypoproteinemic. The decrease in globulins is compatible with failure of passive transfer of immunity. Measurement of IgG on Day 2 confirmed this suspicion. Plasma transfusions were given on Days 2 and 3, resulting in an increase in globulins and measured IgG.
- Hyperbilirubinemia is common during the first week of life and is due to increases in indirect or unconjugated bilirubin. Impaired hepatic function secondary to sepsis may also contribute.

- Liver enzymes are unremarkable. The increases in ALP are typical of a young, growing animal.
- CK is increased due to muscle trauma secondary to delivery and to recumbency of the foal.
- Triglycerides are mildly increased on Day 1. By Day 2, the hypertriglyceridemia is more severe, compatible with the negative energy balance experienced by the foal. Triglycerides gradually returned to normal as the filly began to eat and improve her energy intake.
- The filly was severely hypoglycemic on Day 1 due to failure to nurse and sepsis. By Day 3, she was hyperglycemic. This may occur in response to supplemented fluid therapy or parenteral nutrition. Sick or septic foals may have impaired insulin responses or develop insulin resistance.

The filly improved in strength and began to nurse on her own on Day 4. The foal and mare were discharged from the hospital on Day 10.

8.5.4 PPID

- PPID occurs in aged horses and ponies. Biochemical changes include hyperglycemia with or without increases in liver enzymes.
- Triglyceride levels are variable but marked hyperlipemia may develop with concurrent type 2 diabetes mellitus (Dunkel et al., 2014).

8.5.5 Equine Metabolic Syndrome

- The breed predilection for equine metabolic syndrome includes ponies, Morgan horses, Arabians, Paso Finos, Saddlebreds, Quarterhorses, and Tennessee Walking horses (Frank et al., 2006). Horses are usually obese or have regional adiposity and are at risk for development of laminitis.
- Equine metabolic syndrome is characterized by insulin resistance and animals are hyperinsulinemic (McKenzie, 2011). Blood glucose is often normal, although some horses become hyperglycemic. NEFA are increased due to insulin resistance and impaired suppression of HSL. In studies of fasted horses with insulin resistance but no other complicating factors, triglycerides were increased relative to insulin-sensitive controls but the increases did not always exceed the reference interval (Frank et al., 2006).
- Hyperlipidemia/hyperlipemia may develop spontaneously or secondary to a complicating condition.

References

Aoki T and Ishii M. 2012. Hematological and biochemical profiles in peripartum mares and neonatal foals (heavy draft horse). J Eq Vet Sci 32: 170–176.

Armengou L, Jose-Cunilleras E, Ríos J, Cesarini C, Viu J, and Monreal L. 2013. Metabolic and endocrine profiles in sick neonatal foals are related to survival. J Vet Int Med 27: 567–575.

Axon JE and Palmer JE. 2008. Clinical pathology of the foal. Vet Clin Equine 24: 357–385.

Barsnick RJ and Toribio RE. 2011. Endocrinology of equine neonatal energy metabolism in health and critical illness. Vet Clin Equine 27: 49–58.

Bauer JE. 1983. Plasma lipids and lipoproteins of fasted ponies. Am J Vet Res 44: 379–384.

Bauer JF, Asquith RL, and Kivipelto J. 1989. Serum biochemical indicators of liver function in neonatal foals. Am J Vet Res 50: 2037–2041.

Dunkel B, Wilford SA, Parkinson MJ, Ward C, Smith P, Grahame L, et al. 2014. Severe hypertriglyceridaemia in horses and ponies with endocrine disorders. Eq Vet J 46: 118–122.

Dunkel B and McKenzie HC, III. 2003. Severe hypertriglyceridaemia in clinically ill horses: diagnosis, treatment and outcome. Eq Vet J 35: 590–595.

Frank N. 2011. Equine metabolic syndrome. Vet Clin Equine 27: 73–92.

Frank N, Elliott SB, Brandt LE, and Keisler DH. 2006. Physical characteristics, blood hormone concentrations, and plasma lipid concentrations in obese horses with insulin resistance. J Am Vet Med Assoc 228: 1383–1390.

Frank N, Sojka JE, and Latour MA. 2002. Effect of withholding feed on concentration and composition of plasma very low density lipoprotein and serum nonesterified fatty acids in horses. Am J Vet Res 63: 1018–1102.

Frank N, Sojka JE, and Latour MA. 2003. Effects of hypothyroidism and withholding of feed on plasma lipid concentrations, concentration and composition of very-low-density lipoprotein, and plasma lipase activity in horses. Am J Vet Res 64: 823–828.

Hughes KJ, Hodgson DR, and Dart AJ. 2004. Equine hyperlipaemia: a review. Australian Vet J 82: 136–142.

Jeffcott JB and Field JR. 1985. Current concepts of hyperlipaemia in horses and ponies. Vet Record 116: 461–466.

McKenzie HC. 2011. Equine hyperlipidemias. Vet Clin North Am Equine Pract. 27: 59–72.

Mogg TD and Palmer JE. 1995. Hyperlipidemia, hyperlipemia, and hepatic lipidosis in American miniature horses: 23 cases (1990–1994). J Am Vet Med Assoc 207: 604–607.

Myers CJ, Magdesian KG, Kass PH, Madigan JE, Rhodes DM, and Marks SL. 2009. Parenteral nutrition in neonatal foals: clinical description, complications and outcome in 53 foals (1995–2005). Vet J 181: 137–144.

Naylor JM, Kronfeld DS, and Acland H. 1980. Hyperlipemia in horses: effects of undernutrition and disease. Am J Vet Res 41: 899–905.

Stokol T and Nydam DV. 2005. Effect of anticoagulant and storage conditions on bovine nonesterified fatty acid and β-hydroxybutyrate concentrations in blood. J Dairy Sci 88: 3139–3144.

Tóth F, Frank N, Chameroy KA, and Boston RC. 2009. Effects of endotoxaemia and carbohydrate overload on glucose and insulin dynamics and the development of laminitis in horses. Equine Vet J 41: 852–858.

Tóth F, Frank N, Geor RJ, and Boston RC. 2010. Effects of pretreatment with dexamethasone or levothyroxine sodium on endotoxin-induced alterations in glucose and insulin dynamics in horses. Am J Vet Res 71: 60–68.

Vick MM, Murphy BA, Sessions DR, Reedy SE, Kennedy EL, Horohov DW, et al. 2008. Effects of systemic inflammation on insulin sensitivity in horses and inflammatory cytokine expression in adipose tissue. Am J Vet Res 69: 130–139.

Watson TDG, Burns L, Love S, Packard CJ, and Shepherd J. 1992. Plasma lipids, lipoproteins and post-heparin lipases in ponies with hyperlipaemia. Equine Vet J 24: 341–346.

Yoo IS, Lee HG, Yoon SY, Hong HO, and Lee SR. 2007. Study on changes in racehorses' metabolites and exercise-related hormones before and after a race. Asian-Australasian J An Sci 20: 1677–1683.

Westermann CM, Dorland B, Sain-van der Velden MG de, Wijnberg ID, Breda E van, Graaf-Roelfsema E de, et al. 2008. Plasma acylcarnitine and fatty acid profiles during exercise and training in Standardbreds. Am J Vet Res 69: 1469–1475.

9

Blood Gases
Alonso Guedes

University of Minnesota, Minnesota, USA

9.1 Introduction

Arterial blood gas measurements provide information regarding life-sustaining functions of the cardiopulmonary system. It is useful in assessing oxygenation, ventilation, and acid-base status. These variables are relevant to many clinical settings, but become especially significant when dealing with surgical, emergency and/or critically ill patients. Blood gas measurements can be performed with point-of-care or portable analyzers, which are now very common in veterinary practices, or with central laboratory devices (Wilkins, 2011, Grosenbaugh et al., 1998, Peiro et al., 2010).

9.2 Technical Aspects

9.2.1 Source of Blood

Blood gas analysis of arterial blood is required if the goal is to assess pulmonary function. Mixed venous blood is adequate if the primary goal is to assess acid-base balance or to evaluate if global tissue oxygen demands are being met. Paired arterial and venous samples can be analyzed if the goal is to estimate oxygen extraction ratio.

9.2.2 Collection Sites

Peripheral arteries amenable for sample collection in anesthetized horses include the facial, transverse facial, auricular and metatarsal arteries. In non-anesthetized horses, the transverse facial and carotid arteries are feasible sites for blood collection. Prior hair shaving and application of a topical local anesthetic for ~20 min will facilitate this procedure (Figure 9.1). Antisepsia should be performed prior to sample collection. In newborn foals, the umbilical artery, brachial, median, decubital, and femoral arteries are additional options. Mixed venous blood is collected from a central vessel such as the pulmonary artery, but the jugular vein or cranial vena cava are more practical an clinically acceptable in horses (Magdesian, 2004).

9.2.3 Pre-Analytical Errors

The following precautions should be taken to prevent or minimize pre-analytical errors:

- *Sampling device*: Heparinized plastic or glass syringes, but not plastic vacutainer tubes, are clinically acceptable for blood sampling intended for blood gas measurements (Winkler et al., 1974, Noel et al., 2010). Heparinized plastic vacutainer tubes are acceptable for measurements of bicarbonate, base excess and total carbon dioxide concentrations (Noel et al., 2010).
- *Heparin*: After coating the syringe with heparin, forcefully expel as much of the heparin as possible out of the syringe and needle. Excessive heparin in the syringe (>4% by volume) may significantly change PO_2, PCO_2, base deficit, lactate, and electrolytes (Hopper et al., 2005).
- *Air contamination*: Air bubbles should be promptly removed and the syringe properly capped. Contamination with room air due to either large enough air bubbles or improperly capped syringe may affect the partial pressures of oxygen (PaO_2) and/or carbon dioxide ($PaCO_2$) in the syringe.
- *Storage*: Blood collected into plastic syringes should be analyzed within 10 min of collection, irrespective of storage temperature, to ensure PaO_2 accuracy (Picandet et al., 2007, Deane et al., 2004). If this is not possible, than the glass a syringe should be used and kept in an ice bath and analyzed as within no more than approximately 2 h (Picandet et al., 2007). Accuracy of $PaCO_2$ and pH is well maintained in samples collected in plastic syringes stored for up to 1 h at room temperature (Deane et al., 2004).

Interpretation of Equine Laboratory Diagnostics, First Edition. Edited by Nicola Pusterla and Jill Higgins.
© 2018 John Wiley & Sons, Inc. Published 2018 by John Wiley & Sons, Inc.

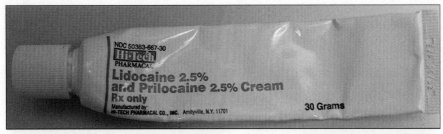

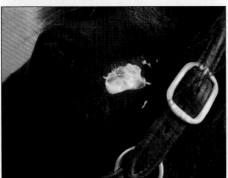
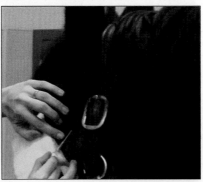

Figure 9.1 Application of a local anesthetic mixture topically to a shaved area to desensitize the skin and facilitate catheterization of the transverse facial artery in an awake horse. After approximately 20 min contact time, the area is scrubbed and the vessel is located via pulse palpation and subsequently punctured using aseptic technique.

9.3 Acid-Base

Biological homeostasis requires maintenance of intracellular and extracellular fluid pH within a narrow range. Plasma pH, rather than pH of other extracellular or intracellular fluids, is relatively easy to measure for clinical assessment of acid-base balance, and either arterial or venous blood can be used for this purpose. A lower than normal plasma pH is termed *acidemia* whereas a higher than normal plasma pH is termed *alkalemia*.

The Henderson-Hasselbach (H-H) equation describes the pH as a function of HCO_3 and $PaCO_2$ such that:

$$pH = 6.1 + \log \frac{HCO_3}{0.03 \times PaCO_2}$$

Where 6.1 is the pKa (negative logarithm of the acid dissociation constant) for H_2CO_3 and 0.03 is the solubility coefficient for CO_2 in plasma (i.e., the factor that relates PCO_2 to the amount of CO_2 dissolved in plasma). This equation predicts that the ratio of dissolved CO_2 ($0.03 \times PaCO_2$) to HCO_3^-, and not their actual concentrations, determines [H^+] and thus pH. It also establishes that a balance between the respiratory and metabolic functions maintains the acid-base status. As such, pH is inversely related to PCO_2 and directly related to HCO_3^-:

$$pH = \frac{HCO_3 \, (metabolic \ component)}{PCO_2 \, (respiratory \ component)}$$

Thus, the two possible acid-base abnormalities (acidemia or alkalemia) can be caused by at least one of four possible acid-base disturbances:

1) Respiratory acidosis: a *rise in* PCO_2 resulting in a *drop in pH* due to a rise in [H^+].

2) Respiratory alkalosis: a *drop in* PCO_2 resulting in a *rise in pH* due to a drop in [H^+].
3) Metabolic acidosis: a *drop in* [HCO_3^-] resulting in a *drop in pH* due to a rise in [H^+].
4) Metabolic alkalosis: a *rise in* [HCO_3^-] resulting in a *rise in pH* due to a drop in [H^+].

The typical physiologic responses to an acid-base disturbance are threefold:

1) *Buffering*: The initial response is to buffer the acid or base created by the systemic abnormality. The predominant buffer in that particular fluid compartment does the buffering. The major extracellular buffer pair is bicarbonate/carbonic acid (HCO_3^-/H_2CO_3). In this open system, bicarbonate reacts with hydrogen ions to form carbonic acid that is subsequently converted to water and CO_2 ($CO_2 + H_2O \Leftrightarrow H_2CO_3 \Leftrightarrow H^+ + HCO_3^-$).
2) *Compensation*: Next, the respiratory system will attempt to compensate for metabolic acid-base abnormalities and the renal system will attempt to compensate for respiratory acid-base abnormalities. Carbon dioxide is eliminated by alveolar ventilation. This compensatory response is typically relatively rapid (minutes). The kidneys regulate the generation and excretion of HCO_3^-. This compensatory response is typically relatively slow (hours).
3) *Correction*: This is typically the last phase and entails rectifying the pathophysiologic process that caused the acid-base abnormality. This may completely eliminate the acid-base disturbance (i.e., correction of a uroabdomen) or at least allow the patient to return to baseline for diseases that have been exacerbated by an acute condition (i.e., pneumonia in a horse with chronic obstructive pulmonary disease).

Age-related differences exist in arterial blood pH in healthy horses such that it is lowest in premature foals (Table 9.1) and highest in geriatric horses (Table 9.2 and Table 9.3) (Aguilera-Tejero et al., 1998, Madigan et al., 1992). Bicarbonate also changes in early life, especially in premature foals, but is stable in the healthy adult (Aguilera-Tejero et al., 1998, Madigan et al., 1992, Rose et al., 1982). The venous PCO_2 ($PvCO_2$) is slightly ($\sim$5 mmHg) higher than arterial PCO_2 ($PaCO_2$) in healthy animals (Arthurs and Sudhakar, 2005), although the difference can be greater in critically ill patients.

Acid-base abnormalities are the result of pathophysiologic processes and not disease entities. The differential diagnosis of any specific acid-base pattern begins with history and physical examination of each individual patient. Simple acid-base abnormalities involve compensatory processes that minimize the effect on pH. For example, acute metabolic acidosis (decreased HCO_3) will trigger respiratory compensation (see expected compensation in Section 9.4 on ventilation) via increased ventilation, resulting in a decrease in $PaCO_2$. This will minimize the change in pH as dictated by the H-H

Table 9.1 Age-related values of arterial blood pH, bicarbonate (HCO_3), base excess (BE), partial pressure of carbon dioxide ($PaCO_2$) and oxygen (PaO_2) in premature foals.

Age	Days of gestation (n)	pH	HCO$_3$ (mmol/l)	BE (mmol/l)	PaCO$_2$ (mmHg)	PaO$_2$ (mmHg)
Birth	270–320 (8)[a]	7.20 ± 0.03	23.4 ± 1.7	−5.4 ± 0.8	66 ± 10	30 ± 4
	320–330 (9)[b]	7.27 ± 0.02	23.9 ± 0.8	−3 ± 1.2	53 ± 2	39 ± 5
1 h	270–320 (4)[a]	7.09 ± 0.04	18.1 ± 2.4	−10.7 ± 2.4	61 ± 3	49 ± 4
	320–330 (8)[b]	7.33 ± 0.02	24.6 ± 0.9	−1.3 ± 0.9	48 ± 3	52 ± 4
1.5–3 h	270–320 (8)[a]	7.06 ± 0.09	19.5 ± 1.5	−8.8 ± 2.0	77 ± 14	45 ± 8
	320–330 (9)[b]	7.36 ± 0.02	26 ± 0.6	0.9 ± 0.6	47 ± 2	65 ± 4
1 d	320–330 (4)[b]	7.30 ± 0.01	20.4 ± 0.2	−5.3 ± 0.6	43 ± 2	57 ± 7
2 d	320–330 (4)[b]	7.34 ± 0.04	21.3 ± 1.9	−3.6 ± 2.6	41 ± 3.4	53 ± 4

a) Pony mares; Induced delivery.
b) Thoroughbred mares; Induced delivery.
Source: Rose (1982). Reproduced with permission of Cambridge University Press.

Table 9.2 Age-related values of arterial blood pH, bicarbonate (HCO_3), base excess (BE), partial pressure of carbon dioxide ($PaCO_2$) and oxygen (PaO_2) in healthy term foals and adult horses.

Age	n	pH	HCO$_3$ (mmol/l)	BE (mmol/l)	PaCO$_2$ (mmHg)	PaO$_2$ (mmHg)	Ref.
Birth	8[c]	7.32 ± 0.12	25.6 ± 0.6	0.2 ± 1.2	53 ± 1.8	43 ± 3.9	(Rose et al., 1982)
	9	7.30 ± 0.02	24 ± 0.8	−0.95 ± 0.8	61 ± 1.5	33 ± 2.5	(Stewart et al., 1984)
0.5 hour	9	7.35 ± 0.01	25 ± 0.7	1.4 ± 0.8	52 ± 1.5	57 ± 1.8	(Stewart et al., 1984)
1 hour	8[c]	7.39 ± 0.01	25.6 ± 0.6	1.5 ± 0.5	44 ± 1.2	78 ± 5.2	(Rose et al., 1982)
1 day	8[c]	7.38 ± 0.009	24.6 ± 0.4	0.3 ± 0.5	43 ± 0.7	85 ± 5.9	(Rose et al., 1982)
2 days	8[c]	7.37 ± 0.01	25.2 ± 0.7	0.3 ± 0.7	44 ± 0.9	82 ± 5.5	(Rose et al., 1982)
4 days	8[c]	7.37 ± 0.01	24.9 ± 1.6	0.6 ± 1.8	44 ± 0.8	86 ± 3.5	(Rose et al., 1982)
7 days	8[c]	7.36 ± 0.01	22.9 ± 1.4	−1.6 ± 1.5	42 ± 2.1	80 ± 7.4	(Rose et al., 1982)
7 (2–11) years[a]	15	–	–	–	43 ± 0.8	98 ± 2.6	(Pacheco et al., 2014)
? (3–8) years[b]	16	7.40 ± 0.005	26.4 ± 0.4	–	43 ± 0.7	102 ± 1.7	(Aguilera-Tejero et al., 1998)
22 (20–28) years[a]	16	–	–	–	43 ± 1.0	99 ± 2.5	(Pacheco et al., 2014)
26.6 (20–45) years[b]	16	7.43 ± 0.007	26.8 ± 0.9	–	42 ± 1.0	90 ± 2.2	(Aguilera-Tejero et al., 1998)

a) Median or
b) mean and range.
c) Thoroughbred mares; Induced delivery at term.

Table 9.3 Age-related values of mixed venous blood[*] pH, bicarbonate (HCO_3), base excess (BE), partial pressure of carbon dioxide ($PvCO_2$) and oxygen (PvO_2) in healthy 11 foals.

Age	Condition	pH	HCO_3 (mmol/l)	BE (mmol/l)	$PvCO_2$ (mmHg)	PvO_2 (mmHg)
2 – 16 h	Upright	–	–	–	49 ± 0.9	35 ± 0.8
	Recumbent		–	–	46 ± 0.8	41 ± 0.7
20 h–4 d	Upright	–	–	–	52 ± 0.9	37 ± 0.5
	Recumbent	–	–	–	48 ± 0.8	42 ± 0.7
5–14 d	Upright	–	–	–	52 ± 0.8	36 ± 0.8
	Recumbent	–	–	–	46 ± 0.5	37 ± 0.6
Birth–14 d	Upright	7.39 ± 0.005	29.6 ± 0.3	5.5 ± 0.3	51 ± 0.5	36 ± 0.4
	Recumbent	7.38 ± 0.004	29.3 ± 0.3	5.0 ± 0.3	52 ± 0.4	41 ± 0.4

[*] Collected from the pulmonary artery.
Source: Madigan (1992).

equation. If this compensation does not occur, then the patient has a mixed (i.e., more than one) acid-base abnormality. Mixed acid-base abnormalities are in general the most common clinical scenarios in critically ill and anesthetized horses.

9.4 Ventilation

The $PaCO_2$ is used to assess alveolar ventilation because CO_2 production is relatively constant under most clinical settings and thus CO_2 elimination is proportional to alveolar ventilation. Higher than normal $PaCO_2$ (hypercapnia) indicates hypoventilation whereas lower than normal $PaCO_2$ (hypocapnia) indicates hyperventilation. The $PaCO_2$ is highest at birth (53–61 mmHg) but rapidly decreases toward adult levels (42–43 mmHg) within hours after birth (Aguilera-Tejero et al., 1998, Rose et al., 1982, Stewart et al., 1984, Pacheco et al., 2014). In healthy foals, body position affects mixed venous $PvCO_2$ at least during the first 2 weeks of life such that it tends to be a 3–8 mmHg higher when the foal is in the upright position compared to the recumbent position (Madigan et al., 1992). Hypoventilation can be caused by central nervous system depression (general anesthesia, head trauma, encephalitis), as compensatory response to metabolic alkalosis, abdominal distension, thoracic wall trauma, neuromuscular dysfunction (diaphragm, intercostal muscles), restrictive pulmonary diseases (pulmonary silicosis/fibrosis, pleural effusion, pneumothorax), and upper airway obstruction.

The precise level of hypercapnia (i.e., high $PaCO_2$) that is considered detrimental is controversial in anesthetized horses. Hypercapnia indicates hypoventilation, and hypoventilation is one of the causes of hypoxemia. In otherwise healthy horses, as long as hypoxemia is not present, hypoventilation to $PaCO_2$ up to 70–80 mmHg may augment cardiac output and tissue perfusion via vasodilation and catecholamine release. Higher $PaCO_2$ levels can cause significant acidemia, predispose to cardiac arrhythmias and increases in intracranial pressure (Khanna et al., 1995, Brosnan et al., 2003). The $PaCO_2$ should be maintained within normal limits (normocapnia) or slightly below normal limits (hypocapnia) in horses with known or suspected increase in intracranial pressure (i.e., intracranial disease or trauma) or with acidemia.

To assess the respiratory contribution to acid-base balance, the typical contribution of changes in $PaCO_2$ to changes in pH should be estimated. In anesthetized horses, the pH will decrease by 0.06–0.07 units (from an assumed neutral pH of 7.4) for each acute increase of 10 mmHg in $PaCO_2$ (from a normal $PaCO_2$ of 40 mmHg) (Blaze and Robinson, 1987). Therefore, a decrease in pH of this magnitude would be expected in cases of acidemia due to acute respiratory acidosis. Similarly, an acute compensatory respiratory response to a metabolic acid-base imbalance should change the pH by approximately this magnitude. If the change in $PaCO_2$ fully accounts for the change in pH, then a simple respiratory acid-base abnormality is likely present. If it doesn't fully account for the change in pH, than a metabolic acid-base disturbance, or more commonly, a mixed acid-base abnormality is present. Below is a simplified algorithm that can be used as a guide to rapidly determine acid-base and oxygenation status of a patient:

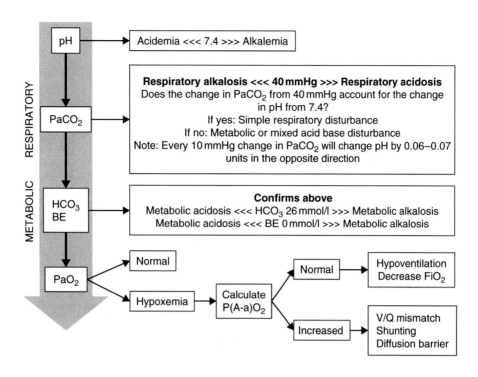

9.5 Oxygenation

The partial pressure of oxygen in arterial blood (PaO_2) is typically used to assess oxygenation, although oxygen content in arterial blood (CaO_2) is probably physiologically more important and will be briefly discussed later in this section. The normal values of PaO_2 in foals and adult horses at different ages are presented in Tables 9.1 and 9.2.

Hypoxemia is present if PaO_2 is less than 80 mmHg and is considered severe if less than 60 mmHg (Magdesian, 2004). Severe hypoxemia occurs frequently in anesthetized horses breathing room air (Figure 9.2). The PaO_2 depends on the fraction of inspired oxygen (FiO_2), alveolar ventilation, ventilation/perfusion (V/Q) matching, and diffusion capacity in the alveolar-capillary interface. As such, hypoxemia may result from disturbances of any of these (i.e., reduced FiO_2, hypoventilation, V/Q mismatch, shunt,

Figure 9.2 Horses under injectable anesthesia breathing a fraction of inspired oxygen (FiO_2) of 21% (room air) frequently become severely hypoxemic ($PaO_2 < 60$ mmHg, Panels A and B). Ventilation ($PaCO_2$) may be normal (Panel A) or slightly decreased (Panels B and C) as evidenced by eucapnia (normal $PaCO_2$) or hypercapnia (increased $PaCO_2$). Increasing FiO_2 to approximately 30% via oxygen insufflation (15 l/min in adult horses) into the airway (nostril or orotracheal tube) will often ameliorate (Panels A and C) and sometimes fully correct (Panel B) hypoxemia. Higher FiO_2 may be needed to fully correct hypoxemia in some horses (Panel C), but it may not be practical in out-of-hospital situations.

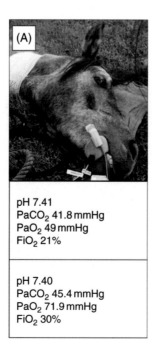
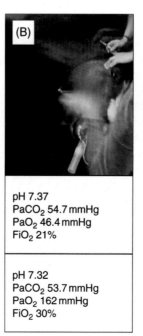
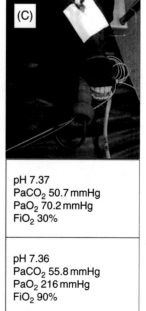

diffusion impairment) although it is more commonly multifactorial (i.e., more than one mechanism involved).

9.5.1 Reduced FiO₂

This is an uncommon cause of hypoxemia. High altitude and iatrogenic ventilation with low FiO_2 are likely the only circumstances where low FiO_2 could be the primary cause of hypoxemia in horses.

9.5.2 Hypoventilation

With hypoventilation, the reduction in alveolar ventilation causes a proportional increase in $PaCO_2$ (i.e., halving alveolar ventilation doubles $PaCO_2$). In other words, the PaO_2 will decrease by a magnitude nearly similar to the increase in $PaCO_2$ as dictated by the alveolar gas equation (with alveolar CO_2 tension being substituted by the arterial CO_2 tension):

$$P_AO_2 = [FiO_2 \times (P_B - P_{H2O})] - [PaCO_2/R]$$

Where: PB, barometric pressure (760 mmHg at sea level); P_{H2O}, partial pressure of water vapor of humidified airway gases (50 mmHg at 38 °C, the horse's normal body temperature); R, respiratory quotient (CO_2 production/O_2 consumption = 0.8). The first part of the alveolar gas equation refers to the partial pressure of inspired oxygen (PiO_2), so it can be re-written as:

$$P_AO_2 = PiO_2 - (PaCO_2/R)$$

At sea level ($P_B = 760$ mmHg), the calculated PiO_2 is approximately 150 mmHg. Assuming a normal $PaCO_2$ of 40 mmHg, the expected P_AO_2 would be approximately 100 mmHg. The expected PaO_2 would be slightly lower because the lung is not a perfect gas exchange unit (i.e., ventilation and perfusion are not perfectly matched). Despite the direct impact of hypoventilation on P_AO_2 and hence PaO_2, increasing the PiO_2 by increasing the FiO_2 (i.e., O_2 supplementation, Figure 9.3) frequently improves hypoxemia due to hypoventilation.

9.5.3 Ventilation/Perfusion Mismatching

This is characterized by an increased scatter of V/Q ratios. It is the most common cause of hypoxemia. Higher perfusion in relation to ventilation (low V/Q ratio) contributes disproportionate amounts of deoxygenated blood to the systemic circulation (i.e., venous admixture). Right to left shunting is an extreme form of low V/Q ratio and in practice it is often difficult to know if hypoxemia is due to true shunt or to increased contribution of areas with low (but not zero) V/Q ratios. Anesthesia and recumbency frequently increases the scatter of V/Q ratios, decreasing significantly the proportion of areas with normal V/Q ratios (Marntell et al., 2005). Increased scatter of V/Q ratios has an appreciable effect on PaO₂ when FiO₂ is in the 21–35% range, thereby contributing to hypoxemia (Lumb, 2000). In these cases, increasing FiO₂ via nasal insufflation with oxygen may ameliorate hypoxemia (Figure 9.3), and may be accompanied by an increase in PaCO₂ (Rush, 2004). Lower perfusion in relation to ventilation (high V/Q ratio) results in alveolar units that are ineffective in CO₂ elimination and O₂ uptake. Alveolar dead space is an extreme form of high V/Q ratio. High V/Q ratios can be caused

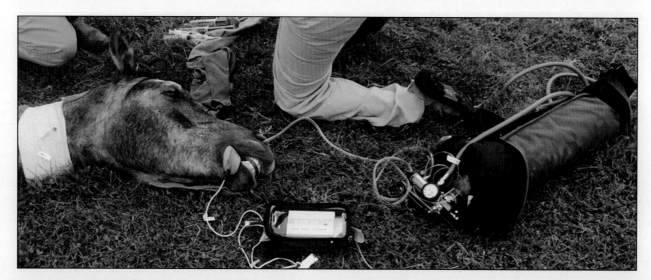

Figure 9.3 Oxygen supplementation can be easily accomplished by using a portable source of oxygen to administer 15 l/min deep into the nostril. This will increase the fraction of inspired oxygen (FiO₂), which frequently offsets the severe hypoxemia commonly observed in anesthetized horses breathing room air (FiO₂ = 21%).

by pulmonary thromboembolism and low pulmonary artery pressure (i.e., shock, inhalation anesthesia) (Marntell et al., 2005, Nyman and Hedenstierna, 1989).

9.5.4 Shunt

Shunt is defined as blood not exposed to ventilated lungs that is added to the systemic circulation. It can result from blood that circulates through unventilated lung regions (i.e., atelectasis, neoplasia, bronchial obstruction) or can be caused by shunting of blood directly from the right to the left side of the circulation (R-L shunt) usually due to congenital cardiac or vascular anomaly (i.e., tetralogy of Fallot, R-L patent ductus arteriosus, atrial or ventricular septal defect). Normally, mean $\pm$ SD shunt fraction is $1 \pm 0.4\%$ in healthy awake, standing horses. This value increases to $5 \pm 5\%$ and $10 \pm 12\%$ at 15 and 25 min of dissociative anesthesia with horses positioned in left lateral recumbency and spontaneously breathing room air. By comparison, at 30 min of anesthesia with halothane delivered in 100% oxygen, shunt fraction in spontaneously breathing horses increases to $19.7 \pm 2.4\%$ and $33.7 \pm 4.6\%$ while in left lateral or dorsal recumbency, respectively. Shunting may be even higher with more prolonged anesthesia and recumbency. Increased in shunt fraction thus contributes significantly to lower than expected PaO_2 during anesthesia (Marntell et al., 2005, Nyman and Hedenstierna, 1989). The magnitude of the shunt fraction will affect the ability of offsetting hypoxemia by increasing FiO_2. The predicted PaO_2 as a function of FiO_2 for different shunt fractions is presented in Table 9.4. In general, increasing FiO_2 is expected to greatly improve PaO_2 with a $\leq 10\%$ shunt fraction, moderately improve PaO_2 with 20% shunt fraction, minimally improve PaO_2 with 30% shunt fraction, and not improve PaO_2 with $\geq 50\%$ shunt fraction (Lumb, 2000).

9.5.5 Diffusion Impairment

Gas exchange between lung and blood depends on the particular gas solubility and pressure gradient across the alveolar-capillary interface, the surface area available for diffusion and the thickness of the alveolar-capillary interface. Hypoxemia due to pure diffusion impairment is rare in veterinary patients. Diffusion impairment more often is a contributor to hypoxemia, along with V/Q mismatch, in conditions such as pulmonary fibrosis, silicosis, interstitial pneumonia, or edema, all of which increase the thickness of the alveolar-capillary interface and/or decrease the available surface area for gas exchange. Increasing the driving pressure across the alveolar-capillary interface by increasing FiO_2 (i.e., oxygen therapy), in addition to

Table 9.4 Approximately predicted arterial oxygen partial pressure (PaO_2, mmHg) in humans* as a function of the inspired oxygen fraction (FiO_2) for different shunt fractions incorporating a factor of V/Q mismatch.

FiO_2 (%)	Shunt fraction (%)					
	0	5	10	20	30	50
21	100	98	70	50	45	35
30	160	120	98	70	55	38
40	240	175	125	80	65	40
50	300	230	160	87	65	40
60	390	290	210	100	70	40
70	475	380	285	130	75	45
80	520	440	340	165	75	50
90	600	520	430	225	88	50
100	>600	585	500	290	110	50

* PaO_2 values are likely similar or worse in horses as the contribution from V/Q mismatch during different shunt fractions are likely greater than in humans.
Source: Lumb (2000). Reproduced with permission of Elsevier.

correcting the thickness of the interface if possible (i.e., reducing edema, inflammation, etc.), can be effective in correcting hypoxemia due to diffusion impairment.

9.6 Arterial Oxygen Content

As mentioned previously, CaO_2 is probably physiologically more relevant than PaO_2 alone. Even though there is a relationship between PaO_2 and CaO_2, as dictated by the oxygen-hemoglobin equilibrium curve, the hemoglobin concentration itself will greatly affect the amount of O_2 carried in arterial blood. Therefore, to more accurately assess oxygenation, it important to know PaO_2, hemoglobin concentration (Hb) and saturation (SaO_2). This will allow calculation of the CaO_2 as:

$$CaO_2 = Hb \times 1.39 \times SaO_2 + (PaO_2 \times 0.003)$$

In a horse with Hb concentration of 10 g/dl, SaO_2 of 98%, and PaO_2 of 97 mmHg, the calculated CaO_2 will be approximately 14 ml/dl. Most (~13.7 ml/dl or 97%) of this O_2 is carried in the bound form and very little (0.3 ml/dl or ~3%) is dissolved in plasma. At the tissue level, the amount of oxygen delivered to them via blood flow (i.e., cardiac output) is also very important and should be taken into consideration when assessing oxygenation. Lastly, calculation of oxygen extraction ratio (OER), which is the percent of oxygen utilized by the tissues in relation to the delivered amount, may be useful in assessing occult oxygen debt. The mixed venous blood oxygen partial pressure (PvO2) and its hemoglobin saturation with oxygen (SvO$_2$) can be obtained via blood gas analysis. Jugular vein blood may be acceptable for clinical purposes, although mixed venous samples obtained from pulmonary artery or right ventricle should be used whenever possible. Other peripheral veins should not be used for blood sampling. The OER can be calculated as:

$$OER\,(\%) = ([CaO_2 - CvO_2] \times 100) \div CaO_2$$

Global oxygen extraction ratio was $18.0 \pm 0.02\%$ in healthy mixed-breed foals age 30–46 h in lateral recumbency (Corley, 2002) and is typically within the 20–30% range in adult horses. Decreases in cardiac output or CaO$_2$ will result in an increased OER such that tissue oxygen demands are met. Assuming normal hemoglobin concentration and quality, the OER can be used as an indirect means of cardiac output. When oxygen delivery decreases below a critical level and/or when oxygen consumption is increased, the OER cannot increase further such that tissue oxygen uptake decreases in parallel with the oxygen supply (i.e., supply-dependent oxygen uptake). The critical oxygen delivery is determined by the maximum global OER, which usually is in the range of 50–60%. When critical OER is exceeded, anaerobic metabolism takes place resulting in the production of lactic acid and metabolic acidosis.

9.7 Summary

Blood gas analyses can be easily performed with point-of-care analyzers. Arterial blood gas analyses are a valuable resource to assess oxygenation, ventilation and acid-base status. If arterial blood cannot be obtained, information regarding ventilation and acid-base may be obtained with analyses of mixed venous blood. It may also give some insight into oxygen consumption.

References

Aguilera-Tejero E, Estepa JC, Lopez I, Mayer-Valor R, and Rodriguez M. 1998. Arterial blood gases and acid-base balance in healthy young and aged horses. Equine Vet J 30: 352–354.

Arthurs GJ and Sudhakar M. 2005. Carbon dioxide transport. Contin Educ Anaesth Crit Care Pain 5: 207–210.

Blaze CA and Robinson NE. 1987. Apneic oxygenation in anesthetized ponies and horses. Vet Res Commun 11: 281–291.

Brosnan RJ, Steffey EP, LeCouteur RA, Imai A, Farver TB, and Kortz GD. 2003. Effects of ventilation and isoflurane end-tidal concentration on intracranial and cerebral perfusion pressures in horses. Am J Vet Res 64: 21–25.

Corley KTT. 2002. Monitoring and treating haemodynamic disturbances in critically ill neonatal foals. Part 1: Haemodynamic monitoring. Equine Veterinary Education 14: 270–279.

Deane JC, Dagleish MP, Benamou AE, Wolf BT, and Marlin D. 2004. Effects of syringe material and temperature and duration of storage on the stability of equine arterial blood gas variables. Vet Anaesth Analg 31: 250–257.

Grosenbaugh DA, Gadawski JE, and Muir WW. 1998. Evaluation of a portable clinical analyzer in a veterinary hospital setting. J Am Vet Med Assoc 213: 691–694.

Hopper K, Rezende ML, and Haskins SC. 2005. Assessment of the effect of dilution of blood samples with sodium heparin on blood gas, electrolyte, and lactate measurements in dogs. Am J Vet Res 66: 656–660.

Khanna AK, McDonell WN, Dyson DH, and Taylor PM. 1995. Cardiopulmonary effects of hypercapnia during controlled intermittent positive pressure ventilation in the horse. Can J Vet Res 59: 213–221.

Lumb A. 2000. Distribution of pulmonary ventilation and perfusion. In: A Lumb (ed.), *Nunn's Applied Respiratory Physiology*, Oxford, UK: Butterworth-Heinemann, pp. 163–199.

Madigan JE, Thomas WP, Backus KQ, and Powell WE. 1992. Mixed venous blood gases in recumbent and upright positions in foals from birth to 14 days of age. Equine Vet J 24: 399–401.

Magdesian KG. 2004. Monitoring the critically ill equine patient. Vet Clin North Am Equine Pract 20: 11–39.

Marntell S, Nyman G, Funkquist P, and Hedenstierna G. 2005. Effects of acepromazine on pulmonary gas exchange and circulation during sedation and dissociative anaesthesia in horses. Vet Anaesth Analg 32: 83–93.

Noel PG, Couetil L, and Constable PD. 2010. Effects of collecting blood into plastic heparinised vacutainer tubes and storage conditions on blood gas analysis values in horses. Equine Vet J Suppl, 91–97.

Nyman G and Hedenstierna G. 1989. Ventilation-perfusion relationhsips in the anaesthetised horse. Eq Vet J 21: 274–281.

Pacheco AP, Paradis MR, Hoffman AM, Hermida P, Sanchez A, Nadeau JA et al. 2014 Age effects on blood gas, spirometry, airway reactivity, and bronchoalveolar lavage fluid cytology in clinically healthy horses. J Vet Intern Med 28: 603–608.

Peiro JR, Borges AS, Goncalves RC, and Mendes LC 2010. Evaluation of a portable clinical analyzer for the determination of blood gas partial pressures, electrolyte concentrations, and hematocrit in venous blood samples collected from cattle, horses, and sheep. Am J Vet Res 71: 515–521.

Picandet V, Jeanneret S, and Lavoie JP. 2007. Effects of syringe type and storage temperature on results of blood gas analysis in arterial blood of horses. J Vet Intern Med 21: 476–481.

Rose RJ, Rossdale PD, and Leadon DP. 1982. Blood gas and acid–base status in spontaneously delivered, term-induced and induced premature foals. J Reprod Fertil Suppl 32: 521–528.

Rush BR. 2004. Respiratory diseases. In SM Reed, WM Bayly and DC Sellon (Eds), *Equine Internal Medicine*, 2nd edn, St. Louis, MO: Saunders, pp. 136–142.

Stewart JH, Rose RJ, and Barko, AM. 1984. Respiratory studies in foals from birth to seven days old. Equine Vet J 16: 323–328.

Wilkins PA. 2011. The equine neonatal intensive care laboratory: point-of-care testing. Clin Lab Med 3: 125–137.

Winkler JB, Huntington CG, Wells DE, and Befeler B. 1974. Influence of syringe materials on arterial blood gas determinations. Chest 66: 518–521.

10

Electrolytes

Krista E. Estell

Department of Medicine and Epidemiology, School of Veterinary Medicine, University of California, California, USA

10.1 Introduction

Abnormalities in electrolyte concentrations are a common occurrence in equine practice and are important to address as they may reflect disease states that result in fluid or electrolyte loss. In particular, gastrointestinal disease and renal insufficiency are common causes of fluid and electrolyte losses in horses. Abnormalities in electrolyte concentrations may also be a result of environmental conditions, prolonged or intense exercise, or may be iatrogenic due to administration of fluids, diuretics, or inappropriately mixed electrolyte supplements and milk replacers. Reference intervals for electrolytes vary between species and laboratories, and as such results should always be interpreted in light of laboratory-specific reference ranges.

10.2 Sample Handling and Analysis

Serum is the most commonly accepted sample for electrolyte analysis, though plasma obtained from blood anticoagulated with sodium or lithium heparin is also routinely used. Sample handling during blood collection, and storage prior to laboratory analysis are important factors in electrolyte interpretation. To prevent hemolysis and changes in electrolyte values, whole blood should not remain at room temperature for longer than 60 min, and serum should be separated from the red blood cells after clot formation and kept refrigerated until analysis is performed. With older chemistry machines that do not use direct ion-selective electrodes, severe lipemia and hyperproteinemia may result in erroneous decreases in electrolyte values as the lipids or proteins account for a large amount of the plasma or serum volume, falsely decreasing the electrolyte concentrations.

10.3 Sodium

When interpreting changes in sodium values, it is important to first determine hydration status. The serum sodium concentration is a reflection of the relative extracellular water volume meaning that changes in hydration can impact sodium balance. Mechanisms of maintaining euvolemia include interactions between the renin-angiotensin-aldosterone system, autonomic nervous system, and hypothalamic-pituitary-adrenal axis and are beyond the scope of this chapter. However, it is important to note that in the normal horse, changes in extracellular fluid volume do not significantly impact sodium concentration. In the normal horse, an increase in sodium concentration results in stimulation of thirst and release of anti-diuretic hormone (ADH) from the hypothalamus. ADH exerts its effects on the kidneys causing increased reabsorption of water in the collecting ducts and excretion of concentrated urine. The normal response to low sodium is the opposite, with inhibition of ADH secretion and excretion of dilute urine.

Due to these normal homeostatic mechanisms, moderate dehydration or electrolyte loss does not greatly impact sodium concentration. However, if changes in hydration status are severe or occur concurrently with loss of electrolytes, extreme fluctuations in sodium concentration can occur. Loss of fluid as a result of diarrhea, reflux, severe sweating, or third-space losses can result in either hyper- or hyponatremia depending on hydration status, the chronicity of the fluid loss, and access to free water. Fluid losses in these conditions are often isotonic as electrolytes and water are being lost concurrently, and does not result in changes in sodium balance until hydration status cannot be maintained, or water intake and renal water retention result in a relative change in total body water.

Sodium imbalances may cause clinical signs ranging from lethargy to obtundation, abnormal mentation, central blindness, and seizures. Caution must be taken in the treatment of dysnatremia, as rapid change in sodium concentration can result in worsening of neurologic dysfunction and damage. The goal for treatment of dysnatremia should be a change in sodium concentration of 0.5–1 mEq/L per hour. Rapid changes in sodium concentration may result in cerebral edema in cases of hypernatremia, and osmotic demyelination in the case of hyponatremia. Slow correction of sodium imbalance can be accomplished by both intravenous and enteral fluid administration and close monitoring of sodium concentration well as neurologic status (Fielding, 2015). If the dysnatremia is resulting in seizures, diazepam (0.1–0.25 mg/kg IV) should be administered in addition to correction of sodium concentration. If neurologic signs worsen during correction of the sodium imbalance, the rate of sodium correction should be slowed to prevent abrupt changes in neuronal cell osmolarity.

10.3.1 Hypernatremia

The most common cause of elevated sodium in the horse is a relative loss of free water that results in hypovolemic hypernatremia (see Box 10.1). An acute loss of fluid (diarrhea, reflux) without water replacement causes increased sodium concentration with concurrent signs of dehydration. Water restriction, particularly during times of high ambient temperature may also result in hypovolemic hypernatremia. Administration of

hypertonic fluids, sodium bicarbonate (enteral or intravenous), and inappropriately mixed milk replacers or electrolyte solutions may cause hypernatremia with a relatively normal hydration status.

10.3.2 Hyponatremia

Hyponatremia is most often caused by loss of sodium-containing fluid (i.e. diarrhea, reflux, excessive sweating) followed by free water intake or retention of water by the renal homeostatic mechanisms described previously (see Box 10.2). Though sodium and water are typically lost in equal amounts, water intake/retention results in a decrease in sodium concentration. If the condition persists untreated, the patient may show clinical signs of dehydration and hypovolemia in spite of a relative free water excess. Rapid accumulation of fluid within a body cavity, as occurs with a ruptured bladder, results in hyponatremia as sodium in the extracellular fluid moves down its concentration gradient into the relatively low sodium fluid in the abdomen. Administration of 5% dextrose in water or excessively diluted milk replacer may also result in hyponatremia. Additionally, some horses with GI discomfort due to enteritis/colitis may drink excessive amounts of water if allowed. Mild to moderate hyponatremia may be found in horses with psychogenic polydipsia with a normal hydration status. These horses are often stall-kept and present for polyuria with no other clinical signs.

Box 10.1 Hypernatremia.

Acute loss of fluid
- Diarrhea, high volume reflux
- Severe sweating
- Third-space fluid loss
  - Drainage of ascites or pleural effusion without volume replacement
- Acute renal insufficiency
  - Diuresis due to severe, persistent hyperglycemia

Water restriction
- No access to water, exacerbated by high ambient temperature
- Iatrogenic
  - Intravenous or oral electrolytes without free water access
  - Inappropriately mixed milk replacer

Dysfunctional Renin Angiotensin Aldosterone System/ Hypothalamic Pituitary Adrenal Axis
- Central or nephrogenic diabetes insipidus
- Mineralocorticoid excess

Box 10.2 Hyponatremia.

Loss of sodium containing fluid
- Diarrhea, reflux
- Excess sweating
- Renal disease
- Adrenal insufficiency

Third-space loss
- Ruptured bladder
- Pleuritis, ascites
  - Rapid, high-volume drainage may result in exacerbation of hyponatremia and hypovolemia

Free water excess
- Iatrogenic
  - 5% dextrose in water
  - Inappropriately mixed milk replacer
- Excessive water drinking
  - Enteritis
  - Psychogenic polydipsia
- HPAA axis abnormalities
  - Inappropriate ADH secretion

10.4 Chloride

Sodium and chloride are the major ions found in the extracellular fluid, and often increase or decrease concurrently in cases of a relative free water deficit. When increases or decreases in chloride occur independently of changes in sodium, acid-base status should be considered. Chloride and sodium are the major ions responsible for the strong ion difference, and have a significant impact on pH according to Stewart's Strong Ion Theory. Full review of acid-base determination is included in Chapter 17, but in summary, the strong ion theory indicates that hydrogen cations and bicarbonate anions (and therefore pH) are dependent variables that can change as a result of increases or decreases in other strong ions. For example, chloride typically has an inverse relationship to bicarbonate: as chloride decreases, bicarbonate increases resulting in a metabolic alkalosis.

10.4.1 Hyperchloremia

Due to the inverse relationship of chloride and bicarbonate, increased chloride concentration occurs with loss of bicarbonate anions in diarrhea or reflux and metabolic acidosis (Box 10.3). Hyperchloremia with normal sodium concentration is a cardinal sign of renal tubular acidosis (RTA). Horses with RTA display non-specific signs of lethargy and inappetance and may have severe electrolyte and acid/base abnormalities with a venous pH of < 7.25, a chloride concentration that may range from 105–120 mEq/L, and a bicarbonate concentration < 15 mEq/L (Aleman and Estell, 2014). RTA occurs when the kidney fails to reabsorb bicarbonate anions, and instead conserves chloride anions to maintain electroneutrality. Type I RTA is more severe, and is a result of failure of the distal tubules to excrete H+. Type I RTA may also result in total body depletion of potassium as K+ cations are excreted instead of H+. Type II RTA is typically self-limiting and is caused by failure of the proximal convoluted tubules to reabsorb bicarbonate anions. When RTA is identified, a full CBC and serum biochemical analysis

with urinalysis should be performed to investigate causes of renal damage or insufficiency. The primary goal of RTA treatment is replacement of bicarbonate and supportive care. Enteral/oral bicarbonate replacement is more effective than IV administration alone, and often both are needed in the early stages of treatment to restore hydration status. Ideally, 50% of the bicarbonate deficit should be replaced within the first 12 h of therapy, with serial monitoring of electrolyte and acid-base status to help guide additional therapy. As a large amount of sodium bicarbonate often needs to be given (100–150 g, q8–12 h; 1 g = 12 mEq) diarrhea may occur, though is typically self-limiting.

Prolonged fluid therapy, particularly in foals, often results in mild to moderate hyperchloremia in horses. Hyperchloremia is most common when saline is used, though all commercially available fluids have a higher concentration of chloride relative to sodium than is physiologic in the horse. As the sodium-chloride difference narrows and chloride increases, a metabolic acidosis typically develops. If bicarbonate is not being lost excessively, the metabolic acidosis can be easily corrected with administration of fluid that does not contain chloride (isotonic sodium bicarbonate).

10.4.2 Hypochloremia

Due to the inverse relationship between bicarbonate and chloride, metabolic alkalosis typically accompanies hypochloremia (see Box 10.4). Low chloride with a normal to acidic pH may occur in horses with diarrhea as excessive loss of chloride relative to sodium may occur, though sodium is often decreased as well. Venous pH is often low in these cases as a result of hypovolemia and lactic acidosis. Hypochloremic metabolic alkalosis is associated with rhabdomyolysis and over-exertion with exhaustion, particularly in high ambient temperatures. Iatrogenic hypochloremia may occur after excessive furosemide administration.

Box 10.3 Hyperchloremia.

With hypernatremia
- Water restriction/free water deficit
- Renal failure
- Diuretic administration
- Hypertonic saline administration
- Dysfunctional RAAS/HPAA

With metabolic acidosis
- Loss of bicarbonate in diarrhea/reflux
- Renal tubular acidosis

Box 10.4 Hypochloremia.

With hyponatremia
- Loss of electrolyte-rich fluid
- Free water excess
  - Iatrogenic
  - Excessive water drinking
  - HPAA axis abnormalities

With metabolic alkalosis
- Rhabdomyolysis
- Exhaustive syndrome

Diuretics
- Furosemide administration

10.5 Potassium

Potassium is one of the most important intracellular cations and maintains the negative cell resting membrane potential that allows the conduction of nerve impulses and muscle contraction. As potassium is an intracellular cation, serum potassium concentrations may not actually represent total body potassium levels. A better idea of intracellular potassium concentrations can be obtained through measurement of erythrocyte potassium, though this measurement may not accurately reflect total body potassium levels in horses (Johnson et al., 1991).

10.5.1 Hyperkalemia

Hyperkalemia due to *in vitro* hemolysis is a common finding, particularly if serum has not been separated from red blood cells within an hour of sampling (Box 10.5). Age-specific reference intervals should be used when interpreting potassium concentration as foals tend to have higher normal potassium concentrations when compared to adults. Mild hyperkalemia is often asymptomatic, but as potassium concentrations increase (>6 mEQ/L), changes in cardiac myocyte membrane depolarization result in characteristic electrocardiogram changes including bradycardia, absent p waves, and tented t waves. If hyperkalemia is allowed to persist untreated, fatal arrhythmia may occur.

Causes of hyperkalemia include failure to excrete potassium-rich urine or movement of potassium from the intracellular space extracellularly. Renal failure, uroabdomen, and urinary outflow obstruction all result in hyperkalemia due to a failure to excrete normal urine. Movement of potassium from the intracellular compartment occurs in severe muscle necrosis seen with exercise induced rhabdomyolysis, immune mediated myositis, nutritional myodegeneration (particularly in foals), and glycogen branching enzyme deficiency. Elevation in potassium concentration can also be seen transiently after anaerobic exercise. Hyperkalemic periodic paralysis (HYPP) results in a transient hyperkalemia as a result of abnormal voltage-gated sodium channels in skeletal muscles. These abnormal channels fail to inactivate when extracellular potassium increases, and continue to pump potassium extracellularly. This results in persistent depolarization of muscle cells and clinical signs that range from muscle fasciculations and third eyelid prolapse to recumbency and laryngeal paralysis. Adrenal insufficiency, which occurs most commonly in neonates, also results in hyperkalemia.

The primary goal of treatment for severe hyperkalemia is movement of potassium from the extracellular to the intracellular space to allow normal membrane depolarization and prevent fatal cardiac arrhythmias. Administration of oral glucose (Karo syrup) by horse owners while waiting for the veterinarian to arrive can be life-saving in cases of HYPP. Administration of glucose results in movement of potassium intracellularly via a glucose/potassium co-transporter. Intravenous dextrose can be administered as up to a 2–5% solution (20–50 mg/ml; 200–500 ml of 50% dextrose in 5 L of fluids) in a potassium-free isotonic fluid such as sodium bicarbonate, saline, or as 5% dextrose in water. Administration of 5% dextrose in water should be used sparingly and with caution as it is not a balanced electrolyte solution. In cases where severe hyperkalemia is suspected, as in an HYPP episode, calcium gluconate (250 ml in 5 L of fluids) should be added to increase the membrane threshold potential for depolarization. Regular insulin (0.01–0.04 IU/kg IV) can be used to enhance intracellular potassium transport, though glucose monitoring must be performed. Long-term treatment of hyperkalemia depends on the underlying etiology; but feeding low-potassium forage in chronic cases and administration of the carbonic anhydrase inhibitor acetazolamide are mainstays of treatment.

10.5.2 Hypokalemia

Mild to moderate decreases in potassium are common in horses with a poor appetite. Potassium loss may also occur from the GI tract as a result of diarrhea, or from the kidneys due to diuretic administration or RTA (Box 10.6). A mineralocorticoid excess from either endogenous production or steroid administration causes a drop in potassium due to decreased renal absorption. In some cases of hypokalemia, potassium may not actually be depleted, but may be sequestered intracellularly due to metabolic alkalosis or administration of glucose or insulin as described previously.

Hypokalemia can be corrected by adding KCl to intravenous fluids, though care should be taken not to administer potassium at a rate greater than 0.5 mEq/kg/h. For the average 500 kg horse, 20–40 mEq of KCl/L

Box 10.5 Hyperkalemia.

Erroneous
- *In vitro* hemolysis
- Prolonged storage

Failure to excrete potassium
- Renal failure
- Uroabdomen
- Urinary outflow obstruction

Extracellular potassium shift
- Rhabdomyolysis
- HYPP
- Transient after anaerobic exercise

Adrenal insufficiency

Box 10.6 Hypokalemia.

Decreased intake
Loss of potassium
- Diarrhea
- Reflux
- Excessive sweating
  - Renal loss
  - RTA
  - Diuretics
  - Mineralocorticoid excess
Intracellular potassium shift
- Alkalosis
- Dextrose administration
- Insulin administration
- Endogenous/exogenous catecholamines

Box 10.7 Hypercalcemia.

Decreased excretion
- Chronic renal failure
Abnormalities in homeostasis
- Primary hyperparathyroidism
- Hypercalcemia of malignancy
- Excess Vitamin D
  - Oversupplementation
  - Plant intoxication

---

of IV fluids (100–200 mEq/5 L over 1 h) is safe and effective at managing hypokalemia. Lite salt and forage that is higher in potassium such as alfalfa and some types of orchard grass hay are effective strategies to manage chronic hypokalemia.

10.6 Calcium

Calcium balance is tightly regulated in horses as it plays an important role in many different organ systems including transmission of nerve impulses, muscle contraction, and hemostasis in addition to acting as a second messenger for cellular communication. Total calcium represents both the active ionized form of calcium and calcium that is albumin bound. As 40–50% of calcium is bound to albumin, changes in protein concentration may result in increases or decreases in calcium concentration, though ionized calcium typically remains the same.

Calcium homeostasis is closely regulated by the parathyroid gland and Vitamin D, and is linked to phosphorus homeostasis. When calcium is low, the parathyroid gland secretes parathyroid hormone (PTH), which results in renal reabsorption of calcium and excretion of phosphorus, increased osteoclastic absorption of both calcium and phosphorus from bone, and increased Vitamin D production by the liver. Vitamin D enhances the absorption of calcium and phosphorus in the gastrointestinal tract, decreases renal excretion of both minerals, and promotes bone calcification. Calcitonin, which is secreted by the thyroid gland when calcium is high, has the opposite physiologic effect of PTH.

10.6.1 Hypercalcemia

As a significant amount of calcium is excreted in urine, chronic renal failure is a common cause of moderate to severe hypercalcemia in horses, particularly if horses are fed calcium-rich diets such as alfalfa hay and feeds that are high in molasses (Box 10.7). Horses with chronic renal failure will also have elevated creatinine and blood urea nitrogen in addition to hyperkalemia and hypophosphatemia.

If renal function is normal, abnormalities in calcium homeostasis should be considered as a cause of hypercalcemia. Ionized and total calcium, phosphorus, PTH, and Vitamin D should be analyzed to determine the underlying cause. Primary hyperparathyroidism occurs infrequently in horses but has been reported in cases of functional parathyroid adenomas. More commonly, hypercalcemia due to an elevation in parathyroid-related peptide (PTHrP) occurs. PTHrp is secreted from various types of neoplastic tumors, and can result in severe hypercalcemia that may occur concurrently with weight loss or lethargy and may be the first clinical sign of disease. Vitamin D intoxication can result in hypercalcemia due to over-supplementation of Vitamin D or ingestion of plants that contain Vitamin D analogs. Plants that have been associated with Vitamin D intoxication in horses include *Cestrum diurnum* (wild jasmine), *Trisetum flavescens* (golden oats or yellow oat grass), and from the Solanaceae family, *Nierembergia veitchii*, *Solanum esuriale*(potato bush, potato weed, queen's nightshade, wild tomato, quena), *S. torvum* (turkey berry), and *S. malacoxylon* (Mello, 2003, Wagstaff, 2008).

Treatment for hypercalcemia is difficult if the inciting cause cannot be treated. Horses with chronic renal failure, for example, should be fed diets that are relatively low in calcium; alfalfa and molasses based feed should be avoided. In cases of primary hyperparathyroidism, identification and removal of the abnormal parathyroid gland may be curative (Tomlinson et al., 2014).

10.6.2 Hypocalcemia

Mild hypocalcemia is typically asymptomatic in horses and occurs commonly with decreased feed intake, and acute renal insufficiency (Box 10.8). Moderate to severe hypocalcemia can occur following prolonged or extreme exercise, transport, or rhabdomyolysis, and sometimes coincides with a decrease in feed intake or a change in

---

Box 10.8 Hypocalcemia.

Decreased feed intake
Hypoalbuminemia
- Ionized calcium is normal
Increased excretion
- Acute renal failure
- Prolonged/extreme exercise
- Prolonged transport
Metabolic alkalosis
- Rhabdomyolysis
Toxins
- Blister beetle (cantharadin) toxicosis
- Oxalate plants
Diuretics
- Furosemide
Abnormalities in homeostasis
- Hypoparathyroidism
- Nutritional secondary hyperparathyroidism

---

feed and a lack of dietary calcium. Clinical signs of moderate to severe hypocalcemia include muscle cramping and synchronous diaphragmatic flutter (discharging of the phrenic nerve due to cardiac muscle contraction) as a result of calcium's role in nerve impulse transmission. Calcium is typically bound to voltage-gated sodium channels, and has a stabilizing effect. When calcium is low, voltage-gated sodium channels are activated by very small increases in membrane potential resulting in the discharge of nerve impulses with relatively little provocation. Abnormalities in calcium homeostasis due to primary and secondary hypoparathyroidsim is rare, but has been reported in horses (Durie et al., 2010, Aguilera-Tejero et al., 2000). Toxic causes of hypocalcemia include blister beetle consumption and resulting cantharadin toxicosis, and consumption of oxalate containing plants. Excessive furosemide administration may also result in hypocalcemia due to increased calcium excretion.

Treatment of hypocalcemia should be considered when ionized calcium is <1.2 mEq/L or clinical signs of hypocalcemia are present. Calcium can be administered as an additive to fluids in the form of 23 calcium borogluconate. An increase in calcium is typically seen at a dose of 100–200 ml/500 kg horse administered as 25 ml/L diluted in polyionic fluids, though more aggressive administration of 250–500 ml diluted to at least a 1:4 ratio in fluids can be administered in severe cases. If higher doses of calcium are used, fluids should be given slowly over 20–30 min and close cardiac monitoring should be performed during administration; treatment should be immediately stopped if bradycardia develops. Calcium levels in horses with clinical signs of hypocalcemia

should be monitored for several days following treatment and these horses should also be supplemented with high calcium containing feed.

10.7 Phosphorus

Phosphorus is primarily found in the bone and teeth, but also plays a role in intracellular energy storage and metabolism in the form of the adenosine phosphates (ATP, ADP, AMP), and extracellularly as a buffer. In plasma, phosphate exists as an inorganic form that is either ionized, complexed to cations, or protein bound, while intracellular phosphorus is organic and unmeasured. Phosphorus homeostasis is closely tied to calcium regulation as described previously, and is regulated by PTH, Vitamin D, and calcitonin.

10.7.1 Hyperphosphatemia

Age-specific reference intervals should be used when interpreting phosphate concentration as growing horses have a high rate of bone turn-over and phosphate is often quite high (Box 10.9). Phosphate may also be increased with *in vitro* or *in vivo* hemolysis. Acute renal insufficiency and decreased glomerular filtration rate is commonly associated with hyperphosphatemia in horses. Hyperphosphatemia has also been associated with exhaustive syndrome after endurance competition. Alterations in phosphorus homeostasis, such as secondary hyperparathyroidism due to excessive dietary intake of phosphate, and Vitamin D toxicity occur less frequently. Additionally, iatrogenic hyperphosphatemia may occur after excessive fleet enema administration to neonatal foals, and hyperphosphatemia has been associated with severe acute tumor necrosis in horses. Treatment of hyperphosphatemia should be directed at addressing the underlying disease process and decreasing dietary phosphate intake. Though literature on treatment of hyperphosphatemia is lacking in horses, fluid

---

Box 10.9 Hyperphosphatemia.

Normal growth and development
Decreased excretion
- Acute renal failure
Prolonged/extreme exercise
Abnormalities in homeostasis
- Nutritional secondary hyperparathyroidism
- Vitamin D intoxication
Excessive administration of phosphorus-containing fleet enemas in the neonate
Hemolysis
Tumor necrosis

Box 10.10 Hypophosphatemia.

Decreased dietary intake
Decreased absorption
- Chronic renal failure
- Large colon resection

Abnormalities in homeostasis
- Hyperparathyroidism
- Pseudohyperparathyroidism (hypercalcemia of malignancy)

Shift to the intracellular space
- Refeeding syndrome
- Endotoxemia, sepsis
- Alkalosis

Box 10.11 Hypermagnesemia.

Excessive administration of magnesium sulfate (Epsom salt).

Box 10.12 Hypomagnesemia.

Decreased feed intake
Prolonged/extreme exercise
Concurrent with colic, ileus, and endotoxemia

---

diuresis and acetazolamide may be helpful in decreasing phosphate concentration. Calcium carbonate may also be useful as it acts as both a phosphate binding agent and increases calcium for absorption (Toribio, 2011).

10.7.2 Hypophosphatemia

Hypophosphatemia is most commonly associated with chronic renal insufficiency in horses as the kidneys lose the ability to reabsorb phosphorous (Box 10.10). Decreased dietary intake is also associated with mildly low phosphate. As phosphate metabolism is regulated by PTH, hyperparathyroidism and elevations in PTHrP can also result in hypophosphatemia. In horses that are re-introduced to feed after starvation, extreme shifts of phosphorus to the intracellular fluid compartment can occur and may result in cell membrane fragility which manifests as rhabdomyolysis and hemolysis in other species, though it has not been well-documented in the horse. Intracellular phosphate shifts are also reported in severe sepsis, endotoxemia, alkalosis, and in horses receiving parenteral nutrition. Other reported causes of hypophosphatemia include excessive magnesium administration and large colon resection (Magdesian, 2015). Treatment is recommended in cases of moderate to severe hypophosphatemia and should be based on phosphorus deficit, though this value can be easily underestimated as most phosphorus exists intracellularly. A maximum dose of 0.24 mmol/kg/day IV in the form of sodium or potassium phosphate is recommended.

10.8 Magnesium

Magnesium is primarily an intracellular cation, which like calcium, exists in both free ionized and albumin-bound forms. Hypermagnesemia occurs infrequently in horses, but is most commonly iatrogenic as a result of excessive magnesium sulfate (Epsom salt) administration via nasogastric intubation (see Box 10.11). Hypomagnesemia is commonly found in horses with decreased feed intake and is most commonly subclinical. Like calcium and phosphate, decreases in magnesium may also occur with exhaustive syndrome following intense or prolonged exercise (see Box 10.12). Additionally, hypomagnesemia may be found concurrently with colic, ileus, endotoxemia, and cardiac arrhythmias in horses, and should be corrected. Dosage of magnesium varies depending on the presence and severity of clinical signs associated with hypomagnesemia. For treatment of ventricular arrhythmias 4 mg/kg of magnesium sulfate IV every 2 min up to a total dose of 50 mg/kg; for subclinical hypomagnesemia or ileus 3–6 mg/kg/h can be administered diluted in fluids as a continuous rate infusion until hypomagnesemia is corrected (van Loon, 2009).

References

Aguilera-Tejero E, Estepa JC, López I, Bas S and Rodríguez M. 2000. Polycystic kidneys as a cause of chronic renal failure and secondary hypoparathyroidism in a horse. Eq Vet J, 32: 167–169.

Aleman M. and Estell K. 2014. Renal tubular acidosis. In BP Smith (ed.) *Large Animal Internal Medicine*. St. Louis, MO: Elsevier.

Durie I, Van Loon G, Hesta M, Bauwens C, and Deprez P. 2010. Hypocalcemia caused by primary hypoparathyroidism in a 3-month-old filly. J Vet Int Med, 24: 439–442.

Fielding CL. 2015. Sodium and water homeostasis and derangements. In CL Fielding and KG Magdesian (eds.) *Equine Fluid Therapy*. Ames, IA: John Wiley & Sons, Inc.

Johnson PJ, Goetz TE, Foreman JH, Vogel RS, Hoffmann WE, and Baker GJ. 1991. Effect of whole-body potassium depletion on plasma, erythrocyte, and middle gluteal muscle potassium concentration of healthy, adult horses. Am J Vet Res, 52: 1676–1683.

Magdesian KG. 2015. Maintenance fluid therapy in horses. In CL Fielding and KG Magdesian (eds.) *Equine Fluid Therapy*. Ames, IA: John Wiley & Sons, Inc.

Mello JRB. 2003. Calcinosis: calcinogenic plants. Toxicon, 41: 1–12.

Tomlinson JE, Johnson AL, Ross MW, Engiles JB, Levine DG, Wisner WA, and Sweeney RW 2014. Successful detection and removal of a functional parathyroid adenoma in a pony using technetium Tc 99 m sestamibi scintigraphy. J Vet Int Med, 28: 687–692.

Toribio RE. 2011. Disorders of calcium and phosphate metabolism in horses. The Veterinary Clinics of North America: Eq Pract, 27: 129–147.

van Loon G. 2009. Management of atrial fibrillation. In NE Robinson and KA Sprayberry (eds.) *Current Therapy in Equine Medicine*. St. Louis, MI: Saunders Elsevier.

Wagstaff JD. 2008. *International Poisonous Plants Checklist: An Evidence Based Reference*, CRC Press.

11

Miscellaneous Solutes

Leslie Sharkey

Department of Veterinary Clinical Sciences, College of Veterinary Medicine, University of Minnesota, Minnesota, USA

11.1 Introduction

Bilirubin, bile acids, ammonia, and lactate are four substances measured in the blood for diagnostic purposes. Serum bilirubin quantitation is usually performed as part of a complete serum biochemical profile, while serum bile acids, ammonia, and lactate are ordered as individual tests, generally based on clinical suspicion for conditions that cause increases in blood content. For each analyte, basic physiologic regulation, recommendations for sample collection and submission, and diagnostic applications and interpretation will be discussed. Unique aspects of equine physiology such as fasting hyperbilirubinemia and gastrointestinal disease associated hyperammonemia present diagnostic challenges for the equine clinician that will be addressed.

11.2 Bilirubin

11.2.1 Physiology

Bilirubin is formed by the degradation of hemoglobin and related proteins by macrophages, occurring at a relatively constant rate in health. Non-covalently bound to albumin as a carrier, unconjugated bilirubin is released from albumin in the hepatic sinusoids and taken up by hepatocytes in a receptor-mediated process. In hepatocytes bilirubin is conjugated to increase water solubility and is transported into the bile caniculi for biliary excretion. A fraction of this conjugated bilirubin slips back into the circulation. A portion of bilirubin is also eliminated via glomerular filtration. Based on these physiological principles, the three main mechanisms for hyperbilirubinemia are increased production due to enhanced cell destruction, particularly of erythrocytes (pre-hepatic cholestasis), failure of hepatocytes to clear bile from the circulation (hepatic cholestasis), and blockage of the biliary system (post-hepatic cholestasis). It is important to note that these mechanisms are not mutually exclusive, and individual horses may have multiple contributing factors to hyperbilirubinemia.

11.2.2 Sample Collection and Methodology

Sample collection for the measurement of serum bilirubin is uncomplicated and conforms to the usual recommendations for the routine serum biochemical profile. Typically, serum bilirubin is reported as a total value, which includes both the unconjugated (indirect bilirubin) and conjugated forms (direct bilirubin). The total bilirubin can be "fractionated," in which the different forms are measured separately. Theoretically, pre-hepatic and hepatic cholestasis should result in a disproportionate increase in unconjugated bilirbubin, while post-hepatic cholestasis would cause increases in the conjugated form. If other laboratory and clinical data (ie evidence of a hemolytic anemia causing pre-hepatic cholestasis) are insufficient to distinguish these processes when there is diagnostic need, fractionation can be requested. In general, if the conjugated bilirubin exceeds approximately 25% of the total, liver disease is a probable cause of the hyperbilirubinemia, and higher values are more specifically suggestive for cholestasis.

11.2.3 Diagnostic Interpretation

Pre-hepatic cholestasis is most frequently the result of increased red cell destruction and is usually associated with significant anemia. With sufficient time for marrow response, hemolytic anemias should be regenerative, however, this can be difficult to assess in horses because reticulocytes are rarely released into the peripheral blood. Examination of a blood film for morphologic abnormalities associated with hemolytic anemia is essential; these include agglutination indicative of immune-mediated red cell destruction, the presence of Heinz bodies and eccentrocytes associated with oxidative damage such as that caused by ingestion of red maple leaves, schistocytes occurring with fragmentation anemias, and red blood cell parasites. Red cell ghosts can be observed with acute intravascular hemolysis, but are not specific as to cause. Hemolyzed plasma and hemoglobinuria characterize acute intravascular hemolysis, and must be distinguished from discoloration of plasma and urine secondary to myoglobinuria associated with muscle damage and from hematuria. With extravascular hemolysis and resolving intravascular events, hyperbilirubinemia and bilirubinuria will predominate. It is important to consider that secondary hypoxia-induced muscle and liver enzyme elevations may accompany acute or severe anemias, possibly complicating data interpretation. Furthermore, liver failure can develop as a complication of equine neonatal isoerythrolysis, and hemolysis can rarely occur as a complication of liver disease in horses, therefore the presence of pre-hepatic cholestasis does not exclude the potential for other causes of hyperbilirubinemia (Boyle et al., 2005, Polkes et al., 2008, Ramaiah et al., 2003).

Causes of hepatic cholestasis in horses include anorexia, liver dysfunction, and sepsis. Fasting hyperbilirubinemia in horses occurs as rapidly as 12 h after food restriction and plateaus in 2 or 3 days, typically not exceeding 10 mg/dl, with a predominance of indirect or unconjugated bilirubin. Anorexia is frequently a cause of hyperbilirubinemia in horses with gastrointestinal disease, which decreases the specificity of hyperbiliuribinemia as an indicator for liver disease and likely contributes to the lack of prognostic significance (Durham et al., 2003, McGorum et al., 1999, Underwood et al., 2010). Neonatal foals have a physiological hyperbiliuribinemia due to immaturity of hepatic processing of bilirubin, however persistent severe hyperbiliuribinemia can result in a syndrome of kernicterus and neurologic damage similar to that described in people (Drivers, 2011, Durán et al., 2009). Post-hepatic cholestasis is relatively rare in the horse compared with many other species, and likely occurs in combination with other forms of cholestasis. It can be associated with hepatocellular swelling, inflammatory and neoplastic infiltration of the liver, and with cholelithiasis.

11.3 Bile Acids

11.3.1 Physiology

Bile acids include a group of related molecules synthesized from cholesterol by hepatocytes and conjugated for excretion in the bile, ultimately to aid in intestinal fat absorption. In the intestine, primary bile acids are chemically modified by bacteria into secondary bile acids.

Both are efficiently absorbed (approximately 90%) into the portal circulation to be returned to the liver for another cycle of biliary excretion in a process referred to as enterohepatic circulation. This process is relatively constant in horses because they consume low fat diets and lack gall bladders, so there is little diurnal variation and sample collection relative to feeding is not a factor. Serum bile acids will be increased when there are too few functional hepatocytes to extract bile acids in the portal circulation, when the portal circulation is abnormal (shunting), and when post-hepatic cholestasis prevents normal transport of bile acids into bile cannaliculi, leading to spillover into the general circulation.

11.3.2 Sample Collection and Methodology

As noted previously, the timing of sample collection for the measurement of serum bile acids is not important in horses, although prolonged fasting (days) may result in elevated serum values. Most commonly used assays use spectrophotometric techniques to measure total bile acids in circulation; lipemia and hemolysis interfere with most assays and should be avoided when possible. Most laboratories will provide interpretive comments specific to their assays to help clinicians understand potential effects of patient data.

11.3.3 Diagnostic Interpretation

Increased serum bile acid concentration is considered to have good positive predictive value for equine hepatopathy based on studies of horses with histologically confirmed liver disease (Durham et al., 2003, McGorum et al., 1999) (see Box 11.1). Sensitivity may be better in chronic liver disease. Nevertheless, serum bile acids were elevated in 28% of 32 surgical colic cases. The majority of these horses had mild to moderate increases and survived, however the two horses with marked elevations were euthanized due to poor prognosis for their surgical disease (Underwood et al., 2010). Healthy foals in the first 6 weeks of life have higher serum bile acid values than adult horses, but non-hepatic illness did not cause additional elevations (Barton and LeRoy, 2007).

11.4 Ammonia

11.4.1 Physiology

Although the term "blood ammonia" is typically used to describe this diagnostic test, at physiological pH, blood ammonium (NH_4^+) rather than ammonia (NH_3^+) predominates. Most ammonium is produced in the intestine through dietary protein digestion and bacterial metabolism.

Box 11.1 Case example of a horse with chronic liver disease.

A 13-year-old Quarter Horse gelding presents with a history of pastern dermatitis progressing to involve white skin on his legs.*

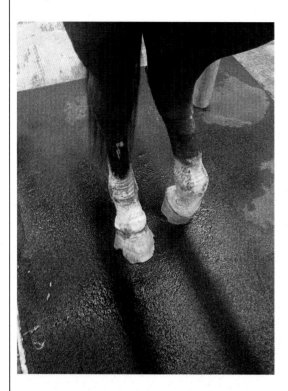

He has a history of winter weight loss. On presentation, the gelding is dull but responsive, dehydrated, and icteric with severe pastern dermatitis. Coagulation times were moderately prolonged. The following abnormalities were present on the serum biochemical profile.

BUN	L	5 mg/dl	(13–23)
Alb	L	1.9 g/dl	(2.9–3.9)
Bili	H	9.3 mg/dl	(0.3–2.0)
ALP	H	661 U/L	(48–148)
GGT	H	811 U/L	(3–18)
SDH	H	32 U/L	(1–7)
AST	H	886 U/L	(162–316)
CK	H	373	(82–303)
Gluc		87 mg/dl	(75–116)
SBA	H	106.0 µmol/L	(<25)

There is evidence of hepatocellular damage (SDH, AST, GGT), cholestasis (Bili, ALP, GGT) and liver dysfunction (low urea, albumin, prolonged coagulation times, and high serum bile acids). The dermatitis was attributed to photosensitization associated with liver disease. A biopsy revealed diffuse marked hepatocellular degeneration and atrophy with megalocytosis and individual cell necrosis, presumed to be chronic exposure to a hepatotoxin. The horse was euthanized due to deteriorating clinical condition and poor prognosis. Type III photosensitization was confirmed as the cause for the skin lesions at necropsy.

*Image courtesy of Dr. Carrie Robbins.

Ammonium is taken up by the portal circulation and delivered to hepatocytes to be used for urea, amino acid, and protein synthesis. Both urea and ammonium undergo renal excretion. Thus, increased ammonium in the blood can be the result of increased intestinal production or decreased hepatic clearance, while decreased renal excretion does not appear to be a clinically significant mechanism for hyperammonemia.

11.4.2 Sample Collection and Methodology

Although standard enzymatic methods are used to measure blood ammonia, diagnostic applications can be limited by fastidious sample collection and handling requirements. Hemolysis causes spurious increases in blood ammonia values and must be avoided. Plasma should be separated from cells immediately after collection and cooled in an ice bath until the assay can be performed, preferably within 1–4 h after collection. Falsely elevated readings can be obtained with delayed separation of cells from plasma due to ammonium production by blood cells, and samples at room temperature will have spurious increases due to degradation of proteins and amino acids in the samples. Decreased values will occur when samples are exposed to air, however, delayed measurement is possible if plasma samples are promptly frozen and kept on dry ice until shortly before analysis. Viable postmortem measurement of ammonia in cerebrospinal fluid and aqueous humor can be performed on samples collected up to 10 h after death for cases in which this diagnostic consideration is delayed (Gilliam et al., 2007).

11.4.3 Diagnostic Interpretation

Blood ammonia is most commonly measured as an indicator of liver dysfunction, typically when the animal has neurologic signs for which hepatic encephalopathy is a differential diagnosis. Horses with histopathologically confirmed liver disease and neurologic signs

---

Box 11.2 Case example of a horse with neurologic signs due to hyperammonemia.

A 4-year-old Quarter Horse mare presented with a history of suspected strangles and neurologic signs and a 2-day history of severe diarrhea. On presentation, the mare was dull and ataxic, dehydrated with hyperemic mucous membranes and had prolonged capillary refill time. Consensual pupillary light reflexes were absent in the right eye, she had a weak panniculus response, and she was unable to prehend food. She had multiple superficial abrasions. Her CBC revealed a degenerative left shift with marked toxic change and relative polycythemia. She was moderately azotemic.

Alb	L	2.7 g/dl	(2.9–3.9)
Bili		1.9 mg/dl	(0.3–2.0)
ALP	H	450 U/L	(48–148)
GGT		12 U/L	(3–18)
SDH	H	16 U/L	(1–7)
AST	H	141 U/L	(162–316)
CK		194	(82–303)
Gluc	H	159 mg/dl	(75–116)
SBA		23.0 μmol/L	(<25)
Ammonia	H	114 μmol/L	(<60)

Increased serum ALP activity and mild secondary hepatocellular damage (SDH, AST) were attributed to gastrointestinal disease. Liver dysfunction was considered unlikely based on normal serum bilirubin, hyperglycemia (likely stress or endotoxemia-related) and serum bile acids, so the hyperammonemia was attributed to the gastrointestinal disease. This mare responded poorly to treatment and was euthanized. Necropsy examination revealed enterocolitis with evidence of multi-organ thrombosis consistent with developing disseminated intravascular coagulation.

---

frequently have elevated blood ammonia, although values may transiently drop into the normal range as clinical signs wax and wane (West, 1996). The degree of elevation does not always correlate with the severity of clinical disease (McGorum et al., 1999). The pathophysiology of hepatic encephalopathy is complex and may involve other factors, such as hypoglycemia, that should also be clinically monitored. Horses are somewhat unique in that primary gastrointestinal disease can manifest as a syndrome of hyperammonemia associated with neurologic signs (Drivers, 2011, Dunkel et al., 2011, Underwood et al., 2010) (see Box 11.2). Both foals and adults typically present with a combination of neurologic and gastrointestinal signs, with a predominance of horses having large intestinal disease (Dunkel et al., 2011). As with hyperammonemia associated with liver dysfunction, the degree of ammonia elevation does not always correspond with clinical signs or severity, although a value of ≥60 μmol/L has been suggested as a diagnostic cut-off based on case reports and one case series. The mechanism for gastrointestinal disease associated hyperammonemia has not been fully established, but increased intestinal permeability to ammonia and overgrowth of ammonia producing bacteria in the gut have been implicated (Drivers, 2011). Rarely, inherited defects of metabolism can cause hyperammonemia (McConnico et al., 1997).

11.5 Lactate

11.5.1 Physiology

Lactate exists in two forms, D-lactate, which is derived from bacterial carbohydrate metabolism, and L-lactate, produced by mammalian cells that can be a marker of hypoxia as well as an important tissue energy source for the heart and brain during shock (Tennant-Brown, 2014). Glycolysis generates pyruvate, which is preferentially converted to lactate in anaerobic conditions, and in some tissues that lack mitochondria such as erythrocytes. Skin, red blood cells, and skeletal muscle produce a baseline amount of lactate that is primarily metabolized by the liver back to pyruvate, and ultimately shunted to the citric acid cycle for gluconeogenesis. Skeletal muscle and renal cortical cells can also metabolize lactate, which can also be excreted in the urine once concentrations are greater than 6–10 mmol/L (Tennant-Brown, 2014).

Box 11.3 Case example of a horse with hyperlactatemia.

An 8-year-old Oldenberg mare presented with a 3-h history of acute colic. On presentation, the mare was quiet, alert, and responsive, but covered in sand and sweat with multiple abrasions. She was tachypneic and tachycardic. Rectal palpation revealed that the large colon extended beyond the pelvic flexure. Her CBC was normal other than a mild relative polycythemia.

Alb		3.6 g/dl	(2.9–3.9)
Bili	H	2.8 mg/dl	(0.3–2.0)
ALP	H	154 U/L	(48–148)
GGT	H	22 U/L	(3–18)
SDH	H	26 U/L	(1–7)
AST	H	415 U/L	(162–316)
CK	H	526	(82–303)
Gluc	H	339 mg/dl	(75–116)
Lactate (presentation)	H	11.15 mmol/L	(<1.5)
Lactate (10 h post)		1.02 mmol/L	(<1.5)

Hyperbilirubinemia and mild increases in hepatocellular (SDH, AST, GGT) and cholestasic enzymes (ALP, GGT) were attributed to colic; muscle damage (AST, CK) was attributed to trauma and poor perfusion. There was a marked stress hyperglycemia. The initial degree of hyperlactatemia was concerning and attributed to poor circulatory status, but the value normalized, suggesting successful management and a better prognosis. Surgical correction of three sites of colonic torsion was performed, and an enterotomy was performed to relieve an impaction of the right dorsal colon. There was a minimal amount of post-surgical diarrhea, but otherwise the mare recovered well.

11.5.2 Sample Collection and Methodology

Point of care analyzers are most practical for the measurement of lactate, and detect L-lactate specifically. Whole blood or plasma may be used; however, sometimes the sample type impacts the results, and results from different analyzers may not be comparable (Nieto et al., 2014). It is thought that unique characteristics of equine erythrocytes have the potential to interfere with the methodology of some analyzers originally developed for human medicine, so it is recommended to use machines that have been specifically validated for diagnostic application in horses. Differences between results obtained from arterial and venous samples are not diagnostically relevant, however, prolonged vessel occlusion, struggling, or increased exertion prior to sampling, and delays in either measurement or separation of plasma from cells can increase values.

11.5.3 Diagnostic Interpretation

Hyperlactatemia is classified as either type A, due to tissue oxygen depletion, or type B, due to other causes. Subtypes of type B hyperlactatemia include B_1 associated with underlying diseases such as sepsis, malignancy, or endocrinopathy, B_2 associated with drugs and toxins, and B_3 associated with congenital metabolic defects. Lactate has been studied as a prognostic indicator and to evaluate response to therapy in horses. Some studies demonstrate that the lactate value at admission has prognostic value, with poorer outcomes when blood lactate exceeds 6–8 mmol/L and a guarded prognosis when values are greater than 8–10 mmol/L, however, there is considerable overlap between survivors and non-survivors (Tennant-Brown, 2014). The underlying presenting condition must also be considered. Data supporting the use of lactate to evaluate response to therapy is more robust, and the prognostic value of an increase or decrease in blood lactate in the face of appropriate therapy is more likely to be accurate than values at admission (Tennant-Brown, 2014) (see Box 11.3). The same general diagnostic patterns are observed in foals as adults, however, the expected values are higher in foals in the first month of life, with reports of up to 4.0 mmol/L in healthy foals in the first few days of life (Tennant-Brown, 2014). While careful attention to the appropriate use of appropriately collected samples with validated instruments can increase the diagnostic and prognostic performance of lactate measurements, the data is best used when integrated with other clinical indicators of patient status.

References

Barton MH and LeRoy BE. 2007. Serum bile acids concentrations in healthy and clinically ill neonatal foals. J Vet Intern Med 21: 508–513.

Boyle AG, Magdesian KG and Ruby RE. 2005. Neonatal isoerythrolysis in horse goals and a mule foal. J Am Vet Med Assoc 227: 1276–1283.

Drivers TJ. .2011. Metabolic causes of encephalopathy in horses. Vet Clin Equine 27: 589–596.

Dunkel B, Chaney KP, Dallap-Schaer BL, Pellegrinit-Masini A, Mair TS, and Boston R. 2011. Putative intestinal hyperammonemia in horses: 36 cases. Eq Vet J 43: 133–140.

Durán MC, Ramírez H, Ramírez A, and Parraguez VH. 2009. Effect of phototherapy on the plasma bilirubin concentration of newborn foals. Vet Record 164: 503–504.

Durham AE, Smith KC, and Newton JR. 2003. An evaluation of diagnostic data in comparison to the results of liver biopsies in mature horses. Eq Vet J 35: 554–559.

Gilliam LL. Holbrook TC, Dechant JE, and Johnson BJ. 2007. Postmortem diagnosis of idiopathic hyperammonemia in a horse. Vet Clin Path 36: 196–199.

McConnico RS, Duckett WM, and Wood PA. 1997. Persistent hyperammonemia in two related morgan weanlings. J Vet Intern Med 11: 264–266.

McGorum BC, Murphy D, Love S, and Milne EM. 1999. Clinicopathologic features of equine primary hepatic disease: a review of 50 cases. Vet Record 145: f134–139.

Nieto JE, Dechant JE, le Jeune SS, and Snyder JR. 2014. Evaluation of 3 handheld portable analyzers for measurement of L-lactate concentrations in blood and peritoneal fluid of horses with colic. Vet Surgery 9999: 1–7.

Polkes AC, Giguére S, Lester GD, and Bain FT. 2008. Factors associated with outcomes in foals with neonatal isoerythrolysis. J Vet Intern Med 22: 1216–1222.

Ramaiah SK, Harvey JW, Giguére S, Franklin RP, and Crawford PC. 2003. Intravascular hemolysis associated with liver disease in a horse with marked neutrophil hypersegmentation. J Vet Intern Med 17: 360–363.

Tennant-Brown B. 2014. Blood lactate measurement and interpretation in critically ill equine adults and neonates. Vet Clin Equine 30: 399–413.

Underwood C, Southwood LL, Walton RM, and Johnson AL. 2010. Hepatic and metabolic changes in surgical colic patients: a pilot study. J of Vet Emerg Crit Care 20: 578–586.

West HJ. 1996. Clinical and pathological studies in horses with hepatic disease. Eq Vet J 28: 146–156.

12

Cardiac Troponin

Anita Varga

Gold Coast Veterinary Service and Consulting, California, USA

12.1 Introduction and Physiology

Troponins are myofibrillar proteins that have an important role in the regulation of the cardiac and skeletal muscle contraction. The troponin complex consists of three different tissue specific isoforms of cardiac troponin; I, T, and C. Troponin I inhibits the actin and myosin interaction, troponin C binds calcium to relieve the inhibition by troponin I, and troponin T binds the complex to tropomyosin. Different troponin isoforms exist in the cardiac and skeletal muscle. Both cardiac troponin I and T are used for the detection of myocardial injury. Cardiac troponin I (cTnI) has only one isoform within the myocardium and is considered as the most specific serum biomarker for the determination of cardiac injury. Previously used classical biomarkers of myocardial damage, such as CK and the isoenzyme of CK (CK-MB), have limited effectiveness in detecting myocardial injury due to their lack of tissue specificity and sensitivity. CK and CK-MB are found in the myocardium, skeletal muscle tissue and gastrointestinal tract and, therefore, are ineffective to detect myocardial injury in the presence of skeletal muscle damage, whereas the measurement of cardiac troponin remains effective (Lazzeri et al., 2008).

The majority of cTnI is present within the sarcomere of the myocyte and between 2.8 and 8.3% of cTnI exists unbound in the cytoplasm (Collinson et al., 2001). Whether this cytosolic component is released into the extracellular space during ischemia rather than after an insult leading to necrosis is under debate (Wu, 2001).

In humans with myocardial injury, two release patterns occur, the transient and persistent release of cTnI. It is postulated that the transient release of troponins occurs from leakage from the cytosolic pool, which results in an early rise of the circulating cTnI concentration. Increased membrane permeability may be generated by reversible oxygen deficits as seen in inflammation or toxic damage that leads to degradation and leakage of free cTnI (Wu, 2001). The transient release is associated with reversible ischemia as it has been demonstrated in a porcine model of ischemic heart disease (Feng et al., 1998).

Irreversible loss of the integrity of cardiac myocytes due to necrosis leads to a prolonged release of increased concentration of cTnI and therefore to a persistent release of cTnI. This liberalization is associated with release from the cytosolic pool combined with a slower release of myofibril-bound troponin complexes, resulting in a sustained elevation of the cTnI concentration (Wu, 2001). In humans, the predominant form of released cTnI is a mixture of proteolytic fragments complexed with TnC. The predominant form of released cTnI in horses is unknown. In ponies, a serum half-life of 0.47 h has been reported and sampling blood within 1–3 h after myocardial insult has been suggested (Kraus et al., 2013). Peak concentration of cTnI occurs around 12–24 h after myocardial injury in humans. While the damaged myocardium is undergoing reperfusion and repair, cTnI is continuously released into the bloodstream. The cardiac troponin concentration can remain elevated for up to 14 days before falling back to pre-injury levels in humans and can, therefore, be used as an indicator of myocardial injury for a longer period of time than other previously used cardiac biomarkers (Babuin and Jaffe, 2005).

The presence of detectable cTnI concentrations has been associated with an increased adverse event rate and increased mortality rate that was shown to be proportional to the magnitude of cardiac troponin release. Horses with colic and elevated cardiac troponin concentration at admission were more likely to have arrhythmias and a negative outcome (Diaz et al., 2014). However, another equine study was unable to show a significant association between increased cTnI concentrations in surviving and non-surviving horses (Nath et al., 2012b).

12.2   Indications

Measurement of cardiac troponins is recommended for the assessment of myocardial injury when viral, bacterial, toxic or nutritional causes of cardiac damage is suspected. For instance, the measurement of cTnI can be useful when managing outbreaks of accidental monensin ingestion. Measuring the troponin concentration will help to detect exposed horses (Divers et al., 2009). Cardiac troponin measurements can also be of benefit when evaluating exercise-induced cardiac dysfunction (Durando et al., 2006, Holbrook et al., 2006).

Any condition that leads to ischemia of the heart muscle such as endotoxemia and shock, as seen in equine acute abdominal diseases (Nath et al., 2012a), can also lead to an increase of blood troponin levels due to the impact of those conditions on the myocardium.

Studies in horses with atrial fibrillation have not shown an increase in cardiac troponin I or T concentrations (McGurrin et al., 2008, Jesty et al., 2009) and therefore measurement of the blood marker in these conditions might not be of any benefit.

12.3   Sample Collection and Handling

Serum, plasma or whole blood can be utilized, depending on the assay used. Heparinized samples can lead to lower measured troponin concentrations, especially in the early phases of myocardial injury (Gerhardt et al., 2000). Heparin interference depends on the immunoassay and brand of collection tubes used as well as the concentration of heparin and troponin within the sample.

Since the release pattern in the equine patient is unknown, serial blood samples are recommended.

Serial measurement is helpful for the evaluation of the progression of myocardial injury, response to treatment and prognosis for survival.

Troponin concentrations in serum samples are stable for at least 12 months if stored at –80°C (Basit et al., 2007). Storage of blood samples at room temperature or refrigerated can have a significant impact on the troponin concentrations recovered within the sample (Varga et al., 2009). Therefore, samples should be tested as soon as possible after collection.

12.4   Immunoassays

No equine-specific cardiac troponin assay is currently available. Due to the high amino acid sequence similarity between equine and human troponin (>90%) (Rishniw and Simpson, 2005), assays that are validated for human cardiac troponin can also be used for equine blood samples. Numerous commercial cTnI assays are available, utilizing different capture and proprietary antibodies with different abilities to measure free or complex forms of cTnI. These differences result in significant and clinical relevant differences between troponin I assays (Collinson and Gaze, 2007). Therefore, the same assay should always be used when the equine patient is re-tested. Establishment of a reference interval of the assay is recommended if no previous study has recorded one. However, healthy horses have very low blood troponin concentrations, often below the detection limit of the assay. Unlike the troponin I assays, there are only a couple of human assay presently available for the measurement of cardiac troponin T. The newer generation cTnT assay has been shown to be of diagnostic value in horses (Van Der Vekens et al., 2015).

References

Babuin L and Jaffe AS. 2005. Troponin: the biomarker of choice for the detection of cardiac injury. CMAJ, 173: 1191–1202.

Basit M, Bakshi N, Hashem M, Allebban Z, Lawson N, Rosman HS, and Maciejko JJ. 2007. The effect of freezing and long-term storage on the stability of cardiac troponin T. Am J Clin Pathol, 128: 164–167.

Collinson PO, Boa FG, and Gaze DC. 2001. Measurement of cardiac troponins. Ann Clin Biochem, 38: 423–449.

Collinson PO and Gaze DC. 2007. Biomarkers of cardiovascular damage and dysfunction – an overview. Heart Lung Circ, 16 Suppl 3: S71–82.

Diaz OM, Durando MM, Birks EK, and Reef VB. 2014. Cardiac troponin I concentrations in horses with colic. J Am Vet Med Assoc, 245: 118–125.

Divers TJ, Kraus MS, Jesty SA, Miller AD, Mohammed HO, Gelzer AR, et al. 2009. Clinical findings and serum cardiac troponin I concentrations in horses after intragastric administration of sodium monensin. J Vet Diagn Invest, 21: 338–343.

Durando MM, Slack J, Reef VB, and Birks EK. 2006. Right ventricular pressure dynamics and stress echocardiography in pharmacological and exercise stress testing. Equine Vet J Suppl, 183–192.

Feng YJ, Chen C, Fallon JT, Lai T, Chen L, Knibbs DR, et al. 1998. Comparison of cardiac troponin I, creatine kinase-MB, and myoglobin for detection of acute ischemic myocardial injury in a swine model. Am J Clin Pathol, 110: 70–77.

Gerhardt W, Nordin G, Herbert AK, Burzell BL, Isaksson A, Gustavsson E, et al. 2000. Troponin T and I assays show decreased concentrations in heparin plasma compared with serum: lower recoveries in early than in late phases of myocardial injury. Clin Chem, 46: 817–821.

Holbrook TC, Birks EK, Sleeper MM, and Durando M. 2006. Endurance exercise is associated with increased plasma cardiac troponin I in horses. Equine Vet J Suppl, 27–31.

Jesty SA, Kraus MS, Gelzer AR, Rishniw M, and Moise NS. 2009. Effect of transvenous electrical cardioversion on plasma cardiac troponin I concentrations in horses with atrial fibrillation. J Vet Intern Med, 23: 1103–1107.

Kraus MS, Kaufer BB, Damiani A, Osterrieder N, Rishniw M, Schwark W, et al. 2013. Elimination half-life of intravenously administered equine cardiac troponin I in healthy ponies. Equine Vet J, 45: 56–59.

Lazzeri C, Bonizzoli M, Cianchi G, Gensini GF, and Peris A. 2008. Troponin I in the intensive care unit setting: from the heart to the heart. Intern Emerg Med, 3: 9–16.

McGurrin MK, Physick-Sheard PW, and Kenney DG. 2008. Transvenous electrical cardioversion of equine atrial fibrillation: patient factors and clinical results in 72 treatment episodes. J Vet Intern Med, 22: 609–615.

Nath LC, Anderson GA, Hinchcliff KW, and Savage CJ. 2012a. Clinicopathologic evidence of myocardial injury in horses with acute abdominal disease. J Am Vet Med Assoc, 241: 1202–1208.

Nath LC, Anderson GA, Hinchcliff KW, and Savage CJ. 2012b. Serum cardiac troponin I concentrations in horses with cardiac disease. Aust Vet J, 90: 351–357.

Rishniw M and Simpson KW. 2005. Cloning and sequencing of equine cardiac troponin I and confirmation of its usefulness as a target analyte for commercial troponin I analyzers. J Vet Diagn Invest, 17: 582–584.

Van Der Vekens N, Decloedt A, Ven S, De Clercq D, and Van Loon G. 2015. Cardiac troponin I as compared to troponin T for the detection of myocardial damage in horses. J Vet Intern Med, 29: 348–354.

Varga A, Schober KE, Walker WL, Lakritz J, and Michael Rings D. 2009. Validation of a commercially available immunoassay for the measurement of bovine cardiac troponin I. J Vet Intern Med, 23: 359–365.

Wu AH. 2001. Increased troponin in patients with sepsis and septic shock: myocardial necrosis or reversible myocardial depression? Intensive Care Med, 27: 959–961.

13

Vitamin and Mineral Assessment

Carrie J. Finno

Department of Population Health and Reproduction, School of Veterinary Medicine, University of California, California, USA

13.1 Introduction

Horses evolved to a grazing and browsing existence, with primary intakes consisting of grasses containing relatively high concentrations of water ingested over multiple feeding periods throughout the day and night. In contrast, the domesticated horse has restricted feeding times and diets have shifted to dried forages, starch, and protein concentrates. As a result, vitamin and mineral deficiencies commonly develop and may result in a variety of diseases. This chapter will focus on the assessment of vitamin and mineral deficiencies in the horse, with an emphasis on the clinical implications of these deficiencies. Eight macrominerals (calcium, phosphorus, magnesium, potassium, sodium, chloride, sulfur, and chromium), nine trace minerals (copper, zinc, manganese, iron, fluorine, iodine, selenium, cobalt, and nickel), and 14 vitamins are discussed. Each section will give an overview, followed by causes and clinical signs of deficiencies and toxicities and a discussion of how to assess a horse's status for that particular vitamin or mineral.

13.2 Macrominerals

13.2.1 Calcium and Phosphorus

The functions of calcium and phosphorus are considered together due their interdependent role as the main elements providing strength and rigidity of the skeleton. Bone has a calcium:phosphorus ration of 2:1 and acts as a reservoir of both elements. A continual state of flux is maintained, with calcium and phosphorus being removed and re-deposited to enable growth and remodeling of the skeleton. Plasma calcium concentration is tightly regulated due to its role in muscle and nerve function.

Regulation: Two hormones tightly regulate distribution and flux of calcium and phosphorus, functioning antagonistically at the level of the bone, intestinal mucosa, and renal tubules. Parathyroid hormone (PTH) is secreted by the parathyroid glands whereas the parafollicular C cells of the thyroid gland secrete calcitonin. A slight decrease in calcium concentration in the extracellular fluid results in an immediate secretion of PTH (Estepa et al., 1998). Excessive calcium concentrations, such as occurs with a vitamin D toxicity, leads to decreased PTH and secretion of calcitonin, which serves to rapidly decrease plasma calcium concentrations by decreasing osteoclastic and increasing osteoblastic activities. The equine kidney plays a greater role in controlling calcium concentrations in the blood than does the intestinal tract.

Deficiency:

1) Naturally occurring sepsis associated with gastrointestinal disease (Garcia-Lopez et al., 2001, Toribio et al., 2001, Dart et al., 1992) and experimental endotoxemia (Toribio et al., 2005)
2) Vitamin D deficiency in young, growing animals, characterized by defective mineralization of new bone, resulting in painful swelling of the physis and osteochondral junctions.
3) Cantharidin toxicosis due to ingestion of alfalfa-containing products contaminated with blister beetles (*Epicauta* sp.)
4) Hypocalcemic tetany from lactation, especially in draft mares, or transport; concurrent hypomagnesemia common
5) Severe rhabdomyolysis
6) Oxalate toxicity
7) Acute renal failure in the horse (hypocalcemia and hyperphosphatemia)

Toxicity:

1) Chronic renal failure (most common cause)
   The horse is unique in that the kidney, rather than the intestine, is the primary site of calcium regulation. Impaired renal calcium excretion associated with

Interpretation of Equine Laboratory Diagnostics, First Edition. Edited by Nicola Pusterla and Jill Higgins.
© 2018 John Wiley & Sons, Inc. Published 2018 by John Wiley & Sons, Inc.

normal intestinal calcium absorption leads to a peripheral hypercalcemia and hypophosphatemia (Tennant et al., 1982). Hypercalemia is significantly more common in chronic renal failure than acute renal failure in the horse (LeRoy et al., 2011).

2) Primary hyperparathyroidism may occur with pituitary tumors and result in elevated PTH concentrations (concurrent hypophosphatemia)

3) Nutritional secondary hyperparathyroidism (NSHP): increased blood PTH concentration, normal or slightly raised serum phosphate concentrations and slightly depressed serum calcium concentrations

Hyperphosphatemia reduces blood calcium concentration and suppresses PTH's ability to stimulate renal activation of vitamin D, further decreasing digestive absorption efficiency. The typical presentation is fibrous osteodystrophy of the facial bones ("big head") but other clinical signs include a stiff gait or shifting-limb lameness, abnormal mastication with oral dysphagia and upper airway stridor.

4) Hypervitaminosis D due to intoxication with ergocalciferol or cholecalciferol

Ingestion of plants containing 1,25-dihydroxyvitamin D-like compounds (*Solanum malacoxylon, S. sodomaeum, Cestrum diumum, Trisetum flavescens*) causes typical clinical signs of vitamin D intoxication, including hypercalcemia, from increased gastrointestinal absorption and bone resorption. Hyperphosphatemia commonly accompanies hypercalcemia.

5) Humoral hypercalcemia of malignancy; reported with gastric squamous cell carcinoma, adenocortical carcinoma, lymphosarcoma, and ameloblastoma

In addition to hypercalcemia, hypophosphatemia and decreased serum concentration of PTH is often observed.

6) Developmental orthopedic disease from inadequate balance of calcium and phosphorus

Assessment: Calcium is principally an extracellular cation existing as ionized calcium or protein-bound to albumin. Ionized calcium normally constitutes about one-half of the total plasma calcium. The ionized form is physiologically active and its concentration in blood plasma is influenced by acid-base status. Normal reference ranges can be found in Table 13.1. The measurement of ionized calcium is recommended when assessing overall calcium status. If an ionized calcium measurement cannot be assessed, it can be estimated based on total calcium concentrations using the following formula (Payne et al., 1973):

$$\text{Corrected Ca (mmol/L)} = \text{measured calcium (mmol/L)} + 0.02(40 - \text{albumin [g/L]})$$

$$\text{Corrected Ca (mg/dL)} = \text{measured calcium (mg/dL)} + 0.08(4 - \text{albumin [g/dL]})$$

Table 13.1 Normal plasma mineral concentrations in adult horses.

Mineral	Normal plasma concentration (adult horse)
Total calcium	11.2–13.6 mEq/L
Ionized calcium	1.58–1.90 mmol/L
Phosphorus	3.1–5.6 mEq/L
Total magnesium	2.2–2.8 mEq/L
Ionized magnesium	0.47–0.70 mmol/L
Potassium*	2.4–4.7 mEq/L
Sodium	132–146 mEq/L
Chloride	99–109 mEq/L
Sulfur*	140 mg/dL
Copper*	0.5–1.5 mg/L
Zinc*	0.5–2 mg/L
Manganese	0.3–0.9 µmol/L
Iron*	0.6–1.7 mg/L
Total Iron Binding Capacity	200–262 µg/dL
Total Thyroxine (T_4)	6–46 nmol/L
Free Thyroxine (T_4)	6–21 pmol/L
Total Triiodothyronine (T_3)	0.3–2.9 nmol/L
Free Triiodothyronine (T_3)	0.1–5.9 pmol/L
Thyroid-stimulating hormone	0.02–0.97 ng/mL
Selenium	0.09–0.30 mg/L

*Not a reliable indicator of whole-body status
Data from Kaneko JJ, Harvey JW, and Bruss M, (eds) 2008. Clinical Biochemistry of Domestic Animals, 6th Edn. Burlington, MA: Academic Press; Lewis LD (ed.) 1995. Equine Clinical Nutrition: Feeding and Care. Williams & Wilkins Media, PA; and Robinson NE and Sprayberry KA (eds) 2009. Current Therapy in Equine Medicine 6. St. Louis, ME: Saunders Elsevier.

Serum phosphorus concentrations are not always an accurate guide to overall phosphorus status but dietary deficiencies of phosphorus are frequently manifested by hypophosphatemia. Therefore, serum phosphorus concentrations provide a good indicator of dietary phosphorus intake (reference range, Table 13.1). Age-related differences exist in the normal range of serum phosphorus concentrations, with young animals having much higher values than adults.

13.2.2 Magnesium

Magnesium constitutes approximately 0.05% of the body mass, 60% of which is in the skeleton and 30% in the muscle. Between 20–30% of magnesium is bound to mostly albumin and 60% is free (ionized) or bound to phosphorus or other components. Magnesium is an important ion in the blood, acting as a cofactor of many enzyme systems and participating in muscle contractions.

Regulation: Homeostasis is achieved from a balance between gastrointestinal absorption and renal excretion. Although adrenal, thyroid and parathyroid hormones influence status, plasma magnesium concentration has a less potent effect on PTH than does plasma calcium concentration. PTH increases plasma magnesium concentration by increasing absorption from the intestines and renal tubules and resorption from bone. Aldosterone secretion results in a decrease in plasma magnesium concentration due to an increase in urinary magnesium excretion.

Deficiency

1) Common complication associated with equine colic (Johansson et al., 2003).
2) Hypomagnesemic tetany has been reported in lactating mares (Baird, 1971) and in horses during transit (NRC, 2007).

 Hypomagnesemia is associated with loss of appetite, sweating, muscle tremors, ataxia, and the potential for collapse and death.

Toxicity: Magnesium toxicity is rare but may result from over-administration of Epsom salts containing $MgSO_4$. Intravenous administration of magnesium produces muscle relaxation but does not alter consciousness.

Assessment: Measurement of total plasma Mg concentrations can provide a reliable estimate of overall magnesium status in the horse, as changes often parallel changes in ionized Mg (Rosol and Capen, 1996). If a horse has concurrent acid-base alterations, measurement of ionized magnesium may be more accurate. Normal concentrations are provided in Table 13.1.

13.2.3 Potassium

Potassium is involved in maintenance of the acid-base balance and osmotic pressure and is an essential ion for neuromuscular excitation. Between 60 and 75% of whole body potassium resides in the skeletal muscle, with only 5% in the extracellular fluid and not always a reflection of the total body potassium.

Regulation: Potassium is obtained from the diet in horses, with normal potassium intake greatly exceeding daily requirements in the healthy horse. The kidney is the main route of excretion of potassium.

Deficiency:

1) Anorexia
2) Diarrhea
3) Acid-base imbalance; metabolic alkalosis

4) Renal tubular acidosis
5) Administration of diuretics, corticosteroids, sodium bicarbonate, insulin, glucose or catecholamines.

 Hypokalemia is associated with muscle weakness, impaired urine concentration ability and arrhythmias

Toxicity:

1) Uroperitoneum
2) Acid-base imbalance; metabolic acidosis may result in hyperkalemia
3) Hypovolemia and renal failure
4) Hyperkalemic periodic paralysis

 Hyperkalemia is associated with muscle weakness or paralysis, lethargy, bradyarrhythmias

Assessment: As potassium is the major intracellular cation and only 5% is in the extracellular fluid, serum potassium concentrations are not always a reflection of total body potassium. Measurement of erythrocyte potassium concentration has been evaluated as an aid for accurately assessing potassium concentrations in horses; however, experimental studies indicate that the erythrocyte potassium concentration does not always accurately reflect potassium deficits. Therefore, plasma or serum potassium is most commonly assessed. Important considerations when evaluating plasma potassium concentrations include false hyperkalemia due to:

1) Delay in separation of serum or plasma over 6 h
2) *In vitro* hemolysis during sampling
3) Markedly elevated leukocyte or thrombocyte count

13.2.4 Sodium

Sodium is the major extracellular cation and therefore the principal determinant of the osmolarity of extracellular fluid. Sodium is critical for the normal central nervous system function.

Regulation: Sodium excretion via the kidney is controlled by the renin-angiotensin-aldosterone system. Hyponatremia will result in aldosterone secretion.

Deficiency:

1) Loss of sodium-containing fluid (diarrhea, blood loss, fluid drainage)
2) Adrenal insufficiency
3) Sequestration of fluid into a third space (peritonitis, ascites, pleuritis, ruptured bladder)
4) Psychogenic polydipsia
5) Inappropriate anti-diuretic hormone secretion
6) Renal failure

 Hyponatremia is associated with weight loss, ileus, lethargy, tremors, blindness and seizures in foals (Lakritz et al., 1992), polyuria, intravascular hemolysis

Toxicity:

1) Water deprivation
2) Salt poisoning
3) Diabetes insipidus
4) Burns

Hypernatremia is associated with thirst, colic, diarrhea, weakness, paralysis, recumbency, sudden death

Assessment: Serum sodium is an accurate estimate of the extracellular fluid volume as changes in water balance are primarily responsible for changes in serum sodium concentration. Therefore, the hydration status of the patient should always be considered for sodium concentration interpretation. False hyponatremia can occur with hyperlipidemia, hyperproteinemia or hyperglycemia.

13.2.5   Chloride

Chloride is the major extracellular anion and is involved in acid-base balance and osmotic regulation. Chloride concentrations should always be evaluated in conjunction with sodium concentrations.

Hypochloremia/hyperchloremia with proportional changes in sodium
As for hyponatremia/hypernatremia (see previously)
Hypochloremia without proportional decreases in sodium
   1) Metabolic alkalosis (heavy sweating in horses)
   2) Furosemide administration
Hyperchloremia without proportional decreases in sodium
   3) Metabolic acidosis
   4) Renal tubular acidosis

Assessment: Serum chloride concentrations are a reliable indicator of extracellular chloride status. Alterations of serum chloride concentrations are typically associated with proportionate changes in serum sodium concentrations as a result of changes in water balance. Additionally, acid-base status is associated with chloride concentrations, with chloride concentrations varying inversely with bicarbonate concentrations.

13.2.6   Sulfur

Sulfur is a component of sulfur-containing amino acids (methionine, cystine and cysteine) and vitamins (biotin and thiamine). The concentration of sulfur-containing amino acids is highest in hoof and hair, which contain keratin that is 4% sulfur. Most horses meet their sulfur requirements from organic forms of the element, mostly in the amino acids of plant proteins. Little inorganic sulfur is absorbed.

Deficiency: Sulfur deficiency in the horse has not yet been described.

Toxicity: Maximum tolerable sulfur concentrations in the horse have not been defined. Accidental over-ingestion of sulfur in a group of horses led to lethargy, colic, jaundice, and death in 2 out of 12 horses (Corke, 1981).

Assessment: A dietary imbalance is best assessed through a full dietary evaluation. Plasma concentration of total sulfur averages 140 mg/dL, of which 80–90% is as a constituent of plasma proteins. Normal plasma concentrations of inorganic sulfates are 0.9–1.5 mg/dL and responsive to fluctuations in dietary intake (Georgievskii et al., 1982).

13.2.7   Chromium

Chromium is essential for normal carbohydrate metabolism where it stimulates glucose clearance in insulin-sensitive -tissues. Results of chromium supplementation studies have varied widely in the horse (Ott and Kivipelto, 1999, Vervuert et al., 2005, Pagan et al., 1995). Based on its potential to regulate insulin sensitivity, supplementation with chromium and magnesium was evaluated in a group of insulin-resistant horses. There was no apparent effect of the supplement on morphometric measurements or insulin sensitivity in the laminitic obese horses (Chameroy et al., 2011).

13.3   Trace Minerals

13.3.1   Copper

Copper is essential for several Cu-dependent enzymes required in the synthesis and maintenance of elastic connective tissue, mobilization of iron stores, preservation of mitochondrial integrity, melanin synthesis and detoxification of superoxide. The horse is not as susceptible to Cu deficiency as are ruminants, but clinical signs have been described.

Regulation: Copper interacts with many other minerals including molybdenum, sulfate, zinc, selenium, silver, cadmium, iron, and lead. In ruminants, higher molybdenum intakes interfere with copper utilization but much higher levels of molybdenum are tolerated by the horse (Underwood, 1977).

Deficiency:

1) Developmental joint disease (DOD)
   There are a number of nutritional and non-nutritional factors that contributed to the development of DOD. However, a number of studies indicate that copper deficiency in foals is associated with decreased bone density and DOD (Bridges et al., 1984, Hurtig et al., 1990). The incidence of DOD has been

decreased when the amount of copper in the diet was increased (Knight et al., 1987).

2) Anemia and hemorrhage from aorta or uterine artery rupture in aged parturient mares (Stowe, 1968).

Toxicity:

1) Horses are relatively tolerant of high dietary copper concentrations.
2) Very high over-dosages of copper can lead to gastroenteritis, hemolysis, jaundice, and hemoglobinuria (Bauer, 1975).
3) A study describing concentrations of trace minerals in the spinal cord of horses with equine motor neuron disease (EMND) reported that copper concentrations were significantly higher in horses with EMND (Polack et al., 2000).

Assessment: A dietary imbalance is best assessed through a full dietary evaluation. Plasma copper can be used to obtain an estimate of copper status (normal values in Table 13.1); however, high serum copper levels can occur with inflammation, infection or vaccination since 70% of the circulating copper is present in the form of ceruloplasmin, a positive acute phase protein (Suttle et al., 1995). Serum ceruloplasmin activity correlates with serum copper concentration but is not of any additional diagnostic benefit (Bell et al., 1987). Liver and serum copper concentrations may not be correlated in some individuals and liver concentrations are the more dependable value (Suttle et al., 1996). The measurement of copper-zinc superoxide dismutase activity level has been evaluated as a determinant of whole body copper status; however, this is not easily performed in the field. Leukocyte copper concentrations has been used experimentally to assess copper contents (Frape, 2010).

13.3.2 Zinc

Zinc is a cofactor for over 200 enzymes, including alkaline phosphatase, collagenase, and carbonic anhydrase, all of which are required in bone formation.

Deficiency:

1) A dietary zinc deficiency leads to inappetance and an overall decreased growth rate in foals and skin lesions may be apparent.
2) An association between low plasma zinc and *Culicoides* hypersensitivity has been reported; however, it has been determined that the decrease appears to be secondary to the bite of this fly, leading to redistribution between plasma and blood cells (Stark et al., 2001).

Toxicity: The horse is relatively resistant to high zinc intake. However, excess zinc can exacerbate bony lesions induced by low copper diets (Ott and Asquith, 1987).

Zinc and copper compete for many of the same transport mechanisms and excessive zinc intake can lead to copper deficiency, especially where dietary copper is not abundant. Zinc toxicity can also lead to reduced calcium absorption. In addition to lameness and enlarged growth plates of the long bones of the legs, excess zinc can lead to anemia and decreased growth (Willoughby et al., 1972).

Assessment: Plasma zinc concentrations are not a reliable indicator of whole body status, as plasma holds only 10–23% of total blood zinc. A dietary zinc imbalance is best assessed through a full dietary evaluation.

13.3.3 Manganese

Manganese is essential for carbohydrate and lipid metabolism and for the synthesis of chrondroitin sulfate. Therefore, it is required in several stages of cartilage formation. Epiphyseal cartilage and bone matrix formation are compromised by a manganese deficiency.

Deficiency:

1) A severe manganese deficiency can lead to fetal resorption or death at birth whereas lesser deficiencies result in irregular estrous cycles.
2) In other species, manganese deficiencies have been associated with abnormal cartilage development; however, this has not been definitively established in the horse.

Toxicity:

1) Manganese toxicity has not been reported in the horse.
2) Administration of a large dosage of manganese chloride intravenously results in pawing, restlessness, sweating and defecation with no effect on blood pressure in an experimental study (Singh et al., 1992).

Assessment: Plasma manganese provide a reliable indicator of whole body manganese status. Reference ranges are provided in Table 13.1.

13.3.4 Iron

Iron is an integral component of hemoglobin, myoglobin, cytochromes, and many enzyme systems. It is distributed primarily in blood hemoglobin (60%), muscle myoglobin (20%), storage forms (bound to ferritin and hemosiderin), and transport forms (bound to transferrin). Iron absorption decreases with excessive intake of cadmium, cobalt, copper, manganese, and zinc (Underwood, 1977). It has been demonstrated that there is no benefit from iron administration or supplementation in horses during increased exercise (Kirkham et al., 1971).

Deficiency:

1) *Chronic or severe blood loss*; initially a normocytic normochromic anemia but progresses to a microcytic hypochromic anemia if the iron deficiency becomes moderate to severe.
2) *Nutritional deficiency*; experimental studies in foals with no access to pasture and potentially iron deficiency in horses with IBD/alimentary lymphoma.

Toxicity: Iron toxicosis, due to over-supplementation, is much more common than iron deficiency.

Neonatal foals are particularly susceptible to iatrogenic iron overload, leading to liver necrosis and thrombocytopenia (Mullaney and Brown, 1988).

Assessment: Hematocrit and blood hemoglobin concentrations are not sensitive indicators of a horse's iron status as neither decreases until a severe anemia is present and thus a severe iron deficiency has been in existence for a prolonged period. Iron status is assessed reliably by serum ferritin concentration. A decrease in ferritin is the earliest indication of inadequate body iron. Total serum iron concentration is unreliable as it declines during inflammation and tissue injury. Serum total iron-biding capacity, percentage iron saturation, and serum unbound-iron-binding capacity do not adequately represent a horse's iron status.

13.3.5 Fluorine

Fluorine is incorporated into teeth and bone as fluorapatite, increasing bone hardness and decreasing solubility.

Deficiency: None reported

Toxicity: fluorine toxicosis from industrial contamination or excess phosphorus supplements that have not been adequately defluorinated.

Flourosis may lead to discolored teeth, bone lesions, lameness, and unthriftiness (Shupe and Olson, 1971).

Assessment: Diagnosis of fluorosis may be difficult due to an extended interval of time between ingestion of excessive fluoride and the onset of clinical signs of toxicity. Fluoride can be measured in rib or tail bones at necropsy and is normally 400–1200 mg/kg. Urine fluoride can be measured (normally 2–6 mg/L) and a concentration above 15 mg/L is considered significant (Bailey and Garland, 1992). The fluoride concentration in plasma, like urine, rapidly changes with intake.

13.3.6 Iodine

Iodine is required for synthesis of the iodine-containing thyroid hormones triiodothyronine (T_3), reverse T_3, and thyroxine (T_4). In the thyroid glands and in peripheral tissues, T_4 is deiodinated to T_3, which is physiologically more potent. An increase in T_3 or T_4 results in an increase in metabolic rate and consequence oxygen utilization and heat production.

Regulation: With iodine deficiency, an insufficient amount of iodide is available to synthesize an adequate amount of iodine-containing thyroid hormones whereas, with iodine toxicosis, excess iodide inhibits thyroid hormone synthesis and/or release by its direct effect on the thyroid gland. Either case results in a reduced level of thyroid hormones and a subsequent increase in thyroid-stimulating hormone (TSH) secretion, which leads to a thyroid gland hypertrophy (goiter).

Deficiency:

1) *Neonatal goiter*: Pregnant mares are at risk for fetal iodine deficiency and toxicity throughout gestation. Deficient foals will demonstrate enlarge thyroid glands, persistent hypothermia, respiratory distress, and increased susceptibility to infections.
2) Abnormal estrous cycles in iodine deficient mares.

Toxicity:

1) Iodine toxicity can result in abortion and infertility in pregnant mares. At birth, the foal will be hypothyroid. Bony abnormalities, including angular limb deformities and defects of the maxilla/mandible, may develop in the foal in utero due to excessive amount of iodine transported to the placenta (Irvine, 1984).
2) There is an association of hypothyroidism with delayed ossification of carpal and tarsal bones (McLaughlin and Doige, 1982).

In other species, hypothyroidism and goiter may also be caused by ingestion of large amounts of goitrogenic plants, such as kale, white clover, rutabaga, and turnips, which are high in perchlorates, nitrates, or thiocyanates, which interfere with iodide accumulation in the thyroid gland. There are currently no reports of such toxicity in the horse.

Assessment: In foals, plasma T_3 and T_4 concentrations are quite variable and not useful for diagnosis. An increase in plasma T_3 in response to TSH stimulation (5 IU given IV) or thyrotropin-releasing hormone (TRH; 500 µg IM) should lead to doubling or greater of plasma and total T_3 concentrations within 1–3 h and a 16% or greater increase in total T_4 within 3–6 h (Murray, 1990, Shaftoe et al., 1998). In adults, thyroid hormone levels decline with age and excess dietary protein. Serum T_3 concentrations appear to be more accurate than T_4 concentrations in adults as a measure of thyroid status.

13.3.7 Selenium

Selenium forms an integral part of the glutathionine-peroxidase enzyme, which helps to prevent the formation of free radicals and destroys lipid peroxides that form and are released into cells. Selenium and vitamin E function together in protecting cell membranes and enzymes from oxidation-induced damage.

Deficiency:

1) Nutritional myodegeneration (white muscle disease) of foals.
   a) Skeletal form: slower onset characterized by muscular weakness, stiffness, trembling, and recumbency with notably hard and painful muscles on palpation. The tongue may be involved, resulting in dysphagia.
   b) Cardiac form: acute signs of respiratory stress, rapid irregular heartbeat, weakness, and often death in 24 h.
   c) Serum muscle enzymes (creatine kinase, asparate aminotransferase) are typically elevated during the acute phase of myodegeneration.
2) Slower growth rate.

Toxicity:

1) Chronic toxicity leads to hair loss, lameness, bony lesions, abnormal hoof horn.
2) Acute toxicity may lead to "blind staggers" characterized by ataxia, blindness, head-pressing, colic, diarrhea, and sudden death. A recent outbreak of acute selenium toxicosis was reported in polo ponies in Florida that were administered a compounded vitamin and mineral supplement containing toxic levels of selenium (Desta et al., 2011).

Assessment: Whole blood selenium concentrations are preferred over plasma and serum (Maas et al., 1992) and are a good measure of whole body selenium status. Selenium-dependent glutathione peroxidase (GSH-Px) of serum and erythrocytes can also be measured but sample storage time and temperature are critical. At necropsy, liver concentrations are evaluated.

13.3.8 Cobalt

The gastrointestinal microflora of horses uses dietary cobalt in the synthesis of vitamin B12 (cyanocobalamin). Cobalt is required for blood cell formation. There are no known field- or experimentally induced cases of either Co or B12 deficiencies in horses.

13.3.9 Nickel

Dietary concentration of nickel is important in the horse; however, nickel deficiencies have not been reported. Toxicities in humans are mostly confined to pollution from metal industries.

13.4 Vitamins

Normal concentrations for plasma/serum vitamin concentrations in adult horses are listed in Table 13.2.

13.4.1 Fat-Soluble Vitamins: A, D, K, and E

13.4.1.1 Vitamin A

Grazing horses derive their vitamin A from the carotenoid pigments, specifically beta-carotene, present in forage. Fresh pasture often exceeds the vitamin A requirement in horses. Beta-carotene is cleaved by enzymes to retinal in the wall of the small intestine at a ratio of two moles of retinal per mole of beta-carotene. Retinal is then reduced to retinol and absorbed. Some beta-carotene is absorbed intact and transported, bound by high density lipoproteins, to fat, skin, and ovaries. Beta-carotene can

Table 13.2 Normal plasma vitamin concentrations in adult horses.

Vitamin	Sample Type	Normal Concentration (Adult Horse)
Vitamin A	Plasma	See Table 13.3
Vitamin D: 25-OH-D[#]	Serum	11–24 nmol/L
Vitamin D: 1,25(OH)$_2$D	Serum	20–25 pg/mL
Vitamin K	N/A	N/A
Vitamin E	Plasma or serum	2–4 mg/μL
Thiamine (Vitamin B$_1$)[##]	Whole blood	5–23 ng/mL
Riboflavin (Vitamin B$_2$)[##]	Whole blood	110–170 ng/mL
Niacin (Vitamin B$_3$) as nicotinate[##]	Whole blood	3–6 μg/mL
Pantothenic Acid (Vitamin B$_5$)[##]	Whole blood	410–820 ng/mL
Vitamin B$_6$[##]	Plasma	26–33 ng/mL
Biotin[##]	Whole blood	310–665 pg/mL
Folic Acid (Vitamin B$_9$)[##]	Plasma	5–17 ng/mL
Vitamin B$_{12}$[##]	Whole blood	700–1780 pg/mL
Choline[##]	Plasma	112–215 μg/mL
Vitamin C (Ascorbic acid)	Plasma	2–4 μg/mL

N/A = not routinely available

Data from Kaneko JJ, Harvey JW, Bruss ML (eds.) 2008. *Clinical Biochemistry of Domestic Animals*, 6th Edn. Burlington, MA: Academic Press; Lewis LD (ed.) 1995. *Equine Clinical Nutrition: Feeding and Care*. Williams & Wilkins Media, PA; and Robinson NE and Sprayberry KA (eds) 2009. *Current Therapy in Equine Medicine 6*. St. Louis ME: Saunders Elsevier.

[#] Reference range from the Diagnostic Center for Population and Animal Health, Michigan State University.

[##] Baker H, Schor SM, Murphy BD, et al. 1986. Blood vitamin and choline concentrations in healthy domestic cats, dogs and horses. Am J Vet Res 47(7): 1468–1471.

function as an antioxidant and is used to assist in maintaining plasma vitamin A concentration. Retinol from the small intestine is transplanted with chylomicrons to the liver for storage. From the liver, retinol is released as a complex with retinol-binding protein for transport to other tissues for use or excreted in the bile. Vitamin A is important for vision, with specific photoreactive metabolites found in visual pigments within the retina. Vitamin A also plays a role maintaining healthy immune function.

Deficiency:

1) Inadequate intake can lead to a vitamin A deficiency, characterized by anorexia, poor growth, night blindness, keratinization of skin and cornea, infertility and increased susceptibility to infections.
2) Squamous metaplasia of the parotid duct (NRC, 2007).
3) Beta-carotene deficiency in mares not grazing on pasture may impair their reproductive abilities due to the antioxidant effects of beta-carotene in ovarian tissue.

Toxicity:

1) Chronic over-supplementation of vitamin A may result in bone fragility, hyperestosis, Teratogenesis, and increased clotting time.
2) Acute over-supplementation of vitamin A can cause alopecia and ataxia and poor muscle tone (Donoghue et al., 1981).

Assessment: Blood plasma retinol is sustained by hepatic reserves and therefore varies only to a small extent with dietary intake. Plasma vitamin A concentrations in the normal range are poorly correlated with liver stores. Variations in the plasma vitamin A concentration depend upon the plasma concentration of retinol-binding protein (RBP), which is altered by hepatic synthesis and protein intake.

There are two methods that are useful in determining a dietary vitamin A imbalance in horses. These two methods include (1) assessing the percentage of the different fractions making up the plasma vitamin A concentration and (2) a relative dose response test (RDR) (Table 13.3). It is important to note that differences occur within 30 days of the abnormal vitamin A intake whereas clinical signs are often not apparent until hepatic storage is depleted, which may take months to years.

13.4.1.2 Vitamin D

Ultraviolet rays from sunlight convert 7-dehydrocholesterol, which is synthesized by the liver, to vitamin D_3 (cholecalciferol) in the skin. In plants, ergosterol is converted to vitamin D_2, which is ingested by grazing horses and absorbed via chylomicrons into lymphatics. Vitamin D, either ingested or produced in the skin, is transported bound to a specific plasma transport protein to the liver,

Table 13.3 Methods of assessing vitamin A concentrations in the horse.

Vit A. or beta-carotene intake	Percent of Total Plasma Vitamin A			
	Retinol	Retinyl Palmitate	Retinyl Acetate	RDR* (%)
Deficient	45–65	31–45		>10–12
Normal	65–88	12–30	<1–12	<10–12
Excessive	<45	>45		

* RDR defined by: $100(A_{14}-A_0)/A_{14} = RDR\%$ where A_{14} is plasma retinol concentration 14–15 h following feeding 224,152 IU (123.5 mg) retinyl palmitate and A_0 is fasting plasma retinol concentration (Greiwe-Crandell et al., 1995). A dietary deficiency is indicated where RDR% is greater than 10–12%. This test measures the hepatic release of retinol.

where it is stored and converted to 25-hydroxyl vitamin D (25-OH-D). 25-OH-D is transported, bound to the same specific transport protein, to the kidney, where it is hydroxylated to either the most active form, calcitrol $(1,25(OH)_2D)$ if needed or, if not, the less active form $24,25(OH)_2D$ is produced. Calcitrol maintains plasma calcium concentrations by working in conjunction with PTH at the level of the bone and intestine. Additionally, calcitrol inhibits proliferation and induces differentiation of many cell types

Regulation: A number of factors influence which form of vitamin D is produced, including plasma concentrations of calcium, phosphorus, PTH and $1,25(OH)_2D$.

Deficiency:

1) Rickets and osteomalacia have not been reported in ponies or horses (El Shorafa et al., 1979).
2) Irregular growth plates may occur.

Toxicity: Most common of all vitamin toxicosis; cumulative effect. Toxicosis can result from administration of excessive vitamin D or plants containing vitamin D glycosides

Clinical signs associated with vitamin D toxicity are decreased exercise tolerance, hyperphosphatemia, weight loss and inappetence, polyuria and polydipsia, azotemia, osteopetrosis with subsequent osteopenia, and widespread soft tissue calcification (Harrington, 1982, Harrington and Page, 1983).

Assessment: The 25-OH-D assay is the best method for determining vitamin D status of an individual horse. Both 25-OH-D and $1,25(OH)_2D$ will be assessed.

13.4.1.3 Vitamin K

Vitamin K is an essential cofactor for the activation of several blood clotting factors, including factors II (prothrombin), VII, IX, and X. Additionally, there are various proteins that require vitamin K for their activation. The natural form of vitamin K (K_1) is highest in green leafy plants and is absorbed, like the other fat-soluble vitamins, from the intestine into lymphatics bound to chylomicrons. Vitamin K_2 is produced by bacteria in the gastrointestinal tract of all animals in varying amounts. Vitamin K_3 is synthetic. Both vitamin K_1 and K_3 are converted to hydroquinone, the active form, in the liver. In most species, vitamin K_3 is excreted in the kidney whereas vitamin K_1 is excreted through the feces. Only a small amount of vitamin K is stored in the body. Therefore, deficiency can develop within 1–3 weeks.

Deficiency: In the horse, there have been no documented cases of vitamin K deficiency from extensive intestinal resection and decreased absorption of fat-soluble vitamins or chronic liver disease, as has been reported in humans. The most common cause of vitamin K deficiency in horses is caused by vitamin K antagonist administration:

1) Dicoumarol ingestion (sweet clover hay); pregnant mares especially susceptible
2) Warfarin administration
3) Accidental ingestion of rodenticides (first and second generation)

Clinical signs associated with vitamin K deficiency include susceptibility to hemorrhage (epistaxis, hematomas in tissues, hemoarthrosis) and weakness)

Toxicity:

1) Acute renal tubular nephrosis (colic signs, painful urination, hematuria, azotemia) (Rebhun et al., 1984).
2) Rapid irregular heart beat.

Assessment: In an emergency situation, vitamin K deficiency can be suspected with increased prothrombin time (PT) and activated partial thromboplastin time (aPTT) and suspected clinical signs. To measure vitamin K concentrations directly, serum concentrations can be assessed via high performance liquid chromatography using fluorometric detection.

13.4.1.4 Vitamin E

There are eight forms of naturally occurring vitamin E; however, d-alpha-tocopherol is the most active form in the body. Vitamin E is absorbed across the intestine and travels bound to chylomicron to the liver, where the RRR-alpha-tocopherol stereoisomer is selected for transport to the other body tissues, bound to very low density lipoproteins. Vitamin E is essential for normal neuromuscular function by acting as a potent antioxidant but can also modulate the expression of certain genes and inhibit platelet aggregation. A recent review of vitamin E and associated equine disorders is suggested for further reading (Finno and Valberg, 2012).

Deficiency:

1) Neuroaxonal dystrophy/equine degenerative myeloencepalopathy (NAD/EDM). NAD/EDM occurs in multiple breeds with most cases demonstrating clinical signs 6–12 months of age. Although the pathophysiology is not completely defined, there is strong evidence of a genetic component whose expression is highly influenced by vitamin E deficiency during the first year of life (Finno et al., 2013). Low serum α-tocopherol has been described in most, but not all, affected foals.

   Clinical signs: Clinical signs include symmetric ataxia that is often more severe in the pelvic limbs than the thoracic limbs, abnormal base-wide stance at rest, and proprioceptive deficits. In some reports, hyporeflexia of the cervicofacial and cutaneous trunci is described in addition to an absent laryngeal adductor reflex (Mayhew et al., 1987). Horses with NAD/EDM that survive to 2–3 years of age commonly exhibit lifelong, stable neurologic deficits.

2) Vitamin E deficiency myopathy (VEM) (Bedford et al., 2013): A subset of horses with vitamin E deficiency may develop clinical signs solely related to muscle atrophy and weakness without evidence of damage to motor nerves. These horses of a wide variety of breeds have been diagnosed with a VEM. Whether VEM is an entity unto itself or a predecessor to development of EMND is not yet known.

   Clinical signs: Horses present with loss of muscle mass, toe dragging, poor performance, weakness and muscle fasciculation.

3) EMND is an acquired neurodegenerative disorder affecting motor nerves supplying highly oxidative type 1 muscle fibers. EMND is associated with low plasma concentrations of vitamin E and a dietary deficiency of vitamin E of at least 18 months duration (Divers et al., 1994).

   Clinical signs: Horses with EMND show signs of generalized muscle wasting, muscle fasciculations, shifting of weight between hindlimbs, low head carriage in some cases and prolonged recumbency.

Toxicity: Unlike other fat-soluble vitamins, excess vitamin E is relatively nontoxic. High intakes of vitamin E can interfere with utilization of other fat-soluble vitamins and have been demonstrated to induce coagulopathy in other species.

Assessment: Serum alpha-tocopherol concentrations are an adequate measure of total body alpha-tocopherol status in healthy horses. Samples should be light-protected, kept chilled, and serum should be removed as quickly as possible. A wide variability in individual serum alpha-tocopherol concentrations over a 72-h time period has been reported (Craig et al., 1989). However, deficient horses have a larger fluctuation in serum alpha-tocopherol than non-deficient horses, presumably from rapid recirculation of alpha-tocopherol between the liver and plasma (Vanschandevijl et al., 2008). Therefore, one sample can gain insight into an animal's overall status (adequate, marginal or deficient). If a sample is marginal (between 1.5–2 µg/mL), an additional sample should be taken and an average calculated (Finno and Valberg, 2012).

In the case of VEM, serum alpha-tocopherol concentrations may be within the normal range but the muscle tissue is deficient (Bedford et al., 2013). In these cases, it may be warranted to measure alpha-tocopherol in muscle biopsy samples. At necropsy, fresh liver is the best tissue to assess whole body vitamin E status.

13.4.2 Water-Soluble Vitamins: B-complex and C

13.4.2.1 Thiamine (Vitamin B₁)

Thiamine, like all B vitamins and vitamin K, is produced by varying amounts of bacteria in the gastrointestinal tract. Thiamine is rapidly absorbed with decreasing efficiency with increasing amounts ingested and excess amounts absorbed are rapidly excreted in the urine. These methods of thiamine limitation protect against thiamin toxicosis. Thiamine is converted to its active coenzyme form, thiamine pyrophosphate (TPP) in the liver and kidney. Thiamine plays an important role in carbohydrate metabolism and in nerve transmission.

Deficiency: A dietary deficiency of thiamine in horses appears to be relatively uncommon or not recognized unless the following events occur:

1) Disruption of the intestinal flora by prolonged oral antimicrobial therapy
2) Decreased intake with prolonged inappetance
3) Intestinal parasitism, as strongyles and coccidia are reported to compete for thiamine (McDowell, 1989)
4) Ingestion of thiamine antagonists such as amprolium, or thiaminase-containing plants such as bracken fern, horsetail, or yellow starthistle.

Toxicosis: Thiamine toxicosis can occur due to parenteral over-administration and may result in transient signs of excitement.

Assessment: A horse's thiamine status is best determined by measuring transketolase activity in red blood cells or other tissues and by the percent stimulation of that activity by exogenous TPP.

13.4.2.2 Riboflavin (Vitamin B₂)

The dietary intake requirement of riboflavin is not high as it is synthesized in varying amounts by microbes in the gastrointestinal tract of all animals. Excess riboflavin is excreted in the urine as there is little storage in the body. In circulation, riboflavin functions in metabolic oxidation-reduction reactions as two enzymes: flavin mononucleotide and flavin adenine dinucleotide.

Deficiency/Toxicity: Not reported in horses to date.
Assessment: Not routinely performed.

13.4.2.3 Niacin (Vitamin B₃)

Niacin consists of equal vitamin activity of nicotinic acid and nicotinamide. Nicotinic acid is converted to nicotinamide in the intestinal mucosa. Nicotinamide is absorbed or produced from tryptophan and incorporated into the pyridine nucleotides nicotinamide adenine dinucleotide (NADH) and nicotinamide adenine dinucleotide phosphate (NADPH). NADH participates in electron transfer to the mitochondrial electron transport chain necessary for energy metabolism. Additionally, nicotinamide has critical roles in the metabolism of carbohydrates, lipids, and amino acids. Excess is excreted in the urine.

Deficiency/Toxicity: Not reported in horses to date.
Assessment: Not routinely performed.

13.4.2.4 Pantothenic Acid (Vitamin B₅)

Pantothenic acid is a constituent of many coenzymes. It is widely distributed in many plant and animal tissues. Excess is excreted in the urine.

Deficiency/Toxicity: Not reported in horses to date.
Assessment: Not routinely performed.

13.4.2.5 Pyridoxine (Vitamin B₆)

Vitamin B₆ includes three forms of pyridoxine (pyridoxine, pyridoxal and pyridoxamine) that have equal vitamin activity on a molar basis. The active forms of pyridoxine are involved in most reactions of amino acid metabolism, lipid, and GABA metabolism, and the synthesis of epinephrine and norepinephrine. Excess pyridoxine is excreted in the urine.

Deficiency/Toxicity: Not been reported in horses to date.

Assessment: Plasma vitamin B₆ is affected by protein intake. Therefore, urinary vitamin B₆ and its major metabolite, 4-pyridoxic acid (PA) have been used in other species as indicators of vitamin B₆ status (Leklem, 1990). Additional measures of vitamin B₆ status include plasma pyridoxal 5-phosphate (PLP), a tryptophan load test or measurement of erythrocyte alanine transaminase are assessed in people (Leklem, 1990) but have not yet been evaluated in horses.

13.4.2.6 Biotin (Vitamin B₇ or Vitamin H)

Biotin is a sulfur-containing vitamin widely distributed in plant and animal tissues. In adult horses, biotin is synthesized by microorganisms in the colon (Carroll et al., 1949). Biotin functions as a coenzyme in reactions involved in gluconeogenesis and the synthesis of glycerol. Biotin supplementation may have a beneficial effect on horses' hooves.

Deficiency/Toxicity: Not been reported in horses to date.
Assessment: Not routinely performed.

13.4.2.7 Folic Acid (Vitamin B₉)

Folic acid is synthesized and absorbed in the horse's cecum and colon (Carroll et al., 1949).

The main form of folic acid in animal and plant tissues contains several glutamate molecules. Both folic acid and vitamin B_{12} are required for red blood cell synthesis. The majority of body folate is stored in the liver as 5-methyltetrahydrofolates. Excretion of folates occurs mainly through the bile, unlike most other B vitamins.

Deficiency/Toxicity: Not been reported in horses to date. As a treatment of equine protozoal myeloencephalitis (EPM), pyrimethamine and sulfonamides work synergistically to block folic acid synthesis. For this reason, this EPM treatment is contraindicated in pregnant mares and long-term use may lead to a folate deficiency anemia.

Assessment: Plasma or serum samples provide an adequate estimate of whole body folic acid status (Table 13.2).

13.4.2.8 Cobalamin (Vitamin B₁₂)

Vitamin B_{12} is only naturally synthesized by microorganisms. Sources for horses therefore are microbial contamination of substances ingested or from microbial production in the colon (Davies, 1971). Cobalt is required for microbial synthesis of vitamin B_{12}. Vitamin B_{12} is required for methionine synthesis and folate entry into cells.

It is utilized in the synthesis of thymidine necessary for DNA synthesis.

Deficiency/Toxicity: Not been reported in horses to date.

Assessment: Whole blood or plasma concentrations provide an accurate estimate of vitamin B_{12} status (Table 13.2).

13.4.2.9 Choline

Choline can be synthesized in the body and is therefore not required in the diet or produced by microbial organisms. Choline synthesis occurs in the liver through methylation of ethanolamine with methyl groups provided from S-adenosyl methionine. Choline functions as a component of the neurotransmitter acetylcholine, phatidyl choline (lecithin), which is important for cell membrane structure, and betaine, which forms methionine and creatine.

Deficiency/Toxicity: Not been reported in horses to date.

Assessment: Plasma concentrations provide an accurate estimate of choline status (Table 13.2).

13.4.2.10 Vitamin C (Ascorbic Acid)

Although vitamin C is available as many forms, only ascorbic acid has significant biologic activity in mammals. In horses, ascorbic acid is synthesized from glucose in the liver. Ascorbic acid functions as an antioxidant, scavenging free radicals within aqueous solutions. Vitamin C is necessary for the synthesis of norepinephrine, tyrosine, lysine and proline, including hydroxyproline, and is therefore required for normal collagen formation.

Deficiency/Toxicity: Unlike humans, the horse is able to synthesize vitamin C and therefore vitamin C deficiencies have not been identified in the horse. There have been no reports of vitamin C toxicosis in horses.

Assessment: Plasma vitamin C concentrations provides a reliable assessment of whole body vitamin C status (Table 13.2).

References

Bailey EMJ and Garland T. 1992. Industrial toxicants. In NE Robinson (ed.), *Current Therapy in Equine Medicine 3*. Philadelphia: WB Saunders, pp. 358–359.

Baird JH. 1971. Lactation tetany (eclampsia) in a Shetland pony mare. Aust Vet J, 47: 402.

Bauer M. 1975. Copper sulfate poisoning in horses. Vet Arch, 45: 257–267.

Bedford HE, Valberg SJ, Firshman AM, Lucio M, Boyce MK, and Trumble TN. 2013. Histopathologic findings in the sacrocaudalis dorsalis medialis muscle of horses with vitamin E-responsive muscle atrophy and weakness. J Am Vet Med Assoc, 242: 1127–1137.

Bell JU, Lopez JM, and Bartos KD. 1987. The postnatal development of serum zinc, copper and ceruloplasmin in the horse. Comp Biochem Physiol A Comp Physiol, 87: 561–564.

Bridges CH, Womack JE, Harris ED, and Scrutchfield WL. 1984. Considerations of copper metabolism in osteochondrosis of suckling foals. J Am Vet Med Assoc, 185: 173–178.

Carroll FD, Goss H, and Howell CE. 1949. The synthesis of B-vitamins in the horse. J Anim Sci, 8: 290.

Chameroy KA, Frank N, Elliott SB, and Boston RC. 2011. Effects of a supplement containing chromium and magnesium on morphometric measurements, resting glucose, insulin concentrations and insulin sensitivity in laminitic obese horses. Equine Vet J, 43: 494–499.

Corke MJ. 1981. An outbreak of sulphur poisoning in horses. Vet Rec, 109: 212–213.

Craig AM, Blythe LL, Lassen ED, Rowe KE, Barrington R, and Slizeski M. 1989 Variations of serum vitamin E, cholesterol, and total serum lipid concentrations in horses during a 72-hour period. Am J Vet Res, 50: 1527–1531.

Dart AJ, Snyder, JR, Spier SJ, and Sullivan KE. 1992. Ionized calcium concentration in horses with surgically managed gastrointestinal disease: 147 cases (1988–1990). J Am Vet Med Assoc, 201: 1244–1248.

Davies ME. 1971. The production of vitamin B 12 in the horse. Br Vet J, 127: 34–36.

Desta B, Maldonado G, Reid H, Puschner B, Maxwell J, Agasan A, et al. 2011. Acute selenium toxicosis in polo ponies. J Vet Diagn Invest, 23: 623–628.

Divers TJ, Mohammed HO, Cummings, JF, Valentine BA, De Lahunta A, Jackson CA, and Summers BA. 1994. Equine motor neuron disease: findings in 28 horses and proposal of a pathophysiological mechanism for the disease. Equine Vet J, 26: 409–415.

Donoghue S, Kronfeld DS, Berkowitz SJ, and Copp RL. 1981. Vitamin A nutrition of the equine: growth, serum biochemistry and hematology. J Nutr, 111: 365–374.

El Shorafa WM, Feaster JP, Ott EA, and Asquith RL. 1979. Effect of vitamin D and sunlight on growth and bone development of young ponies. J Anim Sci, 48: 882–886.

Estepa JC, Aguilera-Tejero E, Mayer-Valor R, Almaden Y, Felsenfeld AJ, and Rodriguez M. 1998. Measurement of parathyroid hormone in horses. Equine Vet J, 30: 476–481.

Finno CJ, Famula T, Aleman M, Higgins RJ, Madigan JE, and Bannasch DL. 2013. Pedigree analysis and exclusion of alpha-tocopherol transfer protein (TTPA) as a candidate gene for neuroaxonal dystrophy in the American Quarter Horse. J Vet Intern Med, 27: 177–185.

Finno CJ and Valberg SJ. 2012. A comparative review of vitamin E and associated equine disorders. J Vet Intern Med, 26: 1251–1266.

Frape D. (ed.) 2010. *Equine Nutrition and Feeding*. Oxford, UK: Blackwell Publishing.

Garcia-Lopez JM, Provost PJ, Rush JE, Zicker SC, Burmaster H, and Freeman LM. 2001. Prevalence and prognostic importance of hypomagnesemia and hypocalcemia in horses that have colic surgery. Am J Vet Res, 62: 7–12.

Georgievskii VI, Annenkov BN, and Samokhin VT. (eds) 1982. *Mineral Nutrition in Animals*, London: Butterworth, and Co.

Greiwe-Crandell KM, Kronfeld DS, Gay LA, and Sklan D. 1995. Seasonal vitamin A depletion in grazing horses is assessed better by the relative dose response test than by serum retinol concentration. J. Nutr. 125: 2711–276.

Harrington DD. 1982. Acute vitamin D2 (ergocalciferol) toxicosis in horses: case report and experimental studies. J Am Vet Med Assoc, 180: 867–873.

Harrington DD and Page EH. 1983. Acute vitamin D3 toxicosis in horses: case reports and experimental studies of the comparative toxicity of vitamins D2 and D3. J Am Vet Med Assoc, 182: 1358–1369.

Hurtig MB, Green SL, and Dobson H. 1990. Defective bone and cartilage in foals fed a low-copper diet. Proceedings from the 35th Annual Meeting of the American Association of Equine Practitioners. 637–644.

Irvine CH. 1984. Hypothyroidism in the foal. Equine Vet J, 16: 302–306.

Johansson AM, Gardner SY, Jones SL, Fuquay LR, Reagan VH, and Levine JF. 2003. Hypomagnesemia in hospitalized horses. J Vet Intern Med, 17: 860–867.

Kirkham WW, Guttridge H, Bowden J, and Edds GT. 1971. Hematopoietic response to hematinics in horses. J Am Vet Med Assoc, 159: 1316–1318.

Knight DA, Weisbrode SE, and Schmall LM. 1987. Copper supplementation and cartilage lesions in foals. Proceedings from the 32nd Annual Meeting of the American Association of Equine Practitioners. 191–194.

Lakritz J, Madigan J, and Carlson GP. 1992. Hypovolemic hyponatremia and signs of neurologic disease associated with diarrhea in a foal. J Am Vet Med Assoc, 200: 1114–1116.

Leklem JE. 1990. Vitamin B-6: a status report. J Nutr, 120 Suppl 11: 1503–1507.

LeRoy B, Woolums A, Wass J, Davis E, Gold J, Foreman JH, et al. 2011. The relationship between serum calcium concentration and outcome in horses with renal failure presented to referral hospitals. J Vet Intern Med, 25: 1426–1430.

Maas J, Galey FD, Peauroi JR, Case JT, Littlefield ES, Gay CC, et al. 1992. The correlation between serum selenium and blood selenium in cattle. J Vet Diagn Invest, 4: 48–52.

Mayhew IG, Brown CM, Stowe HD, Trapp AL, Derksen FJ, and Clement SF. 1987. Equine degenerative myeloencephalopathy: a vitamin E deficiency that may be familial. J Vet Intern Med, 1: 45–50.

McDowell LR. (ed.) 1989. *Vitamins in Animal Nutrition*. San Diego, CA: Academic Press.

McLaughlin BG. and Doige CE. 1982. A study of ossification of carpal and tarsal bones in normal and hypothyroid foals. Can Vet J, 23: 164–168.

Mullaney TP and Brown CM. 1988. Iron toxicity in neonatal foals. Equine Vet J, 20: 119–124.

Murray MJ. 1990. Hypothyroidism and respiratory insufficiency in a neonatal foal. J Am Vet Med Assoc, 197: 1635–1638.

Nutritional Research Council (NRC) 2007. *Nutrient Requirements of Horses*, Washington, DC.

Ott EA and Asquith RL. 1987. The influence of trace mineral supplementation on growth and bone development of yearling horses. Proceedings of the Equine Nutritional and Physiological Society Symposium, pp. 185–192.

Ott EA and Kivipelto J. 1999. Influence of chromium tripicolinate on growth and glucose metabolism in yearling horses. J Anim Sci, 77: 3022–3030.

Pagan JD, Rotmensen T, and Jackson SG. 1995. The effect of chromium supplementation on metabolic response to exercise in Thoroughbred horses. Proceedings of the 14th Equine Nutrition and Physiology Society, Ontario, CA, pp. 96–101.

Payne RB, Little AJ, Williams RB, and Milner JR. 1973. Interpretation of serum calcium in patients with abnormal serum proteins. Br Med J, 4: 643–646.

Polack EW, King JM, Cummings JF, Mohammed HO, Birch M, and Cronin T. 2000. Concentrations of trace minerals in the spinal cord of horses with equine motor neuron disease. Am J Vet Res, 61: 609–611.

Rebhun WC, Tennant BC, Dill SG, and King JM. 1984. Vitamin K3-induced renal toxicosis in the horse. J Am Vet Med Assoc, 184: 1237–1239.

Rosol TJ and Capen CC. 1996. Pathophysiology of calcium, phosphorus, and magnesium metabolism in animals. Vet Clin North Am Small Anim Pract, 26: 1155–1184.

Shaftoe S, Schuk MP, and Chen CL. 1998. TSH response test in 1-day old foals. Equine Vet Sci, 8: 310–312.

Shupe JL and Olson AE. 1971. Clinical aspects of fluorosis in horses. J Am Vet Med Assoc, 158: 167–174.

Singh RK, Kooreman KM, Babbs CF, Fessler JF, Salaris SC, and Pham J. 1992. Potential use of simple manganese salts as antioxidant drugs in horses. Am J Vet Res, 53: 1822–1829.

Stark G, Schneider B, and Gemeiner M. 2001. Zinc and copper plasma levels in Icelandic horses with Culicoides hypersensitivity. Equine Vet J, 33: 506–509.

Stowe HD. 1968. Effects of age and impending parturition upon serum copper of thoroughbred mares. J Nutr, 95: 179–183.

Suttle N, Small J, and Jones D. 1995. Overestimation of copper deficiency in horses? Vet Rec, 136: 131.

Suttle NF, Small JN, Collins EA, Mason DK, and Watkins KL. 1996. Serum and hepatic copper concentrations used to define normal, marginal and deficient copper status in horses. Equine Vet J, 28: 497–499.

Tennant B, Bettleheim P, and Kaneko JJ. 1982. Paradoxic hypercalcemia and hypophosphatemia associated with chronic renal failure in horses. J Am Vet Med Assoc, 180: 630–634.

Toribio RE, Kohn CW, Chew DJ, Sams RA, and Rosol TJ. 2001. Comparison of serum parathyroid hormone and ionized calcium and magnesium concentrations and fractional urinary clearance of calcium and phosphorus in healthy horses and horses with enterocolitis. Am J Vet Res, 62: 938–947.

Toribio RE, Kohn CW, Hardy J, and Rosol TJ. 2005. Alterations in serum parathyroid hormone and electrolyte concentrations and urinary excretion of electrolytes in horses with induced endotoxemia. J Vet Intern Med, 19: 223–231.

Underwood EJ. (ed.) 1977. *Trace Elements in Human and Animal Nutrition*, New York and London: Academic Press.

Vanschandevijl K, Nollet H, Deprez P, Delesalle C, Lefere L, Dewulf J, and Van Loon G. 2008. Variation in deficient serum vitamin E levels and impact on assessment of the vitamin E status in horses. Vlaams Diergeneeskunidig Tijdschrift, 78: 28–33.

Vervuert I, Cuddeford D, and Coenen M. 2005. Effects of two levels of chromium supplement on selected metabolic responses in resting and exercising horses. Pferdeheilkunde, 21: 109–110.

Willoughby RA, Macdonald E, McSherry BJ, and Brown G. 1972. Lead and zinc poisoning and the interaction between Pb and ZN poisoning in the foal. Can J Comp Med, 36: 348–359.

14

Toxicologic Diagnostics

Robert H. Poppenga

California Animal Health and Food Safety Laboratory System and Department of Molecular Biosciences, School of Veterinary Medicine, University of California at Davis, California, USA

14.1 Introduction

Intoxications or suspected intoxications of horses occur less often than for other species, but are frequently more time consuming and challenging to manage (Hovda, 2015). In many cases, animals are found dead without any evidence of prior illness. Histories can be incomplete, while at the same time horse owners, veterinarians, trainers, and feed mills push for a quick answer. A rapid response is often necessary if multiple animals are affected or at risk and to help guide case management for symptomatic animals that are still alive. If feed is a suspected source for toxicant exposure, regulatory actions might be necessary and rapid collection and testing of representative samples is critical.

In cases where the history or clinical signs suggest a specific toxicologic etiology, testing can be specific as well. In other cases where a specific toxicant is not evident, sophisticated screening approaches can be employed to search for unknown toxicants. It is important to note that there are no single analytical procedures that can screen for all potential toxicants. Irrespective of whether specific tests or screening methods are undertaken, it can take several days to generate results.

Finding a chemical in a sample does not necessarily mean that it is the cause of the problem. A complete toxicologic investigation, including a thorough history, description of clinical signs, clinicopathologic testing, including a postmortem examination, collection of appropriate samples, and analytical testing should be undertaken in a careful and systematic manner. Proper documentation of sample collection and processing is crucial because the potential for litigation is high in poisoning cases. An established relationship with an accredited diagnostic laboratory providing advanced testing and a board-certified toxicologist to help guide testing and interpret results will increase the chances of making a correct diagnosis. In many cases, animal owners and veterinarians prematurely conclude that a toxicant is responsible for illness or death when an immediately obvious cause for the illness or death is not evident.

In cases in which a horse is presented to a clinic for evaluation, it might be prudent for the veterinarian to visit the premise where the animal is kept and to help the owner identify hazards or conditions consistent with toxicant exposure. Consultation with other experts such as extension agents who can identify potentially poisonous plants might be necessary.

14.2 History

An accurate history is the starting point for any disease investigation and ensures that appropriate samples are obtained for analysis. Owners often suspect malicious or accidental poisoning in cases where apparently healthy animals suddenly become sick or die. Irrespective of whether an owner suspects poisoning or not, veterinarians need to remain neutral observers until a thorough and systematic investigation is conducted.

One of the most difficult aspects of obtaining an accurate history relates to feeding and feed management. Details regarding the introduction of new feeds should be obtained. The sources of all feed components should be determined. Details concerning feed mixing need to be assessed. If feed mixing occurs off-site, it is important to determine if feeds for other species are also mixed at the facility. If so, inadvertent contamination with potentially toxic feed additives could occur.

Feed should be examined closely for quality and the presence of unusual feed components or foreign material. Samples of feed, both as purchased and as fed, should be obtained and stored appropriately. Dry feeds can be placed in paper bags and stored at ambient temperatures while moist feeds should be refrigerated or frozen pending submission for testing.

Interpretation of Equine Laboratory Diagnostics, First Edition. Edited by Nicola Pusterla and Jill Higgins.
© 2018 John Wiley & Sons, Inc. Published 2018 by John Wiley & Sons, Inc.

Hay and pasture should be examined for the presence of weeds or other contaminants such as blister beetles or clippings from plants such as oleander. The presence of mold growth can be an important finding in grains or forages, although the presence of molds in feeds is often incidental to the actual problem and the absence of obvious mold growth does not rule out a possible mycotoxin problem.

Obtaining representative feed samples for testing can be a challenge, particularly when large amounts of feed are present, since many toxicants can be localized to a restricted portion of the available feed (Carson, 1999). Unfortunately, in some cases, contaminated feed might have been already consumed and therefore unavailable for testing. It is important to keep in mind that diagnostic laboratories typically process only a few grams of sample to be tested; these few grams might have come from several tons of suspect feed.

While intoxication from contaminated water is infrequent, sources should be described and examined for the presence of foreign material or algal growth. In addition, bedding should be inspected for foreign material or plants (e.g., black walnut shavings).

The approach to questioning an owner is critical to avoid overlooking important historical facts. General questions can be asked initially with more specific questions to follow. General questions include whether or not medications, feed additives, or pesticides are present on the property, and if so, whether any had been used recently. Are there any trash or junk piles accessible to animals? Have there been any construction projects undertaken recently? Has there been any movement of animals into a new environment? If pesticides are in use on a premise, determine the active ingredients in products, who last used the products, and which animals might have had exposure or access to storage areas.

Any samples collected in the field need to be properly labeled with unique identification that should include (but not necessarily be limited to) the sample type, location that the sample was collected, and a date. Feed samples should be labeled with lot numbers or manufacturing dates.

14.3   Clinical Signs

Live animals should be evaluated thoroughly and clinical signs accurately described and reported to diagnostic laboratory personnel. The list of toxic differentials can be refined based upon the clinical symptomatology. When possible, the sequence of onset of clinical signs should be provided. The time frame from when the animal was last noted to be normal to the onset of clinical signs should be determined, as well as the cessation, continuation, and duration of signs.

Although pathognomonic signs for specific toxicants are infrequent, some signs might be. For example, horizontal hoof cracks and loss of mane and tail hair is highly suggestive of chronic selenosis. The sudden onset of hypersalivation might be consistent with exposure to slaframine. Unfortunately, many clinical signs are nonspecific. For example, anorexia, colic, and depression can be associated with toxicants as diverse as blister beetles, oleander, or certain drugs.

14.4   Clinicopathologic Testing

One of the most useful approaches to determining a toxic etiology is to identify which organ system or systems are primarily affected. While clinical signs are useful in this regard, they can be misleading. Routine and more specialized clinicopathologic testing helps to identify affected organs such as the liver, kidneys or heart and perhaps narrow the list of differentials to hepatotoxicants, nephrotoxicants, or cardiotoxicants.

If at all possible, dead animals should be brought to an appropriate state diagnostic laboratory for a complete postmortem examination conducted by a board-certified pathologist. This is particularly important if the animal is insured or future litigation is possible. A list of accredited state diagnostic laboratories can be found at the American Association of Veterinary Laboratory Diagnosticians website at www.aavld.org. It is always a good idea to call the diagnostic laboratory prior to sending animals to discuss the case with diagnostic laboratory personnel.

If it is not possible to submit whole animals, a field necropsy should be performed. Consultation with diagnostic laboratory personnel is also recommended before a field necropsy is performed to discuss the case and determine what samples should be collected and how samples should be processed and stored prior to submission. In the absence of specific recommendations, extra samples should be taken to assure that useful samples have been obtained. Samples that are not used can be discarded later. It is always better to have more samples than you think will be needed rather than not having sufficient amounts for appropriate testing or not having them at all.

Often necropsy results will show specific lesions that confirm a presumptive diagnosis or lead to a different path of inquiry. For example, hepatic lesions consisting of megalocytosis, periportal fibrosis, and biliary hyperplasia strongly suggests pyrrolizidine alkaloid intoxication.

Alternatively, no or only general postmortem lesions can be present. The lack of lesions can be helpful as well, since many toxicants do not cause lesions. If financial constraints are of concern, it is always better to start with a through gross and microscopic pathologic examination before extensive toxicology testing is performed. Samples for toxicologic testing can be stored for extended periods of time and analyzed after initial postmortem findings are evaluated. Appropriate documentation of field necropsy results is essential. Consideration should be given to taking pictures of any suspected gross lesions.

14.5 Analytical Testing

Diagnostic laboratories vary in terms of their toxicologic testing capabilities. The list of tests offered by individual diagnostic laboratories can generally be accessed through their respective websites. In situations where a specific analyte is of interest, but a test is not found, it is useful to call the laboratory since diagnosticians are often aware of other laboratories that offer the test of interest. Toxicologic testing can be as simple as visual inspection (e.g., examining forages for weeds or blister beetles) to sophisticated mass spectrometry techniques.

Targeting screening using a variety of analytical approaches is common. For example, screens designed to detect ionophores in feeds generally include four or more specific compounds. Screens for organophosphorus or carbamate insecticides might include several dozen different compounds. Modern analytical approaches can detect multiple metals in a single sample. This avoids the need to test for individual metals and lessens the chance of missing the presence of a potentially toxic metal. Contrary to common perceptions, it is possible to screen samples for a broad array of chemicals in cases in which there is insufficient information to suggest exposure to a specific toxicant. Screening techniques generally rely on mass spectrometry in which the mass spectra or unique "fingerprints" for an unknown compound are compared to commercial or laboratory-specific libraries of known mass spectra.

In many cases, the detection of any amount of a potential toxicant is sufficient for a diagnosis. For example, the qualitative detection of oleandrin or cantharidin in a urine sample is most likely significant. In other cases, it is critical to determine the quantity of a chemical of interest in the sample being tested. Quantification is particularly important when testing feed samples since that is essential information for doing an exposure assessment to see of a potentially toxic dose of a chemical was ingested.

Common antemortem samples for toxicologic testing include urine, serum or plasma, whole blood, and stomach contents (see Box 14.1). Common postmortem samples include liver, kidneys, urine, brain, and stomach or GI contents. Knowledge regarding the time of onset of clinical signs vs. the time of sample collection

antemortem or time to death can be critical to selecting the most important samples for testing. If an animal dies within a few minutes to a few hours after onset of clinical signs or is found dead without warning, analysis of stomach contents is often performed first. If an animal has been symptomatic for longer than a day, it is unlikely that any toxicant will remain in the stomach. In such cases analysis of urine might be more appropriate. Testing often focuses on samples obtained from sites of exposure (e.g., skin or GI contents), sites of metabolism or excretion (e.g., liver, kidneys, or urine), or sites of accumulation (e.g., fat or bone). While other samples such as hair or feces might be useful, in most situations they are not typically tested.

Attention needs to be paid to the optimal amount of a sample required for analysis. Although advances in analytical techniques have resulted in the need for smaller sample sizes, the failure to submit a requested amount can decrease the test sensitivity substantially. For example, if a given test requires 1 g of liver, but only 0.5 g is available, the sensitivity of the test can decrease by half (e.g., if a toxicant can be detected at 1 ppm or greater with 1 g of sample, it might only be detected at 2 ppm or greater if 0.5 g is provided). The other consideration is that for a given case, multiple tests might need to be performed to address toxicants on a differential list. There is nothing more frustrating to everyone involved in an unsolved case than running out of samples to perform additional analytical tests.

Box 14.1 Samples and amounts that are recommended for toxicologic analysis.

Feed samples 500 g, make sure that they are representative

Plants	Entire plant
Water	1 liter in clean container
Whole blood	5–10 ml
Serum	5–10 ml
Urine	As much as is available
GI contents	100 g or more from each GI segment
Liver	100–200 g
Kidney	100–200 g
Brain	Right or left half
Fat	100 g

Except for dry feed or plant samples, all samples should be refrigerated. If a delay in testing, GI contents, tissues, and fluids should be frozen.

Source: Puschner and Galey (2001). Reproduced with permission of Elsevier.

Although many tests routinely take a few days to 2 or 3 weeks to perform, some laboratories might offer STAT analyses. In some cases, particularly those involving multiple animals or feed contamination, laboratory testing is prioritized to provide test results as quickly as possible.

Lastly, given the likelihood of litigation for many poisoning or suspected poisoning cases, it is critical that documentation is complete and that a paper trail can be retrospectively followed, perhaps years after the event. For this reason, appropriate chain-of-custody procedures should be followed for every sample.

14.6 Selecting a Laboratory

No single laboratory can perform all possible toxicologic analyses. For this reason, it is recommended that veterinarians become familiar with several qualified laboratories. Minimum expectations of a qualified laboratory include (Osweiler, 1999):

- A written schedule of fees and services
- Information about quality control programs and accreditation with recognized certifying agencies (e.g., AAVLD)
- Information about the qualifications of staff
- Availability of trained individuals for phone consultation before and after testing
- Use of modern analytical equipment including various mass spectrometry platforms (i.e., GC/MS, LC/MS, and ICP/MS)
- Instructions in the collection and preservation of samples
- Interpretation of test results
- Whenever possible, information on normal or expected values for the tests performed

14.7 Diagnostic Considerations for Specific Equine Toxicants

Acer rubrum (red maple) leaves, either wilted or dried, can cause oxidative damage to red blood cells resulting in methemoglobin formation, Heinz bodies, and a hemolytic anemia (Alward et al., 2006). Intoxications are reported more frequently in the Eastern United States where red maples are common. Gallotannins and free gallic acid, found in *Acer rubrum* leaves, are believed to be metabolized in the ileum of horses by microbial flora to a potent oxidizing agent, pyrogallol (Agrawal et al., 2013).

A diagnosis of *Acer rubrum* intoxication relies on signs consistent with a hemolytic anemia and confirmation, when possible, of ingestion of wilted or dried leaves. In cases in which a tree limb has fallen and the leaves have begun to wilt, evidence of leaf consumption is useful. This is not possible when wilted leaves are consumed after they have fallen from the tree in the fall. However, there might be evidence of leaves in the stomach contents from horses that die. It is possible to test serum or urine samples for pyrogallol to confirm exposure, but the presence of this compound also occurs following ingestion of oak buds, leaves, or acorns. In addition, few laboratories offer such testing.

Aflatoxins are produced by *Aspergillus* species in grains such as corn, cottonseed, and peanuts under certain environmental conditions. Aflatoxins include aflatoxins B_1, B_2, G_1, and G_2 with B_1 being the most toxic (Osweiler, 2001). Aflatoxins are metabolized in the liver to reactive epoxides, which interact with cell DNA, RNA, and proteins to cause hepatocyte damage and death. Depending on the dose and duration of exposure, acute or chronic intoxications occur. Chronic intoxications result in severe liver fibrosis and ultimate liver failure. Signs and clinical findings associated with acute or chronic aflatoxicosis are not specific since many other liver diseases can produce a similar clinical picture.

Aflatoxicosis is not commonly diagnosed in horses. Contaminated corn is the most likely source for exposure. Unfortunately, the occurrence of aflatoxins in a given feedstuff is uneven and failure to obtain a representative feed sample can easily result in negative or misleading test results. Therefore, it is recommended that multiple samples be obtained from different areas of the feed, placed together and thoroughly mixed to obtain a composite sample. Approximately one pound of sample should be submitted for testing. Some laboratories test for all four aflatoxins, while others test only for aflatoxin B_1. Acute hepatotoxicity can be caused by feed concentrations in the parts per million range (ppm), while chronic hepatotoxicity can be caused by concentrations in the parts per billion range (ppb).

Botulinum toxin, produced by *Clostridium botulinum*, causes a gradually progressive and bilateral muscular weakness and paralysis in horses characterized by dysphagia and eventual recumbency (Whitlock and McAdams, 2006, Johnson et al., 2014, 2015). There are several strains of botulinum toxin (A-F) with horses primarily affected by strains A, B, and C.

Botulinum toxin is a potent neurotoxin that impairs acetylcholine neurotransmission at neuromuscular junctions. The onset and progression of signs is dose dependent with small doses of the toxin causing clinical signs up to 10 or more days after exposure and large doses causing clinical signs and death with 8 h. Botulinum spores are ubiquitous in the environment and botulinum toxin can be elaborated in improperly fermented forages (pH > 4.5) (Johnson et al., 2010).

Ideally, detection of preformed toxin in serum or GI contents confirms a diagnosis, but the extremely sensitivity of horses to the toxin often precludes its detection by available methods. Currently, the mouse bioassay and ELISA testing are available for toxin testing. Often, neither is sufficiently sensitive to detect toxin in samples from horses. Only 20% of samples from foals and rare samples from adult horses are positive for the toxin using the mouse bioassay (Whitlock and Adams, 2006). Therefore, testing of suspect feedstuffs is recommended as well. Identification of spores in feedstuffs or GI contents is possible, but generally not as useful since testing can take several weeks to complete. However, identification of spores along with consistent clinical signs helps to confirm the diagnosis. Newer techniques, including mass spectrometry detection of the toxin and quantitative real-time PCR assays for detection of neurotoxic genes of *Clostridium botulinum* hold promise as sensitive diagnostic techniques of the future (Johnson et al., 2014, Wang et al., 2015).

Cantharidin is a vesicant toxin produced by a number of "blister" beetles (*Epicauta* and *Pyrota* spp.). Toxicosis results from the ingestion of baled alfalfa hay or other alfalfa feeds containing dead beetles. As a vesicant, canthardin causes irritation, vesicle formation and ulcerations, or erosions throughout the GI tract and bladder (Hellman and Edwards, 1997). Hypocalcemia, hypomagnesemia, renal failure and cardiac abnormalities have been described.

A diagnosis typically relies on a history of feeding alfalfa and visual detection of dead beetles in suspect forage, consistent clinical signs, and analysis of forage samples, beetles, or urine for the toxin. The detection of any concentration of cantharidin would be considered significant. Identification of beetles might require the expertise of an entomologist; checking with state extension specialists can help to identify appropriate individuals.

Fescue toxicosis occurs in pregnant mares and is associated with ingestion of endophyte-infected tall fescue (*Festuca arundinacea* Schreb.) post gestation day 300 (Blodgett, 2008). The endophyte is a fungus (*Neotyphodium coenophialum*) that lives in a mutualistic relationship with the plant tissues. The endophyte produces ergot peptide alkaloids with ergovaline being the most significant. Ergot peptides are dopamine agonists causing decreased prolactin secretion which affects milk production, lipogenesis, immunity, and reproductive hormones.

Intoxication can be confirmed by testing pasture or hay samples for ergovaline. Ergovaline concentrations > 200 ppb on a dry weight bases are considered to be significant. The presence of the endophyte can be assessed by microscopic examination of stained plant tissue or ELISA testing by plant pathology laboratories.

Fumonisin mycotoxins are produced by the fungus *Fusarium verticilloides* and cause equine leukoencephalomalacia (ELEM or moldy corn disease). Several fumonisins have been isolated with fumonisin B_1 being the most important (Volmer, 2008). ELEM is a disease primarily associated with the feeding of contaminated corn and it occurs sporadically when environmental conditions, such as drought followed by cool and moist conditions during corn pollination and kernel formation, are conducive for toxin production.

Horses are the most sensitive species. Fumonisins cause a rapidly fatal neurological disease with characteristic CNS lesions consisting of softening and necrosis of cerebral white matter. Neurotoxicity is the most common form of intoxication, although hepatotoxicity has been reported following ingestion of lower fumonisin concentrations for longer periods of time.

Fumonisins inhibit ceremide synthase, a sphingolipid metabolizing enzyme resulting in accumulation of sphingosine and sphinganine and disruption of sphingolipid-dependent processes.

A diagnosis most often relies on the presence of characteristic CNS lesions and detection of potentially toxic fumonisin concentrations in a representative feed sample. The minimum dietary concentration of total fumonisins associated with ELEM is approximately 8–10 ppm on an as fed or wet weight basis ingested for approximately 30 days (Volmer, 2008). The Food and Drug Administration suggests that corn and corn by-products intended for use in horse feeds should not contain more than 5 ppm total fumonisins (fumonisins B_1, B_2, and B_3) on a dry weight basis and such feed should constitute no more than 20% of the diet on a dry matter basis (www.fda.gov/Food/GuidanceRegulation/GuidanceDocumentsRegulatoryInformation/ucm109231.htm).

Ionophore feed additives such as monensin, lasalocid, salinomycin, and narasin are common livestock feed additives used to increase productivity or control certain diseases such as coccidiosis. Equids are especially sensitive to the cardiotoxic effects of these compounds. For example, the LD_{50} for horses is 2–3 mg/kg body weight compared to an LD_{50} for cattle of 22–80 mg/kg body weight. Depending on the dose ingested, death can be within hours to days or weeks.

A diagnosis of intoxication most often relies on detection of an ionophore in a representative feed sample at a toxic concentration, along with compatible clinical signs (tachycardia, ataxia, depression, anorexia, and profuse sweating) and the presence of cardiac lesions (Hall, 2001, Bautista et al., 2014). Unfortunately, representative feed samples are often unavailable and cardiac lesions are not pathognomonic and can be subtle to absent (Peek et al., 2004, Bautista et al., 2014). Clinical pathologic changes are non-specific in intoxicated animals, although increased serum concentrations of troponin I can help narrow the differential list to a cardiotoxin.

Detection of an ionophore in antemortem or postmortem biological specimens can confirm exposure, but in the absence of other information cannot be used to diagnose intoxication. Gastrointestinal contents, heart, liver, urine, and serum have been used to detect monensin, but tissue concentrations are variable and dependent on dose and time since exposure to sample collection. In one case involving multiple horses, detectable monensin concentrations in stomach contents were 1 ppm in a horse that died 12 h post-exposure, 6 ppm in a horse that died 48 h post-exposure, to a non-detectable concentration in a horse that died 4 days post-exposure (Bautista et al., 2014). Heart concentrations were 45 ppb and 5.2 ppb in the 12- and 48-h deaths, respectively. Heart concentrations were higher than concentrations in liver, serum, and urine collected at the same time. Ideally, as with most suspected intoxications, multiple samples should be tested, but economics often limits the amount of testing that is done. Irrespective of the ultimate number of samples that are tested, multiple samples should be collected and stored.

Antemortem, a minimum suite of testing might include feed and serum testing, along with indications of cardiac function such as ECGs and troponin I. Postmortem testing would include feed and heart tissue testing and histopathologic demonstration of compatible cardiac lesions.

Nerium oleander (oleander) is a highly toxic plant and where it grows intoxication of animals is frequent. As few as 10–20 leaves are potentially lethal for horses (Renier et al., 2013). The primary toxin in oleander, oleandrin, damages the heart via inactivation of Na + -K+ ATPase in plasma membranes of cardiomyocytes. Clinical signs of intoxication include colic, lethargy, anorexis, diarrhea, and tachycardia, and cardiac arrhythmias such as third degree AV block, bundle branch block, and ventricular fibrillation.

A diagnosis of intoxication is often made following known ingestion of the plant with subsequent onset of compatible clinical signs. Unfortunately, evidence of consumption is commonly absent. Interestingly, in one case series, even though oleander was known to be present on the property, approximately half of the owners or caretakers believed that it was impossible that their animal had ingested oleander (Renier et al., 2013). Exposure can occur when oleander leaves contaminate hay. Oleander leaves are generally easy to detect in forage if a representative sample is available for inspection. Clinical pathologic changes are non-specific.

In cases in which evidence of consumption is absent, but compatible clinical signs are present, it is possible to detect oleandrin in a variety of samples. Antemortem,

serum or plasma, stomach fluid or urine samples can be tested. Postmortem, stomach, or cecal contents, liver, or urine can be tested. If death is rapid, analysis of stomach contents is preferred. If death is delayed, analysis of cecal contents is preferred. In some cases, it might be advisable to test both samples since one or the other might be negative. Quantification of the amount of oleandrin in a sample is not necessary since its presence or absence is the primary diagnostic criteria. Whenever possible, examination of stomach contents for the presence of oleander leaves and histopathologic examination of the heart is recommended.

Pyrrolizidine alkaloids (PAs) are a large group of structurally similar molecules found in a number of plant species. Alkaloid composition and concentrations are variable among plants and differ based upon plant part and maturity. Some PAs are hepatotoxic while others are not. Common PA-containing plant genera in the USA include *Senicio*, *Amsinckia*, *Cynoglossum*, and *Crotalaria*. Intoxication of horses occurs following ingestion of PA-containing plants in pastures, paddocks, or forage. Acute intoxications are rare due to the large amount of ingested plant material that would be required. Chronic intoxication is much more common with clinical signs potentially occurring weeks to months after ingestion. This makes a diagnosis difficult since identification of PA-containing plants, particularly in hay, is often not possible so long after initial exposure.

PAs interfere with hepatocyte replication resulting in hepathocytomegaly and necrosis with bile duct proliferation and fibrosis (Robinson and Gummow, 2015). Pyrroles alkylate double-stranded DNA, thus inhibiting cell mitosis and resulting in megalocytosis. As megalocytes die they are replaced by fibrous connective tissue. Pyrroles bind to cellular constituents in lung and kidney tissues as well. Most affected horses suffer from a chronic delayed form of intoxication with subtle clinical signs of chronic weight loss and debilitation due to hepatic insufficiency (Curran et al., 1996). In the chronic delayed form, the onset of clinical signs can be rather abrupt despite exposure and liver dysfunction being chronic and progressive.

Although non-specific, elevations of GGT are consistent. Prolonged BSP clearance times and elevated bile acid concentrations are also common. A presumptive diagnosis often depends on characteristic liver lesions noted from a liver biopsy or postmortem examination. Some work has been done to detect pyrrole metabolites in blood or other tissues or PA adducts in tissues as a means to confirm exposure, but such testing is not widely available and has not been shown to be useful to diagnose chronic delayed intoxications. Identification of PA-containing plants on a premise or in feed is the most common way to confirm exposure. A diagnosis of intoxication

Table 14.1 Testing considerations for selected equine toxicants.[1]

Toxicant	Preferred sample type	Alternative sample types	Considerations
Acer rubrum (red maple)	Specific testing is not available	Generally not useful	A diagnosis relies on typical signs of hemolytic anemia along with confirming exposure to red maple Examination of stomach contents for red maple leaves
Aflatoxins	Representative feed sample	Generally not useful	Lack of representative feed sample at the time of exposure often precludes detection of aflatoxin concentrations consistent with intoxication
Blister beetle (cantharidin)	Representative forage sample GI contents and urine	Generally not useful	Identification of blister beetles in forage samples or testing for cantharidin Analysis of GI contents and urine for cantharidin
Botulinum toxin	Serum or GI contents	Feed materials	Detection of preformed toxin in serum or GI contents is definitive, but extreme sensitivity of horses often precludes detection of the toxin by available methods Identification of toxin or spores in feed or GI contents can be useful, but delay in test completion makes results useful retrospectively
Algal toxins (anatoxin-a and microcystins)	GI contents or water samples	Generally not useful	Detection of toxin in water samples or in GI content samples Water samples which include algal cells (bloom material) should be collected Identification of algal species in water or GI samples can help guide specific toxin testing.
Fescue	Forage samples	Generally not useful	Ergovaline concentrations in pasture or hay samples > 200 ppb dry weight Endophyte presence can be determined qualitatively by staining plant stems or using ELISA techniques
Fumonisin mycotoxins	Representative feed sample	Generally not useful, serum to test for altered sphinganine to sphingosine ratio	Testing for fumonisins in feed samples is available from many diagnostic laboratories Sphinganine and sphingosine analysis using serum samples is not generally available
Ionophores	Represenative feed samples Stomach contents	Tissues such as heart and liver	Ideally feed samples are tested to confirm exposure to toxic concentrations Representative feed samples are often unavailable Testing stomach contents or tissues can confirm exposure but not intoxication
Juglans nigra (black walnut)	Bedding samples	Generally not useful	Detection of black walnut shavings in bedding samples Most often done using microscopy
Lead toxicosis	Whole blood samples antemortem or liver or kidney samples postmortem	Generally not useful	Whole blood lead concentrations ≥ 0.35 ppm or liver or kidney lead concentrations ≥ 10 ppm (wet weight) are diagnostic for acute intoxications Tissue concentrations as low as 5 ppm is consistent with chronic intoxication
Nerium oleander (oleander)	Serum or urine samples antemortem, GI contents or liver samples postmortem		Detection of oleandrin in any sample is significant Several samples of GI contents should be collected, since testing of only one (i.e., stomach or cecal contents) might miss the presence of the toxin Examination of stomach contents for presence of characteristic leaves is useful
Pyrrolizidine alkaloid (PA) toxicosis	Representative feed samples	Stomach contents	Identification of PA-containing plants in forage or feed samples critical Representative feed samples are often unavailable given the slow progression of disease Measurement of PA in feed samples is possible and often necessary in processed feeds (e.g., hay cubes) A diagnosis often relies on consistent liver lesions (from liver biopsies or postmortem sample)

(Continued)

Table 14.1 (Continued)

Toxicant	Preferred sample type	Alternative sample types	Considerations
Quercus spp. (oak)	Urine or GI contents	Plant material	Measurement of pyrogallol in urine or GI contents Qualitative measurement that confirms exposure only
Selenium	Whole blood and liver samples	Hair	Whole blood and liver selenium concentrations < 1 ppm usually rule out selenosis Whole blood and liver concentrations > 1 ppm might indicate exposure to excessive selenium but do not prove selenosis
Slaframine	Representative forage samples	Generally not useful	Detection of slaframine in forage samples Analysis not widely available Confirmation of *Rhizoctonia leguminicola* on forage by plant pathologist
Taxus spp. (Japanese or English yews)	Stomach contents	Generally not useful	Testing for alkaloids in stomach contents is possible Visual or microscopic detection of leaves on stomach contents can confirm exposure

1 Diagnoses rely on not only analytical testing but consideration of other historical, clinical, and postmortem findings.

is best made by confirming exposure to a PA-containing plant in conjunction with compatible antemortem clinical pathologic abnormalities and liver biopsy lesions or postmortem liver lesions. In some cases, contamination of alfalfa cubes has occurred in which it is difficult to identify a PA-containing plant. In such cases, it is possible to test for the presence of hepatotoxic PAs using gas chromatography – mass spectrometry.

Slaframine is a fungal toxin produced by *Rhizoctonia leguminacola*. The fungus causes "black patch," a sporadic disease of clovers and other legumes (Wijnberg et al., 2009). Infestation normally occurs on plants during wet, humid weather where temperatures range from 25–29 °C. The plant disease appears as dark spots or concentric rings on affected leaves and stems. Intoxication most frequently occurs following consumption of affected pasture or second-cutting forage. Drying of plants decreases the concentration of slaframine over time.

Slaframine is an agonist for muscarinic receptors responsible for regulation of secretory glands. Typically, rapid onset of profuse salivation is the only sign noted. Once animals are removed from affected forage recovery occurs within 1–3 days. A diagnosis is generally made based upon the rapid onset of hypersalivation in con-

junction with feeding legume forages. It might be possible to test forages for the presence of slaframine, but the availability of testing is limited. A plant pathologist can confirm the presence of the plant disease. Extension agents should be consulted if such expertise is desired.

Taxus spp. (Japanese or English yews) are popular ornamental shrubs that contain toxic alkaloids known as taxines A and B (Tiwary et al., 2005). Following ingestion, the plants are most often associated with sudden death due to interference with cardiac depolarization, which results in bradycardia, arrhthymias, and diastolic cardiac arrest. Horses are considered to be more susceptible to intoxication than most other species.

A diagnosis of intoxication is usually based on evidence of consumption of the plant, either through careful observation of yew plants accessible to horses or finding characteristic yew leaves in stomach contents. Visual identification without microscopy is possible, but more extensive mastication by horses might make microscopic identification in stomach contents necessary. Identification of taxines in GI contents is also possible and their detection provides proof of exposure, but relatively few laboratories offer the analysis.

Other select equine toxicants can be found in Table 14.1.

References

Agrawal K, Ebel JG, Altier C, and Bischoff K. 2013. Identification of protoxins and a microbial basis for red maple (*Acer rubrum*) toxicosis in equines. J. Vet. Diagn. Invest. 25: 112–119.

Alward A, Corriher, CA, Barton MH, et al. 2006. Red maple (*Acer rubrum*) leaf toxicosis in horses: a retrospective study of 32 cases. J. Vet. Int. Med., 20: 1197–1201.

Bautista AC, Tahara J, Mete A, et al. 2014. Diagnostic value of tissue monensin concentrations in horses following toxicosis. J. Vet. Diagn. Invest 26(3): 423–427.

Blodgett DJ. 2008. Fescue toxicosis. In JP Lavoie and KW Hinchcliff (eds). *Blackwell's Five Minute Veterinary Consult: Equine*. 2nd Edn. Wiley-Blackwell: Ames, IA, pp. 326–327.

Carson TL. 1999. Investigating feed problems. In JL Howard and RA Smith (eds). *Current Veterinary Therapy 4: Food Animal Practice*. Philadelphia: W.B. Saunders, pp. 238–239.

Curran JM, Sutherland RJ, and Peet RL. 1996. A screening test for subclinical liver disease in horses affected by pyrrolizidine alkaloid toxicosis. Aust Vet J, 75(3): 236–240.

Hall JO. 2001. Toxic feed constituents in the horse. Vet Clin North Am Eq Prac, 17(3): 479–489.

Hellman RG and Edwards WC. 1997. Clinical features of blister beetle poisoning in equids: 70 cases (1983–1996). J AM Vet Med Assoc., 211(8): 1018–1021.

Hovda LR. 2015. Disorders caused by toxicants. In: BP Smith (ed.), *Large Animal Internal Medicine*, 7th Edn, St. Louis: Elsevier, pp. 1578–1616.

Johnson AL, McAdams SC, and Whitlock RH. 2010. Type A botulism in horses in the United States: a review of the past ten years (1998–2008). J vet Diag Invest., 22: 165–173.

Johnson AL, McAdams-Gallagher SC, and Sweeney RW. 2014. Quantitative real time PCR for detection of neurotoxin genes in Clostridium botulinum types A, B and C in equine samples. Veterinary J 199: 157–161.

Johnson AL, McAdams-Gallagher SC, and Aceto H. 2015. Outcome of adult horses with botulism treated at a veterinary hospital: 92 cases (1989–2013). J Vet Int. Med., 29: 311–319.

Osweiler GD. 1999. Using diagnostic resources for toxicology. In JL Howard and RA Smith (eds), *Current Veterinary Therapy 4: Food Animal Practice*, Philadelphia: W.B. Saunders, pp. 235–237.

Osweiler GD. 2001. Mycotoxins. Vet Clin N Am: Eq Prac., 17(3): 547–566.

Peek SF, Margues FD, and Morgan J. 2004. Atypical acute monensin toxicosis and delayed cardiomyopathy in Belgian draft horses. J Vet Int Med., 18: 761–764.

Puschner B and Galey FD. 2001. Diagnosis and approach to poisoning in the horse. Vet Clin N Am Eq Pract., 17(3): 399–409.

Renier AC, Kass PH, Magdesian KG, et al. 2013. Oleander toxicosis in equids: 30 cases (1995–2010). J Am Vet Med Assoc., 242(4): 540–549.

Robinson B and Gummow B. 2015. A field investigation into a suspected outbreak of pyrrolizidine alkaloid toxicosis in western Queensland. Prevent Vet Med., 118: 378–386.

Tiwary AK, Puschner B, Kinde H, et al. 2005. Diagnosis of Taxus (yew) poisoning in a horse. J Vet Diag Invest., 17: 252–255.

Wang D, Krilich J, Baudys J, et al. 2015. Enhanced detection of type C botulinum neurotoxin by the Endopet-MS assay through optimization of peptide substrates. Bioorg and Medic Chem 23: 3667–3673.

Whitlock RH and McAdams S. 2006. Equine botulism. Clin Tech Eq. Pract., 5: 37–42.

Wijnberg ID, van der Ven PJ, and Fink-Gremmels Gehrmann J. 2009. Outbreak of salivary syndrome on several horse farms in the Netherlands. Vet. Rec., 164: 595–597.

Volmer PA. 2008. Fumonisins. In JP Lavoie and KW Hinchcliff (eds), *Blackwell's Five Minute Veterinary Consult: Equine*. 2nd Edn. Ames, IA: Wiley-Blackwell, pp. 326–327.

15

Therapeutic Drug Monitorings
K. Gary Magdesian

Department of Medicine and Epidemiology, School of Veterinary Medicine, University of California, California, USA

15.1   Clinical Background

Therapeutic drug monitoring (TDM) consists of measurement of plasma or serum concentrations of drug for therapeutic and safety purposes. There are two purposes for TDM: (1) Ensure therapeutic concentrations consistent with efficacy, and (2) Ensure safety, particularly for those drugs with a narrow therapeutic index. Therapeutic index is the ratio of the "adverse event EC50" to the "therapeutic effect EC50," where EC50 is the effective concentration of the drug that yields 50% of the maximal response.

TDM is indicated because of marked inter-individual variability in pharmacokinetics of certain drugs among patients. It is most useful when attempting to avoid toxicity of drugs with narrow therapeutic indices, when it is difficult to detect the clinical end point of therapy, when the therapeutic range is narrow, and when target ranges have been validated in the species of interest. Unfortunately, very few drugs have therapeutic targets specifically validated for use in horses. Most are extrapolated from humans, which can be dangerous for drugs with marked species differences in pharmacokinetics.

In addition, it is important to become familiar with laboratory specific therapeutic ranges, as results may vary with the specific assay used, such as ELISA or radioimmunoassay.

15.2   Tests Available

The most common drugs for which TDM is performed in horses are the aminoglycosides. TDM is available for additional drugs as well:

1) Aminoglycosides: amikacin and gentamicin
2) Bromide (potassium or sodium)
3) Digoxin
4) Phenobarbital
5) Phenytoin
6) Quinidine
7) Theophylline

15.3   Sample Collection and Submission

TDM should be performed at steady state in most instances. Steady state concentrations occur after 4–5 half-lives of the specific drug. For drugs with dosing intervals far exceeding their half-lives and do not accumulate, such as aminoglycosides, there is no steady state period achieved and each dose is independent of preceding doses, for the most part. Besides the aminoglycosides, all of the drugs listed above should be sampled at steady state, unless loading doses are used, for TDM. With loading doses, sampling for TDM should be done at the end of the loading dose, after one half-life to ensure the loading concentrations are maintained, and again at steady state. It should be noted that bromide has a very long half-life in horses. Potassium bromide has a half-life of $75 \pm 14\,h$ $(3.1 \pm 0.6\,days)$, and sodium bromide has a half-life of $126\,h$, or $5.2\,days$ (Raidal and Edwards, 2008, Fielding et al., 2003). Therefore, steady state for these drugs would be reached at approximately 12–15 and 21–26 days, respectively.

Sample collection includes serum or plasma, depending on the laboratory requirements. The samples should be spun, with serum or plasma removed. The serum or plasma should be stored in plastic tubes for aminoglycosides (aminoglycosides bind to glass), glass for digoxin, and then refrigerated until shipped with overnight delivery while kept cool. Serum separator tubes should not be used, as many drugs can bind to the silicone gel. Laboratories should be consulted as to optimal tube type for the other drugs, depending on assay used.

TDM of aminoglycosides consists of running peak and trough concentrations. The purpose of the peak is to

Interpretation of Equine Laboratory Diagnostics, First Edition. Edited by Nicola Pusterla and Jill Higgins.
© 2018 John Wiley & Sons, Inc. Published 2018 by John Wiley & Sons, Inc.

ensure concentrations consistent with efficacy, whereas the purpose of the trough is to ensure safety.

For any drug, peak concentrations should be taken early after administration and prior to significant elimination of the drug, but after the distribution phase has been completed. For aminoglycosides, peaks are generally measured 30–60 min after IV administration. The author prefers a 60-min peak to ensure that the distribution phase has been completed, however some clinicians interpret 30-min peaks. Either is fine, as long as this is done with consistency for the clinician to become accustomed with results and uses similar interpretation among horses or foals.

For other drugs, peak concentrations are generally measured at 1–2 h post dosing for orally administered drugs, except for those with slow absorption. For example, peaks for phenobarbital can be measured at 2–5 h post-administration.

Trough concentrations are usually taken just prior to the next dose, especially when it is important for the lowest plasma concentration to still be within the therapeutic range, as for anticonvulsant medications. When the trough concentration is allowed to be sub-therapeutic, and needs to be below specific concentrations in order to avoid toxicity, then the trough is measured to ensure safety, as for aminoglycosides. In this case, troughs are measured at 20–24 h (just before the next dose), as is done for aminoglycosides to ensure that concentrations are consistent with lack of accumulation within the renal tubules. If pharmacokinetic parameters such as half-life are desired to be calculated, then a third plasma or serum sample should be obtained at a few hours (5–8 h) after administration, because the 20–24-h trough samples are often below the limit of quantification of the assay for aminoglycosides and therefore cannot be used in pharmacokinetic analyses.

Single sample TDM can be used for drugs which must remain within the therapeutic range throughout the dosing interval, and when the peak concentration is not critical. This sample would be taken just before the next dose, to evaluate the lowest plasma concentration. This ensures that the minimum plasma concentration is still therapeutic.

15.4 Possible Results

The results obtained from TDM analysis will be presented as serum or plasma concentrations of drug. Each of the drugs has specific targets for TDM. Some of these targets are based on data from horses, whereas many are extrapolated from human and small animal pharmacology. As such, they must be interpreted with caution and in light of clinical and clinicopathological findings.

15.4.1 Therapeutic Drug Monitoring of Aminoglycosides

1) Amikacin results (use plastic tubes):
   a) *Peak*
      Optimally, the peak concentration should be 8–10× the minimum inhibitory concentration (MIC) of the offending microbe whenever a culture is present. For example, if the MIC is 2 μg/mL, then the desired peak concentration should be ≥ 16–20 μg/mL.
      If no MIC is available, then a target peak of ≥ 40 μg/mL should be used for the 1 h peak. If a 30-minute peak is used, then a concentration of ≥ 53–60 μg/mL has been recommended (Bucky et al., 2004, Palmer, 2014).
   b) *Trough*
      The optimal trough concentration for amikacin has not been worked out for horses. Recent recommendations include a trough concentration of < 2 μg/mL. The author prefers to sample the trough concentration at 20 h post-administration, to ensure a minimum of a 4 h interval to allow for tubular cells to evacuate accumulated aminoglycosides.

   Because amikacin is administered once daily and is not intended to accumulate, TDM can be monitored after the first dose (i.e., it never achieves steady state).

2) Gentamicin (use plastic tubes):
   a) *Peak*
      Optimally, the peak should be 8–10× the MIC of the offending microbe whenever a culture is present. If no MIC is available, then a target peak of ≥ 20 μg/mL should be used for the 1 h peak concentration. If a 30-min peak is used, then a concentration of ≥ 30–40 μg/mL has been recommended (Palmer, 2014, Bauquier et al., 2015, Burton et al., 2012).
   b) *Trough*
      The optimal trough concentration for gentamicin has not been worked out for horses and is based on experience and data in humans. Recent recommendations include a trough concentration of < 1 μg/mL. The author prefers to sample the trough concentration at 20 h post-administration, rather than just before the next daily dose (i.e., 24 h mark), to ensure a minimum of a 4-h interval which would allow for tubular cells to evacuate accumulated aminoglycosides.

   Because gentamicin is administered once daily and is intended not to accumulate, TDM can be monitored after the first dose (i.e., it never achieves steady state).

15.4.2 Other Drugs

Most TDM targets have been extrapolated from other species. Others have been modified from those in humans based on experience. Therefore, horses or foals treated with these medications should be monitored closely for clinical efficacy and safety, rather than simply relying on TDM.

1) Bromide (Na or K): The therapeutic target is 1.0–1.5 mg/mL (this can be measured anytime once steady state is achieved, which occurs at 12–15 days for KBr and 21–26 days for NaBr.)
2) Digoxin: The therapeutic range is 0.5–1.5 ng/mL (use glass tubes). Measure peak [1 h] and trough [just before next dose] (Jesty, 2014).
3) Phenobarbital: The therapeutic range is 14–45 μg/mL (peak at 2 h post oral administration, trough just before next dose). In the author's experience, many horses are controlled in terms of seizures with plasma concentrations below 14 μg/mL. Therefore, clinical efficacy, defined as abolition of seizures without excessive sedation, is likely more important than solely relying on plasma concentrations. Further, the half-life of phenobarbital can be quite prolonged in neonatal foals, therefore trough concentrations are quite important.
4) Phenytoin: Therapeutic concentrations are recommended as 5–10 μg/mL as "total" phenytoin, measured 2 h after oral administration. Toxic plasma concentrations are > 10 μg/mL (Sleeper, 2015, Wijnberg and Ververs, 2004).
5) Quinidine: The therapeutic range is 2–5 μg/mL. Toxicity occurs at concentrations > 5 μg/mL (Jesty, 2014).
6) Theophylline: The therapeutic range is 5–12 μg/mL. Toxicity occurs at concentrations > 15–20 μg/mL. Erythromycin and enrofloxacin may inhibit the metabolism of theophylline (Mazan and Ceresia, 2015).

15.5   Interpretation

1) Gentamicin:
   a) *Peak goals*
      i) 10× MIC of the offending microbe at 1 h, Or if no culture is available:
      ii) 30-min peak goal: ≥ 30–40 μg/mL (Bauquier et al., 2015, Burton et al., 2012)
      iii) 60-min peak goal: ≥ 20 μg/mL
   b) *Trough goals*
   c) Trough < 1 μg/mL at 20–24 h</LSL>
2) Amikacin:
   a) *Peak goals*
      iv) 10× MIC of the offending microbe at 1 h, Or if no culture is available:
      v) 30-min peak goal: ≥ 53–60 μg/mL
      vi) 60-min peak goal: ≥ 40 μg/mL
   b) *Trough goals*
      <2 μg/mL at 20–24 h
3) Bromide (Na or K): The therapeutic range is 1.0–1.5 mg/mL
4) Digoxin: The therapeutic range is 0.5–1.5 ng/mL
5) Phenobarbital: The therapeutic range is 14–45 μg/mL
6) Phenytoin: The therapeutic range is 5–10 μg/mL as "total" phenytoin; Toxic plasma concentrations are >10 μg/mL (Sleeper, 2015, Wijnberg and Ververs, 2004).
7) Quinidine: The therapeutic range is 2–5 μg/mL. Toxicity occurs at concentrations >5 μg/mL (Jesty, 2014).
8) Theophylline: The therapeutic range is 5–12 μg/mL. Toxicity occurs at concentrations >15–20 μg/mL.

15.6   Case Example

A 12-year old Quarter Horse gelding was treated for a protein-losing enteropathy. Because of marked neutropenia and immature neutrophilia (bands) on the complete blood count, the horse was treated with gentamicin in order to protect against bacterial translocation. Because there was no isolate from which to target desired peak concentrations (8–10× MIC), a target of ≥20 μg/mL was used. The horse was treated with 7 mg/kg of gentamicin IV once daily (q 24 h).

A 1-h post-administration peak gentamicin concentration was 20.5 μg/mL. A 20-h post trough concentration was <0.3 μg/mL. The peak and trough concentrations were within targets.

References

Bauquier R, Boston RC, Sweeney RW, Wilkins PA, and Nolen-Walston RD. 2015. Plasma peak and trough gentamicin concentrations in hospitalized horses receiving intravenously administered gentamicin. J Vet Intern Med 29: 1660–1666.

Bucky EP, Giguere S, MacPherson M, and Davis R. 2004. Pharmacokinetics of once-daily amikacin in healthy foals and therapeutic drug monitoring in hospitalized equine neonates. J Vet Int Med 18: 729–733.

Burton AJ, Giguere S, Warner L, Alhamhoom Y, and Arnold RD. 2012. Effect of age on the pharmacokinetics of a single daily dose of gentamicin sulfate in healthy foals. Eq Vet J 1–5.

Fielding CL, Magdesian KG, Elliott DA, Craigmill AL, Wilson WD, and Carlson GP. 2003. Pharmacokinetics and clinical utility of sodium bromide (NaBr) as an estimator of extracellular fluid volume in horses. J Vet Int Med 17: 213–217.

Jesty S. 2014. Cardiovascular system. In JA Orsini and TJ Divers (eds), *Equine Emergencies Treatment and Procedures*, St Louis, MO: Elsevier Saunders, p. 131.

Mazan MR and Ceresia ML. 2015. Clinical pharmacology of the respiratory system. In C Ole, B Benz, L Maxwell (eds), *Equine Pharmacology*, Ames: Wiley-Blackwell, p. 167.

Palmer J. 2014. Update on the management of neonatal sepsis in horses. Vet Clin Equine 30: 317–336.

Raidal SL and Edwards S. 2008. Pharmacokinetics of potassium bromide in adult horses. Aust Vet J, 86: 187–193.

Sleeper M. 2015. Equine cardiovascular clinical pharmacology. In C Ole, B Benz, L Maxwell (eds), *Equine Pharmacology*, Ames: Wiley-Blackwell, p. 286.

Wijnberg ID and Ververs FFT. 2004. Phenytoin sodium as a treatment for ventricular dysrhythmia in horses. J Vet Int Med 18: 350–353.

16

Red Blood Cells
Jed Overmann

Veterinary Clinical Sciences Department, College of Veterinary Medicine, University of Minnesota, Minnesota, USA

16.1 Introduction

Circulating red blood cells (RBCs) along with their precursors in the bone marrow are collectively referred to as the erythron. Alterations in the erythron such as anemia and erythrocytosis are common in clinical practice. As a result, it is important for the equine clinician to be familiar with the laboratory diagnostics used to evaluate the erythron, understand interpretation of results, and to be able to reach a conclusion or develop a diagnostic plan based on the combination of laboratory data, clinical history, and physical exam findings.

16.2 Laboratory Diagnostics

Always vitally important for the generation of quality laboratory data is appropriate sample collection and handling, and the reader is referred to Chapter 1 for a full discussion. The mainstay in evaluation of the erythron is the complete blood count (CBC), which should include both numeric data (i.e., that generated by an automated hematology analyzer) and morphologic assessment (ie microscopic evaluation of a peripheral blood smear). In some cases, however, additional diagnostics are needed to more fully assess the RBC population and to determine an underlying cause for an anemia, erythrocytosis, or other RBC abnormality.

16.2.1 CBC

- *Hematocrit (HCT), RBC count, and hemoglobin (Hgb) concentration*: The HCT is the percentage volume of blood occupied by RBCs. When reported as part of a CBC this is most often a calculated value determined from the RBC count and mean cell volume (MCV). A spun HCT or packed cell volume (PCV) is determined by centrifugation of a microhematocrit tube. The RBC count and Hgb concentration are values that are directly measured by automated hematology analyzers. HCT, RBC count, and Hgb concentration tend to increase and decrease together since they are all indicators of the RBC content of blood.

- *MCV*: The MCV is the average volume of an RBC and is directly measured by most hematology analyzers. An increased MCV can be seen in some cases of regenerative anemia, while a decreased MCV may indicate iron-deficiency anemia and is also described as an age-related change in foals (Grondin and DeWitt, 2010).

- *Mean cell hemoglobin (MCH) and mean cell hemoglobin concentration (MCHC)*: These values are derived from the RBC count, Hgb concentration, and MCV and describe the hemoglobin content or concentration of RBCs. MCHC is typically considered more useful compared to MCH, as cell size is taken into consideration in the calculation of MCHC. An increased MCHC is generally an artifact due to causes such as hemolysis (pathologic or *in vitro*), lipemia, icterus, or the presence of large number of Heinz bodies. Decreased MCHC can be seen with iron-deficiency anemia.

- *Red cell distribution width (RDW)*: The RDW is reported on some CBCs and is a measure of variation in the volume of RBCs in a patient. It most often represents the coefficient of variation in measured RBC volumes used to determine the MCV. Increased numbers of small and/or large RBCs will increase the RDW. RDW may be increased in some cases of regenerative anemia, but is not a reliable indicator.

- *RBC morphology*: The following are either common or diagnostically important RBC morphologies that are assessed through evaluation of a peripheral blood film.
  - *Rouleaux*: This is the stacking of RBCs in a somewhat linear formation often described as appearing like "stacks of coins." Rouleaux is common in blood from healthy horses, but can be enhanced by hyperproteinemia (Figure 16.1A).

Interpretation of Equine Laboratory Diagnostics, First Edition. Edited by Nicola Pusterla and Jill Higgins.
© 2018 John Wiley & Sons, Inc. Published 2018 by John Wiley & Sons, Inc.

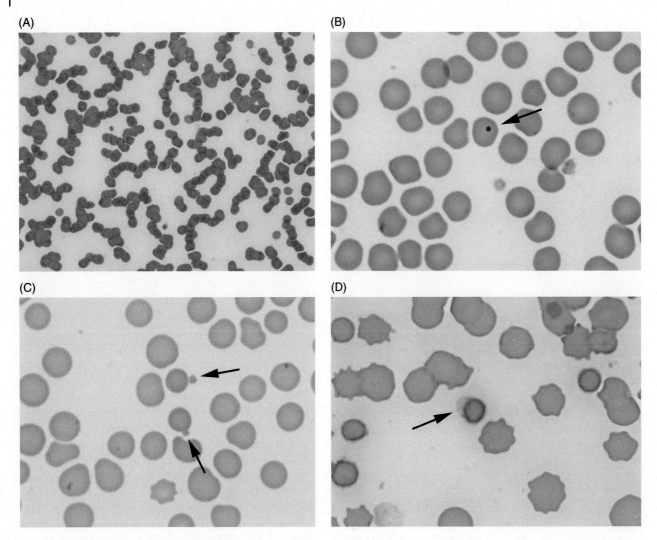

Figure 16.1 (A–D) Equine peripheral blood films. Modified Wright-Giemsa stain. (A) Rouleaux. (B) RBC containing a Howell-Jolly body. (C) Two RBCs with Heinz bodies. (D) Eccentrocyte.

- *Agglutination*: Agglutination is the result of antibody mediated bridging of RBCs and is seen in some cases of immune-mediated hemolytic anemia. True agglutination should be confirmed (and differentiated from prominent rouleaux or other non-specific RBC association) by means of a saline dilution test. The saline dilution test is accomplished by diluting whole blood with saline (generally at 1:2 or 1:4) and evaluating a wet preparation. Rouleaux will disperse with dilution, while true agglutination should persist.
- *Howell-Jolly bodies and anisocytosis:* Howell-Jolly bodies are small, dark, round nuclear fragments in RBCs, and anisocytosis describes variation in the size of RBCs. Small numbers of Howell-Jolly bodies and mild anisocytosis can be normal findings on equine blood films (Figure 16.1B).
- *Heinz bodies:* Heinz bodies are the result of oxidative damage and represent precipitated Hgb attached to the RBC membrane. With Romanowsky-type stains

they often appear as a rounded, pale pink to red projections from the RBC membrane (Figure 16.1C). The presence of Heinz bodies can be confirmed with a new methylene blue stain where they will appear as dark, round, refractile inclusions. Heinz bodies have been reported in horses due to ingestion of oxidants such as dried red maple leaves, onion, and garlic (Pierce et al., 1972, Pearson et al., 2005, Alward et al., 2006). RBCs that contain Heinz bodies are more susceptible to both intravascular and extravascular hemolysis.

- *Eccentrocytes*: Eccentrocytes form from partial fusion of RBC membranes as a result of oxidative damage (Figure 16.1D). Causes listed for Heinz body formation can also cause eccentrocytes. In addition, eccentrocytes have been described with glucose-6-phosphate dehydrogenase deficiency, flavin adenine dinucleotide deficiency as well as suspected *Pistacia* spp. ingestion (Harvey, 2006, Walter et al., 2014).

– *Infectious agents:* Infectious agents causing anemia such as *Babesia caballi* and *Theileria equi* are sometimes identified by peripheral blood film review. False negative results with these organisms, however, are not uncommon due to a low percentage of parasitized RBCs (Wise et al., 2014).

Coombs' Test: see Chapter 41.
Blood Typing/Cross-matching: see Chapter 47.

16.3 Effects of Age, Breed, Sex, and Physiologic Factors

A more complete discussion of the effects of age, breed, sex, and physiologic factors on laboratory evaluators of the erythron can be found elsewhere (Grondin and DeWitt, 2010). Some of the more common and significant factors are discussed here, however. "Hot-blooded" breeds (e.g., Arabian and Thoroughbred) have higher HCT, RBC count, and Hgb concentration when compared to "Cold-blooded" horses (e.g., draft breeds and some ponies). HCT in foals is relatively higher at birth, drops over the next 24h, then continues to decrease slowly over the next few weeks (though generally staying within the lower end of adult reference intervals). MCV in foals is high at birth and then decreases over the next several months. Some minor differences in laboratory evaluators of the erythron have been described between adult male and female horses, though these are likely of limited significance. Mares in late pregnancy and in the first few weeks postpartum may have decreasing HCT and Hgb concentrations (Grondin and DeWitt, 2010). Pain, excitement, or strenuous exercise can result in increased HCT due to splenic contraction (see relative erythrocytosis due to splenic contraction), whereas administration of sedatives and tranquilizers can lead to decreases in HCT due to splenic pooling of RBCs.

16.4 Anemia

Anemia is defined as a decrease in the HCT, RBC count, or Hgb concentration below established reference intervals. Clinical signs of anemia can include lethargy, weakness tachypnea, tachycardia, and pale mucous membranes. Whenever the equine clinician is presented with an anemic patient, the goal is to integrate the constellation of laboratory results, clinical history, and physical exam findings to identify a likely underlying pathophysiologic mechanism for the anemia.

16.4.1 Regenerative

A regenerative anemia is one in which there is a bone marrow response to either loss or destruction of RBCs.

Horses are somewhat unique in that they do not typically release reticulocytes into circulation in regenerative responses as do most other domestic species. As a result, it is more difficult to identify an anemia as regenerative in the horse because typical indicators of regeneration such as a reticulocyte count or degree of polychromasia on a peripheral blood film can't be used. It should be noted, however, that there are some reports of polychromasia and circulating reticulocytes in anemic horses (O'Neil, 2014). A regenerative response in the horse is most often evaluated by monitoring for an increase in HCT over time. Increases in MCV and RDW are seen in some cases of regenerative anemia, but are not consistently elevated. Bone marrow sampling can be performed to directly assess the marrow response if deemed clinically necessary. It generally takes about 4 days following an episode of blood loss or hemolysis for the bone marrow response to begin, and full recovery of HCT from severe blood loss or hemorrhage may take a few months. The regenerative response to hemolysis is often considered to be stronger than that seen with blood loss, possibly due to recovery of iron needed for Hgb synthesis in the case of hemolysis.

- *Blood loss:* Following significant acute hemorrhage, splenic contraction may cause the HCT to be transiently elevated above pre-hemorrhage values, and HCT and total protein concentration will not decrease until compensatory mechanisms cause redistribution of fluid into the vasculature. Decreases in total protein concentration may become evident 4–6h after hemorrhage, while anemia may not be apparent for 12h and the HCT may continue to decrease until 48h after the bleeding event. Chronic blood loss (e.g., gastrointestinal bleeding due to ulcer or neoplasia) can result in an iron-deficiency anemia typified by a decreased MCV and MCHC. In addition, visually hypochromic RBCs and small numbers of RBC fragments may also be seen on review of peripheral blood films. Iron-deficiency anemia is typically regenerative, but if prolonged may become poorly regenerative to non-regenerative. Total protein concentration may be decreased, but in some cases is within reference interval due to increased production offsetting losses. An iron panel can be helpful in confirming iron deficiency. Note that iron-deficiency anemia has also been described in foals due to low dietary intake of iron.
- *Hemolysis*: Hemolysis can be the result of a number of underlying causes including oxidative damage, immune-mediated disease, infectious diseases, iatrogenic (e.g., administration of hypotonic fluids or dimethyl sulfoxide (DMSO) at higher concentrations) and rarely liver failure (Ramaiah, 2003). Hemoglobinemia and hemoglobinuria would support an intravascular hemolytic process, while icterus and hyperbilirubinemia

are typical of extravascular hemolysis. Note that hemoglobinuria should be differentiated from myoglobinuria and hyperbilirubinemia due to causes other than hemolysis (e.g., liver disease) should be considered. RBC morphology such as Heinz bodies and/or eccentrocytes would support oxidative damage, while RBC agglutination, a positive Coombs' test, or flow cytometric identification of RBC surface associated antibody would support an immune-mediated hemolytic process. Diagnostics for infectious causes of hemolytic anemia such as equine infectious anemia virus, *Babesia caballi* and *Theileria equi* are discussed elsewhere.

16.4.2 Non-Regenerative

A non-regenerative anemia is characterized by a lack of bone marrow response. Anemia of inflammation, due to underlying infection, neoplasia, or tissue injury, is the most common cause of a mild to moderate non-regenerative anemia. Other causes of non-regenerative anemia include anemia of chronic renal failure, leukemia, lymphoma, and aplastic pancytopenia. Evaluation of bone marrow is indicated to assess an unexplained, persistent, non-regenerative anemia, especially when other cytopenias are present (Figure 16.2).

16.5 Erythrocytosis

Erythrocytosis is characterized by increases in HCT, RBC count, and Hgb concentration and can be relative or absolute in nature. In relative erythrocytosis, the increases are not reflective of a true increase in total body RBC mass, but are the result of changes in plasma volume or redistribution of RBCs into circulation. Absolute erythrocytosis, in contrast, is the result of a true increase in RBC mass. Causes of relative erythrocytosis are much more common than absolute, and should be considered or ruled out first (Figure 16.3).

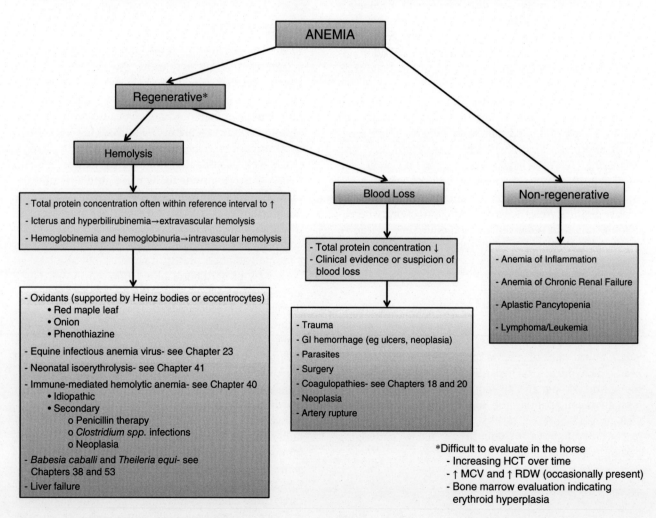

Figure 16.2 Diagnostic approach to anemia.

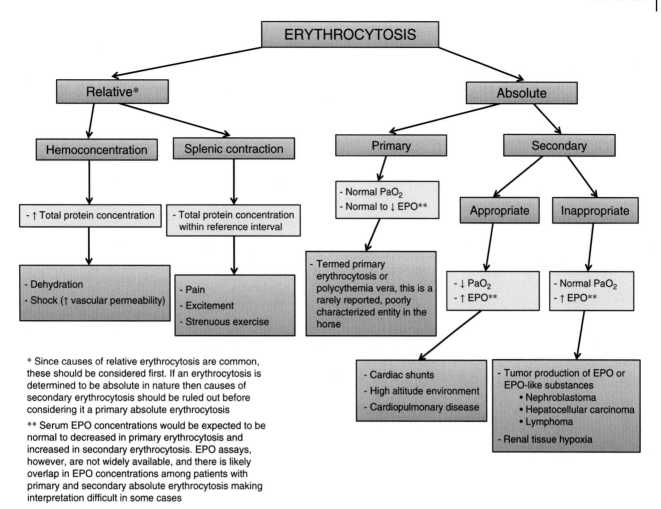

ERYTHROCYTOSIS

Relative*

Hemoconcentration
- ↑ Total protein concentration
- Dehydration
- Shock (↑ vascular permeability)

Splenic contraction
- Total protein concentration within reference interval
- Pain
- Excitement
- Strenuous exercise

Absolute

Primary
- Normal PaO$_2$
- Normal to ↓ EPO**
- Termed primary erythrocytosis or polycythemia vera, this is a rarely reported, poorly characterized entity in the horse

Secondary

Appropriate
- ↓ PaO$_2$
- ↑ EPO**
- Cardiac shunts
- High altitude environment
- Cardiopulmonary disease

Inappropriate
- Normal PaO$_2$
- ↑ EPO**
- Tumor production of EPO or EPO-like substances
  • Nephroblastoma
  • Hepatocellular carcinoma
  • Lymphoma
- Renal tissue hypoxia

* Since causes of relative erythrocytosis are common, these should be considered first. If an erythrocytosis is determined to be absolute in nature then causes of secondary erythrocytosis should be ruled out before considering it a primary absolute erythrocytosis

** Serum EPO concentrations would be expected to be normal to decreased in primary erythrocytosis and increased in secondary erythrocytosis. EPO assays, however, are not widely available, and there is likely overlap in EPO concentrations among patients with primary and secondary absolute erythrocytosis making interpretation difficult in some cases

Figure 16.3 Diagnostic approach to erythrocytosis.

16.5.1 Relative Erythrocytosis

- *Hemoconcentration*: Dehydration causes a reduction in plasma volume and effectively concentrates the RBCs and proteins in circulation. Thus, total protein concentration is often increased in these cases in addition to HCT. Clinical signs of dehydration may also be present to support this interpretation. Increased vascular permeability, as can be seen with shock, results in increased movement of fluid from the intravascular to extravascular space and is another mechanism that can result in a relative erythrocytosis due to hemoconcentration.

- *Splenic contraction*: Pain, excitement, or strenuous exercise can result in epinephrine mediated contraction of the spleen, which results in movement of high HCT splenic blood into circulation. This is a transient change and values will normalize in 40 min to a few hours. Total protein concentration is often within reference interval in these cases.

16.5.2 Absolute Erythrocytosis

- *Primary*: In other species this is considered a chronic myeloproliferative disease (primary erythrocytosis or polycythemia vera) in which production of RBCs is autonomous and requires little to no erythropoietin (EPO). Primary erythrocytosis is not well characterized in the horse and only rare reports exist (McFarlane, 1998).

- *Secondary appropriate*: This condition results from chronic systemic hypoxia which causes increased EPO mediated production of RBCs. Chronic hypoxia in these cases may be due to causes such as cardiopulmonary disease, cardiac shunts, or high altitude environment.

- *Secondary inappropriate*: In this instance there is increased EPO in the absence of systemic hypoxia. In horses, this has been reported with tumor secretion of EPO or EPO-like substances (e.g., hepatoblastoma, hepatocellular carcinoma, and lymphoma) (Roby et al., 1990, Lennox et al., 2000, Koch et al., 2006, Axon et al., 2008). Renal pathology causing localized tissue hypoxia should also be considered.

References

Alward A, Corriher CA, Barton MH, et al. 2006. Red maple (*Acer rubrum*) leaf toxicosis in horses: a retrospective study of 32 cases. J Vet Intern Med, 20: 1197–1201.

Axon JE, Russell CM, Begg AP, et al. 2008. Erythrocytosis and pleural effusion associated with a hepatoblastoma in a Thoroughbred yearling. Aust Vet J, 86: 329–333.

Grondin TM and DeWitt SF. 2010. Normal hematology of the horse and donkey. In DJ Weiss and KJ Wardrop (eds), Schalm's Veterinary Hematology, 6th Edn. Ames, IA: Wiley-Blackwell, pp. 821–828.

Harvey JW. 2006. Pathogenesis, laboratory diagnosis, and clinical implications of erythrocyte enzyme deficiencies in dogs, cats, and horses. Vet Clin Pathol, 35: 144–156.

Koch TG, Wen X, and Bienzle D. 2006. Lymphoma, erythrocytosis, and tumor erythropoietin gene expression in a horse. J Vet Intern Med, 20: 1251–1255.

Lennox TJ, Wilson JH, Hayden DW, et al. 2000. Hepatoblastoma with erythrocytosis in a young female horse. J Am Vet Med Assoc, 216: 718–721.

McFarlane D, Sellon DC, and Parker B. 1998. Primary erythrocytosis in a 2-year-old Arabian gelding. J Vet Intern Med 12: 384–388.

O'Neil E, Horney B, and Burton S. 2014. What is your diagnosis? Blood smear from a foal. Vet Clin Pathol, 43: 287–288.

Pearson W, Boermans HJ, Bettger WJ, et al. 2005. Association of maximum voluntary dietary intake of freeze-dried garlic with Heinz body anemia in horses. Am J Vet Res, 66: 457–465.

Pierce KR, Joyce JR, England RB, et al. 1972. Acute hemolytic anemia caused by wild onion poisoning in horses. J Am Vet Med Assoc, 160: 323–327.

Ramaiah SK, Harvey JW, Giguère S, et al. 2003. Intravascular hemolysis associated with liver disease in a horse with marked neutrophil hypersegmentation. J Vet Intern Med 17: 360–363.

Roby KA, Beech J, Bloom JC, et al. 1990. Hepatocellular carcinoma associated with erythrocytosis and hypoglycemia in a yearling filly. J Am Vet Med Assoc, 196: 465–467.

Walter KM, Moore CE, Bozorgmanesh R, et al. 2014. Oxidant-induced damage to equine erythrocytes from exposure to *Pistacia atlantica*, *Pistacia terebinthus*, and *Pistacia chinensis*. J Vet Diagn Invest, 26: 821–826.

Wise LN, Pelzel-McCluskey AM, Mealey RH, et al. 2014. Equine piroplasmosis. Vet Clin Equine, 30: 677–693.

17

Leukocytes
Jed Overmann

Veterinary Clinical Sciences Department, College of Veterinary Medicine, University of Minnesota, Minnesota, USA

17.1 Introduction

Leukocytes or white blood cells (WBCs) are routinely evaluated to screen for processes such as inflammation or hematopoietic neoplasia or to monitor for progression or resolution of disease. The ability to interpret individual abnormalities and patterns of abnormalities present in the leukocyte populations is important to the equine clinician, and when findings are integrated with physical exam, clinical history, and other laboratory results (e.g., serum chemistry profile, urinalysis, etc.) they can provide valuable diagnostic information.

17.2 Leukocyte Production and Kinetics

Leukocytes are a heterogeneous group consisting of morphologically and functionally distinct cell types that include the neutrophil, eosinophil, basophil, monocyte, and lymphocyte. Neutrophils, eosinophils, and basophils are collectively referred to as granulocytes. Production of granulocytes and monocytes occurs in the bone marrow, whereas lymphocyte production in the adult animal takes place primarily in lymphoid tissues, such as lymph node and spleen.

As neutrophil precursors mature in the bone marrow they go through a series of morphologically distinct stages. Eventually they progress to the segmented neutrophil stage where they populate the bone marrow storage pool and are available for release into circulation. The segmented neutrophils in the bone marrow storage pool are released first during times of increased demand, however, less mature cells (e.g., band neutrophils) can be released if the storage pool is depleted. Once neutrophils are in circulation they can be found in either the circulating pool or marginated pool. The circulating pool consists of cells freely flowing in the vasculature and is the

population assessed when acquiring a sample for a complete blood count (CBC). The marginated pool consists of those neutrophils temporarily adhered to endothelial cells. In health, these two pools contain approximately equal numbers of leukocytes (Carakostas et al., 1981). Shifts between the circulating and marginated neutrophil pools are important mechanisms that drive neutrophilia or neutropenia in some cases. The half-life of neutrophils in circulation is about 10.5 h, after which they migrate into tissues (e.g., sites of inflammation, or in health, respiratory and GI tissues) (Carakostas et al., 1981).

Eosinophils, basophils, and monocytes produced in the bone marrow are released into circulation where they reside in similar pools as those described for neutrophils before migrating into tissues. Monocytes, once in the tissues, have the capacity to differentiate into a variety of subtypes of cells of the mononuclear phagocyte system.

Lymphocytes produced in lymphoid tissues can enter blood where they are distributed into circulating and marginated pools. Lymphocytes that enter tissues may recirculate via lymphatics.

17.3 Laboratory Diagnostics

Laboratory evaluation of leukocytes is primarily accomplished by means of a CBC. Information on the CBC describing the leukocyte populations is collectively referred to as the leukogram and should include a total leukocyte concentration, leukocyte differential including absolute concentrations of each leukocyte type, and morphologic assessment of leukocytes. Proper sample acquisition and handling are critical for generation of quality laboratory data, and the reader is referred to Chapter 1 for a full discussion. The preferred sample for analysis in most cases is EDTA anticoagulated whole blood and it is ideal if sending blood to a reference lab for analysis to also include unstained freshly prepared blood films.

Interpretation of Equine Laboratory Diagnostics, First Edition. Edited by Nicola Pusterla and Jill Higgins.
© 2018 John Wiley & Sons, Inc. Published 2018 by John Wiley & Sons, Inc.

- *Total leukocyte concentration:* This value is typically generated by an automated hematology analyzer. Manual counts using a hemocytometer are sometimes performed when an automated count is not readily available.
- *Leukocyte differential and absolute concentrations:* While some hematology analyzers provide automated leukocyte differentials, a manual differential based on microscopic evaluation of a peripheral blood film is considered the "gold standard" and is the basis for the leukocyte differential and absolute concentrations provided by most academic and reference laboratories. When performing CBCs in-house on a point of care hematology analyzer, microscopic assessment of the leukocyte differential is advised (Flatland et al., 2013).
- *Microscopic evaluation of a peripheral blood film:* As indicated before, this is the gold standard for determining the leukocyte differential. In addition, the blood film can be evaluated for other important morphologic or diagnostic findings such as the presence of band neutrophils, toxic changes, atypical cells/blasts, and presence of infectious organisms (e.g., *Anaplasma phagocytophilum*).

17.4 Leukocyte Morphology and Interpretation of Abnormal Values

17.4.1 Neutrophils

Neutrophils have relatively clear cytoplasm that can contain dust-like pink granules depending on the stain that is used. Nuclei are segmented and nuclear chromatin is clumped (Figure 17.1A). Abnormal neutrophil morphology identified by review of a peripheral blood film may include toxic changes and a left shift. *Toxic changes* are identified by increased cytoplasmic basophilia, foamy appearing cytoplasm, Döhle bodies, and rarely other alterations such as toxic granulation or increased cell size (Figure 17.1B–C). Together these changes are graded subjectively and typically reported on a 1+ to 4+ scale. Toxic changes are observed in neutrophils during times of increased production and their presence is most often associated with inflammation. A *left shift* is defined as the presence of increased numbers of nonsegmented neutrophils in circulation. Most often these nonsegmented neutrophils consist of band neutrophils (Figure 17.1B–C). Left shifts are most often seen associated with significant inflammation in which the bone marrow storage pools of segmented neutrophils have been depleted and thus earlier forms are being released into circulation in an attempt to keep up with peripheral demand. In severe inflammatory processes, in addition to band neutrophils, small numbers of earlier neutrophil precursors such as metamyelocytes and myelocytes may occasionally be seen. A left shift is termed "degenerative" when the nonsegmented neutrophils outnumber the segmented neutrophils, a condition that is associated with a guarded prognosis since this is usually seen with severe inflammation. Toxic changes and left shifts are often seen concurrently. Pelger-Huët anomaly is an asymptomatic congenital condition that results in hyposegmentation of granulocyte nuclei and thus may mimic the appearance of a severe left shift (Grondin et al., 2007). Infectious organisms, notably *Anaplasma phagocytophilum* can be identified in circulating neutrophils during review of peripheral blood films. *Anaplasma phagocytophilum* morulae appear as variably sized, granular, blue-gray inclusions within the cytoplasm of neutrophils (Figure 17.1D).

Neutrophilia

- *Inflammation*: Inflammation is a common cause of neutrophilia and while this is often elicited by an infectious process, immune-mediated disease, surgery, neoplasia, or tissue trauma may also result in a neutrophilia. A left shift and/or toxic changes would support the interpretation of inflammation; however, these features may not always be present, especially if the process is chronic or mild in nature (i.e., situations where bone marrow production and release of neutrophils may keep up with peripheral demand). It should also be noted that inflammatory processes can be present in horses with normal neutrophil concentrations. In these cases, the identification of a left shift, toxic changes, or increased fibrinogen concentration would be helpful in supporting the presence of inflammation.
- *Corticosteroid effects*: Increased corticosteroids are another common cause of neutrophilia and can result from either endogenous release as can be seen with systemic illness or pain, or with administration of an exogenous source. Corticosteroids mediate a neutrophilia through increased release of bone marrow storage pools of mature neutrophils and a shift of neutrophils from the marginated pool to the circulating neutrophil pool. The leukocytosis and neutrophilia are generally moderate and a left shift and toxic change should be absent. Lymphopenia and potentially eosinopenia are also seen due to corticosteroid effects.
- *Epinephrine effects*: Epinephrine effects or a "physiologic leukocytosis" are seen secondary to pain, excitement, or vigorous exercise, which results in catecholamine induced hemodynamic changes that cause neutrophils in the marginated pool to shift to the circulating pool. Neutrophilia is generally mild to moderate and a left shift and toxic changes are absent. A moderate lymphocytosis is also seen in many cases. The leukocytosis is transient and values will normalize in 30 min to an hour once the stimulus is removed. Epinephrine effects are seen

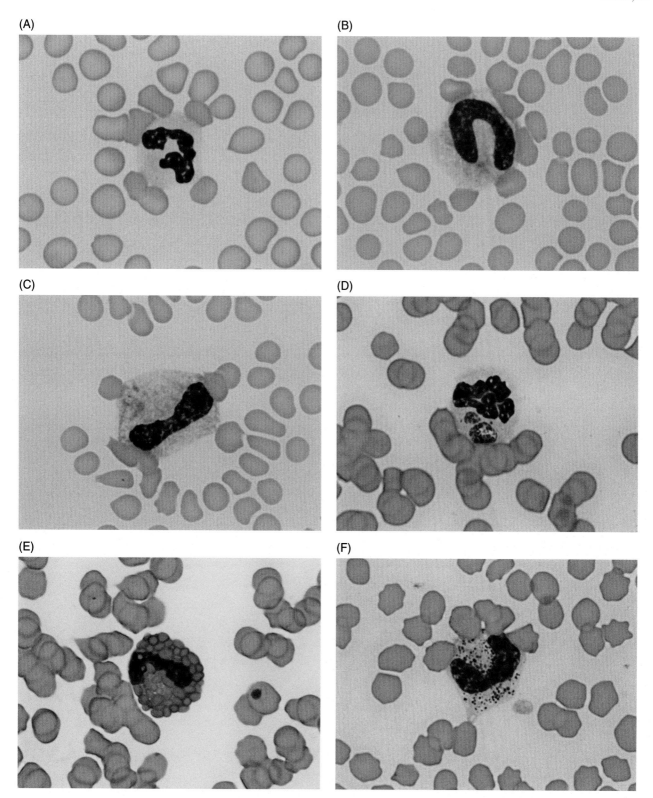

Figure 17.1 (A–I) Peripheral blood films. Equine leukocytes. Modified Wright-Giemsa stain. (A) Segmented neutrophil. (B–C) Toxic band neutrophils. (D) Morulae of *Anaplasma phagocytophilum* in a neutrophil. (E) Eosinophil. (F) Basophil.

(G)

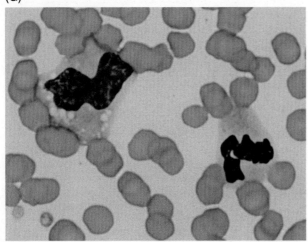

(H)

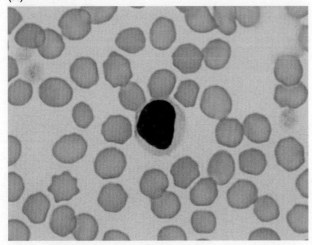

(I)

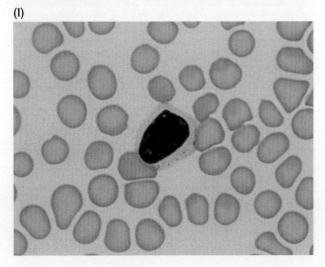

Figure 17.1 (Cont'd) (G) Monocyte (left) and segmented neutrophil (right). (H) Small lymphocyte. (I) Small lymphocyte with cytoplasmic granules.

especially in young, hot-blooded horses and those animals that are not used to being handled.

Neutropenia

- *Inflammatory neutropenia*: Neutropenia can be seen with severe acute inflammatory processes which result in an overwhelming tissue demand and depletion of bone marrow storage pools of neutrophils. Endotoxemia can also result in neutropenia due to a rapid shift of neutrophils from the circulating to marginated neutrophil pools. Toxic changes and a left shift of variable severity may be present. The persistence or worsening of neutropenia, toxic changes, or left shift would be associated with a guarded or unfavorable prognosis.
- *Other*: Other causes of neutropenia include *Anaplasma phagocytophilum* infection, alloimmune neonatal neutropenia, and myelophthisis (e.g., leukemia, lymphoma) (Muñoz et al., 2009, Meyer et al., 2006, Wong et al., 2012; Siska et al., 2013). Bone marrow aspiration and core biopsy would be indicated in cases of persistent unexplained neutropenia, especially when accompanied by other unexplained cytopenias.

17.4.2 Eosinophils

Equine eosinophils have a very characteristic appearance with large reddish-orange cytoplasmic granules that may distort the cellular borders and somewhat obscure the lobulated nucleus (Figure 17.1E).

Eosinophilia: In general, eosinophilia is not common in the horse and when present tends to be relatively mild. Many animals with parasitic infections/infestations, lack a peripheral eosinophilia, but it can occasionally be present (Jain, 1986). Parasites with a tissue migration phase may be more likely to induce a peripheral eosinophilia. Hypersensitivity reactions and idiopathic causes have also been described (Jain, 1986, Schumacher et al., 2000, Bell et al., 2008). Finally, it should also be noted that significant tissue infiltration of eosinophils can be present in the absence of peripheral eosinophilia.

Eosinopenia: Eosinopenia is difficult to identify in the horse as eosinophil concentrations in healthy animals are low. Eosinopenia, however, is described to be a component of a corticosteroid mediated leukogram and may also be seen with acute inflammatory processes.

17.4.3 Basophils

Basophils have a lobed nucleus and clear to light blue cytoplasm that contains variable numbers of purple granules (Figure 17.1 F). Nuclei are often somewhat hyposegmented compared to neutrophil nuclei.

Table 17.1 Common leukogram patterns.

Pattern	Total WBC concentration	Neutrophils	Left shift	Toxic change	Lymphocytes	Monocytes	Comments
Inflammation	↑	↑	+/-	+/-	See comments	WRI-↑	Lymphocytes may be ↓ in acute inflammation or WRI to ↑ with chronic inflammation. Left shift and toxic change may be absent especially in mild or chronic inflammatory processes
Overwhelming inflammation/ Endotoxin	↓	↓	+/-	+/-	WRI-↓	WRI	Persistence or worsening of neutropenia, left shift, and toxic change suggest a guarded to unfavorable prognosis
Epinephrine effects	↑	↑	-	-	↑	WRI-↑	Leukocytosis is mild to moderate. Transient change.
Corticosteroid effects	↑	↑	-	-	↓	WRI	Leukocytosis is mild to moderate. Eosinopenia may also be a component, but is difficult to detect

WRI = Within reference interval

Basophilia: Rare in horses and when present is often associated with causes of eosinophilia such as hypersensitivity reactions.

Basopenia: Considered clinically insignificant and is difficult to identify as healthy animals have very few circulating basophils.

17.4.4 Monocytes

Monocytes have a variably shaped nucleus (e.g., oval, lobed, horse-shoe shaped, or irregular) and gray-blue cytoplasm with fine azurophilic granules (Figure 17.1G). A few clear vacuoles may also be seen in the cytoplasm of some cells.

Monocytosis: May be seen with inflammation or tissue necrosis.

Monocytopenia: Considered clinically insignificant, and is difficult to identify as healthy animals have relatively few circulating monocytes.

17.4.5 Lymphocytes

The majority of lymphocytes seen in peripheral blood are small (i.e., smaller than neutrophils), but small numbers of larger lymphocytes may also be present. Small lymphocytes have a round, dark-staining nucleus, clumped chromatin, and small amounts of basophilic cytoplasm (Figure 17.1H). A minority of lymphocytes may have small numbers of magenta granules visible within their cytoplasm (Figure 17.1I). Larger lymphocytes tend to have more cytoplasm and a lighter-staining nucleus with a less clumped chromatin pattern. Reactive lymphocytes are characterized by morphologic features such as increased amounts of cytoplasm, increased cytoplasmic basophilia, perinuclear clearings, and irregular nuclear shapes. The presence of reactive lymphocytes suggests antigenic stimulation in a patient.

Lymphocytosis: The most common cause of lymphocytosis in the horse is due to epinephrine mediated effects,

but increases due to antigenic stimulation or lymphoid neoplasia may also occasionally be seen.

Lymphopenia: Corticosteroid effects (endogenous or exogenous) and acute infection or inflammation are more common causes of lymphopenia. Though an uncommon cause of lymphopenia, decreased lymphocyte concentrations may be seen with severe combined immunodeficiency syndrome in Arabian foals and common variable immunodeficiency (Crismand Scarratt, 2008, Flaminio et al., 2009).

17.5 General Considerations

- Reference intervals are often established using a range of breeds and ages, though some labs may provide more specific reference intervals (e.g., hot-blooded vs cold-blooded).

- Leukocytosis of up to 20,000 WBCs/µL is common and considered mild to moderate, 20,000–30,000 WBCs/µL is marked, and >30,000 WBCs/µL is relatively uncommon and considered extreme.

- CBC data provide a description of leukocyte populations at a single point in time. Serial testing is important in some cases to monitor for progression or resolution of abnormalities.

- Common leukogram patterns in the horse include inflammatory neutrophilia and neutropenia, epinephrine effects, and corticosteroid effects. General findings for these patterns are summarized in Table 17.1. More than one process or pattern can be present in some patients.

- Hematopoietic neoplasia (e.g., leukemia and lymphoma) is relatively uncommon in the horse, but would be suspected when atypical cells/blasts are present in circulation and/or when extremely high leukocyte concentrations are encountered. Concurrent cytopenias (e.g., anemia, thrombocytopenia, neutropenia) may also be seen in these cases due to myelophthisis and disruption of the bone marrow microenvironment.

References

Bell SA, Drew CP, Wilson WD, et al. 2008. Idiopathic chronic eosinophilic pneumonia in 7 horses. J Vet Intern Med, 22: 648–653.

Carakostas MC, Moore WE, and Smith JE. 1981. Intravascular neutrophilic granulocyte kinetics in horses. Am J Vet Res, 42: 623–625.

Crisman MV and Scarratt WK. 2008. Immunodeficiency disorders in horses. Vet Clin N Am Equine, 24: 299–310.

Flaminio MJBF, Tallmadge RL, Salles-Gomes COM, et al. 2009. Common Variable Immunodeficiency in horses is characterized by B cell depletion in primary and secondary lymphoid tissues. J Clin Immunol, 29: 107–116.

Flatland B, Freeman KP, Vap LM, et al. 2013. ASVCP Guidelines: Quality assurance for point- of-care testing in veterinary medicine, Available online at: www.asvcp. org/pubs/qas/index.cfm (retrieved December 16, 2014).

Grondin TM, DeWitt SF, and Keeton KS. 2007. Pelger-Huët anomaly in an Arabian horse. Vet Clin Pathol, 36: 306–310.

Jain NC. 1986. *Schalm's Veterinary Hematology*. 4th Edn. Philadelphia, PA: Lea & Febiger.

Meyer J, Delay J, and Bienzle D. 2006. Clinical, laboratory, and histopathologic features of equine lymphoma. Vet Pathol, 43: 914–924.

Muñoz A, Riber C, Trigo P, et al. 2009. Hematopoietic neoplasias in horses: myeloproliferative and lymphoproliferative disorders. J Equine Sci 20: 59–72.

Schumacher J, Edwards JF, and Cohen N. 2000. Chronic idiopathic inflammatory bowel diseases of the horse. J Vet Intern Med, 14: 258–265.

Siska WD, Tuttle RE, Messick JB, et al. 2013. Clinicopathologic characterization of six cases of equine granulocytic anaplasmosis in a nonendemic area (2008–2011). J Equine Vet Sci, 33: 653–657.

Wong DM, Alcott CJ, Clark SK, et al. 2012. Alloimmune neonatal neutropenia and neonatal isoerythrolysis in a Thoroughbred colt. J Vet Diagn Invest, 24: 219–226.

18

Platelets

Jed Overmann

Veterinary Clinical Sciences Department, College of Veterinary Medicine, University of Minnesota, Minnesota, USA

18.1 Platelet Production and Kinetics

Platelets are membrane bound cytoplasmic fragments of megakaryocytes. The functions of platelets are varied, but are primarily associated with hemostasis, coagulation, and maintenance of vascular integrity. Each megakaryocyte in the bone marrow has the capacity to release several thousand platelets into circulation over time. The production of platelets (i.e., thrombopoiesis) is largely regulated by thrombopoietin, but other growth factors and cytokines also play a role. Once released into circulation, platelets circulate for approximately 5–9 days before being removed by macrophages in the spleen and liver. A small portion of platelets are also removed from circulation in health due to their involvement in the maintenance of vascular integrity (George, 2000). Approximately 30% of all platelets are transiently sequestered in the spleen. Thus, splenic contraction can result in increased platelet counts due to redistribution of these sequestered platelets. Alternatively, splenic enlargement may result in a decreased platelet count.

18.2 Laboratory Diagnostics

Critical to the generation of quality laboratory data is appropriate sample collection and handling and the reader is referred to Chapter 1 for a full discussion. Of particular relevance to laboratory diagnostics assessing platelets is venipuncture technique. Platelet activation during venipuncture is common, especially with difficult or traumatic draws. As detailed next, this can significantly affect laboratory values for some parameters.

- *Platelet count*: Initial evaluation of platelets generally begins with a platelet count which is effectively a platelet concentration and represents the number of platelets per unit volume of blood. This value is most often generated by an automated hematology analyzer as part of a complete blood count (CBC), but manual methods may occasionally be used. Thrombocytopenia is defined as a platelet count below reference interval, whereas a thrombocytosis is a platelet count above reference interval. Platelet counts (especially those that are decreased) should always be confirmed by evaluation of a peripheral blood film.

- *Mean platelet volume* (MPV): Some automated hematology analyzers report a mean platelet volume which represents the average platelet volume in a sample. The presence of large platelets in circulation is generally associated with increased thrombopoiesis, often in response to a thrombocytopenia or increase utilization of platelets. If enough large platelets are released into circulation this may raise the MPV above the reference interval. Thus, an increased MPV may be an indicator of increased thrombopoiesis, but should be interpreted in light of other laboratory results. If platelet clumping is present, the MPV may not be accurate and interpretation should be avoided. Artifactual increases in MPV may also be seen with delayed sample processing.

- *Plateletcrit* (PCT): The PCT represents the percentage volume of blood occupied by platelets. It is a value reported by some automated hematology analyzers and is most often calculated based on the platelet count and MPV. The plateletcrit may be a better indicator of total platelet mass compared to the platelet count.

- *Peripheral blood film evaluation*: Evaluation of a peripheral blood film is important in assessment of platelets and should be done to confirm the accuracy of platelet counts (see Figure 18.1). First, the blood film should be assessed for the presence of platelet clumps by scanning the feathered edge and body of the blood film. Platelet clumping tends to cause a decrease in the platelet count (i.e., pseudothrombocytopenia) and is commonly seen due to platelet activation during venipuncture. EDTA-mediated platelet clumping has also been described in

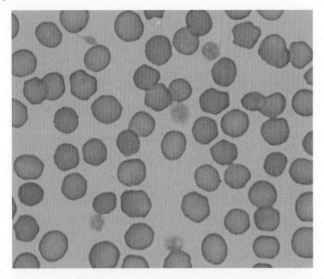

Figure 18.1 Five equine platelets. Peripheral blood film. Modified Wright-Giemsa stain.

the horse (Hinchcliff et al., 1993). An estimate of the platelet count can be determined from a peripheral blood film to further confirm values from automated analyzers, or to provide a quick estimate if access to a platelet count is limited or delayed (see Table 18.1). Finally, peripheral blood film evaluation allows for assessment of platelet morphology. Increased numbers of large platelets (i.e., greater than the diameter of a red blood cell) suggests increased thrombopoiesis.

- *Platelet function testing*: Bleeding time (e.g., template bleeding time or cutaneous bleeding time) is an *in vivo* test that can be used to assess platelet function. This test is performed by creating a standardized superficial wound with the use of a small automated blade device

Table 18.1 Estimating platelet count from a peripheral blood film.

If platelet clumping is absent on a blood film, an estimate of the platelet count can be determined by first assessing the average number of platelets per field using a 100× oil objective.

To find the average number of platelets per 100× oil objective field, 8–10 fields in the monolayer area of the blood film should be evaluated.

To convert the average number of platelets per 100× oil objective field to an estimated platelet count (platelets/µL), multiply by 15,000–20,000
Example: (Average of 10 platelets per 100× oil objective field) × (15,000–20,000) = Estimated platelet count of 150,000–200,000/µL

If platelet clumping is present on a blood film, the estimated platelet count can likely be interpreted as a minimum value, but will underestimate the true value.

As a general rule, finding 6–10 platelets on average per 100× oil objective field on a peripheral blood film indicates an adequate platelet count

---

and recording the time for bleeding to cease. Platelet function defects, as well as thrombocytopenia and von Willebrand disease (vWD) can cause increases in bleeding times. While bleeding time testing is accessible and relatively easy to perform, the template bleeding time as been shown to have relatively poor reproducibility and a wide reference interval, thus limiting its diagnostic utility (Segura and Monreal, 2008). Other techniques for evaluating platelet function such as platelet function analysis (PFA-100), platelet aggregometry, and flow cytometry may be of limited use in clinical practice as these tests are only offered by specialized labs and testing may need to be performed relatively shortly after sample collection.

- *von Willebrand factor assays*: see Section 18.5.

18.3 Thrombocytopenia

Thrombocytopenia is defined as a platelet count below reference interval and is caused by one or more of three basic mechanisms. Those mechanisms are (1) increased platelet consumption or destruction, (2) decreased platelet production, and (3) platelet redistribution. More specific causes of thrombocytopenia are often grouped by the major mechanism driving the decrease in platelets. Equine patients that present with thrombocytopenia most often have clinical signs associated with the underlying cause of the thrombocytopenia as opposed to signs directly related to the low platelet count. Abnormal clinical bleeding, however, does occur in some patients and is most likely in those with platelet counts <10,000–20,000 µL. Inflammatory processes may further predispose a thrombocytopenic patient to hemorrhage (Goerge et al., 2008). Clinical signs are typical of a defect in primary hemostasis and are similar regardless of the underlying cause of the thrombocytopenia. Clinical signs include petechiae and ecchymoses of mucous membranes and skin, epistaxis, melena, hyphema, hematuria, and prolonged bleeding from injection or venipuncture sites.

Increased platelet consumption or destruction: Some causes of increased platelet consumption and destruction include immune-mediated thrombocytopenia, disseminated intravascular coagulation (DIC), sepsis, neonatal alloimmune thrombocytopenia, severe blood loss, snake bite envenomation, severe extensive burns, trauma, and vasculitis. Provided sufficient time, a bone marrow response to thrombocytopenia would be expected in cases of increased peripheral consumption or destruction of platelets. An increased MPV or identification of increased numbers of large platelets on a peripheral blood film would be supportive and may be seen in some cases.

- *Immune-mediated thrombocytopenia* is often characterized by a severely decreased platelet count and can be primary (i.e., idiopathic) or secondary to a variety of processes including bacterial or viral infections, neoplasia, or drug therapies (Sellon et al., 2000, McGurrin et al., 2004, McGovern et al., 2011). Laboratory diagnostics for immune-mediated thrombocytopenia are discussed in more detail in Chapter 42.

- *DIC* causes consumption of platelets leading to variably decreased platelet counts and can be the result of a number of underlying causes such as sepsis, inflammation, colic, severe trauma, or disseminated neoplasia. In addition to a consistent clinical presentation and thrombocytopenia, increased coagulation times and evidence of increased fibrinolysis would be supportive of DIC (see Chapters 20 and 21).
- *Neonatal alloimmune thrombocytopenia* has been reported in foals and is the result of ingestion of colostrum that contains antiplatelet antibodies (see Chapter 43) (Buechner-Maxwell et al. 1997).
- Platelet counts are often within reference interval in cases of *blood loss*; however, severe blood loss can occasionally result in a mild to moderate thrombocytopenia.
- Many *snake venoms* contain substances that induce platelet aggregation. One retrospective study found an association between the degree of thrombocytopenia and severity of envenomation (Fielding et al., 2011, McCleary and Kini, 2013).

Decreased platelet production: A variety of bone marrow disorders can result in thrombocytopenia by causing a decrease in production of platelets. Leukemia, lymphoma, multiple myeloma, and myelofibrosis can all cause thrombocytopenia by infiltration of the bone marrow space and disruption of the hematopoietic microenvironment (Angel et al., 1991, Meyer et al., 2006, Muñoz et al., 2009). Aplastic pancytopenia, either idiopathic or secondary to drugs, toxin, or infectious agents results in severe generalized bone marrow hypoplasia with replacement of this space by fat. Finally, immune-mediated damage of megakaryocytes may occur as version of immune-mediated thrombocytopenia. Bone marrow aspirate and core biopsy would be indicated to assess for these causes and would be warranted in a horse with a persistent unexplained thrombocytopenia, especially when accompanied by unexplained neutropenia and anemia.

Platelet redistribution: Splenomegaly due to a number of underlying causes (e.g., splenic congestion, lymphoma, leukemia, etc.) can result in thrombocytopenia due to "pooling" of platelets within the spleen. Total platelet mass in the patient is not decreased in these cases, rather there has been a redistribution of platelets from the peripheral circulation into the spleen. Severe hypothermia may also cause redistribution of platelets to the spleen.

Multifactorial or unknown: For some specific causes of thrombocytopenia, multiple mechanisms contribute to the development of a low platelet count in a patient. In other instances, the exact mechanism or mechanisms driving the thrombocytopenia associated with a disease or process are poorly defined or unknown.

- Thrombocytopenia is a common feature of *equine infectious anemia* (EIA) due to infection with the lentivirus equine infectious anemia virus. Experimental evidence suggests that decreased platelet production through an indirect suppressive effect on megakaryocytes is a major mechanism in the development of the thrombocytopenia. In addition, decreased platelet life-span mediated by both immune-dependent and immune-independent mechanisms also contribute (Crawford et al., 1996).
- *Equine granulocytic anaplasmosis* is caused by infection with the tick transmitted bacterium *Anaplasma phagocytophilum* and is associated with thrombocytopenia. Multiple mechanisms likely play a role; however, these remain largely unexplained. Several mechanisms for the thrombocytopenia have been postulated including immune-mediated destruction, increased removal by the spleen, and decreased production, however, some of these mechanisms are not supported by experimental studies (Borjession et al., 2001, Granick et al., 2008). Evaluation of a peripheral blood film can aid in a definitive diagnosis in some cases by identification of organisms within the cytoplasm of neutrophils (see Chapter 17).
- A variety of other infectious agents in the horse have been associated with thrombocytopenia such as *equine arteritis virus, Venezuelan equine encephalitis virus, Theileria equi*, and *Babesia caballi*.
- Thrombocytopenia associated with *neoplasia* may be multifactorial in some cases with increased platelet consumption or destruction, decreased production, and altered platelet distribution all being contributing factors (Figure 18.2).

18.4 Thrombocytosis

Thrombocytosis is defined as a platelet count above the established reference interval. Major causes of thrombocytosis may be characterized as physiologic, reactive, or spurious. One additional consideration is essential thrombocythemia or primary thrombocythemia which is a clonal disorder that in people is classified as a chronic myeloproliferative disease. It primarily affects megakaryocytes and results in marked thrombocytosis and megakaryocytic hyperplasia in the bone marrow. This entity has not

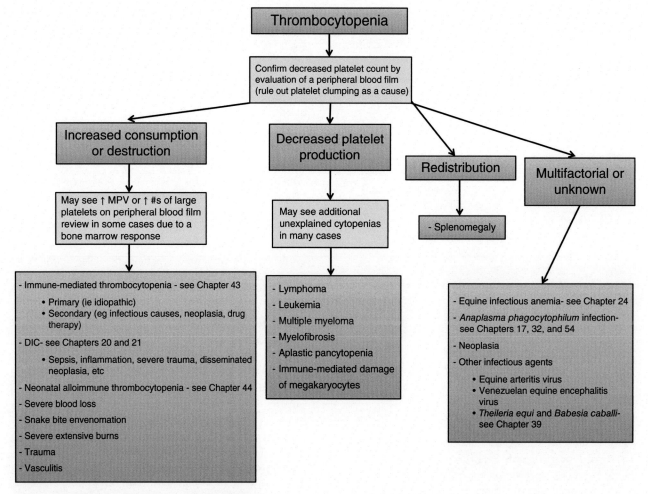

Figure 18.2 Diagnostic approach to thrombocytopenia.

been well described in the horse, however, there are rare reports of persistent marked thrombocytosis of unexplained cause in horses (Sellon et al., 1997) (Figure 18.3).

Physiologic: Pain, excitement, or strenuous exercise can result in epinephrine mediated contraction of the spleen which redistributes platelets within the spleen into circulation causing a transient thrombocytosis. Additional changes due to epinephrine mediated affects that may be evident on a CBC might include erythrocytosis, leukocytosis, neutrophilia, and lymphocytosis. Physiologic thrombocytosis is a relative one as total body platelet mass has not increased, there is just a redistribution of platelets from the spleen into circulation. Thrombocytosis may also be seen post-splenectomy due to lack of sequestration.

Reactive: A reactive thrombocytosis is characterized by increased platelet production from cytokine stimulation. This can be due to a number of underlying causes such as inflammation, neoplasia, or rebound from thrombocytopenia. Inflammatory causes of reactive thrombocytosis are common in the horse and increased platelet production is largely mediated by elevated levels of the inflammatory cytokine IL-6, though other cytokines also play a role (Sellon et al., 1997). Other laboratory abnormalities such as leukocytosis and hyperfibrinogenemia may also accompany inflammatory processes. Rebound thrombocytosis may be seen for a period following recovery from thrombocytopenia (e.g., recovery from immune-mediated thrombocytopenia). Thrombocytosis in other species is sometimes associated with iron-deficiency anemia (e.g., chronic blood loss) and could be a consideration if other clinical and laboratory findings are suggestive (see Chapter 16).

Spurious: Some hematology analyzers can occasionally misclassify components of a blood sample such as red blood cell or white blood cell fragments or cellular debris as platelets. Evaluation of a peripheral blood film to verify automated platelet counts can potentially identify these errors, especially when pronounced.

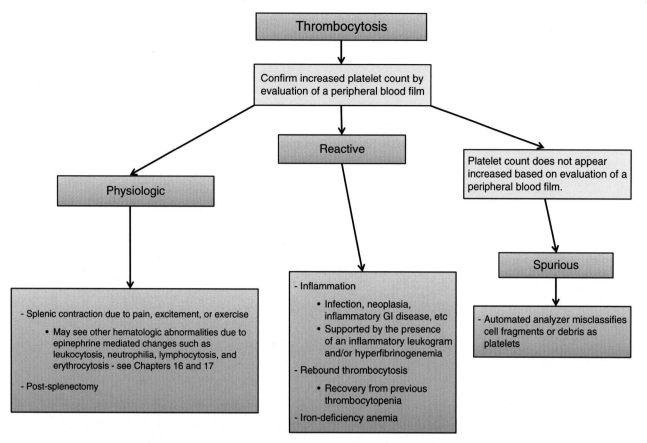

Figure 18.3 Diagnostic approach to thrombocytosis.

18.5 Von Willebrand Disease and Platelet Dysfuntion

Von Willebrand disease (vWD) or platelet dysfunction can result in clinical signs of abnormal bleeding tendencies typical of a defect in primary hemostasis (e.g., epistaxis, hematuria, GI hemorrhage, etc.). Initial diagnostics should be aimed at eliminating thrombocytopenia and coagulation factor deficiencies as a cause for the bleeding as these are more common causes of hemorrhage. Thus, vWD or platelet dysfunction disorders would be of primary concern in a patient that is exhibiting consistent clinical signs in spite of a platelet count and coagulation times (e.g., PT, PTT) that are within reference intervals. A prolonged bleeding time (e.g., template bleeding time) would be expected in cases of vWD or platelet dysfunction.

Von Willebrand Disease (vWD): vWD has been described in the horse and is the result of quantitative and functional defects in von Willebrand factor (vWF). vWF is a protein found in plasma, platelets, and in the subendothelial extracellular matrix and is required for platelet adhesion to subendothelial collagen at sites of vascular injury. If preliminary testing is consistent with vWD (see Section 18.2) then the next step would be determination of vWF concentration. vWF concentration can be measured in plasma and is often referred to as vWF antigen (vWF:Ag). A decreased vWF:Ag concentration would be expected in vWD. Additional assays such as vWF-ristocetin cofactor activity and vWF collagen-binding activity can be used to evaluate vWF function and are helpful in differentiating subtypes of vWD. Type 1 and type 2 vWD have been identified in the horse (Brooks 2008). Type 1 vWD is a quantitative deficiency in vWF:Ag concentration with a proportional decreased in vWF function, whereas type 2 vWD has a disproportionate decrease in vWF function along with decreased vWF:Ag concentration.

Platelet dysfunction: Glanzmann's thrombasthenia is a rare inherited platelet disorder that has been described in the horse. Platelet dysfunction is the result of an absence or marked reduction of the platelet fibrinogen receptor (i.e., glycoprotein complex IIb-IIIA) which is important for platelet aggregation (Livesey et al., 2005). A platelet function defect has also been described in thoroughbreds (Norris et al., 2006). Acquired platelet dysfunction has been associated with a variety of causes including uremia, liver disease, increased fibrin degradation products (FDPs), hyperproteinemia, antiplatelet antibodies, and drugs (e.g., nonsteroidal anti-inflammatory agents) (Fry, 2010).

References

Angel KL, Spano JS, Schumacher J, et al. 1991. Myelophthisic pancytopenia in a pony mare. J Am Vet Med Assoc, 198: 1039–1042.

Borjession DL, Simon SI, Tablin F, et al. 2001. Thrombocytopenia in a mouse model of human granulocytic ehrlichiosis. J Infect Dis, 184: 1475–1479.

Brooks MB. 2008. Equine coagulopathies. Vet Clin N Am Equine, 24: 335–355.

Buechner-Maxwell V, Scott MA, Godber L, et al. 1997. Neonatal alloimmune thrombocytopenia in a Quarter horse foal. J Vet Intern Med, 11: 304–308. Crawford TB, Wardrop KJ, Tornquist SJ, et al. 1996. A primary production deficit in the thrombocytopenia of equine infectious anemia. J Virol, 70: 7842–7850.

Fielding CL, Pusterla N, Magdesian KG, et al. 2011. Rattlesnake envenomation in horses: 58 cases (1992–2009). J Am Vet Med Assoc, 238: 631–635.

Fry MM. 2010. Acquired platelet dysfunction. In DJ Weiss and KJ Wardrop (eds), *Schalm's Veterinary Hematology*, 6th Edn. Ames, IA: Wiley-Blackwell, pp. 626–631.

George JN. 2000. Platelets. Lancet, 355: 1531–1539.

Goerge T, Ho-Tin-Noe B, Carbo C, et al. 2008. Inflammation induces hemorrhage in thrombocytopenia. Blood, 111: 4958–4964.

Granick JL, Reneer DV, Carlyon JA, et al. 2008. Anaplasma phagocytophilum infects cells of the megakaryocytic lineage through sialylated ligands but fails to alter platelet production. J Med Microbiol, 57: 416–423.

Hinchcliff KW, Kociba GJ, and Mitten LA. 1993. Diagnosis of EDTA-dependent pseudothrombocytopenia in a horse. J Am Vet Med Assoc, 203(1): 715–1716.

Livesey L, Christopherson P, Hammond A, et al. 2005. Platelet dysfunction (Glanzmann's thrombasthenia) in horses. J Vet Intern Med, 19: 917–919.

McCleary RJR and Kini RM. 2013. Snake bites and hemostasis/thrombosis. Thromb Res, 132: 642–646.

McGovern KF, Lascola KM, Davis E, et al. 2011. T-cell lymphoma with immune-mediated anemia and thrombocytopenia in a horse. J Vet Intern Med, 25: 1181–1185.

McGurrin MKJ, Arroyo LG, and Bienzle D. 2004. Flow cytometric detection of platelet-bound antibody in three horses with immune-mediated thrombocytopenia. J Am Vet Med Assoc, 224: 83–87.

Meyer J, Delay J, and Bienzle D. 2006. Clinical, laboratory, and histopathologic features of equine lymphoma. Vet Pathol 43: 914–924.

Muñoz A, Riber C, Trigo P, et al. 2009. Hematopoietic neoplasias in horses: myeloproliferative and lymphoproliferative disorders. J Equine Sci 20: 59–72.

Norris JW, Pratt SM, Auh JH, et al. 2006. Investigation of a novel, heritable bleeding diathesis of Thoroughbred horses and development of a screening assay. J Vet Intern Med, 20: 1450–1456.

Segura D and Monreal L. 2008. Poor reproducibility of template bleeding time in horses. J Vet Intern Med, 22: 238–241.

Sellon DC, Levine JF, Palmer K, et al. 1997. Thrombocytosis in 24 horses (1989–1994). J Vet Intern Med, 11: 24–29.

Sellon DC, Spaulding K, Breuhaus BA, et al. 2000. Hepatic abscesses in three horses. J Am Vet Med Assoc, 216: 882–887.

19

Blood Proteins and Acute Phase Proteins

Jed Overmann

Veterinary Clinical Sciences Department, College of Veterinary Medicine, University of Minnesota, Minnesota, USA

19.1 Introduction

Serum and plasma protein concentrations are commonly evaluated as a part of routine laboratory diagnostics. Understanding the basic mechanisms that drive changes in these values is important to the equine practitioner. Proteins in the serum and plasma consist of albumin and globulins. Albumin and the majority of globulins are produced by hepatocytes with a major exception being immunoglobulins that are produced by B cells and plasma cells. Plasma differs from serum in that plasma contains fibrinogen and clotting factors, whereas serum does not. Thus, total protein concentration derived from plasma will be slightly higher than that from serum.

19.2 Protein Measurement

19.2.1 Refractometry

Total protein concentration is often measured by use of a hand-held refractometer, as this is a quick and inexpensive way to screen for hyper- or hypoproteinemia. Measurement of protein concentration by this device is based upon the principle that the degree of light refraction in the plasma or serum is proportional to the concentration of solids (most of which are proteins) and that changes in refraction are due solely to changes in protein concentration. Other substances, however, especially at high concentrations can contribute to the degree of light refraction and falsely increase the total protein concentration reading by refractometry. Substances most likely to cause errors include glucose, urea, cholesterol, and lipoproteins (George, 2001). High concentrations of plasma glucose (700 mg/dL) and blood urea nitrogen (300 mg/dL) were reported to increase total protein concentration readings by refractometry by 0.6 g/dL (Silvermann and Christenson, 1994). Hemolysis does not appear to falsely increase refractometry readings and

hyperbilirubinemia of up to 41.5 mg/dL did not interfere with refractometry measurement of total protein concentration (Gupta and Stockham, 2014).

19.2.2 Biuret Reaction and BCG Dye-Binding Reaction

These methods are used to measure total protein (Biuret) and albumin (BCG dye-binding) concentrations in serum samples and are the values generally reported as part of a serum chemistry panel. Both are based on spectrophotometric measurement of color change with binding of reagents directed at peptide bonds (Biuret) or albumin (BCG dye-binding). The globulin concentration reported on most serum chemistry panels is a calculated value derived from subtracting the albumin concentration from the total protein concentration.

19.2.3 Serum Protein Electrophoresis

Serum protein electrophoresis (SPE) allows for separation of serum proteins into albumin, α_1-globulin, α_2-globulin, β_1-globulin, β_2-globulin, and γ-globulin fractions due to differential migration of these proteins through a matrix to which an electrical field is applied (Riond et al., 2009). Migration occurs at different rates based on the size and charge of individual proteins. Following electrophoretic separation, proteins are stained and proportions of each fraction can be determined from a densitometer tracing. SPE is most often performed to investigate an abnormal (generally elevated) globulin concentration (see Section 19.5.2 on hyperglobulinemia).

19.3 Interpretation of Abnormal Protein Concentrations

Knowledge of total protein concentration along with albumin and globulin concentrations (present on most serum chemistry panels) is helpful in prioritizing the

Interpretation of Equine Laboratory Diagnostics, First Edition. Edited by Nicola Pusterla and Jill Higgins.

underlying mechanism(s) driving an abnormal protein concentration. Certain mechanisms tend to produce certain patterns, though with some there is significant overlap and, in general, interpretation of abnormal protein concentrations becomes more difficult when multiple mechanisms are occurring simultaneously.

19.4 Decreased Protein Concentrations

19.4.1 Panhypoproteinemia

Panhypoproteinemia refers to a decreased total protein concentration with both decreased albumin and globulin concentrations.

- *Blood loss*: A common cause of panhypoproteinemia. With hemorrhage, red blood cells, albumin, and globulins are all lost. Following redistribution of fluid from the interstitial space into the vasculature, the remaining whole blood elements are effectively diluted and anemia develops along with decreases in total protein, albumin, and globulin concentrations.
- *Peritonitis and Pleuritis*: Protein exudation associated with severe acute peritonitis or pleuritis results in loss of proteins into these body cavities. With time, the globulin concentration may normalize due to inflammation
- *Hemodilution*: Excess administration of intravenous fluids or fluid accumulation associated with congestive heart failure.
- *Protein-Losing Enteropathy* (PLE): see discussion under Section 19.4.2 on hypoalbuminemia
- *Dermal losses*: Especially when severe and extensive, burns (thermal or chemical) or other exudative skin lesions can result in non-selective losses of both albumin and globulins. With time, the globulin concentration may normalize due to inflammation.

19.4.2 Hypoalbuminemia

Hypoalbuminemia can be seen with a total protein concentration that is increased, decreased, or within reference interval.

- *PLE:* PLE is a term used to describe gastrointestinal (GI) diseases where increased GI losses of protein and inability to absorb result in hypoproteinemia. This term encompasses a number of diseases including, granulomatous enteritis, GI neoplasia (e.g., lymphoma), acute enterocolitis, equine proliferative enteropathy (EPE) due to *Lawsonia intracellularis* infection, lymphoplasmacytic enteritis, idiopathic eosinophilic enterocolitis, intestinal histoplasmosis, GI parasitism, and so on

(Schumacher et al., 2000, Taylor et al., 2006, Frazer, 2008, Pusterla and Gebhart, 2013). Multiple mechanisms play a role including lymphatic blockage, increased mucosal permeability, exudation due to inflammation or ulcers, and blood loss. Hypoproteinemia due to hypoalbuminemia is a common finding. Globulin concentration may be within reference interval or decreased (see Section 19.4.1 on panhypoproteinemia).

- *Peritonitis and Pleuritis*: see Section 19.4.1 on panhypoproteinemia.
- *Protein-Losing Nephropathy* (PLN): Glomerular damage leads to selective renal losses of some proteins (notably albumin) based on their size and charge. Hypoproteinemia generally accompanies hypoalbuminemia in cases of PLN.
- *Liver failure*: Albumin is produced by hepatocytes and thus hypoalbuminemia can be seen with liver failure. A few studies in horses, however, have shown that hypoalbuminemia is only seen in a minority of cases (Parraga et al., 1995, Durham et al., 2003). One study found only 13% of horses with severe liver disease had hypoalbuminemia and only 5% had hypoproteinemia (Parraga et al., 1995).
- *Starvation/malnutrition*: Hypoalbuminemia can occur in these states when protein catabolism exceeds protein production.
- *Dermal losses*: see discussion under Section 19.4.1 on panhypoproteinemia
- *Inflammation*: Albumin is a negative acute phase protein. Thus, with ongoing inflammation albumin production by the liver is decreased and can result in a mild hypoalbuminemia. Development of hypoalbuminemia due to this mechanism alone generally requires ongoing inflammation of several days to a few weeks.
- *Hyperglobulinemia*: Hypoalbuminemia associated with hyperglobulinemia (e.g., multiple myeloma) may be due to multiple factors including altered production of albumin as a result of inflammation and increased oncotic pressure

19.4.3 Hypoglobulinemia

- *Failure of Passive Transfer* (FPT): FPT in neonatal foals results in hypoglobulinemia from lack of intake or absorption of maternal antibodies (primarily IgG) in colostrum. Hypoproteinemia may also be present. A variety of methods are available to specifically evaluate IgG concentrations in neonatal foals such as single radial immunodiffusion, enzyme-linked immunosorbent assays, latex agglutination, glutaraldehyde coagulation, zinc sulfate turbidity, and turbidemetric immunoassays. See Chapter 45 for a more complete discussion of FPT.

- *Immunodeficiencies*: Primary immunodeficiency disorders such as severe combined immunodeficiency (SCID) in Arabian foals, agammaglobulinemia, common variable immunodeficiency, and so on, could potentially lead to hypoglobulinemia through decreased production of γ-globulins. These are relatively rare conditions (Crisman and Scarratt, 2008).

19.5 Increased Protein Concentrations

19.5.1 Panhyperproteinemia

Panhyperproteinemia refers to an increased total protein concentration with increased albumin and globulin concentrations.

- *Dehydration*: This is a relatively common cause of hyperproteinemia. As dehydration develops and the water content of plasma decreases, proteins (both albumin and globulins) are effectively concentrated. Dehydration can be the result of GI or third space water loss, renal loss, cutaneous loss, or decreased access to water. Physical exam findings supportive of dehydration may also be present along with erythrocytosis.

19.5.2 Hyperglobulinemia

Total protein concentration is often elevated (i.e., hyperproteinemia) concurrently in cases of hyperglobulinemia, but total protein concentration can be within reference interval in some instances.

- *Inflammation*: This is a common cause of hyperglobulinemia and results from increased production of a variety of globulins including acute phase proteins and immunoglobulins. Increases in immunoglobulins are characteristic of chronic inflammatory processes such as hepatitis, infection, immune-mediated disease, neoplasia, and so on. SPE results in these cases will typically show a broad-based peak in the γ-globulin region indicating a polyclonal gammopathy. Polyclonal gammopathies are the result of production of immunoglobulins from a heterogeneous population of plasma cells, a process driven by antigenic stimulation. This is in contrast to a monoclonal gammopathy (see the Neoplasia section next).
- *Neoplasia*: Production of a homogenous immunoglobulin product by a neoplastic plasma cell (e.g., multiple myeloma) or lymphocyte (e.g., lymphoma) population is a relatively uncommon, but documented cause of hyperglobulinemia (Traub-Dargatz et al., 1985, Edwards et al., 1993, Pusterla et al., 2004). Hyperglobulinemia can be marked in some cases, but this is not a consistent feature. SPE in reported cases has revealed a narrow based monoclonal spike present in the α₂, β, or γ-globulin regions. Immunoelectrophoresis can be subsequently performed to identify the immunoglobulin class or isotype if a monoclonal gammopathy is identified. Total protein concentration is generally increased in these cases due to the hyperglobulinemia and albumin concentration is often reported to be decreased. Monoclonal gammopathy of unknown cause has also been reported in the horse (Kent and Roberts, 1990).

19.6 Acute Phase Proteins

Acute phase proteins (APP) are a heterogeneous group of proteins, primarily produced by hepatocytes, whose plasma concentrations change as part of the acute phase response. The acute phase response is a component of the innate immune system and is a general response to infection, trauma, inflammation, or stress which is mediated by proinflammatory cytokines (Cray, 2012). Measurement of APP are of interest clinically as an early detector of inflammation or infection or to monitor progression or resolution of disease. APP are classified as either positive APP or negative APP. Concentrations of positive APP increase as part of the acute phase response, while concentrations of negative APP decrease. Most APP are positive APP, but a notable exception is albumin which is a negative APP. Major positive APP are those that have very low concentrations in health, but significantly increase (i.e., 10–1000-fold) as part of the acute phase response. Major positive APP also increase relatively rapidly (i.e., within 24–48 h) after an inciting event and tend to normalize relatively quickly with the removal of the stimulus. Moderate acute phase proteins are those that have higher concentrations in healthy animals and show a more modest increase (i.e., 2–10-fold) as part of the acute phase response (Cray, 2012). The most commonly evaluated APP in the horse are the major positive APP serum amyloid A (SAA), and the moderate positive APP fibrinogen and haptoglobin.

19.6.1 Fibrinogen

Fibrinogen concentration has long been evaluated as a marker of inflammatory disease in the horse and can be increased (i.e., hyperfibrinogenemia) with either localized or systemic inflammatory processes (Borges et al., 2007, Hooijberg et al., 2014). Increases tend to be relatively modest in comparison to other APP such as SAA and interpretation is also complicated in some cases by the fact that fibrinogen can be consumed in localized or disseminated coagulation, thus masking increases due to inflammation. In spite of this, fibrinogen concentration is commonly measured due to the relative ease and low cost of doing so. Fibrinogen concentration is most often measured semiquantitatively by a heat-precipitation method. This is accomplished by calculating the difference in total protein concentration in plasma as measured by refractometry before and after precipitation and removal of fibrinogen. This method is relatively insensitive to small changes in fibrinogen concentration. Other methods for determination of fibrinogen concentration (e.g., Clauss method, immunoassay) are offered by some labs. It should be noted that dehydration should be considered when interpreting fibrinogen concentration as it can cause a mild increase. Dehydration and loss of plasma volume will tend to concentrate fibrinogen as well as other plasma proteins. As mentioned earlier, fibrinogen concentration can be decreased (i.e., hypofibrinogenemia) due to localized or disseminated coagulation or increased fibrinogenolysis. The heat-precipitation method, however, cannot be used to detect hypofibrinogenemia.

19.6.2 Serum Amyloid A (SAA)

SAA has been evaluated as a marker of infection or inflammation in a variety of conditions in horses. Elevated SAA concentrations have been documented in horses with conditions such as colic, acute viral and bacterial infections, guttural pouch infections, lymphoma, anaplasmosis, hepatitis, experimentally induced aseptic arthritis, lipopolysaccharide-induced arthritis, naturally acquired infectious arthritis, and induced bacterial placentitis (Hulten et al., 1999, Vandenplas et al., 2005,

Jacobsen 2006a, 2006b, Belgrave et al., 2013, Canisso et al., 2014, Hooijberg et al., 2014). Vaccination, surgery, and long distance endurance rides have been associated with increased SAA concentration (Jacobsen et al., 2009, Andersen et al., 2012, Cywinska et al., 2012). SAA is regarded as a relatively sensitive indicator of inflammation or tissue injury in the horse, especially when compared to other markers of inflammation such as leukocyte count or fibrinogen concentration and measurement of SAA is also considered to be useful for monitoring disease and response to therapy in some instances (Jacobsen and Andersen, 2007). A number of methods have been used to measure SAA concentrations in the horse including single radial immunodiffusion, ELISA, slide reversed passive latex agglutination, electroimmunoassay, automated latex agglutination immunoturbidometric assay, and an automated turbidometric immunoassay.

19.6.3 Haptoglobin

Mild elevations in haptoglobin concentrations have been reported in inflammatory processes in the horse including surgery, induced non-infectious arthritis, and placentitis (Kent and Goodall, 1991, Hulten et al. 2002, Canisso et al., 2014). Horses with colic may have increased, decreased or normal serum haptoglobin concentrations (Pihl et al. 2013, Dondi et al. 2015). A primary function of haptoglobin is to bind free hemoglobin in circulation with subsequent removal of this hemoglobin-haptoglobin complex. This is a proposed mechanism to potentially explain the decreased haptoglobin concentrations in some horses with colic.

References

Andersen SA, Petersen HH, Ersboll AK, et al. 2012. Vaccination elicits a prominent acute phase response in horses. Vet J, 191: 199–202.

Belgrave RL, Dickey MM, Arheart KL, et al. 2013. Assessment of serum amyloid A testing of horses and its clinical application in a specialized equine practice. J Am Vet Med Assoc, 224: 113–119.

Borges AS, Divers TJ, Stokol T, et al. 2007. Serum iron and plasma fibrinogen concentrations as indicators of systemic inflammatory diseases in horses. J Vet Intern Med, 21: 489–494.

Canisso IF, Ball BA, Cray C, et al. 2014. Serum amyloid A and haptoglobin concentrations are increased in plasma of mares with ascending placentitis in the absence of changes in peripheral leukocyte counts or fibrinogen concentration. Am J Reprod Immunol, 72: 376–385.

Cray C. 2012. Acute phase proteins in animals. Prog Mol Biol Transl Sci, 105: 113–150.

Crisman MV and Scarratt WK. 2008. Immunodeficiency disorders in horses. Vet Clin N Am- Equine, 24: 299–310.

Cywinska A, Szarska E, Gorecka R, et al. 2012. Acute phase protein concentrations after limited distance and long distance endurance rides in horses. Res Vet Sci, 93: 1402–1406.

Dondi F, Lukacs RM, Gentilini F, et al. 2015. Serum amyloid A, haptoglobin, and ferritin in horses with colic: Association with common clinicopathologic variables and short-term outcome. Vet J. 205(1): 50–55.

Durham AE, Newton JR, Smith KC, et al. 2003. Retrospective analysis of historical, clinical, ultrasonographic, serum biochemical and haematological data in prognostic evaluation of equine liver disease. Equine Vet J, 35: 542–547.

Edwards DF, Parker JW, Wilkinson JE, et al. 1993. Plasma cell myeloma in the horse. A case report and literature review. J Vet Intern Med, 7: 169–176.

Frazer ML. 2008. *Lawsonia intracellularis* infection in horses: 2005–2007. J Vet Intern Med, 22: 1243–1248.

George JW. 2001. The usefulness and limitation of hand-held refractometers in veterinary laboratory medicine: An historical and technical review. Vet Clin Path, 30: 201–210.

Gupta A and Stockham SL. 2014. Refractometric total protein concentrations in icteric serum from dogs. J Am Vet Med Assoc, 244: 63–67.

Hooijberg EH, van den Hoven R, Tichy A, et al. 2014. Diagnostic and predictive capability of routine laboratory tests for the diagnosis and staging of equine inflammatory disease. J Vet Intern Med, 28: 1587–1593.

Hulten C, Gronlund U, Hirvonen J, et al. 2002. Dynamics in serum of the inflammatory markers serum amyloid A (SAA), haptoglobin, fibrinogen and α_2-globulins during induced noninfectious arthritis in the horse. Equine Vet J, 34: 699–704.

Hulten C, Tulamo RM, Suominen MM, et al. 1999. A non-competitive chemiluminescence enzyme immunoassay for the equine acute phase protein serum amyloid A (SAA)-a clinically useful inflammatory marker in the horse. Vet Immunol Immunop, 68: 267–281.

Jacobsen S and Andersen PH. 2007. The acute phase protein serum amyloid A (SAA) as a marker of inflammation in horses. Equine Vet Educ, 19: 38–46.

Jacobsen S, Halling-Thomsen M, and Nanni S. 2006a. Concentrations of serum amyloid A in serum and synovial fluid from healthy horses and horses with joint disease. Am J Vet Res, 67: 1738–1742.

Jacobsen S, Niewold TA, Halling-Thomsen M, et al. 2006b. Serum amyloid A isoforms in serum and synovial fluid in horses with lipopolysaccharide-induced arthritis. Vet Immunol Immunop, 110: 325–330.

Jacobsen S, Vedding Nielsen J, Kjelgaard-Hansen M, et al. 2009. Acute phase response to surgery of varying intensity in horses: A preliminary study. Vet Surg, 38: 762–769.

Kent JE and Goodall J. 1991. Assessment of an immuno-turbidimetric method for measuring equine serum haptoglobin concentrations. Equine Vet J, 23: 59–66.

Kent JE and Roberts CA. 1990. Serum protein changes in four horses with monoclonal gammopathy. Equine Vet J, 22: 373–376.

Parraga ME, Carlson GP, and Thurmond M. 1995. Serum protein concentrations in horses with severe liver disease: A retrospective study and review of the literature. J Vet Intern Med, 9: 154–161.

Pihl TH, Andersen PH, Kjelgaard-Hansen M, et al. 2013. Serum amyloid A and haptoglobin concentrations in serum and peritoneal fluid of healthy horses and horses with acute abdominal pain. Vet Clin Path, 42: 177–183.

Pusterla N and Gebhart C. 2013. *Lawsonia intracellularis* infection and proliferative enteropathy in foals. Vet Microbiol, 167: 34–41.

Pusterla N, Stacy BA, Vernau W, et al. 2004. Immunoglobulin A monoclonal gammopathy in two horses with multiple myeloma. Vet Rec, 155: 19–23.

Riond B, Wenger-Riggenback B, Hofmann-Lehmann R, et al. 2009. Serum protein concentrations for clinically healthy horses determined by agarose gel electrophoresis. Vet Clin Path, 38: 73–77.

Schumacher J, Edwards JF, and Cohen ND. 2000. Chronic idiopathic inflammatory bowel diseases of the horse. J Vet Intern Med, 14: 258–265.

Silvermann LM and Christenson RH. 1994. Amino acids and proteins. In CA Burtis and ER Ashwood (eds), *Tietz Textbook of Clinical Chemistry*, 2nd Edn. Philadelphia, PA: WB Saunders, pp. 625–734.

Taylor SD, Pusterla N, Vaughan B, et al. 2006. Intestinal neoplasia in horses. J Vet Intern Med, 20: 1429–1436.

Traub-Dargatz J, Bertone A, Bennett D, et al. 1985. Monoclonal aggregating immunoglobulin cryoglobulinemia in a horse with malignant lymphoma. Equine Vet J, 17: 470–473.

Vandenplas ML, Moore JN, Barton MH, et al. 2005. Concentrations of serum amyloid A and lipopolysaccharide-binding protein in horses with colic. Am J Vet Res, 66: 1509–1516.

20

Clotting Times (aPTT and PT)

SallyAnne L. Ness[1] and Marjory B. Brooks[2]

[1] *Hospital for Animals, College of Veterinary Medicine, Cornell University, New York, USA*
[2] *The Comparative Coagulation Laboratory, Animal Health Diagnostic Center, College of Veterinary Medicine, Cornell University, New York, USA*

20.1 Clinical Background

Coagulation screening tests are traditionally categorized into tests of primary hemostasis (platelet plug formation), secondary hemostasis (fibrin clot formation), or fibrinolysis (clot breakdown). Secondary hemostasis may be further characterized *in vitro* as two distinct series of activation reactions, the intrinsic and extrinsic pathways, which converge at the common pathway to produce thrombin and subsequently transform soluble plasma fibrinogen into an insoluble fibrin clot.

Activated partial thromboplastin time (aPTT) evaluates the intrinsic and common pathways of secondary hemostasis. It is diagnostically similar to activated clotting time (ACT) but unlike the ACT, is less influenced by platelet abnormalities or hematocrit. Prothrombin time (PT) evaluates the extrinsic and common pathways and their ability to convert fibrinogen to fibrin. PT is often used to detect vitamin K deficiency or monitor vitamin K antagonist anticoagulants, for example, warfarin, brodifacoum, and so on.

20.2 Test(s) Available

Both aPPT and PT are used as screening tests to identify abnormalities in the intrinsic, extrinsic, and/or common coagulation pathways. Both tests involve the addition of specific coagulation-activating reagents to citrated plasma and subsequent measurement of the time to clot formation. The PT reaction is initiated by the addition of tissue factor and calcium to the test sample, while the aPTT reaction is initiated by the addition of phospholipid and negatively charged contact particles followed by calcium.

20.3 Sample Collection and Submission

Blood for aPTT and PT should be collected via minimally traumatic venipuncture into tubes containing sodium citrate (3.2 or 3.8%) anticoagulant (blue top tube). A complete draw into a vacutainer tube results in the appropriate ratio of one part citrate to nine parts blood. Plasma should be separated from cells, placed in a plastic or siliconized glass tube, and shipped chilled with an ice pack in an insulated container.

20.4 Interpretation

APTT and PT values that exceed 120% of the upper end of normal reference range are considered abnormal, however, different reagents and assay configurations influence sensitivity to detect mild factor deficiencies. In general, factor activities <30% of normal result in prolonged clotting times. APTT prolongation is observed with deficiencies in factors V, VIII, IX, X, XI, XII, prothrombin (factor II), or fibrinogen. PT prolongation is observed with deficiencies in factors V, VII, X, prothrombin, or fibrinogen. It is important to note that low fibrinogen concentrations, as is observed in consumptive coagulopathies such as disseminated intravascular coagulation (DIC) or hepatic synthetic failure, will affect the common pathway and result in prolongation of both aPTT and PT. Rodenticides that interfere with vitamin K recycling, for example, warfarin, brodifacoum, inhibit vitamin K dependent factors II, VII, IX, and X result in prolongation of both PT and aPTT, but do not influence fibrinogen. Short or fast clotting times in the aPTT and PT are generally not diagnostically useful.

Interpretation of Equine Laboratory Diagnostics, First Edition. Edited by Nicola Pusterla and Jill Higgins.
© 2018 John Wiley & Sons, Inc. Published 2018 by John Wiley & Sons, Inc.

(A)

(B)

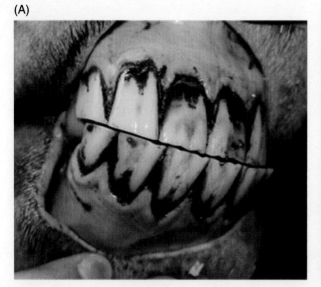
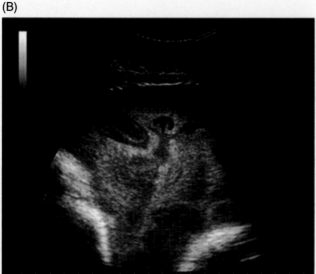

Figure 20.1 Clinical presentation of a mare after consumption of a vitamin K antagonist rodenticide. Spontaneous hemorrhage from the gingiva (A) as well as sonographic evidence of hemoabdomen (B) were observed.

20.5 Case Example

Signalment: 2-year-old Quarter Horse mare, found down in pasture. Upon further investigation, an open bag of rodenticide pellets containing brodifacoum was found in the pasture where the mare had been observed grazing.

Case Details: On presentation, the mare exhibited signs of spontaneous hemorrhage at the nares, gingiva, and vulva (Figure 20.1A). Abdominal ultrasound revealed hemoabdomen (Figure 20.1B). Clotting times revealed marked PT and aPTT prolongation (twice the upper end of normal range) with a normal fibrinogen value.

Interpretation: Given the probable history of brodifacoum consumption, the mare was treated for presumptive vitamin K antagonist toxicity with subcutaneous vitamin K_1 and supportive care. Consultation with the Animal Poison Control Center regarding the duration of action of the rodenticide in question dictated that treatment be continued for 8 weeks. The mare made a full recovery.

Further Reading

Brooks MB. 2008. Equine coagulopathies. Vet Clin N Am-Equine, 24: 335–355.

EClinPath: Coagulation Assays, College of Veterinary Medicine, Cornell University, Ithaca, NY.

Comparative Coagulation Laboratory: Animal Health Diagnostic Center, College of Veterinary Medicine, Cornell University, Ithaca, NY. https://ahdc.vet.cornell.edu/sects/Coag/

Epstein KL. 2014. Coagulopathies in horses. Vet Clin N Am-Equine, 30: 437–452.

21

Antithrombin
SallyAnne L. Ness[1] and Marjory B. Brooks[2]

[1] Hospital for Animals, College of Veterinary Medicine, Cornell University, New York, USA
[2] The Comparative Coagulation Laboratory, Animal Health Diagnostic Center, College of Veterinary Medicine, Cornell University, New York, USA

21.1 Clinical Background

Antithrombin (AT) is a plasma serine protease inhibitor (SERPIN) produced by the liver that inactivates factor IIa (thrombin) and factor Xa, thereby preventing active coagulation complex assembly and subsequent conversion of fibrinogen to fibrin. AT serves as the primary physiologic anticoagulant in circulation, and deficiencies are associated with systemic hypercoagulability and thrombophilia. Unfractionated and low molecular weight heparins acts by markedly potentiating AT inhibitory activity (by 2000–4000-fold in humans).

Hereditary AT deficiencies have not been identified in horses. Acquired deficiencies most often occur secondary to protein-losing enteropathies and nephropathies, consumptive coagulopathies, and hemorrhage. The molecular weight of AT (58 kDa) is slightly less than that of albumin (66 kDa), and thus, horses suffering from hypoalbuminemia secondary to protein loss are often assumed to also be losing AT. In the hypercoagulable stages of disseminated intravascular coagulation (DIC), AT inhibitory activity is often is less than 60–70% of normal.

21.2 Test(s) Available

Commercial human chromogenic substrate assays have been adapted to measure equine AT inhibitory activity (inhibition of factors IIa or Xa). Results are reported as a percent activity of a human or equine plasma standard.

21.3 Sample Collection and Submission

Blood for AT activity should be collected via minimally traumatic venipuncture into tubes containing sodium citrate (3.2 or 3.8%) anticoagulant (blue top tube).

A complete draw into a vacutainer tube results in the appropriate ratio of one part citrate to nine parts blood. Plasma should be separated from cells, placed in a plastic or siliconized glass tube, and shipped chilled with an ice pack in an insulated container.

21.4 Interpretation

Horses with AT activities below normal may display hypercoagulability and prothrombotic tendencies. In horses, this frequently manifests as jugular or distal limb vein thrombosis. Whole blood and/or fresh frozen plasma contain AT; however, volume overload limits the ability of transfusion to restore normal levels in patients with ongoing loss or consumption.

21.5 Case Example

Signalment: 4-year old Thoroughbred gelding presented for colitis

Case Details: This gelding was initially treated with high volumes of intravenous isotonic crystalloid fluids to restore hydration and replace losses to diarrhea. While overall hydration status improved with treatment, the gelding rapidly developed dependent pitting edema in the limbs and ventral abdomen as well as complete thrombosis of the catheterized jugular vein. Bloodwork at that time revealed hypoalbuminemia and below-normal AT activity.

Interpretation: Severe colonic inflammation has led to loss of both albumin and AT into the intestinal lumen, resulting in low systemic oncotic pressure and hypercoagulability, respectively. Administration of isotonic crystalloid fluids without concurrent colloid support has

Interpretation of Equine Laboratory Diagnostics, First Edition. Edited by Nicola Pusterla and Jill Higgins.
© 2018 John Wiley & Sons, Inc. Published 2018 by John Wiley & Sons, Inc.

resulted in the development of dependent edema, while AT deficiency and endotoxin-mediated platelet activation has resulted in jugular vein thrombosis. The gelding was treated with fresh frozen plasma as well as synthetic colloids and made a full recovery.

Further Reading

Brooks MB. 2008. Equine coagulopathies. Vet Clin N Am-Equine, 24: 335–355.

Comparative Coagulation Laboratory: Animal Health Diagnostic Center, College of Veterinary Medicine, Cornell University, Ithaca, NY. https://ahdc.vet.cornell.edu/sects/Coag/

Dallap BL. 2004. Coagulopathy in the equine critical care patient. Vet Clin N Am-Equine, 20: 231–251.

22

Fibrin and Fibrinogen Degradation Products (FDPs)

SallyAnne L. Ness[1] and Marjory B. Brooks[2]

[1] Hospital for Animals, College of Veterinary Medicine, Cornell University, New York, USA
[2] The Comparative Coagulation Laboratory, Animal Health Diagnostic Center, College of Veterinary Medicine, Cornell University, New York, USA

22.1 Clinical Background

Fibrin and fibrinogen degradation products (FDPs) are the end products of primary fibrinogenolysis (cleavage of fibrinogen and non-crosslinked fibrin) or secondary lysis of cross-linked fibrin clots. Elevated FDP concentrations indicate either fibrinogenolysis or fibrinolysis, and may be observed in horses with DIC, severe inflammatory processes and hemorrhagic disorders. Measurement of FDPs has been largely replaced in practice by D-dimer assays, which detect specific, domains of cross-linked fibrin, and are more specific indicators of plasmin's action on fibrin rather than fibrinogen.

22.2 Test(s) Available

Latex agglutination tests designed for human samples have been evaluated in horses and were found to have unacceptably low sensitivity (<40%) (Stokol et al., 2005). Commercial assays for D-dimers demonstrate higher sensitivity and specificity, and have largely replaced FDP measurement in clinical practice.

22.3 Sample Collection and Submission

Blood for FDP or D-dimer measurement should be collected via minimally traumatic venipuncture into tubes containing sodium citrate (3.2 or 3.8%) anticoagulant (blue top tube). A complete draw into a vacutainer tube results in the appropriate ratio of one part citrate to nine parts blood. Plasma should be separated from cells, placed in a plastic or siliconized glass tube, and shipped chilled with an ice pack in an insulated container.

22.4 Interpretation

FDPs and D-dimer will be elevated in response to any process that activates the coagulation cascade and results in clot formation and subsequent fibrinolysis. Nonspecific increase in FDPs may also be observed in response to elevated fibrinogen levels. FDPs and D-dimer have been found to be elevated following colic surgery and in horses suffering from inflammatory gastrointestinal disease. Elevated FDPs and/or D-dimer concentrations are one of the hallmarks of disseminated intravascular coagulation (DIC), which is characterized by initial hypercoagulability and thrombosis, followed in some patients by excessive fibrinolysis and clotting factor depletion, and ultimately death due to thrombosis and/or hemorrhage.

Reference

Stokol T, Erb HN, De Wilde L, et al. 2005. Evaluation of latex agglutination kits for detection of fibrin(ogen) degradation products and D-dimer in healthy horses and horses with severe colic. Vet Clin Path, 34(4): 375–382.

Further Reading

Brooks MB. 2008. Equine coagulopathies. Vet Clin N Am-Equine, 24: 335–355.

Comparative Coagulation Laboratory: Animal Health Diagnostic Center, College of Veterinary Medicine, Cornell University, Ithaca, NY. https://ahdc.vet.cornell.edu/sects/Coag/

Dallap BL. 2004. Coagulopathy in the equine critical care patient. Vet Clin N Am-Equine, 20: 231–251.

Epstein KL. 2014. Coagulopathies in horses. Vet Clin N Am-Equine, 30: 437–452.

23

Coagulation Factors

SallyAnne L. Ness[1] and Marjory B. Brooks[2]

[1] Hospital for Animals, College of Veterinary Medicine, Cornell University, New York, USA
[2] The Comparative Coagulation Laboratory, Animal Health Diagnostic Center, College of Veterinary Medicine, Cornell University, New York, USA

23.1   Clinical Background

Hereditary coagulation factor deficiencies are relatively uncommon in horses, but should be suspected in patients with evidence of abnormal bleeding and abnormal values for screening tests of the intrinsic, extrinsic, or common pathways (i.e., prolongation of PT, aPTT and/or ACT), after more common causes of coagulopathy (e.g., vitamin K antagonism, DIC, hepatic synthetic failure, etc.) have been ruled out. In general, factor activities <30% of normal result in prolonged clotting times. APTT prolongation is observed with deficiencies in factors V, VIII, IX, X, XI, XII, prothrombin (factor II), prekallikrein, or fibrinogen. PT prolongation is observed with deficiencies in factors V, VII, X, prothrombin, or fibrinogen.

- *Hemophilia A and B*: Horses affected by hemophilia A or hemophilia B are deficient in factors VIII and IX, respectively, and generally present as foals with excessive bleeding from minor wounds and hemarthrosis involving multiple joints. Both genetic disorders are X-linked, with male animals being clinically affected and females acting as silent carriers. Hemophilia has been reported in Thoroughbreds, Standardbreds, Quarter Horses, and Tennessee Walking Horses. Acquired, presumably autoimmune hemophilia A has also been reported in a Thoroughbred mare with evidence of anti-factor VIII antibodies. In these patients, the aPTT (intrinsic pathway) is prolonged, while PT and fibrinogen levels are normal. Von Willebrand factor (VWF) is a large plasma glycoprotein that acts as a factor VIII carrier protein and has a major role in supporting platelet adhesion. Von Willebrand disease refers to quantitative or functional deficiencies of VWF and this hemostatic defect has been reported in

Thoroughbreds and Quarterhorses. Mild to moderate factor VIII deficiency occurs in patients with von Willebrand's disease due to factor VIII's short plasma half-life in the absence of von Willebrand factor.
- *Autosomal Factor Deficiencies:* Deficiencies of autosomal coagulation factors (fibrinogen and factors II, V, VII, X, XI, XII) occur less frequently in horses than hemophilia. Severity of clinical signs is generally related to the degree of factor deficiency. Multiple concurrent factor deficiencies have also been reported. Genetic deficiencies in prekallikrein, a factor that participates in contact activation to initiate the intrinsic pathway *in vitro*, have been reported in families of Belgians and miniature horses. Factor deficiencies cause specific prolongation of coagulation screening tests, often performed in response to spontaneous hemorrhage or excessive bleeding after surgery or trauma. Definitive diagnosis is based on functional assays of specific factors.

23.2   Test(s) Available

There are currently two methods to measure specific clotting factor activities: clot endpoint assays and chromogenic assays. Clotting assays are based on the ability of patient plasma to correct the prolonged clotting times of a plasma with a known factor deficiency, while chromogenic assays are based on the ability of factors in the test plasma to cleave specific chromogenic substrates. Assays are currently available for measuring equine factors II, V, VII, VIII, IX, X, XI, and XII; however, it is advisable to contact the coagulation laboratory for consultation prior to submitting samples for specialized coagulation tests (coagulation factors, von Willebrand

Interpretation of Equine Laboratory Diagnostics, First Edition. Edited by Nicola Pusterla and Jill Higgins.
© 2018 John Wiley & Sons, Inc. Published 2018 by John Wiley & Sons, Inc.

factor, antibody-coated platelet assays, etc.) since human assays may require modification for horses.

- *Clotting assays*: These assays test the ability of the patient's plasma to normalize the prolonged clotting time (using a modified PT or aPTT) of specific factor-deficient plasma. For example, if patient plasma is added to factor VIII deficient plasma and the prolonged APTT does not correct, the results indicate a factor VIII deficiency, or hemophilia A. The degree of deficiency can then be quantified by comparing the clotting time of the patient plasma in factor-deficient plasma to a standard curve produced from the serial dilution of a plasma standard pooled from normal animals. The activity of the coagulation factor being measured is typically reported as a percentage activity as compared to the plasma standard.
- *Chromogenic assays*: These assays test the ability of a specific factor or cofactor in the test plasma to cleave or enhance cleavage of a chromogen-linked peptide substrate. The peptide substrate, upon cleavage, produces a colored product. The intensity of color change is proportional to the activity of the factor being measured. Like clotting assays, factor activity can be reported as a percentage activity compared to that of a pooled same-species plasma standard. Several chromogenic assays for coagulation factors, inhibitors, and components of the fibrinolytic system have been validated for horses. These chromogenic assays avoid the use of

human specific factor-deficient plasmas; however, chromogenic assays are generally more expensive than clot endpoint assays.

23.3 Sample Collection and Submission

Blood for clotting factor measurement should be collected via minimally traumatic venipuncture into tubes containing sodium citrate (3.2 or 3.8%) anticoagulant (blue top tube). A complete draw into a vacutainer tube results in the appropriate ratio of one part citrate to nine parts blood. Plasma should be separated from cells, placed in a plastic or siliconized glass tube, and shipped chilled with an ice pack in an insulated container.

23.4 Interpretation

In general, factor activities >50% are considered sufficient for normal hemostasis. Animals with specific factors <30% may demonstrate clinical signs of hemorrhage, however, the exact clinical manifestation will be largely dependent on the identity and severity of the factor deficiency, as well as whether a single factor or multiple factors are involved. Severely affected animals often have residual factor activities of <1% and die within a few days of birth because of uncontrolled umbilical hemorrhage.

Further Reading

Brooks MB. 2008. Equine coagulopathies. Vet Clin N Am-Equine, 24: 335–355.

Comparative Coagulation Laboratory: Animal Health Diagnostic Center, College of Veterinary Medicine, Cornell University, Ithaca, NY. https://ahdc.vet.cornell. edu/sects/Coag/

EClinPath: Coagulation Assays, College of Veterinary Medicine, Cornell University, Ithaca, NY. www.eclinpath. com/hemostasis/tests/screening-coagulation-assays/

Goer RJ, Jackson ML, Lewis KD, et al. 1990. Prekallikrein deficiency in a family of Belgian horses. J Am Vet Med Assoc, 197: 741–745.

Henninger RW. 1988. Hemophilia A in two related quarter horse colts. J Am Vet Med Assoc, 193: 91–94.

Hinton M, Jones DR, Lewis IM, et al. 1977. A clotting defect in an Arab colt foal. Equine Vet J, 9: 1–3.

Littlewood JD, Bevan SA, and Corke MJ. 1991. Haemophilia A (classic haemophilia, factor VIII deficiency) in a Thoroughbred colt foal. Equine Vet J, 23: 70–72.

Mills JN and Bolton JR. 1983. Haemophilia A in a 3-year-old thoroughbred horse. Aust Vet J, 60: 63–64.

Norton EM, Wooldridge AA, Stewart AJ, et al. 2016. Abnormal coagulation factor VIII transcript in a Tennessee Walking Horse colt with hemophilia A. Vet Clin Pathol, 45: 96–102.

Rathgeber RA, Brooks MB, Bain FT, and Byars TD. 2001. Clinical vignette. Von Willebrand disease in a Thoroughbred mare and foal. J Vet Intern Med, 15: 63–66.

Turrentine MA, Sculley PW, Green EM, et al. 1986. Prekallikrein deficiency in a family of miniature horses. Am J Vet Res, 47: 2464–2467.

Winfield LS and Brooks MB. 2014. Hemorrhage and blood loss-induced anemia associated with an acquired coagulation factor VIII inhibitor in a Thoroughbred mare. J Am Vet Med Assoc, 244: 719–723.

24

Equine Infectious Anemia Virus

Sandra D. Taylor

Department of Veterinary Clinical Sciences, College of Veterinary Medicine, Purdue University, Indiana, USA

24.1 Introduction

Equine infectious anemia virus (EIAV) is a lentivirus that causes persistent infection in equids worldwide. This enveloped virus is a member of the Retroviridae family, and infects monocytes/macrophages, dendritic cells, and occasionally endothelial cells (Maury et al., 2005). EIAV causes persistent infection by several mechanisms, including genetic variation through error-prone reverse transcriptase, structural resistance to neutralizing antibodies, integration of proviral DNA into host cell chromatin, and innate resistance to host proteins that inactivate retroviruses (Issel et al., 2014). EIAV is transmitted mechanically by Tabanidae insects, including horse flies and deer flies. The insect acquires EIAV on its mouth parts by drawing blood from a painful bite, which leads to interruption of feeding and potential transmission to a second equine host. Transmission can also occur from blood/plasma transfusions, multi-use needles or syringes and contaminated veterinary equipment.

After a 1–4-week incubation period, acutely infected horses typically develop fever, lethargy, inappetance, and thrombocytopenia. In severe cases, anemia and epistaxis may occur. Most horses clinically recover from the acute stage of infection as the adaptive immune response controls viremia. Following the initial clinical episode, recrudescence of viremia with novel viral quasispecies corresponds with recurrence of clinical disease. This typically occurs during the first year post-infection, followed by a long period of quiescence that is associated with immune control and inapparent carrier status (Montelaro et al., 1984, Sellon et al., 1994). Stress or immunosuppression may allow resurgence of viremia and lead to a chronic stage of infection, which is characterized by weight loss, edema, ataxia, anemia, and thrombocytopenia.

Currently, there is no effective vaccine against EIAV. Options for infected horses include lifelong segregation of 200 m from other equids or euthanasia.

24.2 Diagnostic Testing

Current diagnostic tests for EIAV rely on serologic detection of anti-EIAV antibodies. Given that EIAV exposure and subsequent antibody production correlates to lifelong infection, the presence of serum antibodies against EIAV confirms infection. Two serologic testing strategies are approved for diagnostic testing in the US, including the agar gel immunodiffusion (AGID) test (i.e., Coggins test), and enzyme-linked immunosorbent (ELISA) assays (Burki and Rossmanith, 1990, Coggins et al., 1972). The AGID test detects antibodies against the p26 capsid protein, while the ELISA tests detect antibodies against the gp45 envelope glycoprotein or the p26 capsid protein. ELISA tests that are currently approved by the U.S. Department of Agriculture (USDA) include the competitive ELISA (C-ELISA) from IDEXX Laboratories, Inc., the synthetic fusion protein (FP II)-ELISA from Centaur, Inc., the modified sandwich ELISA from Veterinary Medical Research and Development (VMRD), and the ViraCHEK® ELISA from Synbiotics Corporation. Although there is reportedly good correlation between AGID and ELISA results, the AGID test is relatively insensitive and may yield a false negative result, while the ELISA tests are relatively non-specific and may yield a false positive result (Burki and Rossmanith, 1990). A national surveillance program for EIAV in Italy found that 17% of equids that tested negative on AGID testing were confirmed positive by ELISA (Issel et al., 2013). Because false negative results are more catastrophic than false positive results, it has been suggested that a

Box 24.1 Serological interpretation.

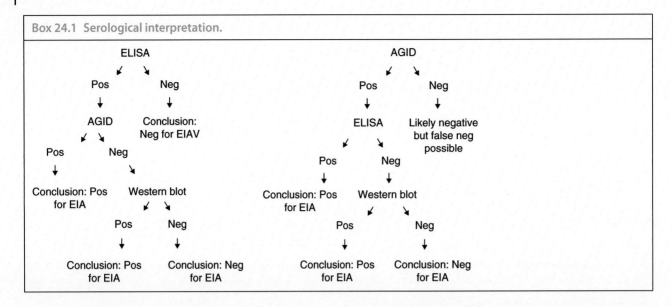

three-tiered program be implemented for EIAV testing that takes advantage of the highly sensitive ELISA tests and the highly specific AGID test (Scicluna et al., 2013). In this scheme, equids would be screened for EIAV using an ELISA test. Positive cases would be confirmed using the AGID test; if results were contradictory between the ELISA and AGID tests, an immunoblot confirmation (Western blot) would be performed at a specific laboratory such as the National Veterinary Services Laboratory or the University of Kentucky (Alvarez et al., 2007, Issel et al., 2013). Although this approach has recently been proposed for optimal serologic testing for EIAV, it has yet to be implemented worldwide. A summary of serological interpretation can be found in Box 24.1.

Several studies have shown efficacy of polymerase chain reaction (PCR) in detecting EIAV genetic material, but there are no commercially available PCR tests at this time (Capomaccio et al., 2012, Cappelli et al., 2011, Dong et al., 2012, Nagarajan and Simard, 2001, Quinlivan et al., 2007).

The USDA Animal and Plant Health Inspection Service requires that certain categories of equids be tested for EIAV, including equids being entered into exhibitions or competitive events, equids being moved interstate, equids changing ownership, and equids entering horse auctions or sales markets (USDA 2007). Results of ELISA tests can be obtained within 1–3 h, while the AGID test requires no less than 24 h. Thus, the more expedient ELISA may be requested for imminent travel purposes.

References

Alvarez I, Gutierrez G, Ostlund E, Barrandeguy M, and Trono, K. 2007. Western blot assay using recombinant p26 antigen for detection of equine infectious anemia virus-specific antibodies. Clin Vaccine Immunol, 14: 1646–1648.

Burki F and Rossmanith E. 1990. Comparative evaluation of the agar gel immunodiffusion test and two commercial ELISA kits for the serodiagnosis of equine infectious anemia. Zentralbl Veterinarmed B, 37: 448–458.

Capomaccio S, Willand ZA, Cook SJ, Issel CJ, Santos EM, Reis JK, and Cook RF. 2012. Detection, molecular characterization and phylogenetic analysis of full-length equine infectious anemia (EIAV) gag genes isolated from Shackleford Banks wild horses. Vet Microbiol, 157: 320–332.

Cappelli K, Capomaccio S, Cook FR, Felicetti M, Marenzoni ML, Coppola G, et al. 2011. Molecular detection, epidemiology, and genetic characterization of novel European field isolates of equine infectious anemia virus. J Clin Microbiol, 49: 27–33.

Coggins L, Norcross NL. and Nusbaum SR. 1972. Diagnosis of equine infectious anemia by immunodiffusion test. Am J Vet Res, 33: 11–18.

Dong JB, Zhu W, Cook FR, Goto Y, Horii Y, and Haga T. 2012. Development of a nested PCR assay to detect equine infectious anemia proviral DNA from peripheral blood of naturally infected horses. Arch Virol, 157: 2105–2111.

Issel CJ, Cook, RF, Mealey RH, and Horohov DW. 2014. Equine Infectious Anemia in 2014: Live with It or eradicate It? Vet Clin North Am Equine Pract, 30: 561–577.

Issel CJ, Scicluna MT, Cook SJ, Cook RF, Caprioli A, Ricci I, et al. 2013. Challenges and proposed solutions for more accurate serological diagnosis of equine infectious anaemia. Vet Rec; 172: 210.

Maury W, Thompson RJ, Jones Q, Bradley S, Denke T, Baccam P, et al. 2005. Evolution of the equine infectious anemia virus long terminal repeat during the alteration of cell tropism. J Virol, 79: 5653–5664.

Montelaro RC, Parekh B, Orrego A and Issel CJ. 1984. Antigenic variation during persistent infection by equine infectious anemia virus, a retrovirus. J Biol Chem, 259: 10539–10544.

Nagarajan MM and Simard C. 2001. Detection of horses infected naturally with equine infectious anemia virus by nested polymerase chain reaction. J Virol Methods, 94: 97–109.

Quinlivan M, Cook RF, and Cullinane A. 2007. Real-time quantitative RT-PCR and PCR assays for a novel European field isolate of equine infectious anaemia virus based on sequence determination of the gag gene. Vet Rec, 160: 611–618.

Scicluna MT, Issel CJ, Cook FR, Manna G, Cersini A, Rosone F, et al. 2013. Is a diagnostic system based exclusively on agar gel immunodiffusion adequate for controlling the spread of equine infectious anaemia? Vet Microbiol, 165: 123–134.

Sellon DC, Fuller FJ, and McGuire TC. 1994. The immuno-pathogenesis of equine infectious anemia virus. Virus Res, 32: 111–138.

USDA. 2007. Equine Infectious Anemia: Uniform Methods and Rules. Washington D.C.: USDA.

25

Equine Influenza Virus

Beate Crossley and Ashley Hill

California Animal Health and Food Safety Laboratory, Department of Medicine and Epidemiology, School of Veterinary Medicine, University of California, California, USA

25.1 Clinical Background

Equine Influenza is a highly contagious RNA virus that can largely be managed by vaccination, however, vaccine efficacy may be compromised by the antigenic drift and resulting emergence of variant subtypes that is characteristic of all influenza viruses (Myers and Wilson, 2006, Daly et al., 2011). Influenza A subtype H3N8 currently circulates nearly globally in the horse population (Cullinane et al., 2010). The incubation period for equine influenza can be less than 24 h in naïve horses, with disease characterized by fever, lethargy, nasal discharge, and coughing (OIE Terrestrial Manual, 2012). Although the disease is self-limiting and most horses recover without complication over a period of a few weeks, secondary infections such as bacterial pneumonia can be problematic. Viremia is rare but possible, and can result in inflammation of skeletal and cardiac muscle, encephalitis, and limb edema. Immunologically naïve and sero-negative horses are at highest risk of contracting and spreading the infection when exposed to actively infected and virus-shedding horses. Young, aged, and stressed horses are at greatest risk for developing viremia and resulting consequences. Persistent or intermittent shedding of virus from subclinically infected horses is not believed to occur (Cullinane et al., 2010, Myers and Wilson, 2006).

25.2 Serological Tests Available

Two serological tests for detecting antibodies to Equine Influenza virus are recognized by the World Organization for Animal Health (OIE); Hemagglutination Inhibition (HI) and Single Radial Hemolysis (SRH) (Morley et al., 1995). Complement fixation (CF) and serum virus neutralization (SVN) tests are occasionally used, although are not widely available. Laboratories will generally offer a panel of influenza subtypes, including influenza strains typically represented in vaccines (e.g., H3N8 Influenza viruses such as A/eq/Miami/63, A/eq/Kentucky/81, A/eq/Ohio/2003, and A/eq/Richmond/1/07, as well as a subtype associated with more recent or circulating non-vaccine H3N8 influenza virus).

25.3 Sample Collection and Submission

Whole blood is collected without additives into a syringe or evacuated tube. If not using a serum-separator tube, the blood clot is allowed to retract prior to decanting clean serum into a sterile tube for transport to the laboratory. Care should be taken when collecting the blood and separating the serum to prevent hemolysis, to the extent possible, from contaminating the test sample. The serum can be delivered chilled or frozen to the laboratory using standard biological specimens shipping procedures.

Acute serum samples should be obtained during the febrile stage of infection (within 24 h of onset of clinical disease) and paired convalescent serum should be collected approximately 2–3 weeks later (Zimmerman and Crisman, 2008, Myers and Wilson, 2006).

25.4 Possible Results

The HI, CF, and SVN test results report antibody values in titers, using two- or 10-fold serial dilution of the test sample to identify the highest dilution of sera with detectable influenza virus antibodies. The SRH measures a zone of hemolysis around a central well containing the test sample, with larger diameter equating to a higher concentration of influenza antibody (Zimmerman and Crisman, 2008).

Interpretation of Equine Laboratory Diagnostics, First Edition. Edited by Nicola Pusterla and Jill Higgins.
© 2018 John Wiley & Sons, Inc. Published 2018 by John Wiley & Sons, Inc.

25.5   Interpretation and Case Examples

Interpretation of influenza serology, regardless of the test method used, requires comparison of the horse's antibody response, either to itself over time (acute and convalescent samples) or to the animal's own antibody profile by testing for multiple subtypes including H3N8 vaccine strains, plus an H3N8 field strain of the Influenza virus. Antibody to influenza virus can be detected for several months post-vaccination or post-infection to virus (Carman et al., 1997). Maternally-derived colostral antibodies are is typically not detected in foals.

Acute and convalescent titers: The paired acute and convalescent samples should be tested at the same time by the laboratory to minimize interpretation error based on routine inter-assay variability. A doubling in size of the SRH ring or a four-fold change in titer is interpreted as seroconversion indicative of active infection:

- Negative: no detectable titer or SRH ring.
- Positive with lack of seroconversion (residual antibody from vaccination or past infection): titer with less than a four-fold change or less than doubling in measureable SRH ring. For example, an acute titer 128 and convalescent titer of 256; SRH ring acute 1.0 mm and convalescent 1.5 mm.
- Positive with seroconversion (active infection): four-fold change in titer or doubling of SRH ring. For example: acute titer 8 and convalescent >32; acute 64 and convalescent >256. SRH ring acute 1.0 mm and convalescent 15.3 mm.

Influenza virus panel: A single serum sample can provide useful results if the sample is tested to detect antibody to a panel of influenza viruses.

- Negative: no detectable titer or SRH ring.
- Non-vaccinated, infected horses will typically have antibody to the subtype they were infected to (H3N8 recently circulating), and little to no cross-reactivity with the other viruses in the panel.
- Vaccinated, non-infected horses will typically have similar titer (SRH ring) and antibody toward the vaccine H3N8 strain(s), and a >4-fold lower antibody titer to the H3N8 recently circulating virus/viruses caused by serologic cross-reaction to the similar H3N8 antigens.
- Vaccinated, infected horses will typically have antibody detectable to all three (or more) influenza viruses in the panel, with the highest titer to the recently circulating influenza virus.

References

Carman S, Rosendal S, Huber L, Gyles C, McKee S, Willoughby RA, et al. 1997. Infectious agents in acute respiratory disease in horses in Ontario. J Vet Diagn Invest, 9: 17–23.

Cullinane A, Elton D, and Mumford J. 2010. Equine influenza – surveillance and control. Influenza Other Respir Viruses., 4: 339–344.

Daly JM, MacRae, S, Newton JR, Wattrang E and Elton DM. 2011. Equine influenza: A review of an unpredictable virus. Vet J, 189: 7–14.

Morley PS, Hanson LK, Bogdan JR, Townsend HGG, Appleton JA, and Haines DM. 1995. The relationship between single radial hemolysis, hemagglutination inhibition, and virus neutralization assays used to detect antibodies specific for equine influenza viruses. Vet Microbio, 45: 81–92.

Myers C and Wilson WD. 2006. Equine influenza virus. Clin Tech Equine Practice, 5: 187–196.

OIE. 2012. Chapter 2.5.7. Equine influenza. OIE Terrestrial Manual 2012: 1–14

Zimmerman KL and Crisman MV. 2008. Diagnostic equine serology. Vet Clin N Am-Equine, 24: 311–334.

26

Alpha-Herpesviruses (EHV-1, EHV-4)

Beate Crossley and Ashley Hill

California Animal Health and Food Safety Laboratory, Department of Medicine and Epidemiology, School of Veterinary Medicine, University of California, California, USA

26.1 Clinical Background

Equine herpesvirus-1 and -4 are ubiquitous alphaherpes viruses, with estimates that 80–90% of horses are infected prior to 2 years of age, and up to 80% of infected horses develop latent infection (Kydd et al., 2006). EHV-1 and EHV-4 are closely-related genetically and antigenically. (Allen et al., 2004) Respiratory infections of horses with EHV-1 and EHV-4 are often subclinical, however, both viruses can cause outbreaks of severe upper respiratory disease in horse populations. Infection generally occurs in horses between weaning and two years of age (Allen, 2002). Clinical respiratory disease is more commonly associated with EHV-4, while respiratory infection with EHV-1 is more likely to progress beyond the respiratory tract and can cause abortion, neonatal foal mortality, myeloencephalopathy, peracute pulmonary vasculitis, and uveitis/chorioretinitis (Allen, 2002, Allen et al., 2004).

26.2 Serological Tests Available

Serum virus neutralization (SVN) is the most common serologic test for EHV-1/4 antibody, however, Complement fixation (CF) and ELISA are also recognized tests in the international community. SVN and CF testing cannot distinguish between EHV-1 and the closely-related EHV-4. Antibody values are reported in titers, using two-fold serial dilution of the test sample to identify the highest dilution of sera with detectable antibody to EHV-1/4. ELISA tests can be formatted to distinguish EHV-1 from EHV-4 (Carman et al., 1997, Allen et al., 2004), or to measure antibody subclasses IgM versus IgG, allowing to determine the acuteness of the infection (Zimmerman and Crisman, 2008). There is, however, no national or international standard for EHV ELISA tests, and correlation of results between different laboratories and manufacturers is not available. ELISA

results are generally reported as optical density or a transformed value calculated from the optical density of the test sample compared to a negative sample, with increasing optical density or ELISA value translating to increased detection of EHV-1/4 antibody.

26.3 Sample Collection and Submission

Whole blood is collected without additives into a syringe or evacuated tube. If not using a serum-separator tube, the blood clot is allowed to retract prior to decanting clean serum into a sterile tube for transport to the laboratory. Care should be taken when collecting the blood and separating the serum to prevent hemolysis, to the extent possible, from contaminating the test sample. The serum can be delivered chilled or frozen to the laboratory using standard biological specimens shipping procedures.

Acute serum samples should be obtained as soon as possible following onset of clinical disease (1–3 days), and paired convalescent serum should be collected approximately 2–4 weeks later.

26.4 Possible Results

Serology is not the preferred diagnostic test for EHV-1/4 infections due to the high incidence of EHV-1/4 infection and persistence of EHV-1/4 antibodies in the normal horse population. Detectable antibodies in a single serum sample cannot be used to diagnose or differentiate recent infection from past infection or vaccination. (OIE *Terrestrial Manual*, 2008) Lack of detectable antibodies can be used to rule out EHV-1/4 as a differential diagnosis in adult horses, however, should not be used to rule out EHV-4 in young horses. Seroconversion, measured by a four-fold or greater change in titer between acute and convalescent samples is sometimes interpreted as evidence of active/recent infection, however, repeated infection or reactivation to EHV-1/4 in the horse can result in seroconversion or increase in antibody levels without evidence of infection or clinical disease. Herd-based testing for EHV-1/4 "outbreaks" may be possible by testing clinically affected horses and comparing titer levels to cohorts in the same herd without evidence of respiratory disease.

26.5   Interpretation and Case Examples

26.5.1   Individual Animal

- Negative for antibody to EHV-1/4 by ELISA, CF, or SVN can be used to rule out infection in adult horses. A negative antibody response for EHV-1/4 cannot reliably be used to eliminate EHV-1/4 from the differential diagnosis in young horses.
- Positive results, regardless of titer or ELISA value are not considered typically diagnostic for a single sample.

CF and ELISA, which detect the IgM subclass of antibody, have value in identifying acute infection to EHV-1/4.

- Positive with seroconversion measured as > 4-fold change in titer is interpreted as recent infection to EHV-1/4, however, recent infection in previously vaccinated horses may result in seroconversion in the absence of clinical disease.

26.5.2   Herd-Based Testing in the Face of a Respiratory Disease Outbreak

A minimum of five samples from clinically-affected horses in the affected barn/premises, are paired with an equal or greater number of samples collected from horses in the same environment but not showing clinical disease. The group of samples is tested at the same time.

- The titer values or geometric mean titers are analyzed in a "case-control" approach, comparing the titers of clinically ill horses to those of apparently healthy horses, and assessing for a statistical difference between the two groups of horses.

References

Allen GP. 2002. Respiratory infections by equine herpesvirus types 1 and 4. In: *Equine Respiratory Diseases*, (eds) P. Lekeux. Ithaca, New York: International Veterinary Information service (www.ivis.org).

Allen GP, Kydd JH, Slater JD et al. 2004. Equid herpesvirus 1 and equid herpesvirus 4 infections. In JAW Coetzer and RC Tustin (eds), *Infectious Diseases of Livestock*. Cape Town, South Africa: Oxford University Press, Ch. 76, pp. 829–859.

Carman S, Rosendal S, Huber L, Gyles C, McKee S, Willoughby RA, et al. 1997. Infectious agents in

acute respiratory disease in horses in Ontario. J Vet Diagn Invest, 9: 17–23.

Kydd JH, Townsend HG, and Hannant D. 2006. The equine immune response to equine herpesvirus-1: the virus and its vaccines. Vet Immun immunop, 111: 15–30.

OIE. 2008. Chapter 2.5.9. Equine rhinopneumonities, OIE Terrestrial Manual, pp. 894–903.

Zimmerman KL and Crisman MV. 2008. Diagnostic equine serology. Vet Clin N Am-Equine, 24: 311–334.

27

Equine Rhinitis Viruses (ERAV, ERBV)

Beate Crossley and Ashley Hill

California Animal Health and Food Safety Laboratory, Department of Medicine and Epidemiology, School of Veterinary Medicine, University of California, California, USA

27.1 Clinical Background

Equine Rhinitis viruses are RNA viruses in the picornavirus family, found in two distinct genera, Equine Rhinitis virus A (ERAV) is a member of the genus aphtovirus, and Equine Rhinitis virus B (ERBV) is in the genus erbovirus (Horsington et al., 2011). Equine Rhinitis virus B currently includes three serotypes. (Horsington et al., 2013b) While ERAV and ERBV serotypes 1 and 2 have been reported worldwide, reports of ERBV serotype 3 to date are limited to Australia, Japan, and the United Kingdom.

The clinical manifestations of Equine rhinoviruses are not well defined. The viruses have been isolated from healthy horses as well as from horses with respiratory disease (Carman et al., 1997). Equine rhinitis viruses are thought to contribute to disease length and severity during co-infections with other viral and bacterial pathogens (Diaz-Mendez et al., 2010). Most ERAV infections are subclinical (Kriegshaeuser et al., 2005), with clinical ERAV infections generally including acute, 1–3 days febrile response (up to 41.4°C), anorexia, serous nasal discharge that later becomes mucopurulent, coughing, swollen mandibular lymphnodes, pharyngitis, and bronchitis (Diaz-Mendez et al., 2014). The high concentrations of ERAV shed in urine have likely contributed to the rapid spread of ERAV in the horse population.

ERBV infection is seldom associated with clinical signs, however, the virus has been recovered from horses showing fever, serous nasal discharge, anorexia, coughing, lymphadenitis, edema of legs, and swollen, painful lymphnodes of head and neck (Diaz-Mendez et al., 2010). Foals typically are infected between 4–6 months of age, and multiple cycles of infection followed by virus clearance and re-infections are seen (Black et al., 2007).

27.2 Serological Tests Available

There are no internationally-standardized serological tests for the equine rhinitis viruses. Serum virus neutralization assays have been used historically to detect ERAV and ERBV-specific antibody in serum samples. ELISA-based assays have been developed to allow for high throughput testing, however, they currently appear less sensitive than the virus neutralization approach. (Horsington et al., 2013a) Western blotting analysis and ELISA approaches are additionally often used in research facilities to detect equine rhinitis viruses and to differentiate ERBV serotypes.

27.3 Sample Collection and Submission

Whole blood is collected without additives into a syringe or evacuated tube. If not using a serum-separator tube, the blood clot is allowed to retract prior to decanting clean serum into a sterile tube for transport to the laboratory. Care should be taken when collecting the blood and separating the serum to prevent hemolysis, to the extent possible, from contaminating the test sample. The serum can be delivered chilled or frozen to the laboratory using standard biological specimens shipping procedures.

Acute serum samples should be obtained as soon as possible following onset of clinical disease (1–3 days), and paired convalescent serum should be collected approximately 2–4 weeks later.

27.4 Possible Results

The SVN test results report antibody values in titers, using two- or 10-fold serial dilution of the test sample to identify the highest dilution of sera with detectable influenza virus antibodies. ELISA results are generally reported as optical density or a transformed value calculated from the optical density of the test sample compared to a negative sample, with increasing optical density or ELISA value translating to increased detection of ERAV or ERBV specific antibody.

27.5 Interpretation and Case Examples

Due to the high prevalence of ERV antibodies in healthy horse populations (Kriegshaeuser et al., 2005), serologic testing for ERV is not frequently used in differential diagnosis of respiratory disease. ERAV seropositivity increases with horse age, with rates of up to 100% having been reported in adult horse populations worldwide. Maternal antibodies are detectable in foals, decaying between 3–9 months of age (Black et al., 2007). Neutralizing antibody typically peaks 2–3 weeks post infection, and can be detected as early as 5–7 days following infection. Antibody seroconversion to equine rhinoviruses in the absence of clinical disease has been associated with environmental contact to other horses, such as entry into training barns.

Dual infections with multiple serotypes of ERBV are not uncommon (Horsington et al., 2013b).

27.5.1 Individual Animal

- Negative for antibody to ERV by SVN or ELISA can be used to rule out infection during clinical disease.
- Positive results, regardless of SVN titer or ELISA value are not considered diagnostic for a single sample as recent from past infection cannot be distinguished.
- Positive with seroconversion measured as >4-fold change in titer suggest recent infection to ERV; however, recent infection may result in seroconversion in the absence of clinical disease.

27.5.2 Herd-Based Testing in the Face of a Respiratory Disease Outbreak

A minimum of five samples from clinically-affected horses in the affected barn/premises, paired with an equal or greater number of samples collected from horses in the same environment but not showing clinical disease should be tested at the same time.

- The titer values or geometric mean titers are analyzed in a "case-control" approach, comparing the titers of clinically ill horses to those of apparently healthy horses, and assessing for a statistical difference between the two groups of horses.

References

Black WD, Wilcox RS, Stevenson RA, Hartley CA, Ficorilli NP, Gilderson JR, and Studdert MJ. 2007. Prevalence of serum neutralizing antibody to equine rhinitis A virus (ERAV), equine rhinitis B virus 1 (ERBV1) and ERBV2. Vet Microbiol, 119: 65–71.

Carman S, Rosendal S, Huber L, Gyles C, McKee S, Willoughby RA, et al. 1997. Infectious agents in acute respiratory disease in horses in Ontario. J Vet Diagn Invest, 9: 17–23.

Diaz-Mendez A, Viel L, Hewson J, Doig P, Carman S, Chambers T, et al. 2010. Surveillance of equine respiratory viruses in Ontario. Can J Vet Res, 74: 271–278.

Diaz-Mendez A, Hewson J, Shewen P, Nagy E, and Viel L. 2014. Characteristics of respiratory tract disease in horses inoculated with equine rhinitis A virus. Am J Vet Res, 75: 169–178.

Horsington J, Gilkerson JR, and Hartley CA. 2011. Identification of mixed equine rhinitis B virus infections leading to further insight on the relationship between genotype, serotype and acid stability phenotype. Virus Res, 155: 506–513.

Horsington, J., Hartley, C.A. and Gilkerson, J.R. (2013b) Seroprevalence study of Equine rhinitis B virus (ERBV) in Australian weanling horses using serotype-specific ERBV enzyme-linked immunosorbent assays. J Vet Diagn Invest, 25: 641–644.

Horsington, J., Lynch, S.E., Gilkerson, J.R., Studdert, M.J. and Hartley, C.A. (2013a) Equine picornaviruses: well known but poorly understood. Vet Microbiol, 167: 78–85.

Kriegshaeuser, G., Deutz, A., Kuechler, E., Skern, T., Lussy, H. and Nowotny, N. (2005) Prevalence of neutralizing antibodies to Equine rhinitis A and B virus in horses and man. Vet Microbiol, 106: 293–296.

28

Interpretation of Testing for Common Mosquito Transmitted Diseases: West Nile Virus and Eastern and Western Equine Encephalitis

Maureen T. Long and Kelli L. Barr

Department of Infectious Diseases and Pathology, College of Veterinary Medicine, University of Florida, Florida, USA

28.1   Introduction

Under consideration in this chapter are viruses that group as alphaviruses, including Eastern, Western and Venezuelan encephalitis (EEE, WEE, and VEE) viruses and the flavivirus, West Nile virus (WNV). These are all transmitted by mosquitoes. While several other mosquito viruses and tick-borne viruses cause CNS infection worldwide in horses (Table 28.1), the clinical features and diagnostic challenges are similar.

28.2   Clinical Background

When clinically apparent disease occurs, in general, the neurologic abnormalities are similar in alphavirus and flavivirus infections in the horse differing mainly by severity of signs and prognosis depending on the infecting virus. A mild to moderate increase in rectal temperature (38.6–39.4 °C [102–103 °F]), anorexia, and depression are the most common initial systemic signs. Particularly in WNV infection, abdominal pain or a colic episode may be the first clinical presentation. Gait abnormalities, including insidious to overt lameness or dragging of a limb, before development of an obvious neurologic syndrome have been reported for most of these viruses. Onset of neurologic signs is frequently sudden and progressive, and the exact course of disease in any one animal is unpredictable. Spinal abnormalities are characterized by ataxia (drunken walk) and paresis (weakness) that can be highly asymmetric in flavivirus infection and generally symmetric for alphaviruses. A common presentation for WNV encephalomyelitis consists of fine and coarse fasciculations of the muscles of the face and neck. Fasciculations can be severe and can involve all four limbs and trunk, affecting normal activities. For both alphaviruses and flaviviruses, horses can have periods of hyperexcitability and apprehension,

sometimes to the point of aggression. Some horses show a change of mentation, and if a state of nonresponsiveness that resembles coma occurs, there is a poor prognosis. In EEEV infection, the animal has become comatose and nonresponsive rapidly compare to all other arboviruses. Overall, the combination, severity, and duration of clinical signs can be highly variable in the more moderate infections such as WNV and WEEV while VEEV is highly variable. In the naïve horse, EEEV infection has a >95% mortality rate. Time to recumbency, coma, and death is less than a week even with aggressive supportive care. In WEEV and WNV infected horses, the mortality rate is 40–50%. For WNV, after initial clinical signs abate, about 30% of horses experience a recrudescence in signs within the first 7–10 days of apparent recovery. In WEEV, VEEV, and WNV infected horses, there can be significant improvement within one to two weeks, and full recovery within 1–6 months can be expected in 90% of patients. Mild to moderate residual weakness and ataxia can occur, with long-term loss of the use of one or more limbs an infrequent sequela. Mild to moderate, persistent fatigue on exercise has also been observed.

28.3   Important Risk Factors

Having an accurate history is essential for accurate test interpretation. The three biggest factors in correct interpretation include vaccination history, geographic location, and age of animal.

28.3.1   Vaccination History

- Primary emphasis should always be on obtaining immunization history since proper immunization will essentially eliminate these arboviruses.
  - Most horses that are diagnosed with EEEV are either not vaccinated or are partially vaccinated. In

Interpretation of Equine Laboratory Diagnostics, First Edition. Edited by Nicola Pusterla and Jill Higgins.
© 2018 John Wiley & Sons, Inc. Published 2018 by John Wiley & Sons, Inc.

Table 28.1 Most common or known alphaviruses, flaviviruses, and bunyaviruses that cause encephalomyelitis in horses.

Virus species	Geographic location	Equine syndrome
Alphavirus		
Eastern equine encephalitis virus	N/S/C America, Carribean	Encephalomyelitis
Western equine encephalitis virus	N/S America	Encephalomyelitis
Venezualen equine encephalitis virus	C/S America, Carribean	Encephalomyelitis
Ross River virus	Australia, Papua New Guinea	Systemic: hemolymphatic Neurologic: ataxia
Semliki Forest virus	East and West Africa	Encephalomyelitis
Flavivirus		
Japanese encephalitis virus	Asia, India, Russia, Western Pacific	Encephalomyelitis
Murray valley virus	Australia, Papua New Guinea	Encephalomyelitis
Kunjin virus	Australia	Encephalomyelitis
St. Louis encephalitis	N/S/C America	Serological only recorded
Usutu	Europe, Africa	Serological only recorded
West Nile	Africa, Middle East, Europe, N/C/S America, Australia	Encephalomyelitis
Louping Ill	Iberian Peninsula, UK	Encephalomyelitis
Powassan	North America, Russia	Encephalomyelitis
Tick-Borne encephalitis	Asia, Europe, Finland, Russia	Encephalomyelitis
Bunyavirus		
California Serogroup: California encephalitis, Jamestown Canyon, La Crosse, Snowshoe hare	North America (US and Canada), parts of eastern Asia	Encephalomyelitis

N = North, S = South, C = Central

the latter, these are either young horses (<3 years of age) or recent arrivals to endemic locales without any or minimal EEEV vaccination.

- Regarding WNV infection, current flavivirus vaccines have excellent immunogenicity and even an annual vaccination that follows a full primary immunization series offers greater than 90% protection, irrespective of vaccine formulation.
- When vaccinated, it is important whether the horse has traveled from locales of low activity (Europe, Northern climates) to those of high or year-round activity (Southern US).

28.3.2 Geographic Considerations

- EEEV and WEEV viruses are separated in North America primarily along the Mississippi River. EEEV activity can occur year round in the southern USA especially during years with limited freezing temperatures. Intense focal activity has been reported in Michigan, Wisconsin, Ohio, Massachusetts, and New Hampshire.
- WEEV is found in western Canada, the USA West of the Mississippi River, Mexico, and South America. WEEV previously isolated in the South and Eastern

USA has been shown to belong to the Highlands J (HJ) virus serogroup.

- VEEV has six antigenically related subtypes that cause large outbreaks, which are not generally found in the USA.
- The South American form of EEEV is now called Madariaga virus (MAD).
  - In 2008 and 2009, large outbreaks have occurred in Central and South America.
  - Very large outbreaks have occurred recently, especially in Brazil.
- Over 50 species of flaviviruses exist (≈53): Japanese encephalitis (JEV), WNV, Kunjin virus (KUN), and Murray Valley encephalitis virus all cause illness in horses.
  - All cross-react on ELISA test formats including IgM and IgG.
  - Since 2010, continued worldwide spread and reemergence of many flaviviruses, especially WNV have occurred.
  - As of 2014, WNV is recognized as having seven lineages with lineage 1 (sublineage 1a, 1b, and 1c) and lineage 2 affecting people and horses. All are detectable in ELISA and PRNT formats with cross-reaction.

Table 28.2 Infectious and non-infectious differential for viral encephalomyelitis.

Infectious causes of neurological disease	Non-infectious causes of neurological disease
Eastern equine encephalitis virus (C)	Trauma (C)
Western equine encephalitis virus (R)	Cervical Vertebral Myeloencephalopathy or Wobblers (C)
West Nile virus (C)	Equine Degenerative Myeloencephalopathy (R)
Equine Herpesvirus 1 (C)	Neoplasia (I; age dependent)
Rabies virus (R)	Hepatoencephalopathy or Liver Failure (C; secondary to infectious and toxic causes)
Pseudorabies virus (R)	Blue Indigo (I: areas of infestation)
Equine infectious anemia virus or Swamp Fever (R)	White Snake Root Poisoning (I; areas of infestation)
Miscellaneous Fungal or Bacterial Infection (C to I dependent upon age)	Moldy Corn Poisoning (I; areas of infestation)
Listeria spp. (R)	Yellow Star Thistle Toxicity (I; area of infestation)
Clostridium botulinum or Botulism (I)	Polyneuritis equi (R)
Sarcocystis neurona or EPM (C)	Organophosphate toxicity (R)
Halicephalobus gingivalis (I)	
Angiostrongylus cantonensis (U)	
Miscellaneous Foreign Diseases: Venezuelan equine encephalitis virus, Borna disease virus, Hendra virus,	

C = Common, High Risk; I = Focal Outbreaks, Intermediate Risk; R = Rare for endemic regions; U = Unknown, emerging disease

28.3.3 Age of Animal

- North American EEEV occurs in primarily young horses.
- The risk of horses exhibiting neurological manifestations and mortality due to WNV increases with age.

28.3.4 Season

- All arboviruses are associated with seasonal mosquito activity.
- Year-round virus transmission and disease can occur in tropical climates.
  - Subtropical climates may have year-round activity with peak activity
    - EEEV infections can be detected as early as March and often peak in July in the Southeastern United States.
    - WNV usually occurs later in the year with peak activity in September extending even through the first 2 weeks of October.

28.4 Clinical Differentials

Although many horses are vaccinated for protection against disease caused by encephalitis causing arboviruses, the incompletely or nonvaccinated horse is always at risk throughout many parts of the world. Clinical signs and antemortem clinical pathologic findings are not specific for mosquito-borne encephalitides. Even in endemic areas where veterinarians frequently see multiple mosquito-born illnesses, it is not possible to diagnose or differentiate between EEEV, WEEV, VEEV, or WNV in the horse with any certainty based on clinical signs and epidemiologic circumstances. Because of its severity, horses affected by EEEV and severe VEEV can resemble many of the very severe infectious and non-infectious brain diseases. West Nile virus and WEEV, when moderate, can include differentials that present as localized spinal abnormalities (Table 28.2).

28.5 Tests Available

Eastern equine encephalitis virus, WEEV, and WNV are reportable diseases, thus it is paramount to obtain a definitive or evidence-based diagnosis for clinical signs of any encephalitis in the horse. This allows institution of effective control measures because of the risk of these viruses to the health and well-being of both humans and equine livestock.

Viral and other encephalitides can cause abnormal cerebrospinal fluid (CSF), which is an important clinical test for the diagnosis of any neurological disease. In particular EEEV is unique in that acute infection frequently results in increased neutrophils in the spinal fluid. These are not toxic and are frequently hypersegmented. In more chronic or in partially vaccinated horses, the

Table 28.3 Summary of known CSF findings for arbovirus diseases.

	Protein	Cells	Cell types	Color
EEEV	▲▲	▲▲	Neutrophils Mononuclear	Normal to mildly turbid
WEEV	▲	▲	Mononuclear	Normal
WNV	N to ▲	N to ▲▲	Mononuclear	Mildly Xanthochromic
KV	▲	N to ▲▲	Mononuclear (some neutrophils)	Mildly Xanthochromic

cellular component may be mononuclear. In WNV, WEEV, and VEEV-infected horses, if the cell counts are abnormal, lymphocytes and monocytes usually predomonate. The protein in this fluid is usually elevated as well (Table 28.3).

28.5.1 Antemortem Testing

Currently, no reliable antemortem diagnostic tests are available to detect virus in clinically affected horses. Serology provides the mainstay of presumptive antemortem diagnosis (Table 28.4). Prompt serological testing is a must for the purposes of accurate diagnosis and reporting of activity. Blood is an inappropriate specimen for virus recovery because circulating virus is no longer present when signs of encephalitis become apparent. In an epidemic situation, however, it might be possible to isolate the virus from nonencephalitic horses and unaffected horses from the same farm concurrent with clinical illness.

Thus, the most reliable way to diagnose these infections is by detection of antibody. During the course of

Table 28.4 Antemortem and postmortem diagnostic tests for detection of arboviruses.

	Antemortem				Postmortem		
	Serology				Serology		
Disease	MAC	NT or PRNT	PCR	VI	MAC	PCR	VI
EEE/WEE	+	*	–	–	**	+	+
VEE	+	*	+	+	**	+	+
WNV	+	*	–	–	**	+	+

+ Useful and indicated

- Not useful or not indicated

* Paired samples in endemic sites with vaccinated animals

** CSF can be collected at the time of death and assayed immediately for clinicopathological abnormalities and MAC ELISA at 1:2 dilution, if positive, intrathecal production likely.

infection, the first antibody produced to infection is IgM for both groups of viruses. In the horse, this response is very crisp, rising sharply during the first few days of clinical neurologic signs and only lasting about 4–6 weeks. Measurement of IgM is at single dilution of 1:400 for WNV, EEEV and other arboviruses in capture ELISA format (MAC). The detection of IgM antibody in CSF (if available) is even more conclusive (dilution must be 1:2). Although the demonstration of specific immunoglobulin M (IgM) antibody (dilution of 1:400) is a highly specific and sensitive method for diagnosis, there can be cross-reactivity of the IgM between alphaviruses (EEEV vs VEEV) and flaviviruses (WNV vs JEV). The confirmatory antibody based test in the nonvaccinated horse is based on serum neutralizing (SN) antibody. An initial sample is taken at the first sign of clinical disease and, in horses that survive, a second sample is obtained 2–4 weeks later. SN antibody is measured in one of two formats, the plaque reduction neutralization test (PRNT) or the microwell (SN) neutralization test. A commonly used screening test is the hemagglutination inhibition (HI) test which uses red blood cells coated with virus to detect antibody. This test should not be used for diagnosis in the horse since it detects both IgM and IgG, has a high degree of cross-reactivity between like viruses, and can have false positive reactions due to nonspecific hemagglutinins.

28.5.2 Postmortem Testing

The viruses EEEV, WEEV, VEEV, and WNV can be isolated or detected after death in brain material of diseased horses by the use of cell cultures, through intracerebral inoculation of suckling mice with infected brain material, and by detection of specific nucleotide sequences using reverse transcriptase–polymerase chain reaction (RT-PCR) technology. Rapid real-time PCR methods performed on clinical specimens have been developed that differentiate between the alphaviruses and flaviviruses. For the alphaviruses and flaviviruses, the CDC protocol utilizes two primer sets.

These primers can also be used on formalin-fixed paraffin embedded tissue (FFPE). Immunohistochemistry can be used to detect virus in formalin-fixed paraffin embedded tissues. In general these techniques are excellent for detection of EEEV in the brain of affected horses. Unfortunately, almost all viral detection methods for WNV infection of horses is less reliable. This is due to comparative viral loads in the brain of horses. EEEV occurs in high amounts in the cortex, midbrain, and hindbrian with limited occurence in the spinal cord. WNV exhibits limited detection of virus overall, however some areas of the brain including the thalamus, hypothalamus, and pons/medulla are most commonly positive. The lumbar spinal cord is also an area in which virus can be detected. Often only a single neuron in a single section of brain tissue will contain virus upon staining with IHC for WNV do an experienced and reliable laboratory must stain several sections of brain and spinal cord.

28.6 Sample Collection and Submission

Antemortem samples should consist of unclotted whole blood for CBC, clotted whole blood for clinicopathological analysis, clotted whole blood for serology, and CSF for clinical pathological analysis and detection of IgM. Plasma is of no use for detection virus in the sick animal, however, stablemates can often have the virus in new encroachments, thus herd testing is of value. However, no virus will be detected in fully vaccinated stablemates. The laboratory which performs the test must be reliable because the E protein, which is detected in the MAC format, requires specialized procedures to provide a conformationally correct protein that reacts accurately with serum samples. If whole virus is used, incorrect inactivation of whole virus or expression of proteins can cause a change in the results of the assay or even pose a biosecurity risk if inadequately inactivated. This problem is further compounded by the fact that MAC ELISA formats are possible for all arboviruses, however with the commercialization of the viral proteins used for these assays, many laboratories, including state laboratories, have discontinued this test format for both EEEV and WNV. The EEEV antigen is exceptionally difficult to obtain commercially even for federal and state laboratories due to federal regulations which restrict the dissemination of the virus. WNV antigen is now commercially made, but prohibitively expensive for underfunded laboratories. Most state diagnostic laboratories, if they do not offer the MAC ELISA within the laboratory, will forward the serum sample to the National Veterinary Services Laboratory (NVSL) in Ames, Iowa. These considerations are very important because lack of test availability at a local laboratory will delay results by several days if not possibly weeks.

In the field necropsy situation, it is advisable to obtain a sample of inner cortex (gray and white matter) as well as hindbrain at the pons and medulla. If spinal cord is available, cervical and lumbar cord both should be submitted. In the case of simultaneous rabies detection, it is important that the arbovirus laboratory receive appropriate samples since the rabies laboratory will request a cross-section of the pons and medulla as well, where high amounts of arbovirus localization occurs. A section from caudal to the medulla or the rostral colliculi should be tested if the pons and medulla is not available. Shipment must conform to legal guidelines using an inner, non-crushable and leak proof primary package surrounded by a box that is certified for handling (https://www.fishersci.com/us/en/home.html).

28.7 Interpretation of Results

Confirmation of WNV infection with encephalitis in horses begins with assessment of (1) whether the horse meets the case definition based on clinical signs, (2) whether the horse resides in an area in which WNV has been confirmed in the current calendar year in mosquito, bird, human, or horse, and (3) vaccination history. Most horses that are clinically apparent with EEEV and WNV have an IgM titer, which remains for 4–6 weeks. The sensitivity and specificity of this test are >80% for both of these infections. With this high sensitivity and specificity in the clinical horse, most arbovirus surveillance and antemortem diagnosis are based on this single test. In the nonvaccinated horse, a four-fold change in paired neutralizing antibody titers is confirmatory of a diagnosis of WNV and/or EEEV infection, although a second sample is rarely obtained for EEEV. Vaccination induces formation of neutralizing antibody to the E protein of the virus, which likely confounds interpretation of the PRNT, thus, the reliance on the PRNT for serologic confirmatory diagnosis of WNV in horses has diminished.

"Vaccine" breaks have been difficult to fully substantiate due to difficulty in obtaining an authentic vaccine history. Anecdotally, based on a decade of arboviral consulting by the author, new ownership without previous adequate vaccination, incomplete primary immunization, and lack of annual consistency of WNV vaccination have been commonly found in further inquiry as an underlying issue in WNV disease in the "vaccinated" horse.

28.8 Case Example

Several serum samples and nasal swabs from horses have been submitted to the local diagnostic laboratory for testing in the face of a small focal febrile illness with

Table 28.5 Testing results for the case example.

Clinical Signs	H1	H2	H3	H4	H5	H6
	Recumbent	Ataxic/Weak/ Febrile	No abnormalities	No abnormalities	Mildly increased temperature	No abnormalities
CSF	Slight increased protein/ mononuclear cells	Slight increased protein/ mononuclear cells	ND	ND	ND	ND
EEEV HI	Positive @5	Negative < 5	Negative < 5	Negative < 5	Negative < 5	Negative < 5
EEEV MAC	Negative @400	Negative @400	Negative @400	Negative @400	Negative @400	Negative @400
WNV MAC	Positive @400	Negative @400	Negative @400	Negative @400	Negative @400	Negative @400
EHV-1 PCR (nasal swab)	Positive for wild type virus	Negative	Negative	Negative	Positive for wild type virus	Negative
EHV-4 PCR	Negative	Negative	Negative	Negative	Negative	Negative

H = horse, ND = not done, @ = reciprocal of the dilution

varied neurological signs involving a group of six horses which recently shipped to a southern US state in the late Fall. These were hunter-jumper mixed breed horses that just arrived from Northern Europe and had received a single injection of WNV vaccine (killed product that requires two initial injections) and no EEEV vaccine before shipping. Arrival was at least 8 weeks prior to the onset of clinical signs. The origin and complete geographic history of these horses is unknown beyond the fact that the horses shipped out of Germany.

28.8.1 Clinical Assessment

Given the fact that multiple horses are affected, the differential diagnoses would consist of an infectious disease, especially those that cause neurological disease. Under consideration would be mostly viral causes because of the concurrent clinical signs. If these horses did not have increased rectal temperatures, one would have to consider non-infectious causes also (Table 28.2).

Serum samples and nasal swabs were sent to various laboratories for testing since no one laboratory in this southern state offered a comprehensive panel for infectious neurological disease. No plasma samples were submitted from these horses and the hospital laboratory performed the CSF analysis. A local University laboratory performed the ELISA for detection of IgM antibody for both EEEV and WNV. The state diagnostic laboratory performed an HI test for EEEV. Yet another private laboratory performed equine herpes virus 1 (EHV-1) testing on the nasal swabs. The federal laboratory performed neutralizing testing on the samples, which takes up to 2 weeks for results; thus the initial results only consisted of the HI-EEEV and the MAC-EEEV and MAC-WNV results for the arboviruses and the PCR for EHVs. At the time of testing, one horse was recumbent, while two others were febrile with one exhibiting weakness and ataxia. The remaining three were normal.

28.8.2 Interpretation of Testing

A common issue for many species-specific diseases and reportable disease testing is lack of comprehensive local testing requiring shipment of samples to regional or federal test laboratories. Analysis of diagnostic test results is best made in the light of clinical findings (Table 28.5). CSF testing consisted of a mononuclear cellularity in the face of ataxia in Horse 1, thus EEEV was considered less likely but was not altogether ruled out. The positive HI test was also not very meaningful given that the MAC-EEEV was negative in all horses and is usually (but not always) positive once a horse demonstrates clinical signs such as ataxia or recumbence. The positive MAC-WNV in Horse 1 was considered the most indicative of recent exposure. One injection of WNV vaccine is not protective and will likely not interfere with the MAC ELISA results, upon exposure so this was considered significant (also considering the length of time since the horses has received any vaccine injection). What is extremely important is that both affected and nonaffected horses were shedding EHV-1 (non-neurotropic). It must be remembered that (1) the non-neurotropic strains of EHV-1 are infectious and (2) can cause neurological signs in horses. However, the CSF was more consistent with WNV; EHV-1 usually has increased protein without significant increase in WBC (Table 28.3). The horses were isolated due to the EHV-1 shedding and deemed WNV suspect and reported to the state department of health.

28.8.3 Course of Disease and Disease Outcome

The recumbent horse was able to rise within 48 hours and both febrile horses recovered uneventfully. Follow-up testing demonstrated seroconversion of H1 and H2 WNV over the course of 4 weeks. All seronegative horses were vaccinated for EEEV and WNV. Follow-up testing at 4 weeks for EHV-1 was negative for virus on all nasal swabs and serum. All horses were released from farm imposed isolation with a third round of nasal swabs at approximately 8 weeks.

29

Streptococcus equi ss *equi*

Ashley G. Boyle

Department of Clinical Studies, New Bolton Center, School of Veterinary Medicine, University of Pennsylvania, Pennsylvania, USA

29.1   Clinical Background

The main surface proteins of the organism *Streptococcus equi* ss *equi* (*S. equi*) are M-like fibrinogen-binding proteins SeM and SzPSe. They are antiphagocytic and highly immunogenic. Indirect enzyme-linked immunosorbent assays (iELISA) detect total immunoglobulin G (IgG) antibodies from the host immune system directed against these surface proteins and were developed to identify "hyperresponder" horses which manifest purpura hemorrhagica complications secondary to strangles vaccination (Pusterla et al., 2003, Sweeney et al., 2005, Davidson et al., 2008).

Serologic tests are not to be used in place of *S. equi* quantitative polymerase chain reaction (qPCR) or bacterial culture for identification of index, active or carrier cases of *S. equi*. *S. equi* serologic tests can be used to detect recent infections (time frame and accuracy depend on the test used), determine the risk of developing purpura hemorrhagic prior to *S. equi* vaccination by identifying horses with existing high level of antibody, support a diagnosis of disseminated *S. equi* abscessation (bastard strangles), and possibly support a diagnosis of existing *S. equi*- associated purpura hemorrhagica (Sweeney et al., 2005). It is debatable whether the serum serologic value portrays the level of current protection as some sources state that most protection against infection is at the mucosal level (Timoney and Eggers, 1985).

29.2   Tests Available

Multiple tests are currently available depending in which country the veterinarian practices. The tests targeting full length SeM surface antigen (IDEXX, Equine Diagnostic Solutions [EDS], and ID.vet) have been criticized for their lack of specificity and cross-reactivity with *Streptococcus zooepidemicus*. As a result, iELISA

assays using surface antigen portions unique to *S. equi* (N-terminal portion of SeM, C-terminal portion of SzPSe, and a portion of SEQ2190) have been developed (see Table 29.1).

29.3   Sample Collection and Submission

All tests are performed on serum shipped and cooled overnight. Check serum volume required with specific laboratory.

29.4   Possible Results

See Tables 29.1 and 29.2.

29.5   Serological Results and Interpretation

- *Whole SeM* (IDEXX, EDS, CSU): See Table 29.2 for detailed interpretations of results. These values do not apply to foals <6 months of age due to maternal antibody interference. *S. equi* carrier status cannot be determined by the SeM ELISA (Davidson et al., 2008). Vaccination status and natural infection play a significant role in serum antibody production resulting in significant overlap in interpretation of results (Table 29.2; Sheoran et al., 1997). Due to the cross-reactivity between SeM and the homolog of SzM, there is the potential for false positive results. No published control studies have been performed examining the sensitivity/specificity of these tests or their true reliability of the association of very high titers with metastatic strangles and especially purpura hemorrhagica. Vaccination is contraindicated in the horse with a titer

Interpretation of Equine Laboratory Diagnostics, First Edition. Edited by Nicola Pusterla and Jill Higgins.
© 2018 John Wiley & Sons, Inc. Published 2018 by John Wiley & Sons, Inc.

Table 29.1 Availability of serologic tests for *Streptococcus equi* ss *equi*. Source: Data from Robinson (2013) and Hobo (2008).

Country	Laboratory	Antigen tested	Cross reactivity	Sensitivity	Specificity	Result
USA	IDEXX, EDS	Whole (full-length) SeM	Homologue SzM from *S. zooepidemicus*	NA	NA	Dilution Value with Pos/Neg cut-off and correlating titers
France	ID.vet	Whole (full length) SeM	Homologue SzM from *S. zooepidemicus*	89.9%[1]	77.0%[1]	Pos/Neg optical density cutoff value
United Kingdom	Animal Health Trust (AHT)	N-terminal recombinant protein fragments of SEQ2190 (antigen A) and SeM (antigen C)	None known	93.3%[1]	99.3%[1]	Pos/Neg optical density cut off value
Japan	Epizootic Research Center, Equine Research Institute, Japan Racing Association	Proline-glutamic acid-proline-lysine antigen with five repetitions (PEPK-5R) C- terminal SzPSe	Minimal cross-reactivity with *S. zooepidemicus*	97%[2]	88.9%[2]	Pos/Neg optical density cut off value
USA	Research Colorado State University (research only)	Whole (full length) SeM	Cross- reactivity to SzM antibodies is removed via preincubation of sera with heat-killed *S. zooepidemicus*	NA	NA	Dilution Value with Pos/Neg cutoff and correlating titers

1 (Robinson et al., 2013),
2 (Hobo et al., 2008)

Table 29.2 Interpretation of SeM-specific ELISA (IDEXX, EDS).

Result		Interpretation
Negative		No previous vaccination or infection to *S equi*. Peracute exposure (<7 days).
Positive	1:200–1:400	Recent infection to *S equi* or previous vaccination > 1 year. Retest recommended.
	1:800–1:1,600	Recent infection. *S. equi* infection >6 months, <2 years ago. Vaccination within the last 1 year.
	1:3,200–1:6,400	Recent *S. equi* infection (within 4 to 12 weeks). 1–2 weeks post intramuscular vaccination or 2–4 weeks post intranasal vaccination. Do not vaccinate these horses.
	≥1:12,800	Maybe associated with metastatic abscessation or purpura hemorrhagica. Do not vaccinate these horses.

(Sweeney *et al*, 2005)
Source: Sweeney (2008). Reproduced with permission of American College of Veterinary Internal Medicine.

of ≥ 1:3,200 due to the risk of developing purpura hemorrhagica (Sweeney et al., 2005, Boyle et al., 2009). Older horses, horses other than Thoroughbreds and Warmbloods, and horses vaccinated with the attenuated–live intranasal vaccination Pinnacle (Zoetis) were likely to have an SeM-specific antibody titer of ≥ 1:1,600 when 188 healthy horses were sampled (Boyle et al., 2009). When examining SeM–specific antibody titers in both healthy and *S. equi* convalescent horses, horses with a history of clinical strangles disease logically were more likely to have titers of ≥ 1:3,200 (Boyle et al., 2012). Titer response will vary amongst individuals and titers ≥ 1:3,200 have been documented for up to 20 months post natural *S. equi* outbreak. Therefore, vaccination for *S. equi* is not recommended within 2 years of an outbreak without determining the SeM ELISA titer for the specific animal (Boyle et al., 2012).

- *Whole SeM* (ID.vet): When compared to the antigen A and antigen C combination assay (AHT), this serological assay had lower sensitivity and specificity (see Table 29.1) using a *S. equi* naïve Icelandic population as the true negatives and UK horses known to be positive via bacterial culture as the true positives (Robinson et al., 2013).

- *PEPK-5R*: This test reportedly has less cross-reactivity with *S. zooepidemicus* than the whole SeM test, but previous *S. equi* vaccination does affect the interpretation of the results, thus requiring additional research (Hobo et al., 2006, 2008, 2010).

- *Combined SEQ2190 (antigen A) and SeM (antigen C)* (Animal Health Trust iELISA): This test has the

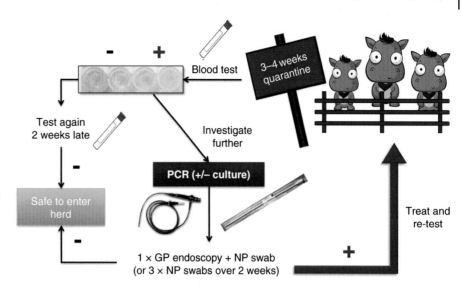

Figure 29.1 The combined SEQ2190 (Antigen A) and SeM (Antigen C) serology can be used in unvaccinated horses to prescreen new animals prior to introduction into the herd. If an asymptomatic horse tests negative on serology, it is recommended that the horse be retested 2 weeks later before introducing the animal into the new herd. If the new arrival is positive on serology, then guttural pouch lavage qPCR and endoscopic examination is warranted. If guttural pouch examination is not possible, then three nasopharyngeal washes over a 2-week period should be performed, though this is not ideal (Robinson et al., 2013). *Source:* Waller (2013). Reproduced with permission of Elsevier.

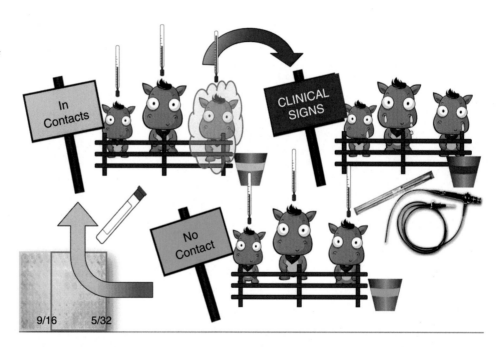

Figure 29.2 The combined Antigen A and C serology can also be utilized in the control of outbreaks. Guttural pouch lavage and endoscopy should be performed on all previously clinical animals three weeks post the resolution of clinical signs. The asymptomatic nonexposed and exposed groups are then tested at that time with the combined iELISA assays to identify who requires additional screening via guttural pouch lavage and endoscopy to find subclinical carriers from these two groups (Robinson et al., 2013). *Source:* Waller (2013). Reproduced with permission of Elsevier.

benefit of no cross-reactivity with *S. zooepidemicus*. At the time of writing (March 2016) it is currently only available in Europe. This test reliably detects a positive seroconversion within two weeks of *S. equi* infection, as well as in persistently infected animals (Robinson et al., 2013). Therefore, this test can be used to prescreen new animals prior to introduction into the herd (Figure 29.1). If an asymptomatic horse tests negative on serology, it is recommended that the horse be retested 2 weeks later before introducing the animal into the new herd. If the new arrival is positive on serology, then guttural pouch lavage qPCR and endoscopic examination is war-

ranted. If guttural pouch examination is not possible, then three nasopharyngeal washes over a 2-week period should be performed, though this is not ideal. The combined Antigen A and C serology can also be utilized in the control of outbreaks (Figure 29.2). Guttural pouch lavage and endoscopy should be performed on all previously clinical animals three weeks post the resolution of clinical signs. The asymptomatic nonexposed and exposed groups are then tested at that time with the combined iELISA assays to identify who requires additional screening via guttural pouch lavage and endoscopy to find subclinical carriers from these

---

Box 29.1 Clinical indications to use SeM and SEQ2190 serology

Uses of Whole SeM Serology

Yes:

To determine the safety of future vaccination and associated risk of purpura hemorrhagica.

To identify cases of *S. equi equi* metastatic abscessation or possibly *S. equi equi* associated purpura hemorrhagica.

No:

Should not be used to identify *S. equi equi* carrier status.

Should not be used to identify recent infection to *S. equi equi* (time frame not specific enough) or to identify an index or active case of strangles.

Debatable as to whether serum serology identifies the need for vaccination (i.e., how much immunological protection does the horse currently have?).

Uses of Combined SEQ2190 and SeM

To be used in unvaccinated populations.

Screening tool to identify horses recently exposed (within 2 weeks) to *S. equi equi* or possible carriers of *S. equi equi* prior to introduction to the herd or to identify possible carriers at the end of an outbreak. Serologically negative horses are screened a second time, 2 weeks later, to confirm their negative status. Guttural pouch endoscopy in conjunction with *S. equi equi* PCR and culture is then performed on the serologically positive horses to identify guttural pouch carriers of *S. equi equi*.

---

two groups (Robinson et al., 2013). Unfortunately, all current vaccines will develop an antibody response to these serological assays making the practitioner unable to determine the source of the antibody response if the horses have been previously vaccinated (Waller, 2013).

Serologic tests for *S. equi* target the antiphagocytic surface proteins of the organism can be used to determine the safety to vaccinate for strangles, support *S. equi* metastatic abscessation diagnosis, possibly support *S. equi* associated purpura hemorrhagica diagnosis, and identify recent infection. Cross-reactivity with *Streptococcus zooepidemicus* can result in false positive results. New tests that target different proteins are available in the United Kingdom to increase specificity and can be incorporated into herd prevention management and outbreak control due to increased sensitivity and detection of exposures as recent as 2 weeks (Box 29.1).

29.6 Case Discussions

29.6.1 Whole SeM Serology

A 7-year-old Appendix Quarterhorse gelding presents for intermittent colic and low-grade fevers of unknown origin. Prior medical history is unknown. Minimum database reveals a hyperfibrinogenemia, anemia, and hyperproteinemia characterized by a hyperglobulinemia. A large spherical mass is found on palpation per rectum cranial to the pelvic inlet at arm's length, just left of midline. Ultrasonographic examination per rectum identifies a structure that is 13 cm in diameter with a heterogenous center and a thick capsule. Abdominocentesis reveals an exudate characterized by a high total protein and an increased nucleated cell count. Culture of the abdominal fluid is negative. SeM-specific ELISA serology is greater than 1:12,800 providing a strong case that this intrabdominal mass is a *S. equi equi* abscess most likely associated with a mesenteric lymph node based on its location.

Acknowledgments

Dr. Boyle's research has been supported by Boehringer Ingelheim Advancement in Equine Research Grant, the American Quarter Horse Foundation, the Frances Cheyney Glover Endowment Fund, the Raymond Firestone Research Fund, the International Arabian Foundation, and the University of Pennsylvania Equine Research Endowment Funds.

References

Boyle AG, Smith MA, and Boston RC. 2012. Risk factors for high serum SeM titers after natural outbreaks of *Streptococcus equi equi* in horses. In 9th International Conference of Equine Infectious Disease Abstracts. J Eq Vet Science 32: S3–S95.

Boyle AG, Sweeney CR, Kristula M, Boston RC, and Smith G. 2009. Factors associated with likelihood of horses having a high serum *Streptococcus equi* SeM-specific antibody titer. JAVMA 8: 973–977.

Davidson A, Traub-Dargatz J, Magnuson R, Hill A, Irwin V, Newton R, et al. 2008. Lack of correlation between antibody titers to fibrinogen-binding protein of *Streptococcus equi* and persistent carriers of strangles. J Vet Diagn Invest 20: 457–462.

Hobo S, Niwa H, and Anzai T. 2006. Proline-glutamic acid-proline-lysine peptide set as a specific antigen for the serological diagnosis of strangles. Vet Rec 159: 629–632.

Hobo S, Niwa H, and Anzai T. 2008. Proline-glutamic acid-proline-lysine repetition peptide as an antigen for the serological diagnosis of strangles. Vet Rec 162: 471–474.

Hobo S, Niwa H, Anzai T, and Jones JH. 2010. Changes in serum antibody levels after vaccination for strangles and after intranasal challenge with *Streptococcus equi* subsp. *equi* in horses. J Equine Sci 21: 33–37.

Pusterla N, Watson JL, and Affolter VK. 2003. Purpura haemorrhagica in 53 horses. Vet Rec 153: 118–121.

Robinson C, Steward K, Potts N, Barker C, Hammond T, Pierce K, et al. 2013. Combining two serological assays optimizes sensitivity and specificity for the identification of *Streptococcus equi* subsp *equi* exposure. Vet J 197: 188–191.

Sheoran AS, Sponseller BT, Holmes MA, and Timoney JF. 1997. Serum and mucosal antibody isotype responses to M-like protein (SeM) of *Streptococcus equi* in convalescent and vaccinated horses. Vet Immunol Immunopathol 59: 239–251.

Sweeney CR, Timoney JF, Newton JR, and Hines MT. 2005. *Streptococcus equi* infections in horses: guidelines for treatment, control, and prevention of strangles. J Vet Intern Med 19: 123–134.

Timoney JF and Eggers D. 1985. Serum bactericidal responses to *Streptococcus equi* of horses following infection or vaccination. Equine Vet J 17: 306–310.

Waller AS. 2013. Strangles: Taking steps towards eradication. Vet Micro 167: 50–60.

30

Corynebacterium pseudotuberculosis

Sharon J. Spier and Jennifer Jeske

Department of Medicine and Epidemiology, School of Veterinary Medicine, University of California, California, USA

30.1 Disease Overview

Corynebacterium pseudotuberculosis is a Gram-positive, intracellular, facultative anaerobic bacterium that causes disease in multiple species including horses, goats, sheep, and occasionally cattle, humans, and other species worldwide (Aleman et al., 1996, Spier, 2015). The nitrate-positive biotype causes three clinical disease syndromes in horses, the most prevalent of which is the formation of external abscesses containing copious purulent material and typically located in the pectoral muscles, ventral abdomen, inguinal region, axillary region, sheath, or mammary tissue. Infection in horses is commonly known as "Pigeon fever," due to swelling in the pectoral region resembling a pigeon's breast (Figure 30.1). Less commonly, horses may develop single or multiple internal abscesses in the abdominal cavity, peritonitis, bronchopneumonia, and/or pleuritis. Internal infection is thought to represent <10% of total cases and may occur with or without a previously reported history of external abscess formation. The third and least common disease manifestation in North America is ulcerative lymphangitis, generally involving one hind limb and representing approximately 1% of cases (Aleman et al., 1996, Kilcoyne et al., 2014).

Identification and treatment of external abscesses that result from *C. pseudotuberculosis* infection are often accomplished through physical examination and surgical drainage of abscesses or monitoring of abscess expansion and rupture. Identification and treatment of internal abscesses is more challenging, considering the nonspecific clinical signs and clinicopathologic findings in horses with thoracic or abdominal infections. A combination of physical examination, hematologic testing, advanced imaging, and culture may be needed to confirm infection (Figure 30.2). Ultrasonographic features of hepatic, renal and splenic infection suggestive of, though not pathognomonic for, infection attributable to *C. pseudotuberculosis* have been described (Vaughan et al., 2004, Pratt et al., 2005). Abdominal ultrasonography is useful to evaluate the extent of infection, guide tissue sampling for culture submission, and monitor response to therapy. Research findings regarding the ulcerative lymphangitis form of *C. pseudotuberculosis* infection are more limited, however, aggressive and prolonged treatment with antimicrobial and anti-inflammatory medications is recommended for this form of infection (Spier, 2015).

In North America, clinical disease may occur throughout the year (Kilcoyne et al., 2014). Peak incidence for external infection in California occurs in late summer to early fall when insect vector populations are at their highest numbers (Aleman et al., 1996). A separate study specifically evaluating horses with internal abscesses showed a peak incidence several months later, from November through January (Pratt et al., 2005). Interestingly, a biannual incidence peak pattern has been observed in Texas with a peak incidence earlier in spring in addition to a peak in fall, suggesting different insect vectors or other environmental factors may be responsible for disease spread (Szonyi et al., 2013, Kilcoyne et al., 2014). The soil-dwelling bacterium is believed to be spread by biting flies, contamination of abraded skin, or inhalation, and is long lived in the environment (Spier et al., 2012). The fly vector component of disease transmission may contribute to the observed seasonality of infection. Historically, the highest disease incidence in the United States has been reported in California and Texas although there is increasing frequency of cases in all regions of the United States, Western Canada, and Northern Mexico (Spier, 2008, Kilcoyne et al., 2014).

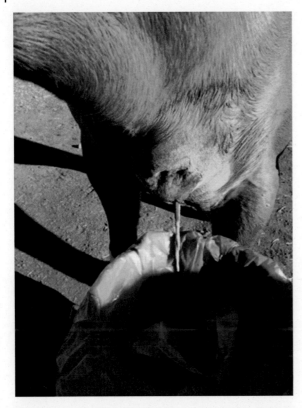

Figure 30.1 Typical pectoral abscess due to *Corynebacterium pseudotuberculosis* infection, which is one of the most common clinical manifestations. Bacterial culture is all that is required to confirm infection.

30.2 Diagnostic Tests

30.2.1 Clinicopathological Findings

Clinicopathologic findings in horses with internal infection are generally indicative of a non-specific, chronic, inflammatory process. Common hematologic findings in horses with internal infection include leukocytosis with neutrophilia, hyperglobulinemia, hyperfibrinogenemia, and anemia.

30.2.2 Culture

Corynebacterium pseudotuberculosis grows well, although slowly, with colonies visible on blood agar within 24–48 h. Culture should be used to confirm all three forms of *C. pseudotuberculosis* infection in horses, though samples for external forms of disease (external abscesses and ulcerative lymphangitis) are most easily obtained. Samples for culture from external lesions may be submitted from aspirates prior to surgical drainage. In horses with internal infection, acquisition of samples for culture may require ultrasound – guided fine needle aspirates or trans-tracheal wash (TTW) depending upon the location of infection. Not all sites of infection

can be safely sampled in the case of internal infection; however, adjunctive tests including clinicopathologic findings (CBC, serum biochemistry, or abdominocentesis) and serology can be used as supportive evidence for diagnosis.

30.2.3 Serology – Synergistic Hemolysis Inhibition Test (SHI Test)

The SHI test, which measures IgG antibodies to an exotoxin of *C. pseudotuberculosis* in serum, can be useful to support a diagnosis of *C. pseudotuberculosis* infection. Serology is most commonly used to support a diagnosis of internal infection when history, clinical and clinical pathologic findings are consistent with chronic inflammation. In cases of suspected internal infection, serology alone should not be used as a definitive diagnostic test. Serology can also be used to support a diagnosis of lymphangitis due to *C. pseudotuberculosis* when culture is not possible.

The basis for the SHI test is the ability of *C. pseudotuberculosis* toxin to produce a zone of hemolysis when serum is applied to a blood agar plate containing erythrocytes sensitized with *Rhodococcus equi* culture broth. If anti-*C. pseudotuberculosis* toxin antibodies are present in the test serum, the hemolysis reaction is neutralized (inhibited) (Knight, 1978) (Figure 30.3). Serial dilutions of serum from the patient and positive and negative control sera are added to separate wells and incubated with *C. pseudotuberculosis* toxin. Absorbent disks are then dipped in each well and placed on a sensitized blood agar plate to be incubated overnight. The endpoint titer is the highest serum dilution for which the disk has no surrounding hemolysis (indicating a sufficient concentration of antibodies against *C. pseudotuberculosis* toxin at that dilution to neutralize hemolytic activity). Any hemolysis surrounding a disk indicates a lack of antibody presence, with a zone of hemolysis measuring <0.5 mm considered doubtful for antibody presence and a zone >0.5 mm considered negative for antibody presence (Knight, 1978).

Reciprocal antibody titer results are expected to be low to non-existent early in the disease process and should increase in the weeks following infection. Re-testing in 2–4 weeks should be considered for horses tested early in the disease process when negative results are obtained, and re-testing can also be used to look for increasing antibody titers in horses with measurable antibody titers early in the disease process. Resolution of the disease can be assessed by monitoring return to normal values on complete blood count, improvement in repeat abdominal ultrasound examinations and decrease in SHI titers. Be mindful that SHI titers will remain elevated for many months, however, due to the long half-life of IgG

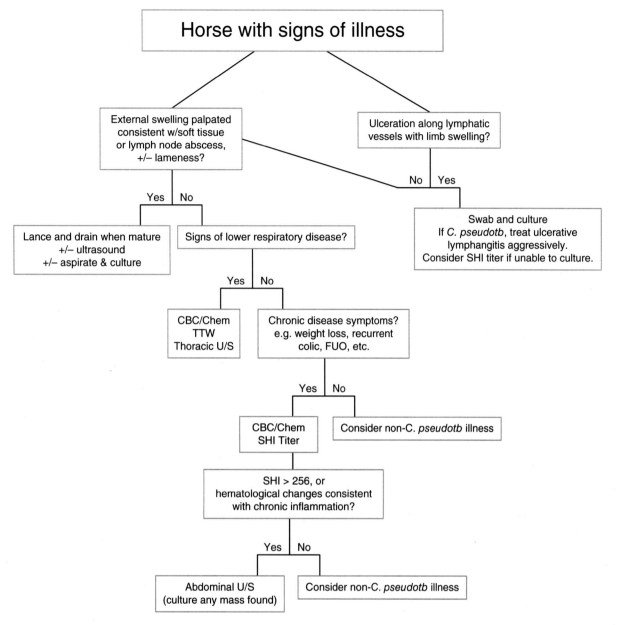

Figure 30.2 Diagnostic flow chart for systemic infection caused by *Corynebacterium pseudotuberculosis*.

(21 days), so return to normal for other parameters may be more useful.

Increased SHI titer results are associated with *C. pseudotuberculosis* infection in horses but not with a specific disease manifestation (Figure 30.4). Considerable overlap in titers exists between horses with external abscesses (e.g., pectoral or ventral abdominal abscesses), internal infection and even exposed herdmates without clinical evidence of infection. As such, the SHI test has its greatest utility in aiding or supporting the diagnosis of internal infection in the absence of external disease. When supportive evidence of chronic inflammation exists, in the absence of external abscessation, SHI titer results of ≥512

are associated with a likelihood ratio of 10.75 as compared to horses with SHI titers <512. That is to say a patient whose SHI titer is measured at ≥512, who does not have external infection, has a post-test odds of *C. pseudotuberculosis* nearly 11 times that of their pre-test odds of disease. When a four-tier titer system is used, titer results of <2 or ≥2 and ≤160 yielded likelihood ratios near zero significantly decreasing post-test odds of disease, while titers ≥256 and ≤1024 or ≥1280 yielded likelihood ratios of 3.76 and 15.99, respectively (Jeske et al., 2013). Horses with titers ≥256 exhibiting clinical signs compatible with internal infection are good candidates for advanced imaging such as abdominal or thoracic ultrasound.

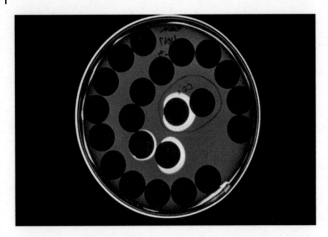

Figure 30.3 Photograph of the SHI serologic test for IgG antibodies to the bacterial exotoxin produced by *Corynebacterium pseudotuberculosis*.

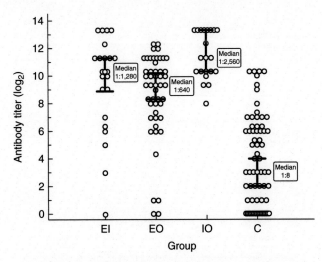

Figure 30.4 Dot plot of log$_2$–transformed anti–*Corynebacterium pseudotuberculosis* toxin antibodies measured via serum SHI testing in 170 horses of various breeds (171 records; 92 cases of *Corynebacterium pseudotuberculosis* infection and 79 controls with no evidence of *C. pseudotuberculosis* infection). Case horses were grouped according to disease location (external abscess only [n = 49], internal abscess only [21], or external and internal abscesses [22]). Bars represent 95% confidence intervals. C = Control. EI = External and internal abscess. EO = External abscess only. IO = Internal abscess only.

Previous reports have shown an association with internal infection in horses with titers ≥512. However, these studies have also pointed out that horses with external abscesses may also have antibody titers ≥512, suggesting that increased titers are indicative of active chronic infection as opposed to internal disease. A tendency toward more modest increases in SHI titers in horses with internal infection causing pneumonia or pleuritis has been reported in comparison to the dramatic increases in titers in horses with internal abscesses in abdominal organs. It is postulated that infection in abdominal organs such as the liver, kidney or spleen result in a delay in clinically apparent symptoms, as compared to when the respiratory system is affected (Aleman et al., 1996, Pratt, 2005, Jeske et al., 2013).

Due to the wide range of overlapping titers between clinical forms of disease and exposure, it is emphasized that SHI test results should always be evaluated in light of the entire clinical and clinicopathologic findings for an individual patient. A diagnosis of internal infection should never be made based upon serologic results without other supportive data.

30.3 Summary

Ideally, bacterial culture should be used to confirm *C. pseudotuberculosis* infection.

The SHI test is useful in identifying systemic infection with *C. pseudotuberculosis*, but a complete clinical evaluation is necessary to establish evidence for an internal infection in horses with concurrent or recently resolved external abscesses, as there is considerable overlap of titers.

Ultrasound imaging is an important and useful diagnostic method for detection of systemic *C. pseudotuberculosis* infection. Although samples from internal organs can be difficult to obtain, ultrasound-guided aspiration of liver and kidney abscesses has yielded material with positive culture results. Pure growth of *C. pseudotuberculosis* in bacterial culture of a fluid or tissue sample provides a definitive diagnosis. Positive culture results may be obtained from tracheal wash fluid, pleural fluid, peritoneal fluid, kidney and liver aspirates, urine, and – less often – blood. Early diagnosis coupled with aggressive and prolonged antimicrobial therapy offers the best prognosis for survival from internal infection.

References

Aleman M, Spier S.J, Wilson WD, et al. 1996. *Corynebacterium pseudotuberculosis* infection in horses: 538 cases (1982–1993). J Am Vet Med Assoc, 209(4): 804–809.

Jeske JM, Spier SJ, Whitcomb MB, et al. 2013. Use of antibody titers measured via serum synergistic hemolysis inhibition testing to predict internal Corynebacterium pseudotuberculosis infection in horses. J Am Vet Med Assoc, 242(1): 86–92.

Kilcoyne I, Spier SJ, Carter CN, et al. 2014. Frequency of *Corynebacterium pseudotuberculosis* infection in horses across the United States during a 10-year period. J Am Vet Med Assoc, 245(3): 309–314.

Knight HD 1978. A serologic method for the detection of *Corynebacterium pseudotuberculosis* infections in horses. Cornell Vet, 68(2): 220–237.

Pratt SM, Spier SJ, Carroll SP, et al. 2005. Evaluation of clinical characteristics, diagnostic test results, and outcome in horses with internal infection caused by *Corynebacterium pseudotuberculosis*: 30 cases (1995–2003). J Am Vet Med Assoc, 227(3): 441–448.

Spier SJ. 2008. *Corynebacterium pseudotuberculosis* infection in horses: An emerging disease associated with climate change? Eq Vet Ed, (20): 37–39.

Spier SJ, Toth B, Edman J, et al. 2012. Survival of *Corynebacterium pseudotuberculosis* biovar equi in soil. Vet Rec 170(7): 180.

Spier SJ. 2015. *Corynebacterium pseudotuberculosis* infection. In KA Sprayberry and NE Robinson (eds), *Current Therapy in Equine Medicine.* 7th edn. St. Louis: Saunders Elsevier Inc., pp. 184–187.

Szonyi B, Swinford A, Clavijo A. et al. 2013. Re-emergence of pigeon fever (*Corynebacterium pseudotuberculosis*) infection in Texas horses: Epidemiologic investigation of laboratory-diagnosed cases. J Vet Eq Vet Sci, (34): 281–287.

Vaughan B, Whitcomb MB, Pratt SM et al. 2004. Ultrasonographic appearance of abdominal organs in 14 horses with systemic *Corynebacterium pseudotuberculosis* infection. In Proceedings of the 50th Annual Convention of the American Association of Equine Practitioners. pp. 63–69.

31

Neorickettsia risticii

Sandra D. Taylor

Department of Veterinary Clinical Sciences, College of Veterinary Medicine, Purdue University, Indiana, USA

31.1 Introduction

Equine neorickettsiosis (EN), formerly known as Potomac horse fever and equine monocytic ehrlichiosis, is caused by the bacterium *Neorickettsia risticii*. Horses typically become infected by ingestion of intermediate hosts that carry *N. risticii*, or ingestion of fresh water containing *N. risticii*. Once in the gastrointestinal tract, *N. risticii* infects and replicates in colonic epithelium as well as monocytes and tissue macrophages. Common clinical signs of EN include anorexia, fever, and diarrhea. Abortion and laminitis may also occur. Common clinicopathological abnormalities in affected horses include hypocalcemia, hyponatremia, hypochloridemia, and neutropenia (Bertin et al., 2013). Available diagnostic tests include serum indirect fluorescent antibody (IFA) testing, serum enzyme-linked immunosorbent assay (ELISA), whole blood or fecal microbial culture, and polymerase chain reaction (PCR) from whole blood or feces. Treatment for EN includes intravenous administration of polyionic fluids to replace fluid and electrolyte losses, and administration of oxytetracycline to eliminate *N. risticii*. Plasma transfusions may be required to replace plasma proteins. Although vaccination may decrease incidence and severity of disease, EN can occur in vaccinated animals (Bertin et al., 2013). Vaccination for EN has been shown to induce low levels of serum antibodies, and vaccine failure has been reported to be as high as 89% (Atwill and Mohammed, 1996, Dutta et al., 1998). In addition, a retrospective evaluation of 44 horses with EN found that 82% of horses were fully vaccinated against *N. risticii* (Bertin et al., 2013). Currently, only one vaccine is available in the United States and contains one strain of inactivated bacterin (Dutta et al., 1998). The prognosis for horses with EN is good; in a population of hospitalized horses diagnosed with EN, the survival rate was 73% (Bertin et al., 2013).

31.2 Diagnostic Testing

To date, there is no reference standard for diagnosis of EN, as no available antemortem test is 100% sensitive or specific, and postmortem changes in the gastrointestinal tract are often non-specific (Bertin et al., 2013, Dutra et al., 2001, Stewart et al., 1995). Of the currently available antemortem tests, PCR for detection of *N. risticii* nucleic acid in horses with compatible clinical signs is highly sensitive and specific for EN and is, therefore, the current standard for diagnosis. Experimental infection of horses with *N. risticii* results in positive PCR results from whole blood and fecal samples (Barlough et al., 1997, Biswas et al., 1994, Mott et al., 1997, Pusterla et al., 2000a, 2000b). In one study, experimentally infected horses that were sampled daily were PCR positive on whole blood from approximately 7–21 days post-infection, and were PCR positive on feces from approximately 14–25 days post-infection (Pusterla et al., 2000b). Given that clinical signs were apparent from approximately 12–20 days post-infection, and that in a clinical scenario, horses are typically tested at the onset of clinical signs, whole blood PCR may be more sensitive than fecal PCR in the early course of disease. It is important to note that in the same study, some horses tested negative on whole blood PCR later in the disease course, but were still PCR positive on feces. Taken together, it is therefore recommended that *both* whole blood and feces are submitted for PCR testing in horses suspected to have EN.

Isolation of *N. risticii* in blood monocytes or tissue macrophages is no longer routinely performed given the time-consuming nature of the test and the lack of necessary reagents at many laboratories. Microbial culture of *N. risticii* does provide a definitive diagnosis of EN, with positive blood culture results obtained up to 28 days following experimental *N. risticii* infection (Mott et al., 1997).

Indirect fluorescent antibody (IFA) testing can be used to detect antibodies against *N. risticii*, but results can be difficult to interpret. A four-fold increase in titer between acute and convalescent sera strongly suggests infection, but failure to seroconvert does not rule out infection (Bertin et al., 2013, Mott et al., 1997, Palmer and Benson, 1994). Affected horses might exhibit high titers at the onset of clinical signs (Mott et al., 1997, Palmer and Benson, 1994), and false positive results are common (Madigan et al., 1995). In addition, vaccination might increase IFA titers, but many vaccinated horses fail to demonstrate a positive IFA titer (Atwill and Mohammed, 1996). A retrospective study of horses diagnosed with EN based on positive whole blood or fecal PCR reported a wide variation in IFA titers among horses, some of which were vaccinated (Bertin et al., 2013). Although PCR is the current diagnostic standard for detecting horses with clinical EN, IFA testing may be useful in chronic cases (>25 days post-infection) in which antigen is no longer detectable, given that IFA titers typically peak 4–5 weeks post-infection (Mott et al., 1997). As noted before, vaccination might increase IFA titers, but positive IFA in an unvaccinated horse might support a diagnosis of EN (Madigan et al., 1995) (Box 31.1).

Indirect and competitive enzyme-linked immunosorbent assays (ELISAs) have been developed to detect IgM or IgG antibodies to *N. risticii*, but these tests are not currently available for commercial use (Dutta et al., 1987, Pretzman et al., 1987, Shankarappa et al., 1989). Comparison of ELISA to IFA in experimentally-infected horses and horses with non-confirmed, naturally occurring EN failed to demonstrate a significant difference in sensitivity or specificity between tests (Dutta et al., 1987, Pretzman et al., 1987, Shankarappa et al., 1989). Given the superior diagnostic ability of PCR to detect infected horses and the cumbersome nature of ELISA testing, use of this test in a clinical setting has become obsolete.

Gross and histologic findings in horses with EN are non-specific, precluding their use in providing a definitive diagnosis of EN. Colonic and cecal walls might be thickened with edema and serosal congestion, and mesenteric lymph nodes might be enlarged (Dutra et al., 2001, Stewart et al., 1995). Diffuse mononuclear inflammatory cell infiltrates might be detected in the colonic and cecal lamina propria of affected horses, and submucosal vascular thrombosis might be observed (Stewart et al., 1995). Electron microscopy, special stains, or PCR may be used to detect *N. risticii* in selected gastrointestinal tissue sections (Dutra et al., 2001, Pusterla et al., 2000b).

31.3 Case Examples

The following case examples are included in a retrospective study investigating EN in 44 horses that presented to a referral institution (Bertin et al., 2013). IFA titers are expressed as the reciprocal of the dilution.

31.3.1 Case #1

- Signalment: 23-year old Pony of America mare
- History: four-day history of lethargy, anorexia and diarrhea. Vaccinated 1 month prior to presentation.
- Diagnostic testing Day 1
  - IFA titer (acute): 10,240
  - PCR of whole blood and feces: positive
  - (Convalescent IFA titer not done)
- Interpretation: PCR confirmed EN. Although recent vaccination could have contributed to the IFA titer, the degree of response suggested acute infection.
- Outcome: developed laminitis in all four feet and was humanely euthanized on Day 3.

31.3.2 Case #2

- Signalment: 12-year old Arabian gelding.
- History: 1-day history of lethargy, anorexia and colic. Unknown vaccination history.
- Diagnostic testing Day 1
  - IFA titer (acute): 80
  - PCR of whole blood and feces: positive
- Diagnostic testing Day 15
  - IFA titer (convalescent): 80
- Interpretation: PCR confirmed EN. The positive IFA titer indicated infection or vaccination, but the

---

Box 31.1 Serological interpretation.

1) Serological result on a single serum sample collected during acute disease
   - Negative result: no infection or recently infected horse that is displaying clinical signs but has not had adequate time for seroconversion
   - Positive result from unvaccinated horse: evidence of recent infection
   - Positive result from vaccinated horse: evidence of recent infection or detection of vaccine-derived antibodies
2) Serological result on acute and convalescent serum samples
   - Negative result: infection with *N. risticii* is unlikely
   - Positive result with no increase in titer: no active infection
   - Positive result with increase in titer (≥4-fold): strongly supports recent infection

vaccination history in this horse was unknown. The lack of increase in the convalescent titer highlights the insensitivity of the IFA test in diagnosing clinical EN.
- Outcome: responded to treatment and discharged on Day 7.

31.3.3 Case #3

- Signalment: 2-year old Thoroughbred filly
- History: 1-day history of anorexia and fever, never vaccinated against EN.
- Diagnostic testing Day 1

- IFA titer (acute): 40
- PCR of whole blood and feces: positive
- Diagnostic testing Day 14
- IFA titer (convalescent): 2,560
- Interpretation: PCR confirmed EN. The low acute IFA titer in this unvaccinated horse was due to infection, but the minimal degree of response was likely due to the acute nature of infection (insufficient time to generate a significant antibody response). The convalescent IFA titer is supportive of recent infection.
- Outcome: responded to treatment and discharged on Day 5.

References

Atwill ER and Mohammed HO. 1996. Evaluation of vaccination of horses as a strategy to control equine monocytic ehrlichiosis. J Am Vet Med Assoc 208: 1290–1294.

Barlough, JE, Rikihisa Y, and Madigan JE. 1997. Nested polymerase chain reaction for detection of *Ehrlichia risticii* genomic DNA in infected horses. Vet Parasitol 68: 367–373.

Bertin FR, Reising A, Slovis NM, Constable PD,. and Taylor SD. 2013. Clinical and clinicopathological factors associated with survival in 44 horses with equine neorickettsiosis (Potomac horse Fever). J Vet Intern Med 27: 1528–1534.

Biswas B, Vemulapalli R, and Dutta SK. 1994. Detection of *Ehrlichia risticii* from feces of infected horses by immunomagnetic separation and PCR. J Clin Microbiol, 32: 2147–2151.

Dutra F, Schuch LF, Delucchi E, Curcio BR, Coimbra H, Raffi MB, et al. 2001. Equine monocytic Ehrlichiosis (Potomac horse fever) in horses in Uruguay and southern Brazil. J Vet Diagn Invest, 13: 433–437.

Dutta SK, Rice RM, Hughes TD, Savage PK, and Myrup AC. 1987. Detection of serum antibodies against *Ehrlichia risticii* in Potomac horse fever by enzyme-linked immunosorbent assay. Vet Immunol Immunopathol, 14: 85–92.

Dutta SK, Vemulapalli R, and Biswas B. 1998. Association of deficiency in antibody response to vaccine and heterogeneity of *Ehrlichia risticii* strains with Potomac horse fever vaccine failure in horses. J Clin Microbiol, 36: 506–512.

Madigan JE, Rikihisa Y, Palmer JE, DeRock E, and Mott J. 1995. Evidence for a high rate of false-positive results with the indirect fluorescent antibody test for *Ehrlichia risticii* antibody in horses. J Am Vet Med Assoc, 207: 1448–1453.

Mott J, Rikihisa Y, Zhang Y, Reed SM, and Yu CY. 1997. Comparison of PCR and culture to the indirect fluorescent-antibody test for diagnosis of Potomac horse fever. J Clin Microbiol, 35: 2215–2219.

Palmer JE and Benson CE. 1994. Studies on oral transmission of Potomac horse fever. J Vet Intern Med, 8: 87–92.

Pretzman CI, Rikihisa Y, Ralph D, Gordon JC, and Bech-Nielsen S. 1987. Enzyme-linked immunosorbent assay for Potomac horse fever disease. J Clin Microbiol, 25: 31–36.

Pusterla N, Leutenegger CM, Sigrist B, Chae JS, Lutz H, and Madigan JE. 2000a. Detection and quantitation of *Ehrlichia risticii* genomic DNA in infected horses and snails by real-time PCR. Vet Parasitol 90: 129–135.

Pusterla N, Madigan JE, Chae JS, DeRock E, Johnson E, and Pusterla JB. 2000b. Helminthic transmission and isolation of *Ehrlichia risticii*, the causative agent of Potomac horse fever, by using trematode stages from freshwater stream snails. J Clin Microbiol 38: 1293–1297.

Shankarappa B, Dutta SK, Sanusi J, and Mattingly BL. 1989. Monoclonal antibody-mediated, immunodiagnostic competitive enzyme-linked immunosorbent assay for equine monocytic ehrlichiosis. J Clin Microbiol 27: 24–28.

Stewart MC, Hodgson JL, Kim H, Hutchins DR, and Hodgson DR. 1995. Acute febrile diarrhoea in horses: 86 cases (1986–1991). Aust Vet J 72: 41–44.

32

Anaplasma phagocytophilum
Janet Foley and Nicole Stephenson

Department of Medicine and Epidemiology, School of Veterinary Medicine, University of California, California, USA

32.1   Introduction

Equine granulocytic anaplasmosis (EGA, formerly equine granulocytic ehrlichiosis) is caused by the tick-transmitted bacterium, *Anaplasma phagocytophilum*, which infects horse, human, and canine leukocytes, causing an acute febrile disease (Pusterla and Madigan, 2007). Epidemiological features are summarized in Box 32.1; these features reflect that the disease is predominantly tick-transmitted and occurs where there is overlap with *Ixodes scapularis,* deer tick, or black legged tick (upper Midwest and northeast, Pusterla and Madigan, 2007) or *I. pacificus*, the western black-legged tick (Pacific northwest, Reubel et al., 1998). Iatrogenic transmission can occur through contaminated blood transfusion (Pusterla and Madigan, 2007). Transplacental transmission has been documented in people and cattle but not horses (Dhand et al., 2007, Pusterla et al., 1997).

Most infected horses manifest no clinical signs and recover without incident, particularly if they are young when first exposed, while more severe disease is typical in older horses (Box 32.1). Death is rare and is usually due injury caused by ataxia or secondary bacterial infection and subsequent disseminated intravascular coagulation. Even with high fever, laminitis is extremely rare. Left untreated, infection is generally left-limiting over 10–14 days (Madigan, 1993).

32.2   Routine Diagnostic Tests

Utility of tests for EGA is described in Table 32.1. CBC abnormalities in infected horses can include leukopenia, characterized by neutropenia and lymphopenia, profound thrombocytopenia, anemia (generally mild), icterus of the serum, and morulae (inclusion bodies) within neutrophils, and less commonly eosinophils and monocytes on routine blood smear. Later in infection,

the horse may develop leukocytosis. Serum chemistry may be normal, but reported abnormalities include hyperbilirubinemia, increased fibrinogen, hypoproteinemia, and increased liver enzymes (Berrington et al., 1996). Results of urinalysis are normal. If imaging is performed, nonspecific abnormalities may include splenomegaly, pulmonary infiltrates, or blood vessel changes characteristic of hypovolemia.

32.3   Specialized Diagnostic Tests

An initial, presumptive diagnosis can be made in an EGA-endemic area on the basis of history and clinical signs combined with characteristic the CBC finding of thrombocytopenia. Specialized, confirmatory diagnostics that can be performed include visualization of morulae within leukocytes on a blood or buffy coat smear, PCR, or serology (Figure 32.1).

32.3.1   Blood or Buffy Coat Cytology (Detection of Morulae)

Detection of multiple morulae inclusions within neutrophils and less commonly eosinophils and monocytes on a peripheral blood smear is a quick and inexpensive confirmatory diagnostic test. Morulae can generally be detected starting 1–2 days after the onset of fever (Franzén et al., 2005, Madigan et al., 1995, Richter et al., 1996). Using a cover slip or two slides, drag the buffy coat across the slide, dry, and then do a Wright-Giemsa stain. *A. phagocytophilum* morulae are stippled, blue-gray to dark blue, pleomorphic inclusions within the cytoplasm of neutrophils and, occasionally, eosinophils and monocytes (Figure 32.2). At the peak of infection (day 12–15), up to 50% of neutrophils can become infected; however, because infected horses are sometimes neutropenic, this may still be hard to detect. A buffy coat preparation can

Interpretation of Equine Laboratory Diagnostics, First Edition. Edited by Nicola Pusterla and Jill Higgins.

be utilized instead and is more sensitive for detection of morulae. The sample is prepared by centrifuging anticoagulated whole blood, removing the plasma, and then placing a single drop of the white cell fraction on top (the buffy coat) on the edge of a slide. A negative result should not rule out the diagnosis of EGA. Additionally, there

---

Box 32.1 Key features of equine granulocytic anaplasmosis epidemiology and clinical presentation.

- Tick-transmitted disease, cases typically occur from late fall through spring when adult tick vectors quest for hosts (Madigan, 1993).
- Should be considered even if there is no documented history of a tick bite if in an endemic area or if there is a history of recent travel (within a few weeks) to an endemic area.
- Incubation period in experimentally infected horses is 8–12 days (Reubel et al., 1998, Richter et al., 1996).
- Associated with fever (38.3–41 °C, 101–108 °C), depression, anorexia.
- More severe clinical signs common in horses over 4 years of age are head pressing against a wall, ataxia, elevated heart rate, anorexia, icterus, limb edema, and petechiation of the nasal mucosa. Rare cardiac involvement with ventricular tachycardia or arrhythmia.
- Confirming the diagnosis is important to rule out other febrile illnesses and in development of a prevention plan for other horses.

---

are other normal features of neutrophils and staining artifacts that can appear superficially similar to morulae, suggesting that examination of the smear by an experienced cytologist is warranted.

32.3.2   Polymerase Chain Reaction (PCR)

See Chapter 54.

32.3.3   Serology

Various serologic diagnostic tests have been developed to detect antibodies to *A. phagocytophilum* and are offered at commercial laboratories. Although IgM antibodies in principle may circulate in blood within a few days of infection, serology for IgM associated with *A. phagocytophilum* is rarely performed because the titer tends to be low, specialized testing protocols would need to be employed, and PCR would still be more sensitive for diagnosis of acute infection. IgG antibodies are usually undetectable in the week or so of infection (Madigan, 1993) and therefore this method of diagnosis is more useful later after infection or even to confirm diagnosis retrospectively. Additionally, a single positive titer may result from previous infection; therefore, a diagnosis can only be confirmed based on serology if there is documented seroconversion from negative to positive or a four-fold increase in paired antibody titers over 2–4 weeks. Early initiation of antibiotic treatment may diminish antibody production, making retrospective serology less sensitive as well. The most

---

Table 32.1 Features and interpretation for various types of diagnostic tests for equine granulocytic anaplasmosis.

Diagnostic test	Advantages	Disadvantages	Interpretation
Response to antibiotic treatment	Quick (12–24 h) and inexpensive	Nonspecific	Not confirmatory, can see response with multiple febrile illnesses
Leukopenia, thrombocytopenia, anemia and elevated liver enzymes	Part of minimum database, suggestive in endemic areas	Nonspecific	Consistent but neither required nor confirmatory
Cytology	Quick and inexpensive	Sensitivity varies depending on timing during course of infection, morulae may be difficult to detect by the untrained observer	Detection of morulae w/in WBCs is confirmatory; however, a negative result does not rule it out
PCR	High sensitivity and specificity, early detection of infection	Blood sample must be taken prior to initiation of antibiotic therapy	A positive result is confirmation of an active infection; however, a negative result does not completely rule out infection
Serology: IFA and ELISA	Quantitative result, can use to make a retrospective diagnosis	Need paired samples 2–4 weeks apart to confirm diagnosis	A 4-fold increase in paired titers over 10–14 days confirmatory of acute infection. Result may be negative early in course of infection. A single positive result could indicate prior infection.

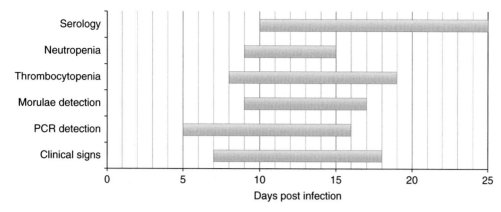

Figure 32.1 Timeline of clinical signs, CBC findings, and diagnostic detection of *A. phagocytophilum* infection in the horse.

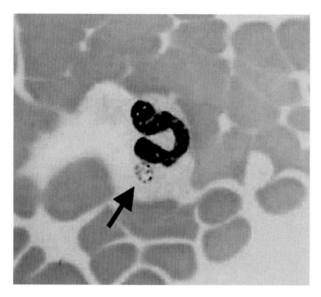

Figure 32.2 *Anaplasma phagocytophilum* morula (arrow) within a neutrophil on a blood smear from a horse with equine granulocytic anaplasmosis (Wright-Giemsa stain, 1000×).

appropriate uses of serology are to retrospectively confirm a diagnosis if PCR testing was negative or not available, or to test for the occurrence of *A. phagocytophilum* infection in a new geographical area or herd of horses.

The most common serological tests for horses for EGA are *indirect immunofluorescence assay* (IFA) and *enzyme-linked immunosorbent assay* (ELISA). For the IFA, serum antibodies bind to antigen that is fixed on wells on a slide and a secondary antibody conjugated to a fluorescein label is then reacted in the well. The wells are evaluated by a laboratory scientist examining the slide under epifluorescent microscopy. The test is made quantitative by performing it using different dilutions of patient serum. A diagnosis can be made if there is a four-fold increase in titer over 2–4 weeks. Because of differences in sensitivity and procedures across laboratories, a standard cut-off for what constitutes a positive test would need to be

determined in each laboratory with a panel of known (gold-standard) positive and negative samples and thus one common cut-off value does not exist.

ELISA is a related technology in that antigen is adhered to 96-well plates, patient serum is incubated in each well with the antigen, and colorimetric detection is used by reacting chemicals conjugated to the secondary antibody. An important difference between IFA and ELISA is that crude antigen is used in IFA (i.e., the pathogen grown within horse cells or cultured cells in a laboratory), while ELISA can be designed using either crude extracted antigen or recombinant purified antigen. In the latter case, any cross-reacting or interfering contaminants in the preparation, such as extraneous proteins to which the horse may have generated antibodies, can be eliminated. However, this typically is not a serious problem for serology for EGA. In principle, the intensity of the color change of ELISA is correlated with the absolute amount of patient anti-*A. phagocytophilum* IgG. As for IFA, specific cutoffs for values considered to be positive need to be determined for each laboratory. Many laboratories also prefer to offer ELISA relative to IFA as there is some subjectivity in interpreting results on IFA while ELISA is read by a machine which reports optical density, minimizing the possibility of user error.

There is a *point-of-care ELISA technology-based test* for canine granulocytic anaplasmosis caused by the same pathogen (SNAP 4Dx Plus Test, IDEXX Laboratories), which is reported to work well for feline samples as well. Its utility for equine diagnostics has not been established.

Western blotting is a possible, more specific test that is available to obtain further information on host antibody responses to various *A. phagocytophilum* proteins. To run a western blot, all of the proteins that the bacteria produce in cell culture are separated by size and charge along a gradient and then transferred to a nitrocellulose membrane. Then patient serum is reacted with the proteins on the membrane, allowing one to determine whether the horse has elaborated antibodies to the major antigen of *A. phagocytophilum,* which is a bacterial surface protein called *msp2,* or any of the other proteins the bacterium produces. The advantage of doing a western blot is that any animal with a true serological response to the bacteria would ordinarily make IgG specifically against the major antigen: if a horse appeared to be ELISA or IFA-positive but the western blot showed reactivity against various proteins that did *not* include *msp2,* one might infer that the IFA and ELISA were false-positive. While western blots have important roles in confirmatory diagnosis of some diseases, for example Lyme disease, rates of false-positive ELISA and IFA tests for EGA are low, making western blot less important for this disease. One caveat is that there are several pathogens related to *A. phagocytophilum* with which horses can be infected, and it is not known whether ELISA and IFA could possibly appear false-positive in a horse infected with one of these other pathogens. For example, people with human monocytic ehrlichiosis, caused by *Ehrlichia chaffeensis,* and dogs with canine monocytic ehrlichiosis, caused by *E. canis,* will sometimes test positive serologically for HGA or CGA, respectively. They do not have specific antibodies to *A. phagocytophilum msp2* but

rather to various proteins elaborated during the course of several diseases, such as heat shock proteins. In this regard, western blot can help identify the specific IgG species that are produced. For horses, the most plausible disease that shares immunological characteristics with EGA is equine neorickettsiosis (formerly Potomac horse fever) caused by the related rickettsial pathogen *Neorickettsia risticii.* Although cross-reaction is theoretically possible, there is no empirical evidence that horses with equine neorickettsiosis or EGA develop antibody responses that obscure serological diagnosis.

32.3.4 Culture

A. phagocytophilum has been propagated *in vitro* in the human neutrophilic leukemia cell line HL-60 (Goodman et al., 1996). However, samples will only test culture-positive if they have not been grossly contaminated with skin fauna, and if have been transported quickly under appropriate conditions to one of the few research laboratories that perform culture. Even in these highly specialized laboratories, culture may not be positive in PCR-positive animals. Thus, culture is impractical and rarely used as a method of clinical diagnosis although it has been utilized in the research setting.

References

Berrington A, Moats R, and Lester S. 1996. A case of *Ehrlichia equi* in an adult horse in British Columbia. Can Vet J, 37: 174.

Dhand A, Nadelman RB, Aguero-Rosenfeld M, Haddad FA, Stokes DP, and Horowitz HW. 2007. Human granulocytic anaplasmosis during pregnancy: case series and literature review. Clin Infect Disease, 45: 589–593.

Franzén P, Aspan A, Egenvall A, Gunnarsson A, Åberg L, and Pringle J. 2005. Acute clinical, hematologic, serologic, and polymerase chain reaction findings in horses experimentally infected with a European strain of *Anaplasma phagocytophilum.* J Vet Int Med, 19: 232–239.

Goodman JL, Nelson C, Vitale B, Madigan JE, Dumler JS, Kurtti TJ, and Munderloh UG. 1996. Direct cultivation of the causative agent of human granulocytic ehrlichiosis. New Eng J Med, 334: 209–215.

Madigan J. 1993. Equine ehrlichiosis. Vet Clin N Am-Eq, 9: 423–428.

Madigan JE, Richter PJ, Kimsey RB, Barlough JE, Bakken JS, and Dumler JS. 1995. Transmission and passage in horses of the agent of human granulocytic ehrlichiosis. J Infect Disease, 172: 1141–1144.

Pusterla N, Braun U, Wolfensberger C, and Lutz H. 1997. Intrauterine infection with *Ehrlichia phagocytophila* in a cow. Vet Rec, 141: 101–102.

Pusterla N and Madigan JE. 2007. *Anaplasma phagocytophilum* infection. In D Sellon and M Long (eds.) *Equine Infectious Diseases.* St. Louis, MI: Saunders Elsevier.

Reubel GH, Kimsey RB, Barlough JE, and Madigan JE. 1998. Experimental transmission of *Ehrlichia equi* to horses through naturally infected ticks (*Ixodes pacificus*) from northern California. J Clin Microbiol, 36: 2131–2134.

Richter PJ, Kimsey RB, Madigan JE, Barlough JE, Dumler JS, and Brooks DL. 1996. *Ixodes pacificus* (Acari: Ixodidae) as a vector of *Ehrlichia equi* (Rickettsiales: Ehrlichieae). J Med Entomol, 33: 1–5.

33

Lawsonia intracellularis
Connie J. Gebhart

Veterinary and Biomedical Sciences, University of Minnesota, Minnesota, USA

33.1 Introduction

Equine proliferative enteropathy (EPE) caused by *Lawsonia intracellularis* has become a commonly diagnosed intestinal disease in horses. Although a common enteric infection in pigs and other animals, infection with *L. intracellularis* was only first reported in horses in 1982. Since then, many sporadic cases and occasional outbreaks on breeding farms have been reported and EPE has become endemic on many farms. Though most of the cases have been reported from the United States, recent reports have shown that this disease has reached a global occurrence with cases also documented in Canada, Europe, South Africa, Japan, Brazil, and Australia. Economic impacts of EPE are now being recognized and these impacts relate to the cost of monitoring, prevention and control, cost of treatment, and losses related to retarded growth or even death of affected weanlings. In fact, affected and recovered Thoroughbred yearlings were reported to sell for 68% of the average price of non-affected yearlings by the same sire.

33.2 *Lawsonia intracellularis*

L. intracellularis is an obligately intracellular, small, curved, gram-negative bacterium that is found within the apical cytoplasm of infected intestinal enterocytes. It causes proliferation of the affected enterocytes, resulting in an adenomatous thickening of the mucosa of the small, and sometimes large, intestine. This hyperplasia of the crypt glands results in malabsorption and decreased growth rate or even weight loss. *Lawsonia intracellularis* can only be grown *in vitro* in cell culture, requiring a specific anaerobic atmosphere and dividing cells for growth.

33.3 Equine Proliferative Enteropathy

Equine proliferative enteropathy typically affects weaned foals less than one year of age and in North America is most often diagnosed between the months of August and February. Although the disease is seen in foals from 2 to 13 months of age, those between 4 and 9 months are most susceptible to infection. Cases of EPE have occasionally been diagnosed in adult animals. The epidemiology of *L. intracellularis* in horses is not well-understood. Transmission likely occurs through ingestion of fecal material from herd mates or other animals. In fact, the disease has been described in numerous species of animals, both domestic and wild, with the presence of intracellular *L. intracellularis* bacteria in proliferating enterocytes of the intestine being a consistent finding.

Clinical signs of EPE are nonspecific and include fever, lethargy, anorexia, peripheral edema, diarrhea, weight loss (or retarded weight gain) and colic. Often, a slight fever is an early feature of the disease in horses. However, the disease can be subclinical in foals and be manifested by a self-limiting and transient decrease of serum total protein concentration along with decreased weight gain as compared to unaffected foals.

Confirmation of a diagnosis of EPE currently is best done by necropsy with demonstration of the typical gross and histological lesions in the intestine. Grossly, lesions are commonly found in the distal jejunum and ileum, but may extend throughout the small and large intestines, depending on severity. Pathologic lesions range from multifocal to confluent regions of mucosal hyperplasia and these hyperplastic mucosal regions can form prominent folds or a corrugated appearance. The affected mucosal surface may also demonstrate variable

Interpretation of Equine Laboratory Diagnostics, First Edition. Edited by Nicola Pusterla and Jill Higgins.
© 2018 John Wiley & Sons, Inc. Published 2018 by John Wiley & Sons, Inc.

Box 33.1 Recommendations for antemortem diagnosis of EPE.

- Measurement of total protein and albumin concentrations
- Abdominal ultrasonography
- qPCR
  qPCR is very specific (100%) and an excellent confirmatory test
  Positive qPCR results support EPE
  Negative qPCR results can be expected if horses are subclinically affected, fecal samples are collected from foals with prior antimicrobial treatment or late in the course of disease
- Serology
  Serology is less specific than qPCR, but is more sensitive
  Detectable *L. intracellularis* antibodies may indicate EPE or subclinical disease
  Negative serology results can be expected in the early stage of the disease, when humoral immune responses are not yet detectable

---

degrees of erosion and/or ulceration. Postmortem confirmation of EPE is made by histologic demonstration of proliferation of crypt epithelial cells with the presence of intracellular *L. intracellularis*, which can be demonstrated by silver staining or immunohistochemistry with *L. intracellularis*-specific antibodies.

An antemortem diagnosis of EPE is challenging, but common findings include hypoproteinemia, thickening of segments of the small intestine observed on ultrasonography and demonstration of *L. intracellularis* shed in the feces by qPCR. A unique but consistent laboratory finding of clinical EPE in foals is hypoproteinemia due to hypoalbuminemia (Box 33.1).

A presumptive antemortem diagnosis of EPE may be made based on the age of the horse, clinical signs, presence of hypoproteinemia, and thickened small intestinal loops on ultrasonographic evaluation. However, other causes of enteropathy and protein loss must be ruled out. Because of the cost and potential side-effects of treatment, laboratory confirmation of a diagnosis should be attempted prior to beginning antimicrobial therapy. Further, successful treatment and prevention of clinical disease in herd mates or on endemic farms requires an accurate and timely diagnosis. However, shedding of *L. intracellularis* by infected horses cannot be detected by culture as the organism is obligately intracellular. Though a few laboratories are able to cultivate the bacterium in a cell culture system with a specific atmosphere, *in vitro* cultivation of *L. intracellularis* is not amenable to routine diagnostics.

qPCR of feces is a very specific (100%) and an excellent confirmatory test for shedding of *L. intracellularis*, but negative qPCR results can be expected if horses are subclinically affected. Also, negative qPCR results may be obtained if the fecal samples are collected from foals with prior antimicrobial treatment or late during the disease timeline, when *L. intracellularis* organisms are no longer shed in the feces.

Serologic tests can also be applied antemortem, but they have the disadvantage of not being able to discriminate between active infection and past-exposure. Further, negative serology results can be expected in the early stage of the disease, when humoral immune responses are not yet detectable. Detectable *L. intracellularis* antibodies may indicate EPE or subclinical infection and, therefore, though serology is less specific than qPCR, it is more sensitive. Therefore, it is recommended to combine both fecal qPCR and serology for laboratory confirmation of a diagnosis of EPE since these assays may have complementary sensitivity and specificity during various time points in the disease or under different disease severities.

33.4 Comparison of Serological Assays

Proliferative enteropathy is also a widespread and economically important disease in pigs; as such, methods currently used for the diagnosis of EPE were first described for detection of this disease in pigs. Serological tests such as an immunoperoxidase monolayer assay (IPMA) and an enzyme linked immunosorbant assay (ELISA) for the detection of *L. intracellularis*-specific antibodies have been described for pigs and applied to horses (Table 33.1). The IPMA is a serologic enzyme immunoassay test commonly used for the diagnosis of viral infections. The obligately intracellular organism *L. intracellularis* infects cell line monolayers *in vitro*; consequently, cell monolayers can be used in the same way as virus-infected cell line monolayers to perform serology with the IPMA. Results are interpreted using an inverted microscope. Reported sensitivity and specificity for this test for diagnosis of porcine proliferative enteropathy is 91% and 100%, respectively. The slide-based immunoperoxidase assay (SIPA) is similar to the IPMA, but performed using cell-free *L. intracellularis* whole cell antigen applied to welled glass slides, allowing results to be viewed using a standard microscope. The ELISA method used for horses incorporates a column chromatography purified *L. intracellularis* antigen.

The increasing interest and demand for better access to EPE serology testing instigated a study to determine

Table 33.1 Characteristics of three serological assays available for detecting humoral IgG for *Lawsonia intracellularis* in foals and horses.

Test	IPMA: ImmunoPeroxidase Monolayer Assay	SIPA: Slide ImmunoPeroxidase Assay	ELISA: Enzyme_Linked ImmunoSorbant Assay
Source	Routinely used for porcine serology testing	Similar to the IPMA	Adapted from porcine test (Wattanaphansak et al., 2008)
Antigen	Uses bacteria grown cell culture monolayers	Uses bacteria placed on glass slides	Uses purified bacteria
Values	Titered from 1:60 to 1:480	Titered from 1:60 to 1:480	Cut-off 55 EU or greater is positive (Page et al., 2011)
Performance	Sensitivity 91%, specificity 100% (Guedes et al., 2002a,b,c)	Sensitivity and specificity similar to IPMA (Pusterla et al., 2011)	More sensitive, but lower specificity

Table 33.2 Number of positive results obtained for each serology test when testing sera from weanling and healthy horses with and without equine proliferative enteropathy. Agreements within each category are shown.

Category/Animal Status	No. tested	IPMA	SIPA	ELISA	Category agreement
EPE-affected weanling	100	*100/100	96/100	98/100	97% Kappa = 0.95
Non-clinical weanling	120	0/120	1/120	8/120	96% Kappa = 0.91
Non-clinical horse	130	11/130	41/130	49/130	81% Kappa = 0.61

*Number positive/number tested

the agreements of the three assays currently in use in the United States for detection of *L. intracellularis* antibodies in weanlings and horses of various ages. Serum samples used in this comparison were collected from weanling foals and horses of various ages. Sera from 100 weanlings submitted for laboratory confirmation of EPE or weanling sera collected from herds with confirmed outbreaks of EPE (clinical signs of EPE with detection of *L. intracellularis* shedding by qPCR from at least one affected animal) were considered EPE positive sera. Sera used were from weanlings with at least two of the following findings: hypoproteinemia, thickened small intestine on ultrasound, peripheral edema, and diarrhea with no other enteric pathogens detected. Sera used from confirmed outbreaks of EPE were from foals that had at least one of these clinical signs of EPE and either had herd mates confirmed to be EPE positive (by necropsy or positive qPCR) or were themselves qPCR positive for *L. intracellularis* in the feces. Sera from 120 normal weanlings, collected from herds with no history of EPE were considered EPE negative sera. In addition, sera from 130 randomly collected healthy adult horses with no signs of EPE and from herds with no history of EPE aged yearling to 27 years were tested. For the IPMA, serum antibody titers were measured in serial 2-fold dilutions of serum from 1:30 to 1:480 using a previously described method but incorporating an anti-equine IgG immunoperoxidase conjugate. Though any positivity or background staining was noted at a titer of 30, a titer of 60 was used as the minimum cutoff value for a horse to be considered seropositive. The SIPA was performed similarly to the IPMA, with the exception that the antigen consisted of *L. intracellularis* grown in cell culture and spotted onto each of 24-well glass slides. Slides were then stained using the same reagents and methods as the IPMA with a titer of 60 used as the minimum cutoff value for a positive result. The ELISA method was performed as previously described using purified cell-cultured antigen bound to 96-well plates with absorbance read in a plate reader. A positive cut-off of 55 ELISA units (EU) or greater was utilized for differentiation of seronegative from seropositive results. The gold standard used for the calculation of sensitivity and specificity of each serology method at each serum titer was either EPE-affected or normal animals according to the criteria defined above. The results of each method, whether from EPE-affected or normal weanlings, agreed in sera samples at the currently used cut-off levels (Table 33.2). For sera from EPE-affected and normal weanlings, the percentage of agreement between the three tests was 97 and 96%, respectively. The total agreement for these two groups of samples was 95%. Sensitivities were 100, 96, and 98%,

Table 33.3 Specificity and sensitivity results of the IPMA, SIPA, and ELISA using different serum dilutions or cut-off units, respectively, from weanlings and healthy horses of various ages.

Category	IPMA titer				SIPA titer				ELISA cut-off	
	1:60	1:120	1:240	1:480	1:60	1:120	1:240	1:480	>55 EU	>110 EU
Weanling Sensitivity	*100	100	90	75	96	90	76	60	98	91
Weanling Specificity	100	100	100	100	98	100	100	100	94	100
Horse Specificity	92	98	99	100	76	87	98	100	73	92

* Percent

Box 33.2 Recommendations for herd monitoring for EPE.

- After initial index case
  Daily examination, monitor temperature and weight gain
  Weekly serology and/or total protein levels
- Endemic herds
  Daily examination, monitor temperature and weight gain
  Bi-monthly to monthly serology and/or total protein levels (post weaning)

---

while specificities were 100, 98, and 94% for the IPMA, SIPA, and ELISA, respectively, for the weanling foal sera. If the cut-off value for a positive for weanlings were changed to 120 for the IPMA and SIPA methods, the resultant sensitivity values would decrease slightly to 90% for the SIPA, while specificities would remain high, approaching 100% for both (Table 33.3). Similarly, if the cut-off for the ELISA were increased from >55 to >110 EU, the sensitivity and specificity for this test for weanlings would change to 91 and 100%, respectively. Agreements for healthy, non-clinical horses are also shown in Table 33.1 and were 81% for these three serology tests. However, if the cut-off values for a positive result for the IPMA and SIPA methods were increased from a titer of 60 to 120, the specificity of these two tests would increase to 98% and 87%, respectively. Likewise, if the cut-off for a positive result for the ELISA was increased to >110 EU, the specificity for this test would increase dramatically from 73 to 92%. In conclusion, the serological testing results for EPE agreed well for the IPMA, SIPA, and ELISA tests for weanlings at the current cut-off values used. However, less agreement was observed in healthy aged horses for these tests, possibly due to background affects from these sera or due to higher baseline levels of *L. intracellularis* antibodies in this population. These discrepancies could be corrected by adjusting the cut-off levels for a positive test for this age group. Further, lower specificity for all three tests for this group of sera may be, in part, due to the presence of subclinically affected animals in the group.

33.5 Diagnostic Recommendations

After diagnosis of an index EPE case in a herd, one should consider screening the remaining weanling population on an affected farm to detect subclinically-affected or early disease in herd mates. This is best achieved by daily clinical monitoring of foals to recognize early signs of disease, including taking rectal temperatures and assessment of weight (calculating daily weight gain). This should be combined with serology and/or measurement of total protein levels every 7–10 days (Box 33.2). qPCR testing of healthy herd mates is not advised in this situation due to the expense of testing and the low rate of positives as healthy herd mates rarely shed detectable levels of *L. intracellularis*. Weanlings that are seropositive or have low total protein levels should undergo further diagnostic testing (such as ultrasound or PCR) to confirm clinical EPE.

Monitoring of an endemic herd follows similar guidelines to those for herds with diagnosed index cases. This includes regular exams, as well as monthly testing by serology and/or total protein levels. This monitoring should begin at least four weeks prior to the historical first detection of clinical cases.

References

Guedes RM, Gebhart CJ, Deen J, et al. 2002a. Validation of an immunoperoxidase monolayer assay as a serologic test for porcine proliferative enteropathy. J Vet Diagn Invest, 14: 528–530.

Guedes RM, Gebhart CJ, Winkelman NL, et al. 2002b. A comparative study of an indirect fluorescent antibody test and an immunoperoxidase monolayer assay for the diagnosis of porcine proliferative enteropathy. J Vet Diagn Invest, 14: 420–423.

Guedes RM, Gebhart CJ, Winkelman NL, et al. 2002c. Comparison of different methods for diagnosis of porcine proliferative enteropathy. Can J Vet Res, 66: 99–107.

Page AE, Slovis NM, Gebhart CJ, et al. 2011a. Serial use of serologic assays and fecal PCR assays to aid in identification of subclinical *Lawsonia intracellularis* infection for targeted treatment of Thoroughbred foals and weanlings. J Am Vet Med Assoc, 238: 1482–1489.

Pusterla N, Gebhart C, and Slovis NM. 2011. How to monitor and prevent the occurrence of Lawsonia intracellularis infection in weanling foals from farms with endemic or sporadic occurrence of equine proliferative enteropathy. 57th Annual Forum of the American Association of Equine Practitioners, November 18–22, 2011, San Antonio, TX, pp. 196–201.

Wattanaphansak S, Asawakarn T, Gebhart CJ, and Deen J. 2008. Development and validation of an enzyme-linked immunosorbent assay for the diagnosis of porcine proliferative enteropathy. J Vet Diagn Invest 20: 170–177.

Further Reading

Duhamel GE and Wheeldon EB. 1982; Intestinal adenomatosis in a foal. Vet Pathol, 19: 447–450.

Frazer ML. 2008. *Lawsonia intracellularis* infection in horses: 2005–2007. J Vet Intern Med, 22: 1243–1248.

Gebhart CJ and Guedes RMC. 2010. *Lawsonia intracellularis* and the proliferative enteropathies. In CL Gyles (ed.), *Pathogenesis of Bacterial Infections in Animals*, 4th Edn. Hoboken, NJ: Wiley-Blackwell Publishing.

Gebhart CJ, Page AE, Kelley M, et al. 2012. A comparative study of serology assays for equine proliferative enteropathy. Am Assoc Equine Pract Annual Meeting.

Jones GF, Ward GE, Murtaugh MP, et al. 1993. Enhanced detection of intracellular organism of swine proliferative enteritis, ileal symbiont intracellularis, in feces by polymerase chain reaction. J Clin Microbiol 31: 2611–2615.

Lavoie JP, Drolet R, Parsons D, et al. 2000. Equine proliferative enteropathy: a cause of weight loss, colic, diarrhoea and hypoproteinaemia in foals on three breeding farms in Canada. Equine Vet J 32: 418–425.

McGurrin MK, Vengust M, Arroyo LG, et al. 2007. An outbreak of *Lawsonia intracellularis* infection in a standardbred herd in Ontario. Can Vet J, 48: 927–930.

McOrist S, Gebhart CJ, Boid R, et al. 1995. Characterization of *Lawsonia intracellularis* gen. *nov.*, sp. *nov.*, the obligately intracellular bacterium of porcine proliferative enteropathy. Int J Syst Bacteriol, 45: 820–825.

Page AE, Stills HF, Chander Y, et al. 2011b. Adaptation and validation of a bacteria-specific enzyme-linked immunosorbent assay for determination of farm-specific *Lawsonia intracellularis* seroprevalence in central Kentucky Thoroughbreds. Equine Vet J, 43 Suppl 40: 25–31.

Pusterla N and Gebhart C. 2009. Equine proliferative enteropathy caused by *Lawsonia intracellularis*. Equine Vet J 21: 183–185.

Pusterla N and Gebhart CJ. 2013. Equine proliferative enteropathy – a review of recent developments. Equine Vet J 45: 403–409.

Pusterla N and Gebhart CJ. 2013. *Lawsonia intracellularis* infection and proliferative enteoopathy in foals. Vet Microbiol 167: 34–41.

Pusterla N, Jackson R, Wilson R, et al. 2009b. Temporal detection of *Lawsonia intracellularis* using serology and real-time PCR in Thoroughbred horses residing on a farm endemic for equine proliferative enteropathy. Vet Microbiol 136: 173–176.

34

Borrelia burgdorferi

Amy L. Johnson[1] and Bettina Wagner[2]

[1] *Department of Clinical Studies – New Bolton Center, University of Pennsylvania School of Veterinary Medicine, Pennsylvania, USA*
[2] *Department of Population Medicine and Diagnostic Science, College of Veterinary Medicine, Cornell University, New York, USA*

34.1 Overview of Lyme Disease in Horses

Infection with *Borrelia burgdorferi*, a tick-borne spirochete and the causative agent of Lyme disease, is commonly recognized in horses in North America and other parts of the world. However, the true incidence of Lyme disease in horses is unknown and difficult to determine. Clinical signs historically attributed to *B. burgdorferi* infection in horses include chronic weight loss, sporadic lameness, stiffness, arthritis, swollen joints, muscle tenderness or wasting, hepatitis, laminitis, a sporadic low-grade fever, abortion, hyperesthesia, behavior changes, uveitis, and encephalitis (Burgess, 1988, Butler et al., 2005, Magnarelli et al., 1988). Several syndromes have been described in the literature, including neuroborreliosis (Burgess and Mattison, 1987, Hahn et al., 1996, James et al., 2010, Imai et al., 2011), uveitis (Priest et al., 2012), and pseudolymphoma (Sears et al., 2012) that have been correlated with infection with *B. burgdorferi*. Clinical signs of Lyme disease are thought to appear several months after infection occurred. However, the causal role of the spirochetes is difficult to confirm in most clinical cases due to challenges in detecting or isolating *B. burgdorferi* from the horse using available diagnostic tests. Thus, the diagnosis of Lyme disease is supported by serological test results confirming the presence of antibodies against *B. burgdorferi*. It is, however, important to note that most infected horses undergo seroconversion without ever developing clinical signs of disease. Some horses display compatible clinical signs and receive a putative diagnosis of Lyme disease based on positive serologic tests when in reality another disease process, such as non-infective osteoarthritis, is the cause of the problem. The inability to know if the horse's disease is caused by *Borrelia* infection using available diagnostic tests, combined with variable clinical manifestations of infection, make diagnosis of clinical Lyme disease

challenging. Therefore, the diagnosis of Lyme disease in horses should always be based on several criteria including (1) clinical signs compatible with Lyme disease, (2) potential exposure to *B. burgdorferi* (via residence in or travel to an endemic area), (3) careful exclusion of all other possible differential diagnoses, and (4) positive serological results confirming infection with *B. burgdorferi* (Divers et al., 2009). Based on these criteria, signs most commonly attributed to Lyme disease in horses are orthopedic problems, behavioral changes, tactile hyperesthesia, and neurological deficits.

34.2 Overview of Serologic Testing

Infection with *B. burgdorferi* can be confirmed with serologic testing (Table 34.1). A positive test result indicates the presence of antibodies against *B. burgdorferi* at the sampling time point and might represent different infection stages depending on test utilized. None of the tests prove causation of current clinical signs or predict whether infection is likely to cause clinical signs in the future. Horses living in an endemic area frequently have antibodies against *Borrelia*. On its own, a positive serologic test indicating infection with the spirochete has a low positive predictive value of disease (Magnarelli et al., 2000, Divers et al., 2012). In fact, many infected horses are able to eliminate or regulate the infection and will never develop Lyme disease. However, with the exceptions of acutely infected or immunocompromised horses, negative test results will have a high negative predictive value. There is no known correlation between magnitude of titer and likelihood of disease. Horses with clinical disease can have low or high positive antibody levels against *B. burgdorferi*. The magnitude of the antibody response seems to be more influenced by the individual's immune response to the spirochetes and the frequency of infection

Interpretation of Equine Laboratory Diagnostics, First Edition. Edited by Nicola Pusterla and Jill Higgins.

Table 34.1 Serologic tests for *Borrelia burgdorferi* infection in horses.

Test	Laboratory	Antibody targets	Interpretation	References
Equine Multiplex Assay	AHDC, Cornell	• 3 recombinant antigens: OspA, OspC, and OspF	• Quantitative; results expressed as median fluorescent intensities (MFIs) • Anti-OspA antibodies – vaccination and/or chronic infection; correlate to antibodies detecting the 31 kDa band on WB • Anti-OspC antibodies – early infection, 3 weeks – 5 months post infection; possibly vaccination if whole bacterins are used; correlate to antibodies detecting 22 kDa band on WB • Anti-OspF antibodies – chronic infection; >7 weeks of infection; correlate to antibodies detecting 29 kDa band on WB	• Wagner et al., 2011 • Wagner et al., 2013
SNAP®4Dx	IDEXX	• Synthetic peptide (C6) that mimics specific Bb antigen (IR6 of VlsE)	• Qualitative; color development visually (subjectively) interpreted • Positive results indicate natural exposure, not vaccination • Anti-C6 antibodies correlate to antibodies that detect the 39 kDa band on WB	• Johnson et al., 2008 • Wagner et al., 2013
WB	CVMDL, UConn	• Whole cell lysate from cultured Bb • Antigens separated by molecular weight	• Qualitative; band pattern visually (subjectively) interpreted • Can give qualitative information regarding vaccination status and infection stage	• Bosler et al., 1988 • Carter et al., 1994 • Dzierzecka and Kita 2002
IFAT ELISA	CVMDL, UConn	• Whole cell lysate from cultured Bb	• Quantitative; results expressed as antibody titer • Positive results must be confirmed by WB • Cross-reactions occur with antibodies against other *Borrelia* or spirochete spp. or against flagella • Will not differentiate vaccinal versus natural exposure antibodies	• Marcus et al., 1985 • Magnarelli et al., 1988 • Bosler et al., 1988 • Magnarelli and Anderson, 1989 • Magnarelli et al., 1997

WB – Western blot; IFAT – indirect fluorescent antibody test; ELISA – enzyme-linked immunosorbent assay; AHDC, Cornell – Animal Health Diagnostic Center, Cornell University College of Veterinary Medicine; CVMDL, UConn – Connecticut Veterinary Medical Diagnostic Laboratory, University of Connecticut; Osp – outer surface protein; Bb – *Borrelia burgdorferi*; IR – immunodominant region; VlsE – Vmp-like sequence, expressed.

than by the presence or absence of clinical disease. Horses in endemic areas generally have higher antibody levels than those in regions where Lyme disease is emerging (BW, unpublished data). Tests that are based on specific recombinant proteins or peptides of *B. burgdorferi* such as the Multiplex assay might assist in interpreting stage of infection and vaccination status. Whole cell lysate assays such as immunofluorescent antibody tests (IFATs) or ELISA tests do not distinguish between infection stages or between infection and vaccination. In addition, whole cell lysate assays often give false positive results because of cross-reactivity with antibodies

against common bacterial structures such as flagellar antigens as evidenced in serological assays developed for dogs (Lindenmayer et al., 1990, Shin et al., 1993) and also experimentally confirmed for horses (BW, unpublished data). Thus, positive test results in whole cell lysate based assays required confirmation by Western blotting (WB). The "Lyme" WB can differentiate antibodies against common, cross-reactive antigens from those that are indicative of infection with *B. burgdorferi* and can assist in determining vaccination status. WB is, however, a subjective method of rather low analytical and diagnostic sensitivity (Wagner et al., 2011).

34.3 Interpretation of Results

34.3.1 General Principles

- A positive serological result for antibodies against *B. burgdorferi* in a horse that has never been vaccinated generally indicates past or present infection. Persistent infection with *B. burgdorferi* induces a long-lasting antibody response as shown in experimental dog and horse models (Appel et al., 1993, Chang et al., 2005, Wagner et al., 2015) and in human, canine and equine patients (Levy et al., 2008, Wagner et al., 2012, 2013). Cross-reacting antibodies against other *Borrelia* or spirochete species can confound interpretation if whole bacterial cell lysate tests are used. A positive result on its own does not confirm that the infection is causing or will cause clinical signs; the diagnosis of Lyme disease always needs to be based on the four criteria discussed previously.
- For the vast majority of cases, a negative result indicates that the horse has not been infected with *B. burgdorferi*, the diagnosis "Lyme disease" should be deleted from the list of differentials, and alternative diagnoses should be pursued. It is considered unlikely that a horse would show clinical signs related to *Borrelia* infection prior to seroconversion. There is currently no experimental infection model that induces clinical signs of disease in horses. However, experimental studies performed in dogs have shown that clinical signs typically occur between 2–5 months after initial infection (Appel et al., 1993). In horses, it is unknown how much time typically elapses between infection and development of clinical signs. There is some accumulated observed, unpublished evidence that the 2–5 months' time frame between infection and the first onset of clinical signs may also be similar in horses, although clinical signs may become evident at a much later time. In a few cases, primarily horses with neurologic or ocular borreliosis, serum results are negative despite severe clinical disease. Some of these horses have negative serum results but compelling evidence of local antibody production in the eye or CNS. If the CNS or eyes become infected, the spirochetes often seem to sequester in these tissues. In addition to the sometimes very high local antibody values, *Borrelia* can often be detected by PCR or histology in the respective tissues. If this happens, the antigenic load can become very low in the periphery causing antibody values to decrease and eventually become negative in serum.
- Although there is limited data regarding kinetics of the anti-*Borrelia* antibody response in experimentally infected horses, antibodies against certain antigens are potentially predictive for early or late

infection stages. These predictions are based on knowledge of spirochete biology, regulation of outer surface protein expression as well as extrapolation from known antibody responses in other species including experimental rodents (Pal et al., 2004, Grimm et al., 2004), dogs (Wagner et al., 2012), and people (Akin et al., 1999). For example, antibodies against outer surface protein C (OspC) are indicative for recent infection due to the expression pattern of this outer surface protein on the spirochetes during and after transmission to the mammalian host, while antibodies against OspF are indicators of chronic infection because OspF appears on the spirochete surface weeks after the host is infected (Akin et al., 1999, Pal et al., 2004, Grimm et al., 2004, Wagner et al., 2012). The clinical significance of infection stage has not yet been determined for horses. However, antibodies to OspC are detectable as early as 3 weeks after infection in dogs (Wagner et al., 2012) and before antibodies to OspF and C6 are measurable in horses (Wagner et al., 2013). Diagnostic data from horses further suggest that antibiotic treatment during the early infection stages results in a faster decline of antibodies and a higher percentage of treated horses that become seronegative after 2–3 months, than treating long-term chronically infected horses (BW, unpublished data).

34.3.2 Specific Situations

- Vaccinated horses: There are no approved Lyme vaccines for use in horses, but some practitioners will immunize horses using canine vaccines. Currently, there are four available canine vaccines. Three (LymeVax®, Zoetis; Duramune®Lyme, Boehringer-Ingelheim; Nobivac®Lyme, Merck) are two-strain bacterins that can induce antibody production against multiple antigens, including all *Borrelia* proteins that are in these whole bacterins (to varying degrees). One (Recombitek®Lyme, Merial) is a recombinant pure non-adjuvanted protein that only includes the OspA antigen. Knowledge of vaccination history will assist in interpreting serologic results. In general, all available tests can only distinguish between vaccination and infection if the recombinant vaccine is used. All other vaccines may interfere, at least transiently, with the ability to diagnose infection with *B. burgdorferi* in serological assays.
- Lyme neuroborreliosis (LNB): A serologic diagnosis of LNB would be best made by documentation of intrathecal antibody production, which in theory could be achieved by submitting paired serum and CSF samples

for quantitative antibody testing. The most accurate results would be obtained by calculation of a specific antibody index or C-value. Unfortunately, there are no validated tests or formulae to determine intrathecal antibody production against *Borrelia* in horses. Although the Multiplex assay is sensitive enough to detect *Borrelia*-specific antibodies in the CSF, challenges include lack of an established optimal serum:CSF cutoff for Lyme testing, the possibility of an abnormal blood-brain barrier permitting passive antibody diffusion into CSF, and effects of sample dilution on measured antibody levels (e.g., the Multiplex assay tests serum at a dilution of 1:400 whereas CSF is generally run undiluted or occasionally at 1:2).

- Post-treatment: Quantitative antibody testing likely allows confirmation of successful clearance of infection but is not necessarily predictive of clinical response. Different experimental infection and treatment studies in dogs have shown that antibody values to *B. burgdorferi* infection markers such as OspF and C6 decline with a short delay after treatment while non-treated, persistently infected dogs maintain long-term antibody values against these proteins (Levy, 2008, Wagner et al., 2015). Similarly, experimentally infected and antibiotic-treated ponies showed a marked decline in ELISA values following successful treatment (Chang et al., 2005). However, naturally infected, antibiotic-treated horses did not all show similar reductions in ELISA values post-treatment, leading investigators to conclude that the value of measuring whole-cell anti-*B. burgdorferi* antibody following antibiotic treatment is unclear and results should not be over-interpreted (Divers et al., 2012). More recent data using the Multiplex assay suggest that antibodies to *B. burgdorferi* OspF and C6 antigens are short-lasting and only maintained long-term if *B. burgdorferi* persists in the circulation. Consequently, if the antigenic load declines the antibodies to these antigens also decline based on their half-life. If infection is eliminated, the antibodies decrease to negative serological test values. This pattern of antibody persistence or decline has been observed for many horses with antibodies to OspF in the past few years (BW, unpublished data). However, since reliable pathogen detection methods are missing for *B. burgdorferi,* definitive proof to confirm that horses that become seronegative have truly eliminated infection is missing. Although persistence of *B. burgdorferi* infection is confirmed for different species including horses and is typically associated with seropositive results, it remains controversial if every seropositive horse is persistently infected.
- Immunocompromised hosts: Sometimes horses with postmortem-confirmed neurologic and/or ocular disease have negative serologic results despite identification

of *Borrelia* in tissue samples. Many of these horses have detectable antibodies against *Borrelia* in samples other than serum (e.g., CSF, aqueous, or vitreous humor), but a few seronegative horses show no evidence of local antibody production against *Borrelia* in these samples using available serological tests. The undetectable or local antibody production might result from the organism's ability to escape immune detection or a compromised host immune response in some horses. One severely neurologically affected horse with equivocal serologic results was confirmed to have hypogammaglobulinemia most likely due to common variable immunodeficiency (CVID) (James et al., 2010), and one of the authors (ALJ) has also diagnosed CVID in horses with neuro-or ocular-borreliosis.

34.4   Available Tests

Several tests have been utilized to detect anti-*Borrelia* antibody production in horses, including an immunofluorescent antibody test (IFAT), enzyme-linked immunosorbent assay (ELISA), Western blot (WB), C6-based in-clinic tests (SNAP®3Dx or 4Dx), fluorescent bead-based assay (Equine Lyme Multiplex assay), and luciferase immunoprecipitation system (LIPS). The last test is not currently commercially available and detects antibodies to the recombinant antigens VOVO (VlsE-OspC-VlsE-OspC), decorin-binding protein A (DbpA), and DbpB (Burbelo et al., 2011). Table 34.1 provides a summary of the available serological testing options that are either performed for horses at accredited diagnostic laboratories or are commercially available and have been shown to provide meaningful results with horse serum. Additional tests that are currently available for dogs include the Quant C6® (Idexx), AccuPlex4® (Antech), and Abaxis ELISA Quantitative Lyme Test® (Abaxis Veterinary Reference Laboratories). To the authors' knowledge, these three tests have not been validated for equine samples and should not be utilized.

34.5   Test Comparisons

The Equine Lyme Multiplex assay was initially validated for equine samples by comparing results to WB testing using a Bayesian model approach, which takes into consideration that no true gold standard exists for Lyme serology. Using the Bayesian model the Multiplex assay showed a higher sensitivity but lower specificity than WB (Wagner et al., 2011).

Additionally, anti-OspF antibody results from combined Equine Lyme Multiplex assay/WB testing were compared to anti-C6 antibody results using the SNAP®4Dx test.

The use of the combined Multiplex/WB results created an artificial gold standard sample set due to the identical test results in both assays. The comparison indicated a high agreement between antibodies against OspF and C6 on Multiplex assay, with 9.4% of samples having discrepant results. When the SNAP® 4Dx test was evaluated using combined Multiplex and WB test results as an artificial gold standard, the SNAP®4Dx testing test showed a small number (~5%) of false positive and negative results (Wagner et al., 2013).

Although the LIPS test is not commercially available, it has been compared to the IFAT using equine samples (Burbelo et al., 2011). Results indicated marked heterogeneity and spectrum of antibody responses in horses against different *B. burgdorferi* antigens, with limited overlap (50%) between IFAT and LIPS testing with three different antigens.

34.6 Summary of Recommendations

Making a diagnosis of Lyme disease in the living horse remains challenging. For horses with compatible clinical signs and potential exposure to *Borrelia*, alternative differential diagnoses should be considered and appropriate diagnostic testing should be performed to confirm or exclude other causes of disease. If serologic analysis confirms *Borrelia* infection and no alternative diagnosis is made, Lyme disease becomes a likely cause of clinical signs. Using a quantitative test (such as the Lyme Multiplex assay) will allow more accurate assessment of local antibody production (e.g., in CSF or ocular fluids) and potentially more accurate diagnosis of neuro- or ocular-borreliosis.

References

Akin E, McHugh GL, Flavell RA, et al. 1999. The immunoglobulin (IgG) antibody response to OspA and OspB correlates with severe and prolonged Lyme arthritis and the IgG response to P35 correlates with mild and brief arthritis. Infect Immun 67: 173–181.

Appel MJG, Allan S, Jacobson RH, et al. 1993. Experimental Lyme disease in dogs produces arthritis and persistent infection. J Infect Dis 167: 651–664.

Bosler EM, Cohen DP, Schulze TL, et al. 1988. Host responses to *Borrelia burgdorferi* in dogs and horses. Ann N Y Acad Sci 539: 221–234.

Burbelo PD, Bren KE, Ching KH, et al. 2011. Antibody profiling of *Borrelia burgdorferi* infection in horses. Clin Vaccine Immunol 18: 1562–1567.

Burgess EC. 1988. *Borrelia burgdorferi* infection in Wisconsin horses and cows. Ann NY Acad Sci 539: 235–243.

Burgess EC and Mattison M. 1987. Encephalitis associated with *Borrelia burgdorferi* infection in a horse. J Am Vet Med Assoc 191: 1457–1458.

Butler CM, Houwers DJ, Jongejan F, et al. 2005. *Borrelia burgdorferi* infections with special reference to horses: a review. Vet Q 27: 146–156.

Carter SD, May C, Barnes A, et al. 1994. *Borrelia burgdorferi* infection in UK horses. Equine Vet J 26: 187–190.

Chang Y-F, Ku Y-W, Chang C-F, et al. 2005; Antibiotic treatment of experimentally *Borrelia burgdorferi*-infected ponies. Vet Microbiol 107: 285–294.

Divers TJ, Mair TS, and Chang Y-F. 2009. Lyme disease in horses. In: TS Mair and RE Hutchinson, (eds). *Infectious Diseases of the Horse*. Cambridgeshire: Equine Veterinary Journal Ltd., pp. 286–292.

Divers TJ, Grice AL, Mohammed HO, et al. 2012. Changes in *Borrelia burgdorferi* ELISA antibody over time in both antibiotic treated and untreated horses. Acta Veterinaria Hungarica 60: 421–429.

Dzierzecka M and Kita J. 2002. The use of chosen serological diagnostic methods in Lyme disease in horses. Part II. Western blot. Pol J Vet Sci 5: 79–84.

Grimm D, Tilly K, Byram R, et al. 2004. Outer-surface protein C of the Lyme disease spirochete: a protein induced in ticks for infection of mammals. Proc Natl Acad Sci USA 101: 3142–3447.

Hahn CN, Mayhew IG, Whitwell KE, et al. 1996. A possible case of Lyme borreliosis in a horse in the UK. Equine Vet J 28: 84–88.

Imai DM, Barr BC, Daft B, et al. 2011. Lyme neuroborreliosis in 2 horses. Vet Pathol 48: 1151–1157.

James FM, Engiles JB, and Beech J. 2010. Meningitis, cranial neuritis, and radiculoneuritis associated with *Borrelia burgdorferi* infection in a horse. J Am Vet Med Assoc 237: 1180–1185.

Johnson AL, Divers TJ, and Chang Y-F. 2008. Validation of an in-clinic enzyme-linked immunosorbent assay kit for diagnosis of *Borrelia burgdorferi* infection in horses. J Vet Diagn Invest 20: 321–324.

Levy SA, O'Connor TP, Hanscom JL, et al. 2008. Quantitative measurement of C6 antibody following antibiotic treatment of *Borrelia burgdorferi* antibody-positive nonclinical dogs. Clin Vaccine Immunol 15: 115–119.

Lindenmayer J, Weber M, Bryant J, et al. 1990. Comparison of indirect immunofluorescent-antibody assay, enzyme-linked immunosorbent assay, and Western immunoblot for the diagnosis of Lyme disease in dogs. J Clin Microbiol 28: 92–96.

Magnarelli LA, Anderson JF, Shaw E, et al. 1988. Borreliosis in equids in northeastern United States. Am J Vet Res 49: 359–362.

Magnarelli LA and Anderson JF. 1989. Class-specific and polyvalent enzyme-linked immunosorbent assays for detection of antibodies to *Borrelia burgdorferi* in equids. J Am Vet Med Assoc 195: 1365–1368.

Magnarelli LA, Flavell RA, Padula SJ, et al. 1997. Serologic diagnosis of canine and equine borreliosis: use of recombinant antigens in enzyme-linked immunosorbent assays. J Clin Microbiol 35: 169–173.

Magnarelli LA, Ijdo JW, Van Andel AE, et al. 2000. Serologic confirmation of *Ehrlichia equi* and *Borrelia burgdorferi* infection in horses from the northeastern United States. J Am Vet Med Assoc 217: 1045–1050.

Marcus LC, Patterson MM, Gilfillan RE, et al. 1985. Antibodies to *Borrelia burgdorferi* in New England horses: serologic survey. Am J Vet Res 46: 2570–2571.

Pal U, Yang X, Chen M, et al. 2004. OspC facilitates *Borrelia burgdorferi* invasion of *Ixodes scapularis* salivary glands. J Clin Invest 113: 220–230.

Priest HL, Irby NL, Schlafer DH, et al. 2012. Diagnosis of *Borrelia*-associated uveitis in two horses. Vet Ophthalmol 15: 398–405.

Sears KP, Divers TJ, Neff RT, et al. 2012. A case of *Borrelia*-associated cutaneous pseudolymphoma in a horse. Vet Dermatol 23: 153–156.

Shin SJ, Chang JF, Jacobson RH, et al. 1993. Cross-reactivity between *B. burgdorferi* and other spirochetes affects specificity of serotests for detection of antibodies to the Lyme disease agent in dogs. Vet Microbiol 36: 161–714.

Wagner B, Freer H, Rollins A, et al. 2011. Development of a multiplex assay for the detection of antibodies to *Borrelia burgdorferi* in horses and its validation using Bayesian and conventional statistical methods. Vet Immunol Immunopathol 144: 374–381.

Wagner B, Freer H, Rollins A, et al. 2012. Antibodies to *Borrelia burgdorferi* OspA, OspC, OspF and C6 antigens as markers for early and late infection in dogs. Clin Vacc Immunol 19: 527–535.

Wagner B, Goodman LB, Rollins A, et al. 2013. Antibodies to OspC, OspF and C6 antigens as indicators for infection with *Borrelia burgdorferi* in horses. Equine Vet J 45: 533–537.

Wagner B, Johnson J, Garcia-Tapia D, et al. 2015. Comparison of effectiveness of cefovecin, doxycycline, and amoxicillin for the treatment of experimentally induced early lyme borreliosis. BMC Vet Res 11: 163.

35

Clostridium difficile
K. Gary Magdesian

Department of Medicine and Epidemiology, School of Veterinary Medicine, University of California, California, USA

35.1 Clinical Background

Clostridium difficile is an anaerobic Gram-positive, spore-forming bacterium associated with diarrhea and enteric diseases in horses, as well as several other species. The disease has been termed *"C. difficile* infection" (CDI). In humans, it has emerged as the most frequently reported nosocomial pathogen in hospitals ("hospital-acquired CDI"). It also occurs outside of hospitals, with 25–33% of *C. difficile* infections acquired in the community (Lessa et al., 2015). Hospital-acquired CDI is associated with antibiotic use and is more severe in older patients. Community acquired CDI, on the other hand, is associated with younger patients and develops without clear exposure to antibiotics or other risk factors (Leffler and Lamont, 2015). Acid suppression as occurs with proton pump inhibitors (e.g., omeprazole) is suspected to be another risk factor for CDI in humans (Leffler and Lamont, 2015) Additional risk factors in humans include advanced age, inflammatory bowel disease, organ transplantation, chemotherapy, chronic kidney disease, immunodeficiency, and exposure to infected people.

Clostridium difficile infection (CDI) may develop as a primary infection, seen most commonly in foals, or as a secondary dysbiosis associated with the administration of antimicrobials in horses of any age. Antimicrobials affect the GI microbiome resulting in reduced colonization resistance, thereby allowing *C. difficile* to take hold and proliferate. The microbe is toxigenic, producing a number of exotoxins. The best studied of these are toxin A (Tcd A, enterotoxin) and B (Tcd B, cytotoxin), toxins that are associated with pathogenicity. Strains that do not produce either of these toxins are considered nonpathogenic.

Clostridium difficile is associated with a wide range of clinical disease. It can be associated with mild, self-limiting diarrhea as well as severe, life-threatening colitis. *C. difficile* has also been associated with anterior enteritis in a small group of horses (Arroyo et al., 2006). It can also be cultured from the feces of horses subclinically, especially in horses on antimicrobials and in foals. While *C. difficile* is not generally considered to be part of the normal flora of adult horses, it can be found in the feces of up to 30% of clinically healthy foals on some farms (Baverud et al., 2003).

The mortality rate of CDI in humans and adult horses varies and has been reported to be 6–20% in humans and up to 24% in horses (Ruby et al., 2009, Leffler and Lamont, 2015, Planche and Wilcox, 2015). Indicators of severe infection include acute kidney injury, severe ileus, abdominal distention, and marked hypoalbuminemia. One notable difference between CDI in humans and horses is that humans may develop recurrent CDI, whereas horses generally do not.

35.2 Tests Available

Available laboratory tests for *C. difficile* infection (CDI) detect either the organism or its toxins (toxin A and/or B). The tests that detect the organism include culture and enzyme immunoassays (EIA) for an antigen found on all isolates of *C. difficile*, "glutamate dehydrogenase" (GDH). GDH is an enzyme constitutively produced in large quantities by *C. difficile*, including both toxigenic and nontoxigenic strains, making it a good marker of the presence of the organism. The tests that detect organism are more often positive than those targeting toxins. Merely the presence of the organism does not define disease, because both nontoxigenic and toxigenic strains can be found subclinically in horses. The detection of toxin (A and/or B) in feces better identifies cases with clinically relevant disease. However, the sensitivity of immunoassay toxin tests varies, and is low in some cases, thereby missing some of the cases. In contrast, PCR analysis alone may be overly sensitive to be used as a standalone test. Therefore, a combination of tests for both organism and toxin maximizes the sensitivity and specificity.

A two-step approach is recommended for diagnosis of the disease.

Step 1: Tests for organism:

1) Culture. This requires anaerobic culture on selective media.
2) GDH immunoassay.

Step 2: Tests for toxins:

1) Toxin immunoassays (usually combined with GDH)
2) Stool cytotoxicity assay
3) PCR for toxin gene sequences

35.2.1 Immunoassays

1) Glutamate Dehydrogenase or "Common Antigen" tests: Glutamate dehydrogenase (GDH) enzyme immunoassay (EIA):

   This test detects a cell wall antigen that is present on all *C. difficile* isolates (Korman, 2015). The turnaround time is <2 h. This is an initial screening test with high sensitivity and high negative predictive value. However, because it alone does not test for toxins, GDH-positive samples must undergo a second, confirmatory test for toxigenic infection. Therefore, many commercial EIA kits include both GDH and toxin tests. The sensitivity of GDH assays is high (>90%) in humans, and was 93% in equine feces as compared to direct fecal culture of toxigenic strains when using the Triage *Clostridium difficile* panel (Biosite, San Diego, CA) (Ruby et al., 2009, Korman, 2015). It also has a high specificity and negative predictive value (Korman, 2015).

2) Toxin enzyme immunoassays (EIA): These are immunoassays that test feces directly for toxins. Many currently available kits test for the presence of either of the major toxins ("toxin A or B"), whereas others evaluate for them separately. These EIAs have high specificity (>95%), but, unfortunately, they have variable sensitivities and in general the sensitivity is not as high as for GDH. In human feces, the sensitivity of EIAs has ranged from 67–83% as compared to stool cell culture cytotoxin assays, long considered to be the gold standard for detection of toxin B. Compared to this stool cytotoxin test, the Techlab *C. difficile* Tox A/B II ELISA (Techlab Inc.; Blacksburg, VA) had a sensitivity of 84% and specificity of 96% (Medina-Torres et al., 2010). Because they can miss toxins, the EIAs are no longer recommended for use as stand-alone tests for diagnosis of CDI (Korman, 2015). Rather, they should be used as part of the two-step diagnosis described previously.

35.2.2 Additional Tests for Toxigenicity

1) Cell cytotoxicity assay: The cytotoxin neutralization assay (CTNA) using cell culture is considered the traditional gold standard test for identification of toxigenic infections. This tests for toxin B in filtrates of feces by evaluating for cytopathic effect on cell cultures. It has a longer turn-around time (24–48 h) and is relatively labor intensive, and has largely been replaced by the EIAs.

2) PCR identification of toxin genes: This is a relatively new diagnostic modality introduced to clinical medicine in terms of diagnostics for CDI. PCR assays target toxins A and B genes (tcdA and tcdB, respectively). The sensitivity of PCR in feces is very high (>90% vs CTNA, >85% compared to culture), as is the specificity (>95%) (Korman, 2015). It has a very high negative predictive value. Questions remain as to its positive predictive value as it can be positive in asymptomatic patients that are shedding toxigenic isolates (Korman, 2015). Many feel that PCR is too sensitive to be relied upon alone for a diagnosis of CDI (Leffler and Lamont, 2015, Polage et al., 2015). Therefore, patients can be misdiagnosed if they are shedding low numbers of toxigenic *C. difficile* yet have another underlying primary disorder. In humans, up to 25% of human patients referred to secondary centers for CDI had alternative diagnoses, such as irritable bowel syndrome (IBS) and inflammatory bowel disease (IBD) (Jackson et al., 2015). Because of this, PCR is not recommended for use as a screening test in horses without diarrhea, because subclinical transiently colonized horses can be positive. In diarrheic horses, it should be used in conjunction with an antigen test as part of a two-step diagnostic. The negative predictive value of PCR is quite high, and a negative result means CDI is very unlikely. In human patients, stool PCR tests remain positive for *C. difficile* for up to 30 days post treatment, so follow-up tests are not indicated in most cases (Surawicz et al., 2000).

35.2.3 Additional Test for Organism

Anaerobic culture: This is the diagnostic gold standard along with the CTNA previously. Because there are nontoxigenic isolates of *C. difficile*, simple culture does not necessarily indicate toxigenicity and only identifies the presence of the microbe. The cultured isolate can then be tested for toxin gene sequences using PCR. The long turn-around time (>3 days) makes it impractical for acute cases of diarrhea, and culture has largely been replaced by GDH immunoassays to detect the organism in feces. However, culture is still necessary when ribotype and antimicrobial susceptibility testing are required, such as during outbreaks or for cases that are refractory to treatment, respectively.

35.3 Recommended Approach for Diagnostic Testing for *Clostridium difficile* Infection

A two-step testing protocol, with initial screening for organism followed by tests for toxins, is recommended:

1) Only clinical cases should be tested. Horses without fever (suspected to be of GI origin), neutropenia, diarrhea or ileus/reflux should not be tested.
2) An EIA with antigen (GDH) and toxin testing should be performed as a two-step process. If both are positive, the diagnosis is supported. If both are negative, the diagnosis is not supported and other etiologies should be pursued.
   A positive GDH test indicates that the organism is present in feces, however it does not necessarily imply toxigenic strains. Therefore, a positive GDH test must be followed up with a confirmatory test, either a fecal toxin EIA or PCR for toxin genes in feces.
3) If antigen is positive, but toxin is negative on the EIA, then PCR should be performed on feces for the toxin gene sequences. If positive, and other etiologies are ruled out, then a diagnosis can be confirmed. If PCR is negative, look for additional causes of diarrhea or ileus.

If PCR is solely relied up, as with a "diarrhea panel" that are offered by many commercial molecular diagnostic laboratories, positive results must be interpreted in light of clinical signs, history, and additional diagnostic tests to rule out other causative agents. A positive GDH EIA makes the finding of positive genes by PCR much more substantive, as it indicates the microbe is present in relatively high concentrations (two-step approach) (Ruby et al., 2009). In human medicine, reliance on PCR alone has resulted in an increase in CDI diagnosis rate by ≥ 50%, with thought that some of these are misdiagnoses (Longtin et al., 2013, Polage et al., 2015). Further studies are needed to define the role of PCR as a sole test for diagnosis of CDI. Therefore, in the meantime, it should only be used in diarrheic or refluxing animals, and optimally used in conjunction with a GDH EIA to establish clinical significance through the two-step approach.

35.4 Sample Collection and Submission

Feces should be tested for horses with diarrhea. Gastric contents can be used for horses with reflux such as those with anterior enteritis.

Additional potential comorbidities or other causes should be ruled out (Table 35.1). *C. difficile* can be present with *C. perfringens*, *Salmonella* spp., and other pathogens (Magdesian et al., 2002).

35.5 Possible Results

Positive Case:
Positive on two steps:

1) Positive GDH on EIA or culture positive
2) Positive toxin A/B on EIA or on fecal PCR

*Note: EIA for GDH and toxins are usually on the same kit

Negative Case:

Negative GDH on EIA *and* negative for toxins on EIA or fecal PCR

35.6 Interpretation

The diagnosis of CDI is based on (Table 35.2):

1) Combination of signs and history
2) Two-step testing:
   a) Microbiological evidence of *C. difficile*:
      i) GDH screen (immunoassay/EIA), OR
      ii) culture
   b) Presence of toxins in feces
      i) Immunoassay for toxins (EIA), OR
      ii) Fecal PCR for toxin genes

*Note: The EIA for GDH and toxins are usually on the same EIA kit.

3) Ruling out cocontributors or other causes

Table 35.1 Common causes of diarrhea in horses.

Infectious causes:

Clostridium difficile
Clostridium perfringens
Salmonella spp.
Coronavirus
Antibiotic-associated dysbiosis
Small strongyle hypobiosis
Neorickettsia risticii
Lawsonia intracellularis
Rotavirus (foal)
Cryptosporidium parvum (foal)

Noninfectious causes:

Sand accumulation
Right dorsal colitis
Toxins
Inflammatory bowel disease
Neoplasia
Food intolerance
Moldy feed
Grain overload
Anaphylaxis

Table 35.2 Algorithm of diagnostic work-up for *Clostridium difficile* infection.

1) Optimal approach with most definitive evidence:

   Use for adult horses with antibiotic-associated diarrhea and in foals with nonspecific diarrhea, including outbreaks
   First step: Run fecal EIA with both GDH and toxin (A or B) assays
   If both GDH and toxin positive = definite evidence for CDI
   If both GDH and toxin negative = look for other cause
   If GDH positive and toxin negative = perform PCR for toxin genes

2) PCR for toxin genes:
   Use for adult horses that are GDH positive and toxin negative on fecal immunoassays
   Use for foals with nonspecific diarrhea
   If positive = suspect case, rule out other causes
   If negative = unlikely to be *C. difficile*

3) Culture:
   Run in conjunction with fecal EIA for GDH and toxin
   If negative EIA, run fecal PCR for toxin genes
   Use for outbreak situations to perform antimicrobial susceptibility to metronidazole
   Can be used for typing of isolates

It should be noted that positive tests must be interpreted in light of other diagnostics. The diagnosis of a horse with enterocolitis should not be solely relied upon a test for *C difficile*. Other agents, including *Salmonella* spp., coronavirus, *Neorickettsia risticii*, *C. perfringens*, and other causes of enterocolitis, should be ruled out (Table 35.1). Some of these may cause comorbidity. For example, horses can be coinfected with *Salmonella* and *C. difficile*, or foals can be coinfected with *C. perfringens* and *C. difficile*.

Testing of horses with normal stool consistency is not recommended. Posttreatment testing is also not strongly recommended, and requires further study in horses. In humans, posttreatment testing has no role in confirming eradication as patients can remain positive for toxins for some time after resolution of diarrhea (Leffler and Lamont, 2015, Sethi et al., 2010).

35.7 Case Example

A 9-year old Thoroughbred mare was presented for diarrhea that developed following a 4-day course of ceftiofur administration. She developed a 104 °F, watery diarrhea, and signs of endotoxemia. A fecal immunoassay (EIA) was positive for both *C. difficile* GDH antigen and toxins A/B. Fecal culture revealed positive growth for *C. difficile*. In this case, the two-step diagnostic criteria have been met, namely identification of the microbe (on EIA or culture) and toxins (on EIA). Five negative cultures for *Salmonella* were also obtained.

References

Arroyo LG, Stampfli HR, and Weese JS. 2006. Potential role of *Clostridium difficile* as a cause of duodenitis-proximal jejunitis in horses. J Med Microbiol, 55: 605–608.

Baverud V, Gustafsson A, Franklin A, Aspan A, and Gunnarsson A. 2003. *Clostridium difficile*: prevalence in horses and environment, and antimicrobial susceptibility. Equine Vet J, 35: 465–471.

Jackson M, Olefson S, Machan JT, and Kelly CR. 2015. A high rate of alternative diagnoses in patients referred for presumed *Clostridium difficile* infection. J Clin Gastroenterol, 50(9): 742–746.

Korman TM. 2015. Diagnosis and management of *Clostridium difficile* infection. Semin Respir Crit Care Med, 36: 31–43.

Leffler DA and Lamont JT. 2015. *Clostridium difficile* infection. New Engl J Med, 372: 1539–1548.

Lessa FC, Mu Y, Bamberg WM, et al. 2015. Burden of *Clostridium difficile* infection in the United States. New Engl J Med, 372: 825–834.

Longtin Y, Trottier S, Brochu G, et al. 2013; Impact of the type of diagnostic assay on *Clostridium difficile* infection and complication rates in a mandatory reporting program. Clin Infect Dis, 56: 67–73.

Magdesian KG, Hirsh DC, Jang SS et al. 2002. Characterization of *Clostridium difficile* isolates from foals with diarrhea: 28 cases (1993–1997). J Am Vet Med Assoc, 220: 67–73.

Medina-Torres CE, Weese JS, and Stampfli HR. 2010. Validation of a commercial enzyme immunoassay for detection of *Clostridium difficile* toxins in feces of horses with acute diarrhea. J Vet Intern Med, 24: 628–632.

Planche T and Wilcox MH. 2015. Diagnostic pitfalls in *Clostridium difficile* infection. Infect Dis Clin N Am 29: 63–82.

Polage CR, Gyorke CE, Kennedy MA, Leslie JL, Chin DL, Wang S, et al. 2015. Overdiagnosis of *Clostridium difficile* infection in the molecular test era. JAMA Intern Med 175: 1792–1801.

Ruby RR, Magdesian KG, and Kass PH. 2009. Comparison of clinical, microbiologic, and clinicopathologic findings in horses positive and negative for *Clostridium difficile* infection. J Am Vet Med Assoc 234: 777–784.

Sethi AK, Al-Nassir WN, Nerandzic MM, Bobulsky GS, and Donskey CJ. 2010. Persistence of skin contamination and environmental shedding of *Clostridium difficile* during and after treatment of *C. difficile* infection. Infect Control Hosp Epidemiol, 31: 21–27.

Surawicz CM, McFarland LV, Greenberg RN, et al. 2000; The search for a better treatment for recurrent *Clostridium difficile* disease: use of high-dose vancomycin combined with *Saccharomyces boulardii*. Clin Infect Dis, 31: 1012–1017.

36

Leptospira spp.

Janet Foley and Mary H. Straub

Department of Medicine and Epidemiology, School of Veterinary Medicine, University of California, California, USA

36.1 Introduction

One of the most challenging diagnostic dilemmas in equine infectious disease is determining how to interpret clinical signs, history, and laboratory test results for horses suspected of having leptospirosis (Box 36.1). Moreover, the risk of leptospirosis is often considerably underestimated in many geographical areas and clinical presentation in most domestic animals may be nonspecific, making it important for a clinician to develop an appropriate index of suspicion for leptospirosis and request supportive testing. In this chapter, we describe history and clinical signs that should alert clinicians to consider further testing for exposure to pathogenic leptospires, we overview the diagnostic modalities available, and we discuss how results of testing should be interpreted towards optimum treatment of horses.

The organism that causes leptospirosis in the horse is typically either *Leptospira interrogans* or *L. kirschneri* though seven other pathogenic *Leptospira* spp. exist (Ko et al., 2009). These fragile spirochete bacteria have a flagellum and an outer membrane containing abundant lipopolysaccharide (LPS) (Cameron, 2015, Haake and Zückert, 2015). Leptospires require a wet environment and may persist for several weeks if water is stagnant, warm (between 10–25 °C), and neutral pH, after being shed in the urine of infected animals (Faine, 2000).

Horses are typically exposed to *Leptospira* by ingestion of wet vegetation or water that has been contaminated by urine of a carrier or reservoir host, after which leptospires penetrate mucous membranes or breaches of skin, although other routes of exposure include contact with aborted fetuses, placentas, uterine discharge, or milk or with water contaminated by any of these materials. Exposure can also occur during mating. The best-characterized reservoir hosts are *Rattus* spp. that

appear to tolerate the infection within renal tubules without developing renal failure or succumbing, and shed infectious leptospires for months (Johnson et al., 2004, Thiermann, 1981). Farm animals, particularly pigs and cattle, are commonly reported to shed *Leptospira* (Adler and de la Peña Moctezuma, 2010) and may be a source of infection to horses. These animals are not reservoirs in the classical sense because they also suffer from abortion and other clinical leptospiral manifestations.

There are currently two distinct classification schemes for leptospires based on serovars and DNA (Box 36.2). These two classification schemes do not correspond; for example, two different leptospires within a serogroup (Pomona, for example) could actually be in two different species of *Leptospira* based on genotype. In fact, serologically identical leptospires have been identified in up to six different species of *Leptospira* (Levett, 2001). This can lead to confusion if the classification scheme being used is not explicitly stated or if results from serological tests are compared to results from DNA-based diagnostic tests.

Although various host species tend to be infected with a suite of serovars typical of that host, there are many instances of serovars originating from one host species and infecting another. Infecting serovars differ depending on geographic location and typically reflect the serovar(s) circulating in local wildlife. In North America, antibodies to serovars Pomona and Grippotyphosa are the most common detected in horses, while antibodies against serovars Bratislava, Hardjo, and Icterohaemorrhagiae have also been reported (Donahue et al., 1995, Timoney et al., 2011, Williams et al., 1994). There is evidence that horses may be a reservoir host for serovar Bratislava (Hines, 2014, Kitson-Piggot and Prescott, 1987), in which case they could be chronically infected and shed leptospires in their urine, but remain clinically healthy.

Interpretation of Equine Laboratory Diagnostics, First Edition. Edited by Nicola Pusterla and Jill Higgins.
© 2018 John Wiley & Sons, Inc. Published 2018 by John Wiley & Sons, Inc.

Box 36.1 Key points in understanding equine leptospirosis.

- Leptospirosis is a bacterial disease cause by *Leptospira* spp. Leptospires are shed in infected animals' urine, can persist in wet environments, and can infect dogs, horses, people, and other animals.
- Leptospirosis sometimes causes liver and kidney failure; equine cases more likely to present with uveitis (or so called "moon blindness"). Infection during pregnancy can lead to late-term abortions or stillbirths. Infection may be subclinical.
- In most species, the incubation period for acute disease ranges from 2 to 30 days. In horses, uveitis typically occurs months after initial infection.
- Diagnosis of active infection is best done by PCR while serology, which is more sensitive than PCR, is useful for confirming cases retrospectively and identifying an outbreak.
- Serology for leptospirosis is complicated by extensive cross-reaction among serovars. Also, exposed horses tend to have extremely high titers that are long-lasting, making it difficult to correlate titer with disease.

Box 36.2 Classification of *Leptospira*

Classification by serovar

- Most widely used and available, most familiar.
- Can be done on a horse that is not actively infected or shedding leptospires.
- Based on the cross-reactivity of patient sera against different *Leptospira* isolates.
- Serovar is defined as a *Leptospira* strain whose homologous rabbit antiserum only agglutinates that particular strain (Faine, 2000).
- Cross-reactivity serovars are grouped into serogroups; there are over 300 serovars grouped into approximately 30 serogroups (Picardeau, 2013).

Classification by genotype

- Rapidly becoming more widely used in the scientific literature.
- Based on DNA homology.
- Requires active shedding of sufficient numbers of spirochetes that their DNA can be detected.
- Has resulted in identification of 21 species of *Leptospira*, with at least nine known to be pathogenic to animals (Ko et al., 2009, Levett, 2015).

36.2 Clinical History and Physical Examination

The most commonly reported equine manifestations of equine leptospirosis are abortion and equine recurring uveitis (ERU) (Box 36.3). There isn't necessarily a characteristic history, with the exception that seroprevalence studies (but not studies of clinical infection) have demonstrated increased risk with age (Barwick et al., 1997, Lees and Gale, 1994) and in some areas, leptospirosis is more likely during wet or warm seasons (Baverud et al., 2009) (Jung et al., 2010). Acute infection covers the spectrum from asymptomatic or very ill, while transplacental transmission may lead to fetal death or chronic disease in the foal (Timoney et al., 2011, Donahue et al., 1995, Hines, 2014). Uveitis is a non-specific finding and can be due to a variety of causes, with *Leptospira* infection being only one (Hines, 2014). Less commonly, kidney or liver disease can occur in horses with leptospirosis.

36.3 Routine Diagnostic Tests

Results of routine diagnostic tests are nonspecific and reflect infection, inflammation, and possibly organ failure, including leukocytosis with neutrophilia, indicators of liver and kidney disease, occasionally hyperbilirubinemia and hyperfibrinogenemia, and isosthenuria on urinalysis. Anterior chamber fluid clinical chemical and cytological analysis is nonspecific for uveitis. Pathology grossly may appear normal or there may be swollen, erythematous and hemorrhagic placentas, or

---

Box 36.3 Clinical signs of equine leptospirosis.

- Acutely infected horses may be asymptomatic or febrile, depressed, anorectic, or icteric.
- Transplacental transmission may lead to fetal resorption, stillbirth, or weak or dying neonates (Timoney et al., 2011).
- Foals that survive transplacental transmission may have weakness, icterus, hematuria, or pneumonia (Donahue et al., 1995, Hines, 2014).
- Uveitis is a non-specific immune-mediated disease caused by *Leptospira* and a variety of other causes.
- Leptospiral uveitis may due to active infection in the eye or be immune response to infection months or years earlier (Hines, 2014).
- *Leptospira*-induced ERU can be unilateral, progress to bilateral, chronic, and result in blindness.
- Less commonly, horses with leptospirosis have icterus or acute renal failure.

renal tubular changes. On histopathology, Gram stain, hematoxylin and eosin, and silver staining could document leptospires.

36.4 Specialized Diagnostic Tests

See Box 36.4.

- MAT: The MAT or Microscopic Agglutination Test is considered the gold standard for serological diagnosis of leptospirosis. Serum samples are screened against a panel of reference serovars representing the locally common serogroups. Results for each serovar are given as titers, though due to cross-reactivity and even paradoxical reactions (where the highest titers are detected to a serogroup different from the infecting one), the results of MAT cannot be used to identify the infecting serovar (Levett, 2001).

- ELISA: Unlike MAT, ELISA (Enzyme-Linked Immunofluorescent Antibody) tests use only a single, genus-specific antigen to detect antibodies in the serum. ELISA tests can be used to detect either IgM or IgG.
- Other serological tests: Other diagnostic tests that can be used to detect antibodies to leptospires are much less commonly encountered in veterinary medicine: these include indirect fluorescent antibody test (IFAT), latex agglutination tests, and slide agglutination tests, among others.
- Polymerase chain reaction (PCR): See Chapter 54.
- Darkfield microscopy: Motile leptospires in fresh fluids such as blood, urine and aqueous humor can sometimes be visualized under darkfield microscopy. Samples can be centrifuged to concentrate leptospires for visualization.
- Staining: An immunohistochemical stain specific for *Leptospira* may be applied to fixed tissues for visualization

Box 36.4 Diagnosis of *Leptospira*.

	Indirect nonspecific diagnosis	Indirect specific diagnosis	Direct diagnosis	Supportive approaches
Methodology	Response to treatment	Serology: microscopic agglutination, less commonly ELISA	PCR, DNA sequencing, multiple-locus strain typing, immunohistochemical (IHC) stain on tissue	Darkfield microscopy, silver stain
Target of test	Horse	Surface antigens on bacterium	Various gene or antigen targets	Bacterium
Performance	Nonspecific, variable	Groups broadly distinct bacteria together but at scale of herd or small geographical area suggests common exposure	Yields confirmation (PCR, culture, IHC) and possible strain-specific identification (MLST, sequencing) of infecting bacterium	Requires very fresh sample (darkfield) and biosafety
Expense	Low	High	Range	Moderate
Best use for test	As indicated for standard of care for patient	Retrospective evaluation of suspect case; Best to test acute and convalescent samples one to four weeks apart; Snapshot of whether multiple horses exposed to same source	PCR on all acute infections; IHC on pathology, other tests for research or further exploration of source	
Interpretation	Some antibiotics are also anti-inflammatory, confounding interpretation; Supports but does not confirm leptospirosis	Four-fold rising titer confirmatory, may be negative in acute disease, very high titer doesn't confirm infection (Poonacha et al., 1993) (Bernard, 1993)	PCR highly sensitive unless horse is currently not shedding (then use serology); IHC very sensitive post-mortem	Both require expertise in interpretation, may have false-positive results
Notes		IgM ELISA may also detect an antibody response slightly sooner after infection than MAT since MAT is less sensitive to IgM (WHO, 2003)		Darkfield often not available, both tests may be superseded (darkfield by PCR, silver stain by IHC)

and confirmation of the organisms. Silver staining can also be used to visualize leptospires in fixed tissues.

- Culture: Leptospires are obligate aerobes which grow best at temperatures between 28–30°C in specialized media. The spirochetes are very slow-growing that limits the usefulness of culture as a diagnostic tool. However, culture is the only way to definitively identify the infecting strain of *Leptospira* spp., which can help determine the source in the case of an outbreak. Samples that can be cultured include blood, urine, aqueous humor, CSF, and internal organs (kidney, liver, lung).

36.5 Response to Therapy

Horses with leptospiral renal failure or hepatitis may be expected to resolve clinical signs when treated with antibiotics. This is not the case with ERU because of the immune component of the disease; thus, failure to respond to antibiotics does not rule leptospirosis as an inciting cause out.

36.6 Herd Health and Public Health Considerations

Leptospirosis is a zoonotic disease shed in the urine of a diversity of domestic animals and wildlife, thus a case in one horse suggests risk to other animals in the same area, including possibly humans. This is supported by research that showed that horses maintained in groups were at greater risk of leptospirosis than horses held singly (Hines, 2014). Confirming the strain type causing infection in a particular horse may seem unnecessary for treatment of an individual horse; however, ultimately, horses and other in-contact animals cannot be well-protected if the source cannot be determined. During acute infection and following leptospiral abortions, horses may shed infectious leptospires in their urine, which could be a source of infection to handlers. Therefore, acutely infected horses should be handled with care and caregivers should wear gloves and protect mucous membranes until the horse has PCR-negative urine or has been treated with appropriate antibiotics for at least 4 days.

References

Adler B and De La Peña Moctezuma A. 2010. *Leptospira* and leptospirosis. Vet Microbiol, 140: 287–296.

Barwick RS, Mohammed HO, Mcdonough PL, and White ME. 1997. Risk factors associated with the likelihood of leptospiral seropositivity in horses in the state of New York. Am J Vet Res, 58: 1097–1103.

Baverud V, Gunnarsson A, Engvall EO, Franzen P, and Egenvall A. 200.) *Leptospira* seroprevalence and associations between seropositivity, clinical disease and host factors in horses. Acta Vet Scand, 51: 1–15.

Bernard WV. 1993. Leptospirosis. Vet Clin N Am-Equine, 9: 435–44.

Cameron C. 2015. Leptospiral structure, physiology, and metabolism. In B. Adler (ed.), *Leptospira and Leptospirosis*. Berlin/Heidelberg: Springer, pp. 21–41.

Donahue JM, Smith BJ, Poonacha KB, Donahoe JK, and Rigsby CL. 1995. Prevalence and serovars of *Leptospira* involved in equine abortions in central Kentucky during the 1991–1993 foaling seasons. J Vet Diagn Invest, 7: 87–91.

Faine S, Adler B, Bolin C, and Perolat P. 2000. *Leptospira and Leptospirosis*, Medisci Press, Melbourne, Australia.

Haake D and Zückert W. 2015. The leptospiral outer membrane. In B. Adler (ed.), *Leptospira and Leptospirosis*. Berlin/Heidelberg: Springer, pp. 187–221.

Hines MT. 2014. Leptospirosis. In DC Sellon and MT Long (eds), *Equine Infectious Diseases*. 2nd edn. St. Louis: W.B. Saunders, pp. 302–311.

Johnson MA, Smith H, Joeph P, Gilman RH, Bautista CT, Campos KJ, et al. 2004. Environmental exposure and leptospirosis, Peru. Emerg Infect Disease, 10: 1016–1022.

Jung BY, Lee KW, and Ha TY. 2010. Seroprevalence of *Leptospira* spp. in clinically healthy racing horses in Korea. J Vet Med Sci, 72: 197–201.

Kitson-Piggot AW and Prescott JF. 1987. Leptospirosis in horses in Ontario. Can J Vet Res, 51: 448–451.

Ko AI, Goarant C, and Picardeau M. 2009. *Leptospira*: the dawn of the molecular genetics era for an emerging zoonotic pathogen. Nature Rev Microbiol, 7: 736–747.

Lees VW and Gale SP. 1994. Titers to *Leptospira* species in horses in Alberta. Can J Vet Res, 35: 636–40.

Levett PN. 2001. Leptospirosis. Clin Microbiol Rev, 14: 296–326.

Levett PN. 2015. Systematics of *Leptospiraceae*. In B. Adler (ed.), *Leptospira and Leptospirosis*. Berlin/Heidelberg: Springer.

Picardeau M. 2013. Diagnosis and epidemiology of leptospirosis. Médecine et Maladies Infectieuses 43: 1–9.

Poonacha KB, Donahue JM, Giles RC, Hong CB, Petrites-Murphy MB, Smith BJ, et al. 1993. Leptospirosis in equine fetuses, stillborn foals, and placentas. Vet Pathol, 30: 362–369.

Thiermann AB. 1981. The Norway rat as a selective chronic carrier of *Leptospira icterohaemorrhagiae*. J Wildlife Disease, 17: 39–43.

Timoney JF, Kalimuthusamy N, Velineni S, Donahue JM, Artiushin SC, and Fettinger M. 2011. A unique genotype of *Leptospira interrogans* serovar Pomona type kennewicki is associated with equine abortion. Vet Microbiol, 150: 349–353.

WHO. 2003. *Human leptospirosis: guidance for diagnosis, surveillance and control.* Geneva: WHO.

Williams DM, Smith BJ, Donahue JM, and Poonacha KB. 1994. Serological and microbiological findings on 3 farms with equine leptospiral abortions. Eq Vet J, 26: 105–108.

37

Fungal Pathogens

Jill Higgins[1] and Nicola Pusterla[2]

[1] Equine Consulting Services-Penryn, California, USA
[2] Department of Medicine and Epidemiology, School of Veterinary Medicine, University of California, California, USA

37.1 Introduction

A suspicion for fungal disease must be established in the equine patient based on clinical signs, geographical location, and exclusion of more common pathogens. From there, a combination of diagnostic procedures must be used to achieve a definitive diagnosis of the exact fungal agent. The detection of fungal organisms by microbiological culture is difficult and slow because of their fastidious growth requirements. Molecular-based assays are used to detect fungal organisms in various biological specimens while immunohistochemistry, fluorescent *in situ* hybridization and PCR are used to diagnose fungal organisms in histopathological sections. Serological testing can be used to support a fungal infection in horses; however, its use is limited and restricted to selected fungal pathogens.

37.2 Diagnostic Testing

37.2.1 Coccidioidomycosis

Coccidioides immitis and *Coccidioides posadasii* are dimorphic soil saprophytes, existing as a mold on culture media and a non-budding spherule in host tissue. They grow in sandy alkaline soils in semiarid climates including portions of California, Arizona, New Mexico, Texas, Nevada, and Utah. Infection usually occurs via inhalation of airborne arthroconidia and subsequently causes initial respiratory tract disease. Lymphohematogenous dissemination can follow, leading to infections in various organs including bone, skin, and abdominal viscera. Very rarely, localized, external infections are thought to occur via transcutaneous inoculation. Reported cases in horses have traditionally been fairly severe and often fatal including cases of interstitial pneumonia, osteomyelitis,

mastitis, abortion, and superficial and internal abscesses (Kramme and Ziemer, 1990, Ziemer et al., 1992, Walker et al., 1993, Stoltz et al., 1994).

A suspected diagnosis of coccidioidomycosis commonly relies on the geographic origin or travel history of the patient, clinical signs, an inflammatory leukogram (hyperproteinemia, hyperfibrinogenemia, leukocytosis, and neutrophilia) and additional diagnostic modalities including body fluid analysis, imaging diagnostics and organ biopsies. A definitive diagnosis is achieved by positive culture, cytologic isolation, or molecular detection of the organism from body fluid samples or tissues. For these reasons, serologic results become very important in making a diagnosis, predicting prognosis, determining likely form of the disease and evaluating response to treatment (Table 37.1). A distinction is made between IgM antibodies (the early precipitin type indicative of recent exposure/infection) and IgG antibodies (the complement fixation type that is present later in the course of the immune response: Pappagianis, 2001). In a seroepidemiologic survey, the seroprevalence of IgG coccidioidal antibodies among 197 healthy adult horses sampled over a 6-month period in a highly endemic area (greater Phoenix, AZ) was 4% (Higgins et al., 2005). All positive horses had a titer of 8 or less and had declining or static titers with each subsequent recheck without ever developing clinical signs. The low prevalence of positive titers in horses in endemic areas makes the diagnostic value of a positive titer, especially a high titer in a clinically ill animal, very strong. Because of the rarity of positive horses in the population, a positive titer in an asymptomatic horse should be taken seriously and rechecked to determine the antibody kinetics. In a retrospective study of 39 clinical equine cases, magnitude of titer was found to significantly correlate with certain forms of the disease, while other forms had overlapping titer distribution (Higgins et al., 2007, Table 37.2).

Table 37.1 Characteristics of relevant equine fungal pathogens.

	Distribution	Useful diagnostics	Veterinary laboratories offering serology in the USA
Coccidioides immitis *Coccidioides posadasii*	Southwestern United States	Culture, PCR and cytology of body fluids Histology of organ biopsies Serology	UCD, UT, CSU, CU, NMDA, MDL
Blastomyces dermatitidis	Mississippi, Missouri, Ohio, Great Lakes region, East Coast, parts of Canada	Culture and cytology of body fluids Histology of organ biopsies Serology	UT, CSU, CU MDL
Histoplasma capsulatum	Ohio, Mississippi, Texas, Virginia, Delaware, Maryland	Culture and cytology of body fluids Histology of organ biopsies Serology	UT, CSU, CU MDL
Cryptococcus neoformans *Cryptococcus gattii*	Worldwide	Culture and cytology body fluids Histology of organ biopsies Capsular antigen detection	UT, CSU, CU, UGA, NMDA, MDL
Aspergillus species	Ubiquitous	Culture, PCR and cytology of body fluids and organ biopsies Histology of organ biopsies Serology	CSU, CU, NMDA

UCD = Coccidioidomycosis Serology Laboratory and Clinical Services, Department of Medical Microbiology and Immunology, www.ucdmc. ucdavis.edu/medmicro/cocci.html; CSU = Colorado State University, Veterinary Diagnostic Laboratories, http://csu-cvmbs.colostate.edu/vdl/Pages/ default.aspx; CU = Cornell University, Animal Health Diagnostic Center, https://ahdc.vet.cornell.edu; MDL = Miravista Diagnostics Laboratory, http://miravistalabs.com; NMDA = New Mexico Department of Agriculture, Veterinary Diagnostic Services, www.nmda.nmsu.edu/vds; UT = University of Tennessee, Veterinary Medical Center, Diagnostic Laboratory Services, https://vetmed.tennessee.edu/vmc/dls/Pages/default.aspx; UGA = University of Georgia, Veterinary Diagnostic Laboratories, www.vet.uga.edu/dlab.

Table 37.2 Distribution of IgG coccidioidal antibody level based on the different forms of the disease in 39 horses diagnosed with coccidioidomycosis.

Disease form	No. horses	Titer range	Geometric mean titer
Pneumonia	6	32–64	51
Pneumonia with effusion	11	64–1,024	226
Disseminated	10	32–512	104
Abortion	6	2–8	4
Osteomyelitis	3	8–32	13
Cutaneous	3	1–32	5

Source: Higgins et al. (2007). Reproduced with permission of Elsevier.

37.2.2 Blastomycosis

Blastomyces dermatitidis is a thermally dimorphic fungus, existing as a mold in room temperature and as a budding yeast-like cell when replicating in the host. It is endemic to the Mississippi, Missouri, and Ohio River basins, the Great Lakes region, the eastern seaboard, and certain areas of Canada (Table 37.1). Infection in susceptible mammals occurs mainly by inhalation and respiratory colonization. Few reports of equine blastomycosis have been made in the literature including a mare with superficial abscesses around the anus, vulva, and udder (Benbrook et al., 1948), a mare and a miniature horse gelding both with fulminating pleuropneumonia and

peritonitis due to this saprophytic soil fungus (Toribio et al., 1999, Dolente et al., 2003) and a mare with systemic blastomycosis (Wilson et al., 2006). Diagnosis in these cases was made based upon positive culture of pleural fluid after 5 days from one horse and histological evidence of budding yeast forms from the cutaneous lesions or affected sites at necropsy in the other two horses. Cultures produced yeasts with germ tube formation and a short-lived mycelial stage after 6 weeks of incubation in one case (Dolente et al., 2003). This confirms that mycelial growth occurs slowly, and the cultures may take several weeks to become positive making it less desirable as an immediate diagnostic test. *Blastomyces* yeasts can be identified on cytologic examination; they are spherical, 15–17 μm with basophilic protoplasm and unstained, uniformly shaped refractile wall, and are often found within multinucleated giant cells. In a retrospective study of 115 dogs, blastomycosis was definitively diagnosed by cytologic or histological examination of fine needle aspirates, fluid samples or biopsies in 80% of the cases, while only 6% were diagnosed on the basis of serology alone with the remaining dogs diagnosed on *post-mortem* (Arceneaux et al., 1998). This may indicate that isolation of this particular organism may be more rewarding than it is for other specific fungal pathogens. In dogs and humans, it is recommended that serologic testing be used only if multiple attempts to identify the organism have failed, due to relative ease of organism isolation as compared to the lack of a serologic test that will yield a diagnosis correctly in all cases (Bradsher, 2003, Kerl, 2003). Serology is available in horses and can be useful as supporting evidence when strongly positive. Despite the rarity of reported equine cases, blastomycosis should be included in differential diagnoses for chronic infections in horses from endemic areas.

37.2.3 Histoplasmosis

Histoplasmosis is seen primarily as an opportunistic infection that can be clinically significant in highly susceptible or immunocompromised animals, while exposure usually results in self-limiting pneumonia in immunocompetent individuals. Horses seem particularly resistant to infection, as the number affected is minimal in proportion to the population exposed (50–73% skin test positive for horses from endemic areas, Rezabek et al., 1993). The highly endemic areas in the United States are the Ohio and Mississippi River valleys, with Texas, Virginia, Delaware, and Maryland being endemic to a lesser degree (Table 37.1). Infection occurs via inhalation or ingestion of the mycelial form, then the tissue form becomes an asexually reproducing intracellular yeast phagocytosed by cells of the reticuloendothelial system throughout the body, causing an affinity for dissemination. Abortion or early neonatal death with interstitial or granulomatous pneumonia and dissemination in fetuses or foals born from clinically healthy mares was the most common presentation in a retrospective study of nine horses (Rezabek et al., 1993). Disseminated histoplasmosis following suspected *Histoplasma* pneumonia in an adult quarter horse mare, possibly immunosuppressed by prolonged administration of corticosteroids, has been reported (Johnston et al., 1995), as has granulomatous pneumonia in a 6-month-old foal who died of the disease (Richman, 1948), a 2-year-old filly successfully treated with amphotericin B for 5 weeks (Cornick, 1990) and an adult horse with *Histoplasma* pneumonia and concurrent *Yersinia* colitis (Katayama

et al., 2001). Diagnosis is based upon visualization of the organism in affected tissues (differentiated from other fungal pathogens by the fact that these organisms are much smaller and are typically clustered within cells of the mononuclear phagocyte system) or positive culture. Serology, using the immunodiffusion assay can be a useful diagnostic adjunct, as the presence of both possible bands of precipitation (M and H) in the AGID test indicates current active infection.

37.2.4 Cryptococcosis

Cryptococcus neoformans is another opportunistic pathogen of immunologically compromised individuals. Unlike other fungal infections, cryptococcosis does not have a defined geographical distribution and veterinary reports have been made worldwide. *C. neoformans* var. *neoformans* (*C. neoformans*) is the most common cause of cryptococcosis in mammalian species and has been associated with bird (particularly pigeon) excreta (Table 37.1). The other variety is *C. neoformans* var. *gattii* (*C. gattii*), and the two are differentiated based on the capsular antigens. It is a yeast-like fungus that replicates by budding and forms a large polysaccharide capsule that appears as a characteristic halo around the cell when stained with India ink. In horses, it has a predilection for the respiratory tract and the central nervous system with reports of meningitis, rhinitis, and pneumonia (Riley et al., 1992, Ainsworth and Hackett, 2004). In a retrospective study, six equine cases of cryptococcal pneumonia were reported, all resulting in euthanasia without attempted treatment (Riley et al., 1992). Nearly all reported horses had an underlying illness (including exercise-induced pulmonary hemorrhage, viral upper respiratory tract infection, and bacterial pneumonia) that may have predisposed them to cryptococcosis. As with many of the other fungal pathogens, there are reported cases of cryptococcal pneumonia in aborted equine fetuses from otherwise healthy mares (Ryan and Wyand, 1991, Blanchard and Filkins, 1992).

As with other fungal organisms, the most reliable method to establish a diagnosis is to directly visualize the organism on cytologic or histopathological evaluation of specimens from affected areas. The organism can be identified by its large heteropolysacchardie capsule (1–30 μm) that does not take up common cytologic stains. Common testing consists of latex agglutination to identify cryptococcal capsular antigens, as opposed to serologic methods used for other fungal infections which test for antibody levels. Antigen detection is useful once the infection has become established and the capsular antigen becomes solubilized in body fluids and is also used to monitor response to treatment, as a positive response is correlated with a decline in antigen level (Kerl, 2003).

37.2.5 Aspergillosis

Aspergillus fumigatus is the most prevalent pathogenic species in this group of ubiquitous molds, although *A. flavus, A. nidulans,* and *A. niger* can also cause disease (Table 37.1). *Aspergillus* grows throughout the environment on stored feeds, old bedding and decaying vegetation. Invasive aspergillosis in immunocompetent animals or humans is rare, but has been documented in horses (Moore et al., 1993, Carrasco et al., 1997). Systemic infection is generally a disease of the immunocompromised patient following profound neutropenia, loss of gastrointestinal mucosal integrity allowing fungal translocation, prolonged use of antimicrobials or corticosteroids, concurrent debilitating disease, and pituitary adenomas with subsequent hyperadrenocorticism.

Ante-mortem diagnosis of aspergillosis is a challenging task due to variety in clinical forms and ubiquitous exposure in horses. Because *Aspergillus* occurs widely as an environmental contaminant, repeated isolation of the organism or histological demonstration of hyphal invasion of tissues is required before invasive disease can be strongly considered. There is now a PCR system for recognition of three major pathogenic *Aspergillus* species (*A. fumigatus, A. niger,* and *A. flavus*) that can be used to confirm repeat isolation of the same fungal species, increasing the likelihood of it being the causal agent, as opposed to detecting multiple different contaminant species (Sugita et al., 2004). Serologic titers of diseased horses do not vary significantly from titers detected in clinically normal horses due to frequent exposure; however, immunoblotting analysis indicates reactivity to low molecular mass antigens with sera from diseased horses but not from normal horses (Guillot et al. 1999). These specific antigens may correspond to those that are released during invasive mycelial growth in tissues, whereas normal horses would react only against conidial antigens (through common exposure). These tests may aid in *ante-mortem* diagnosis, but careful assessment of risk factors, history, and clinical signs are required to develop a degree of suspicion in the first place.

References

Ainsworth DM and Hackett RP. 2004. Fungal pneumonia. In SM Reed, WM Bayly, and DC Sellon (eds), Equine Internal Medicine, 2nd edn. St. Louis: Saunders, pp. 329–331.

Arceneaux KA, Taboada J, Hosgood G, et al. 1998. Blastomycosis in dogs: 115 cases (1980–1995). J Am Vet Med Assoc, 213: 658–664.

Benbrook EA, Bryant JB, and Sanders LZ. 1984. A case of blastomycosis in the horse. J Am Vet Med Assoc, 112: 475–478.

Blanchard PC and Filkins M. 1992. Cryptococcal pneumonia and abortion in an equine fetus. J Am Vet Med Assoc, 201: 1591–1592.

Bradsher RW. 2003. Blastomycosis. In WE Dismukes, PG Pappas and JD Sobel (eds), Clinical Mycology. New York: Oxford University Press, pp. 299–310.

Carrasco L, Tarradas MC, Gomez-Villamandos JC, et al. 1997. Equine pulmonary mycosis due to *Aspergillus niger* and *Rhizopus stolonifer*. J Comp Pathol, 117: 191–199.

Cornick JL. 1990. Diagnosis and treatment of pulmonary histoplasmosis in a horse. Cornell Vet, 80: 97–103.

Dolente BA, Habecker P, Chope K, et al. 2003. Disseminated blastomycosis in a miniature horse. Eq Vet Ed, 15: 139–142.

Guillot J, Sarfati J, de Barros M, et al. 1999. Comparative study of serological tests for the diagnosis of equine aspergillosis. Vet Rec, 145: 348–349.

Higgins JC, Leith GS, Voss ED, et al. 2005. Seroprevalence of antibodies against *Coccidioides immitis* in healthy horses. J Am Vet Med Assoc, 226: 1888–1892.

Higgins JC, Pusterla N, and Pappagianis D. 2007. Comparison of *Coccidioides immitis* serologicical antibody titers between forms of clinical coccidioidomycosis in horses. Vet J, 173: 118–123.

Johnston PF, Reams R, Jakovljevic S, et al. 1995. Disseminated histoplasmosis in a horse. Can Vet J, 36: 707–709.

Katayama Y, Kuwano A, and Yoshihara T. 2001 Histoplasmosis in the lung of a race horse with yersiniosis. J Vet Med Sci, 63: 1229–1331.

Kerl ME. 2003. Update on canine and feline fungal diseases. Vet Clin N Am-(Small Animal), 33: 721–747.

Kramme PM and Ziemer EL. 1990. Disseminated coccidioidomycosis in a horse with osteomyelitis. J Am Vet Med Assoc, 196: 106–109.

Moore BR, Reed SM, Kowalski JJ, et al. 1993. *Aspergillosis granuloma* in the mediastinum of a non-immunocompromised horse. Cornell Vet, 83: 97–104.

Pappagianis D. 2001. Serologic studies in coccidiodomycosis. Sem Resp Infect, 16: 242–250.

Rezabek GB, Donahue JM, Giles RC, et al. 1993. Histoplasmosis in horses. J Comp Pathol, 109: 47–55.

Richman H. 1948. Histoplasmosis in a colt. N Am Vet, 29: 710.

Riley CB, Bolton JR, Mills JN, et al. 1992. Cryptococcosis in seven horses. Aust Vet J, 69: 135–138.

Ryan MJ and Wyand DS. 1981. *Cryptococcus* as a cause of neonatal pneumonia and abortion in two horses. Vet Pathol, 18: 270–272.

Stoltz JH, Johnson BJ, Walker RL, et al. 1994. *Coccidioides immitis* abortion in an Arabian mare. Vet Pathol, 31: 258–259.

Sugita C, Makimura K, Uchida K, et al. 2004. PCR identification system for the genus *Aspergillus* and three major pathogenic species: *Aspergillus fumigatus*, *Aspergillus flavus* and *Aspergillus niger*. Med Mycol, 42: 433–437.

Toribio RE, Kohn CW, Lawrence AE, et al. 1999. Thoracic and abdominal blastomycosis in a horse. J Am Vet Med Assoc, 214: 1357–1359.

Walker RL, Johnson BJ, Jones KL, et al. 1993. *Coccidioides immitis* mastitis in a mare. J Vet Diagn Invest, 5: 446–448.

Wilson JH, Olsen EJ, Haugen EW, et al. 2006. Systemic blastomycosis in a horse..J Vet Diagn Invest,, 18: 614–619.

Ziemer EL, Pappagianis D, Madigan JE, et al. 1992. Coccidioidomycosis in horses: 15 cases (1975–1984). J Am Vet Med Assoc, 201: 910–916.

38

Sarcocystis neurona and *Neospora hughesi*
Amy L. Johnson

Department of Clinical Studies – New Bolton Center, University of Pennsylvania School of Veterinary Medicine, Pennsylvania, USA

38.1 Introduction

Equine protozoal myeloencephalitis (EPM) is likely the most frequently diagnosed infectious neurologic disease of horses in North America. This disease is most often caused by central nervous system (CNS) infection with *Sarcocystis neurona*, although infection with other protozoal species, particularly *Neospora hughesi*, has also been reported (Marsh et al., 1996). Horses are infected with *S. neurona* through consumption of food or water contaminated with opossum feces containing sporocysts. The life cycle of *N. hughesi* is not well-elucidated but vertical transmission likely plays a role (Pusterla et al., 2011). These parasites can affect any part of the CNS, causing highly variable clinical signs that might manifest insidiously or suddenly and subsequently progress slowly or rapidly.

Despite decades of research, EPM remains a diagnostic challenge. Antemortem diagnosis is always presumptive; definitive diagnosis requires postmortem confirmation of protozoal infection by microscopic identification, immunohistochemistry, culture, or PCR. For highest accuracy, diagnosis in the living horse should be based on fulfillment of three criteria: presence of compatible clinical signs referable to the CNS, exclusion of other differential diagnoses, and confirmation of exposure to one of the protozoal parasites through immunologic testing (Furr et al., 2002). Several factors can confound accurate diagnosis. EPM is a great mimicker and can rarely be discounted based on clinical signs, although affected horses are typically not painful or febrile unless comorbidities exist. Many affected horses show general proprioceptive ataxia that is often asymmetric as well as muscle atrophy due to lower motor neuron involvement. However, other horses might show symmetric ataxia or signs consistent with a focal lesion, such as localized muscle atrophy or a single cranial nerve deficit. Additionally, since many neurologic conditions are difficult to diagnose in the living horse, or require expensive or extensive diagnostic testing (potentially with limited availability), ruling out differential diagnosis can be challenging. Finally, a gold-standard laboratory test does not exist, and practitioners are forced to rely on serologic tests, which have several limitations.

38.2 Overview of Serologic Testing

There are several immunologic tests currently in use for EPM diagnosis. All commonly used tests are based on detection of anti-protozoal antibodies in serum and/or cerebrospinal fluid (CSF); different tests identify different antibodies. One of the biggest problems with serologic testing is exposure to the parasite with subsequent seroconversion in the absence of CNS infection. Even if CSF is analyzed, results can be affected by blood contamination or natural diffusion of antibodies from blood to CSF (Furr, 2002).

It is essential to recognize that serology serves as an adjunct to diagnosis and should not be the mainstay. The author discourages performing serologic testing as part of a general health screen or pre-purchase exam due to the very low positive predictive value (PPV; defined here as the proportion of horses with positive results that truly have EPM) when a non-neurologic horse is tested. Likewise, serology should not be used to determine whether or not a horse is neurologic. The presence or absence of neurologic disease is determined by the clinical exam; serology can then help refine the differential diagnoses list for a neurologic horse.

38.3 Interpretation of Results

Several general principles can be used in interpretation of EPM test results.

- If only serum is tested, a positive result indicates exposure to the organism but does not confirm CNS infection. In the author's experience, the magnitude of the titer does not correlate well with whether the horse truly has EPM, and depends more on amount and chronicity of exposure as well as individual variation in immune response.

- A negative serum result usually indicates that the horse has not been exposed to the protozoa and alternative diagnoses should be pursued. However, one important exception is the recently infected horse that is displaying clinical signs but has not had adequate time for seroconversion. Therefore, neurologic horses with a recent onset of compatible clinical signs but negative serum results warrant repeated serologic testing in 10–14 days. If the second test is positive, it confirms recent exposure and increases the likelihood of an EPM diagnosis.

- If only CSF is tested, a positive result is more likely to correlate with an EPM diagnosis than a positive serum result. However, false positive results can occur, either due to blood contamination of the CSF sample or to normal diffusion of antibodies from blood into CSF. Horses with higher serum titers are more likely to have false positive CSF results in both of these circumstances. Cytological analysis of CSF is always recommended, both to quantify blood contamination and to provide additional information regarding the disease process. Small amounts of blood contamination (equivalent to as few as 8 RBCs/μL CSF) might cause false positive results using Western blot (WB) tests (Miller et al., 1999). However, indirect fluorescent antibody test (IFAT) and SnSAG2 enzyme-linked immunosorbent assay (ELISA) results are not impacted until CSF contains >10,000 RBCs/μL (Finno et al., 2007; Furr et al., 2011).

- A negative CSF result usually means that an alternate diagnosis is warranted. The rare exception is the recently infected horse that shows clinical signs prior to having adequate time to generate a detectable antibody response to the parasite. In these rare cases, repeat CSF testing in 10–14 days is likely to yield a positive result.

- Submitting both serum and CSF allows comparison of antibody levels assuming a quantitative test is used, providing evidence for or against intrathecal antibody production, which is expected to occur with CNS infection. Weak positive CSF results in the presence of strong positive serum results are inconsistent with CNS infection. Current evidence suggests that identification of intrathecal antibody production is the most accurate way to diagnose EPM in the living horse. This determination requires use of a calculated C-value, specific antibody index, or serum:CSF reciprocal titer ratio with a well-established cutoff value (Furr et al., 2011, Reed et al., 2013).

38.4   Available Tests

Currently, several types of immunologic tests are commercially available, including Western blot (WB), indirect fluorescent antibody (IFAT), and surface antigen (SAG) ELISAs. The WB is a semiquantitative test for antibodies against merozoite lysate; the IFAT is a quantitative test for antibodies against whole merozoites, and the SAG ELISAs are quantitative tests for antibodies against various immunodominant surface antigens. All tests can be performed on serum or CSF, and none is considered a gold standard. Descriptions of commercially available testing options and reported test performance are shown in Table 38.1 (which lists tests for antibodies against *S. neurona*) and Table 38.2 (which lists tests for antibodies against *N. hughesi*).

38.5   Test Comparisons

Three publications (Duarte et al., 2003, Johnson et al., 2010, 2013) detail direct comparisons between different tests, and three unpublished studies (Saville, 2007, Reed et al., 2010, Renier et al., 2012) have been presented in abstract form. These comparison studies are detailed in Table 38.3; all focused on EPM caused by *S. neurona*. Although none of the studies examined all of the currently available tests, and the types of samples utilized were variable, some general conclusions can be drawn. Testing serum alone yielded less accurate results than testing CSF alone or a serum:CSF titer ratio, generally due to low specificity. One notable exception was the SAG1 ELISA, which showed poor sensitivity. Poor to fair test agreement was observed; samples that were split and submitted to multiple labs often had discrepant results. Three of the six comparison studies evaluated the SAG2, 4/3 ELISA serum:CSF titer ratio; in all three studies this test demonstrated the highest overall accuracy as compared to the WB, IFAT, and SAG1 ELISA. However, the SAG1, 5, 6 ELISA has not yet been evaluated in any comparison study, so its performance is currently unknown.

38.6   Summary of Recommendations

Making a diagnosis of EPM in the living horse begins with a thorough clinical examination to confirm the presence of neurologic signs. Alternative differential diagnoses should be considered and appropriate diagnostic testing performed when applicable. Exposure to protozoal pathogens can be confirmed via serologic analysis. Current evidence suggests that the most accurate indication of

Table 38.1 Commercially available immunologic tests for antibodies against *Sarcocystis neurona*.

Test	Laboratory	Interpretation	Sample	Reported performance		References
				Sensitivity (%)	Specificity (%)	
WB[1]	EDS UC Davis IDEXX	• Band pattern read and interpreted visually (subjective) • Results usually reported as negative, weak positive, low positive, or positive	Serum CSF	89[2], 80[3], 89[4], 90[5] 89[2], 87[3], 83[5]	71[2], 38[3], 87[4], 42[5] 89[2], 44[3], 86[5]	1) Granstrom et al., 1993 2) Granstrom 1997 3) Daft et al., 2002 4) Duarte et al., 2003 5) Morrow (pers. comm. 2014)
mWB[6]	Michigan State	• Similar to standard WB (above)	Serum	100[6]	98[6] *(n.b, negative cases not from North America)*	6) Rossano et al., 2000
IFAT[4]	UC Davis	• Serum positive at ≥1:80 has ≥55% probability* of EPM • Serum negative at ≤1:40 has ≤33% probability* of EPM • CSF positive at ≥1:5 has 92% probability* of EPM	Serum CSF Serum:CSF titer ratio	89[4], 83[7], 94[9], 59[10] 100[7], 92[9], 65[10]	100[4], 97[7], 85[9], 71[10] 99[7], 90[9], 98[10] 98[10]	7) Duarte et al., 2004 8) Duarte et al., 2006 9) Johnson et al., 2010 10) Johnson et al., 2013
SAG1 ELISA[11]	Antech	• Serum positive at ≥1:16 but recommended cutoff ≥1:32	Serum	68[12], 13[9]	71[12], 97[9]	11) Ellison, 2003 12) Hoane et al., 2005a
SAG2, 4/3 ELISA[13]	EDS	• Serum positive for exposure at ≥1:250 • CSF correlates well with EPM if ≥1:40 • Serum:CSF titer ratio very predictive of EPM if ≤100	Serum CSF Serum:CSF titer ratio	30–86 (depending on cutoff)[14], 71[10] 77–96 (depending on cutoff)[14], 88[10] 86 (cutoff ≤50) or 93 (cutoff ≤100)[14], 88[10]	37–88 (depending on cutoff)[14], 50[10] 58–96 (depending on cutoff)[14], 86[10] 96 (cutoff ≤50) or 83 (cutoff ≤100)[14], 100[10]	13) Yeargan and Howe, 2011 14) Reed et al., 2013
SAG1, 5, 6 ELISA[15]	Pathogenes	• Serum positive at ≥1:8, indicating infection	Serum	N/A	N/A	15) Ellison and Lindsay, 2012

WB – Western blot; mWB – modified Western blot; IFAT – indirect fluorescent antibody test; SAG – surface antigen; ELISA – enzyme-linked immunosorbent assay; EDS – Equine Diagnostic Solutions (Lexington, KY); UC Davis – University of California at Davis; EPM – equine protozoal myeloencephalitis; CSF – cerebrospinal fluid
* based on pre-test probability of 10%; see no. 8

Table 38.2 Commercially available immunologic tests for antibodies against *Neospora hughesi*.

Test	Laboratory	Interpretation	Reported performance	References
IFAT	UC Davis	• Serum positive at ≥1:320; negative at <1:40 • CSF positive at ≥1:5	• Serum Se 100%, Sp 100% at cutoff of 1:640 • Serum Se 100%, Sp 71% at cutoff of 1:320 • Se and Sp estimates calculated using samples from experimentally infected horses, not EPM cases	Packham et al., 2002
ELISA	EDS	• Serum positive at ≥1:500 • CSF positive at ≥1:5 • Serum:CSF titer ratio provides most accurate EPM diagnosis	• Serum Se 94%, Sp 95% compared to WB detection antibodies (not EPM cases)	Hoane et al., 2005b

IFAT – indirect fluorescent antibody test; ELISA – enzyme-linked immunosorbent assay; UC Davis – University of California at Davis; EDS – Equine Diagnostic Solutions (Lexington, KY); CSF – cerebrospinal fluid; EPM – equine protozoal myeloencephalitis; Se – sensitivity; Sp – specificity; WB – Western blot
Source: Adapted from Packham et al. (2002) and Hoane et al. (2005b).

Table 38.3 Test comparisons, focusing on EPM caused by *Sarcocystis neurona*.

Reference	Tests (and samples) compared	Sample origin	Results	Author conclusions
Duarte et al., 2003 *J Vet Diagn Invest*	• WB (serum) • mWB (serum) • IFAT (serum)	• Necropsy cases (9 positive, 39 negative)	• Similar Se (89%) for all 3 • Variable Sp (IFAT 100%, WB 87%, mWB 69%)	IFAT accuracy was better than WB tests.
Saville, 2007 *ACVIM forum EPM SIG*	• WB (serum) • mWB (serum) • IFAT (serum) • SAG1 ELISA (serum)	• Experimental cases (1 *S. neurona* positive, 1 *S. fayeri* positive, 2 negative) • Clinical cases (3 positive, 10 negative) • Necropsy case (1 positive)	• Variable for each case; limited agreement between tests	WB and IFAT were most accurate, though IFAT was cross-reactive with *S. fayeri*. mWB tended to have false positive results while SAG1 ELISA tended to have false negative results.
Johnson et al., 2010 *J Vet Intern Med*	• IFAT (serum, CSF) • SAG1 ELISA (serum)	• Necropsy cases (9 positive, 17 negative) • Clinical cases (10 positive, 29 negative)	• Marked difference in Se (IFAT serum 94%, IFAT CSF 92%, SAG1 ELISA serum 13%) • Comparable Sp (IFAT serum 85%, IFAT CSF 90%, SAG1 ELISA serum 97%)	Low Se limited the usefulness of the SAG1 ELISA.
Reed et al., 2010 *ACVIM forum*	• WB (CSF) • IFAT (serum) • SAG1 ELISA (serum) • SAG2, 4/3 ELISA (serum:CSF ratio)	• Necropsy cases (7 positive, 5 negative) • Clinical cases (6 positive, 2 negative)	• Variable Se (SAG2, 4/3 ELISA 90%, WB 90%, IFAT 70%, SAG1 ELISA 55%) • Variable Sp (SAG2, 4/3 ELISA 100%, WB 95%, SAG1 ELISA 90%, IFAT 85%)	SAG2, 4/3 ELISA serum:CSF ratio was the most accurate.
Renier et al., 2012 *ACVIM forum EPM SIG*	• IFAT (CSF) • SAG2, 4/3 ELISA (serum:CSF ratio)	• Necropsy cases (6 positive, 17 negative) *(n.b., 1 positive case due to N. hughesi not S. neurona)*	• IFAT Se (100%) higher than SAG2, 4/3 ELISA Se (83%) • SAG2, 4/3 ELISA Sp (100%) higher than IFAT Sp (82%)	IFAT advantages include testing for *N. hughesi* and use as serum stand-alone test. *(n.b., SAG2, 4/3 ELISA serum:CSF ratio had higher overall accuracy.)*
Johnson et al., 2013 *J Vet Intern Med*	• IFAT (serum, CSF, serum:CSF ratio) • SAG2, 4/3 ELISA (serum, CSF, serum:CSF ratio)	• Necropsy cases (11 positive, 28 negative) • Clinical cases (6 positive, 14 negative)	• SAG2, 4/3 ELISA serum:CSF ratio was most accurate (97%) • IFAT CSF and serum:CSF ratio also had high accuracy (88%)	Serum testing alone was least accurate; more accurate methods should be used. SAG2, 4/3 ELISA serum:CSF ratio was most accurate.

ACVIM – American College of Veterinary Internal Medicine; EPM – equine protozoal myeloencephalitis; SIG – special interest group; WB – Western blot; mWB – modified Western blot; IFAT – indirect fluorescent antibody test; SAG – surface antigen; ELISA – enzyme-linked immunosorbent assay; Se – test sensitivity; Sp – test specificity; CSF – cerebrospinal fluid active CNS infection is obtained via concurrent testing of CSF and serum samples using quantitative tests to allow detection of intrathecal antibody production. The SAG2, 4/3 ELISA serum:CSF titer ratio and *Neospora* ELISA serum:CSF titer ratio are the only tests currently commercially available that provide this information.

References

Daft BM, Barr BC, Gardner IA, et al. 2002. Sensitivity and specificity of western blot testing of cerebrospinal fluid and serum for diagnosis of equine protozoal myeloencephalitis in horses with and without neurologic abnormalities. J Am Vet Med Assoc, 221: 1007–1013.

Duarte PC, Daft BM, Conrad PA, et al. 2003. Comparison of a serum indirect fluorescent antibody test with two Western blot tests for the diagnosis of equine protozoal myeloencephalitis. J Vet Diagn Invest, 15: 8–13.

Duarte PC, Daft BM, Conrad PA, et al. 2004. Evaluation and comparison of an indirect fluorescent antibody test for detection of antibodies to *Sarcocystis neurona*, using serum and cerebrospinal fluid of naturally and experimentally infected, and vaccinated horses. J Parasitol, 90: 379–386.

Duarte PC, Ebel ED, Traub-Dargatz J, et al. 2006. Indirect fluorescent antibody testing of cerebrospinal fluid for diagnosis of equine protozoal myeloencephalitis. Am J Vet Res, 67: 869–876.

Ellison SP, Kennedy T, and Brown KK. 2003. Development of an ELISA to detect antibodies to rSAG1 in the horse. Intern J Appl Res Vet Med, 1: 318–327.

Ellison SP and Lindsay DS. 2012. Decoquinate combined with levamisole reduce the clinical signs and serum SAG 1, 5, 6 antibodies in horses with suspected equine protozoal myeloencephalitis. Intern J Appl Res Vet Med, 10: 1–7.

Finno CJ, Packham AE, Wilson WD, et al. 2007. Effects of blood contamination of cerebrospinal fluid on results of indirect fluorescent antibody tests for detection of antibodies against *Sarcocystis neurona* and *Neospora hughesi*. J Vet Diagn Invest, 19: 286–289.

Furr M. 2002. Antigen-specific antibodies in cerebrospinal fluid after intramuscular injection of ovalbumin in horses. J Vet Intern Med, 16: 588–592.

Furr M, Howe D, Reed S, et al. 2011; Antibody coefficients for the diagnosis of equine protozoal myeloencephalitis. J Vet Intern Med 25: 138–142.

Furr M, MacKay R, Granstrom D, et al. 2002. Clinical diagnosis of equine protozoal myeloencephalitis (EPM). J Vet Intern Med, 16: 618–621.

Granstrom DE, Dubey JP, Davis SW, et al. 1993. Equine protozoal myeloencephalitis: antigen analysis of cultured *Sarcocystis neurona* merozoites. J Vet Diagn Invest, 5: 88–90.

Granstrom DE. 1997. Equine protozoal myeloencephalitis: parasite biology, experimental disease, and laboratory diagnosis. In: Proceedings of the International Equine Neurology Conference, p. 4.

Hoane JS, Morrow JK, Saville WJ, et al. 2005a. Enzyme-linked immunosorbent assays for the detection of equine antibodies specific to *Sarcocystis neurona* surface antigens. Clin Diagn Lab Immunol, 12: 1050–1056.

Hoane JS, Yeargan MR, Stamper S, et al. 2005b. Recombinant NhSAG1 ELISA: a sensitive and specific assay for detecting antibodies against *Neospora hughesi* in equine serum. J Parasitol, 91: 446–452.

Johnson AL, Burton AJ, and Sweeney RW. 2010. Utility of 2 immunological tests for antemortem diagnosis of equine protozoal myeloencephalitis (*Sarcocystis neurona* infection) in naturally occurring cases. J Vet Intern Med, 24: 1184–1189.

Johnson AL, Morrow JK, and Sweeney RW. 2013. Indirect fluorescent antibody test and surface antigen ELISAs for antemortem diagnosis of equine protozoal myeloencephalitis. J Vet Intern Med, 27: 596–599.

Marsh AE, Barr BC, Madigan J, et al. 1996. Neosporosis as a cause of equine protozoal myeloencephalitis. J Am Vet Med Assoc, 209: 1907–1913.

Miller MM, Sweeney CR, Russell GE, et al. 1999. Effects of blood contamination of cerebrospinal fluid on western blot analysis for detection of antibodies against *Sarcocystis neurona* and on albumin quotient and immunoglobulin G index in horses. J Am Vet Med Assoc, 215: 67–71.

Packham AE, Conrad PA, Wilson WD, et al. 2002. Qualitative evaluation of selective tests for detection of *Neospora hughesi* antibodies in serum and cerebrospinal fluid of experimentally infected horses. J Parasitol, 88: 1239–1246.

Pusterla N, Conrad PA, Packham AE, et al. 2011. Endogenous transplacental transmission of *Neospora hughesi* in naturally infected horses. J Parasitol, 97: 281–285.

Reed SM, Howe DK, Morrow JK, et al. 2013. Accurate antemortem diagnosis of equine protozoal myeloencephalitis (EPM) based on detecting intrathecal antibodies against *Sarcocystis neurona* using the SnSAG2 and SnSAG4/3 ELISAs. J Vet Intern Med, 27: 1193–2000.

Reed SM, Howe DK, Yeargan MR, et al., 2010. New quantitative assays for the differential diagnosis of equine protozoal myeloencephalitis (EPM). ACVIM Forum (unpublished).

Renier AC, Morrow JK, Graves A, et al., 2012. Diagnosis of equine protozoal myeloencephalitis using indirect fluorescent antibody testing and enzyme-linked immunosorbent assay titer ratios for *Sarcocystis neurona* and *Neospora hughesi*. ACVIM Forum, EPM SIG (unpublished).

Rossano MG, Mansfield LS, Kaneene JB, et al. 2000. Improvement of western blot test specificity for detecting equine serum antibodies to *Sarcocystis neurona*. J Vet Diagn Invest, 12: 28–32.

Saville WJA. 2007. Comparison of diagnostic tests for EPM run on blinded sera at four different laboratories. ACVIM Forum, EPM SI (unpublished).

Yeargan MR and Howe DK. 2011. Improved detection of equine antibodies against *Sarcocystis neurona* using polyvalent ELISAs based on the parasite SnSAG surface antigens. Vet Parasitol, 176: 16–22.

39

Babesia caballi and *Theileria equi*

Angela Pelzel-McCluskey[1] and Josie Traub-Dargatz[2]

[1] United States Department of Agriculture, Animal and Plant Health Inspection Service, Veterinary Services, Colorado, USA
[2] Colorado State University, College of Veterinary Medicine and Biomedical Sciences, Department of Clinical Sciences, Colorado, USA

39.1 Introduction

Equine piroplasmosis (EP) is a tick-borne apicomplexan hemoprotozoan-caused disease affecting horses, donkeys, mules, and zebras. The causative agents are *Theileria* (formerly *Babesia*) *equi* and *Babesia caballi*. Although the natural transmission of these hemoparasites is via competent tick vectors, transmission can also occur by transfer of blood from infected to naïve horses by iatrogenic means.

Clinical signs of infection in equids range broadly from intravascular hemolysis and associated systemic illness to no clinical abnormalities detectable depending on stage of the disease. Most horses regardless of clinical syndrome exhibit some degree of anemia characterized by decreased packed cell volume, hemoglobin, and erythrocyte count. Peracute and acute signs may include fever, jaundice, anemia, hemoglobinuria, bilirubinuria, digestive or respiratory signs, and occasionally death. Equids with subacute piroplasmosis may have anorexia, lethargy, weight loss, anemia, limb edema, poor performance, increased heart and respiratory rates, and splenomegaly. Equids that survive acute disease inevitably become inapparent carriers and may exhibit no clinical signs of infection yet can serve as reservoirs for transmission to naïve equids (Ueti et al., 2008).

The chronic, inapparent carrier equid presents challenges in diagnosis, eradication, and control measures. Both *T. equi* and *B. caballi* are considered to be etiologic agents of foreign animal disease in the United States and suspicion of infection with either agent is required to be reported to state and federal animal health officials.

39.2 Serological Tests Available

Serological tests for EP focus on detection of the presence of various types of antibodies to *T. equi* or *B. caballi*. Currently available and routinely used EP serological tests include the complement fixation test (CFT), indirect immunofluorescent assay (IFA), and competitive enzyme-link immunosorbent assay (cELISA) for *T. equi* and *B. caballi* separately.

The CFT depends on activation of complement during specific interaction of antibody and antigen. Infected horses seroconvert on the CFT approximately 8–11 days after infection with titers beginning to decline at 2–3 months (Oladosu et al., 1992, Hailat et al., 1997, De Waal et al., 1988, Bruning, 1996). The CFT is a very specific test yet lacks sensitivity in chronic or inapparent phases of infection mainly because some antibodies produced during these phases of infection do not fix complement (Cunha et al., 2006, Knowles et al., 1992, Lewis et al., 2008). Cross-reactivity between *T. equi* and *B. caballi* antibodies when using the CFT has been documented (Donnelly et al., 1982). The CFT can be reliably used in acute cases of infection, whereas results in a non-clinical carrier should be interpreted with caution.

The IFA test is considered to be more sensitive than the CFT during chronic infection (Bruning, 1996). However, the need to dilute serum to improve specificity in IFA test performance reduces sensitivity. Experimentally infected *T. equi* and *B. caballi* horses are first positive to the IFA test at 3–20 days post-infection (Weiland, 1986). The IFA is often used as an adjunct test to aid in analysis of CFT and cELISA results, and it remains one of the prescribed tests for equine piroplasmosis recommend by the World Organization for Animal Health (OIE) (World Organization for Animal Health, 2014).

The cELISA, the other regulatory test approved by the OIE for international horse movement, is considered to be the most sensitive test for chronic or inapparent *T. equi* infection. The cELISA, which detects antibody responses to equine merozoite antigen (EMA) 1 and 2, is validated for detection of antibodies against numerous isolates of *T. equi* found globally (Knowles et al., 1992). The cELISA for *B. caballi* is also routinely used for

Interpretation of Equine Laboratory Diagnostics, First Edition. Edited by Nicola Pusterla and Jill Higgins.

detection of chronic infection or inapparent carriers (Kappmeyer et al., 1999). The currently available *B. caballi* cELISA relies on the recognition of epitopes on rhoptry-associated protein 1 (RAP-1) that are not conserved across all isolates. Both cELISA kits are federally-licensed and approved test kits marketed by VMRD (Pullman, WA) and are not available to general practitioners.

Diagnostics historically used only in a research setting have recently become part of routine diagnosis and surveillance in the USA. A Western blot, or immunoblot test, is currently offered by the National Veterinary Services Laboratories in Ames, Iowa as a confirmatory diagnostic test to the cELISA for *B. caballi*. A Western blot test is also under validation to be used as a means of clearance confirmation in *T. equi*-infected horses treated with imidocarb dipropionate, as it seems to be an early indicator of antibody disappearance posttreatment prior to the percentage inhibition on the cELISA test dropping into the negative range.

39.3 Microscopy and Molecular Assays

In acute, clinical cases of EP, direct microscopy of stained blood smears can be used diagnostically to visualize the presence of *T. equi* and/or *B. caballi* organisms.

Specifically, *B. caballi* merozoites appear pyriform shaped and occur in pairs within erythrocytes (Figure 39.1), while *T. equi* merozoites appear as four pyriform parasites in a Maltese cross formation within erythrocytes (Figure 39.2). In non-clinical horses or in chronic cases of infection, the number of circulating organisms is usually too low to reliably diagnose *T. equi* or *B. caballi* infection by direct microscopy alone and serological assays should be used in these cases to determine the disease status of the equid.

Molecular assays for detection of both *T. equi* and *B. caballi* are also available and consist of either nested or real-time polymerase chain reaction (PCR) tests performed on whole blood samples in EDTA (see also Chapter 51, Molecular Diagnostics for Infectious Pathogens). PCR relies on the amplification and detection of parasite DNA isolated from the peripheral blood of an infected equid. It is a highly sensitive test that when performed as a nested PCR can detect a positive result in an animal with *T. equi* parasitemia as low as 0.000006% (Nicolaiewsky et al., 2001). However, the genetic variation reported between isolates of *T. equi* make the use of this test on a global scale challenging. The validity of the *T. equi* EMA-based nested PCR used in the United States has been questioned in other countries with differing genetic lineage of *T. equi* isolates (Bhoora et al., 2009). Given the variation in PCR methodology, isolate

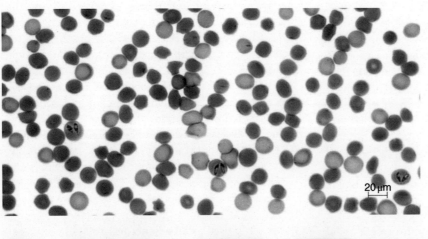

Figure 39.1 *Babesia caballi* merozoites appear pyriform shaped and occur in pairs within erythrocytes. *Source:* courtesy of Dr. Donald Knowles.

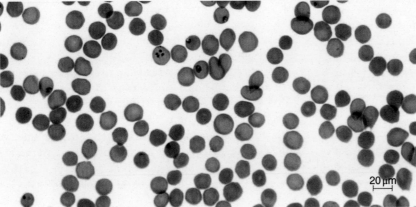

Figure 39.2 *Theileria equi* merozoites appear as four pyriform parasites in a Maltese cross formation within erythrocytes. *Source:* courtesy of Dr. Donald Knowles.

inconsistencies, and the inherent nature of the test, it is unlikely in the near future that PCR will be standardized and used commercially for detection of *T. equi* or *B. caballi*. Due to the sensitivity of the assay, it is currently being used to provide additional diagnostic support in horses confirmed seropositive for EP and as one of several tests to confirm clearance of *T. equi* in horses enrolled in the United States Department of Agriculture (USDA) treatment program.

39.4 Selection of Diagnostic Tests

Selection of the appropriate EP diagnostic test depends upon both the reason for testing and the current stage of infection of the equid being tested. The use of multiple EP assays run in parallel or series may be necessary to correctly determine the infection status of the animal. Given the types of antibody detected by the different serologic assays, the CFT and IFA assays produce positive results earlier in the course of infection than the cELISA test. In the cases of chronically infected animals, the cELISA and the IFA assays will continue to produce positive results, whereas the CFT titers in a chronically-infected animal are usually negative or only intermittently positive at low titers. The reliability of results from direct microscopy on stained blood smears also often depends upon the stage of infection. Higher levels of circulating organisms present during acute or clinical stages of infection lend to a higher likelihood of visualizing the organisms on a stained blood smear, whereas organisms on blood smear during the chronic stages of EP are rarely seen. For diagnosis of acute or clinical cases of EP, a combination of early-reacting serologic assays such as CFT and/or IFA along with direct microscopy on stained blood smears would provide the best chance of confirming or ruling out *T. equi* or *B. caballi* infection. For screening of non-clinical and/or chronically infected equids, serologic testing by cELISA and/or IFA is recommended.

The designated reason for the test also plays a role in selection of diagnostic tests used for EP. For the purposes of importation, for example, the US employs both the cELISA and the CFT to be run in parallel. This provides the best snapshot of the current infection status of the horse presented for import by using both an assay that reliably detects the chronically infected horse (cELISA) and an assay that is capable of detecting a recently exposed horse (CFT) coming from an EP-endemic region. Likewise, the testing of potentially exposed equids associated with the investigation of a confirmed positive horse should also employ testing in parallel using serologic assays to detect both recent exposure (CFT or IFA) and chronic infection (cELISA). For movement testing of non-clinical horses originating

from non-endemic areas, the use of the cELISA test alone has proven to be a reliable and cost-effective method of testing.

Use of either nested or real-time PCR and Western blot testing for *T. equi* in the US has been used mostly for research purposes and limited to follow-up testing of serologic positive or suspect samples and posttreatment testing of previously infected horses. Recently identified challenges of establishing appropriate dilution of samples for PCR testing and potential interference of equine DNA producing occasional false positive results led to the limitations of its current use and PCR testing at this time should not be used for widespread screening or surveillance purposes. However, a series of PCR testing over time has been a valuable tool as an early indicator of successful clearance of *T. equi* after treatment using the high-dose immidocarb dipropionate protocol in the US (Ueti et al., 2012). The *T. equi* Western blot, likewise, has been beneficial posttreatment as an early indicator of antibody dissipation prior to the complete reversion to antibody negative status on the cELISA assay.

The Western blot for *B. caballi*, however, was developed for a different purpose and is currently being used in the US as the confirmatory test for the *B. caballi* cELISA after widespread surveillance testing identified a limited number of false positive reactors on the *B. caballi* cELISA and a confirmatory test was needed (Awinda et al., 2013). Samples testing positive on the *B. caballi* cELISA should be subsequently run on the *B. caballi* Western blot to confirm the result.

39.5 Interpretation of Results

Results of cELISA assays for *T. equi* and *B. caballi* are reported as a percentage inhibition (%I) with results of 40%I or higher considered to be a positive result. Specific to the *T. equi* cELISA, while there is currently no official suspect range of percentage inhibition specified for the cELISA test, *T. equi* percentage inhibitions reported in the 35–39.9%I range should be given additional consideration and supplemental diagnostics may be indicated to determine the actual infection status of the animal. Percentage inhibitions in this range (35–39.9%I) have often been identified in recently infected horses whose cELISA titers are currently rising but not yet in the positive range or in horses who have been previously treated for EP, have cleared the infection, and whose antibody titers are currently coming down from the positive range. Specific to the *B. caballi* cELISA, a modest percentage of false positive results have been previously reported (Awinda et al., 2013) which were correctly differentiated from current infections using the Western blot as a confirmatory test for the *B. caballi* cELISA. It is highly recommended that *B. caballi*-positive results on the cELISA test be confirmed by *B. caballi* Western blot, especially in regions with low prevalence of *B. caballi* infection or in other instances where *B. caballi* exposure is considered unlikely.

Regarding the CFT for either *T. equi* or *B. caballi*, a positive reaction reported at dilutions of 1:5 and higher is considered a positive result. While CFT positive titers for either organism occur more often early in the course of infection, those titers may also persist at low levels or intermittently in chronically infected horses and, thus, the CFT positive result alone cannot be used to determine the current stage of infection as being either acute or chronic. Cases in which the CFT is positive and the cELISA is negative are more likely to be recent or acute cases of infection, especially in the instance when organisms can be visualized on a stained blood smear by microscopy.

Results of the IFA test for either *T. equi* or *B. caballi* are reported by the laboratory as either positive or negative and are subjectively determined based on the brightness or dimness of fluorescent staining observed by the technician in comparison to positive and negative controls. Considering the relative subjectivity in reading the assay results, it is important that an experienced technician perform this interpretation. Similar to the positive CFT test, a positive IFA result often can be seen earlier in the course of infection, but may continue to be regularly or intermittently positive in a chronically affected animal as well.

Results for either the *T. equi* or *B. caballi* Western blot assays are reported by the laboratory as either positive or negative and are based on a technician's visualization of the banding pattern resulting from the sample in comparison to banding patterns of known positive and negative controls. Positive results on either the *T. equi* or *B. caballi* Western blot are indicative of the presence of a multi-banding antibody pattern specific to the organism of interest. While a wide variety of multi-banding patterns have been seen with either organism, there are usually characteristic bands present at specific molecular weights which are conserved across many lineages of *T. equi* or *B. caballi* even though specific genetic lineages of the organisms can produce bands at additional molecular weights that differ slightly from other lineages. For the purposes of *T. equi* posttreatment Western blot testing, a negative result is achieved when the previously strong characteristic bands have begun to fade or have disappeared completely indicating a decrease in the production of specific *T. equi* antibodies which occurs over time after permanent clearance of the organism from the blood. While the time it takes for the Western blot to become negative posttreatment can vary from months to years, the negative Western blot result does generally precede that of a negative result on the cELISA test

posttreatment. In the case of the *B. caballi* Western blot, a negative result is seen as either the absence of any bands or the presence of a single antibody band at 50 kDa (which is typically present in instances of a false positive *B. caballi* cELISA result), rather than the characteristic multi-banding pattern of true *B. caballi* infection.

Results for either nested or real-time PCR are reported by the laboratory as either positive or negative. As noted previously, use of PCR assays for both *T. equi* and *B.caballi* have been limited due to a variety of challenges inherent in the assay. PCR assays have been mainly employed for testing in series on horses with positive results on some other EP diagnostic assay and/or to assess organism clearance from the bloodstream subsequent to EP treatment. Positive PCR results reported on samples tested for one of these purposes is usually a reliable indicator of the presence of DNA belonging to the etiologic agent for EP currently in the bloodstream. A single negative PCR result, however, cannot alone confirm the absence of infection, especially in animals with positive results on other EP assays and which may be experiencing low or undetectable levels of circulating organism. For this reason, posttreatment testing protocols for EP employ the use of a series of PCR results obtained over time on the treated horse to provide a more accurate picture of whether or not organism clearance has been achieved.

Diagnostic interpretation of *T. equi* or *B. caballi* results in the case of foals born to EP-positive mares has some additional considerations than those seen in the adult horse. While transmission of *T. equi* or *B. caballi* from mare to foal either *in utero* or during parturition has been reported (Allsopp et al., 2007), it does not appear to be a common occurrence. To rule out transmission of *T. equi* or *B. caballi* from a known infected mare to her foal, both serologic and molecular assays may need to be used. It should first be recognized that foals born to EP-positive mares acquire antibodies to the requisite EP organism involved upon consumption of the mare's colostrum which causes them to test positive on serologic assays (cELISA, CFT, and/or IFA) until the waning of maternal antibodies post-weaning or several months thereafter. If the disease status of the foal is to be determined while maternal antibodies are still present, then either nested or real-time PCR could be used to provide an indication of the presence or absence of actual infection. For confirmation of the disease status of a foal born to an EP-positive mare, however, it is recommended that serologic testing of the foal occur post-weaning at an age when maternally-derived EP antibodies should have reliably dissipated. At this stage, a truly uninfected foal will revert to seronegative status.

The only reported gold-standard level diagnostic test for either *T. equi* or *B. caballi* infection is transfusion from the subject horse into a recipient splenectomized horse and subsequent monitoring of the recipient for development of clinical signs over 14 days and serologic or other diagnostic evidence of the presence of transferred infection (Ueti et al., 2012). While this method is highly effective for either confirming or ruling out EP infection in the subject horse, it is both expensive and results in the loss of use or death/euthanasia of the recipient horse.

References

Allsopp MTEP, Lewis BD, and Penzhorn BL. 2007. Molecular evidence for transplacental transmission of *Theileria equi* from carrier mares to their apparently healthy foals. Vet Parasitol, 148: 130–136.

Awinda PO, Mealey RH, Williams LBA, et al. 2013. Serum antibodies from a subset of horses positive for *Babesia caballi* by competitive enzyme-linked immunosorbent assay demonstrate a protein recognition pattern that is not consistent with infection. Clin Vacc Immunol, 20(11): 1752–1757.

Bhoora R, Quan M, Qweygarth E, et al. 2009. Sequence heterogeneity in the 18S rRNA gene within *Theileria equi* and *Babesia caballi* from horses in South Africa. Vet Parasitol, 159: 112–120.

Bruning A. 1996. Equine piroplasmosis an update on diagnosis, treatment, and prevention. BVJ, 152: 139–151.

Cunha CW, McGuire TC, Kappmeyer LS, et al. 2006. Development of specific immunoglobulin Ga (IgGa) and IgGb antibodies correlates with control of parasitemia in *Babesia equi* infection. Clin Vacc Immunol, 13: 297–300.

De Waal DT, Van Heerden J, Van den berg SS, et al. 1988. Isolation of pure *Babesia equi* and *Babesia caballi* organisms in splenectomized horses from endemic areas in South Africa. Onderstepoort J Vet Res, 55: 33–35.

Donnelly J, Phipps LP, and Watkins KL. 1982. Evidence of maternal antibodies to *Babesia equi* and *Babesia caballi* in foals of seropositive mares. Eq Vet J, 14: 126–128.

Hailat NQ, Lafi SQ, al-Darraji AM, et al. 1997. Equine babesiosis associated with strenuous exercise: clinical and pathological studies in Jordan. Vet Parasitol, 69: 1–8.

Kappmeyer LS, Perryman LE, Hines SA, et al. 1999. Detection of equine antibodies to *Babesia caballi* by recombinant *B. caballi* rhoptry-associated protein 1 in a competitive-inhibition enzyme-linked immunosorbent assay. J Clin Microbiol, 37: 2285–2290.

Knowles DP Jr, Kappmeyer LS, Stiller D, et al. 1992 Antibody to a recombinant merozoite protein epitope identifies horses infected with *Babesia equi*. J Clin Microbiol, 30: 3122–3126.

Lewis MJ, Wagner B, and Woof JM. 2008 The different effector function capabilities of the seven equine IgG subclasses have implications for vaccine strategies. Mol Immunol, 45: 818–827.

Nicolaiewsky TB, Richter MF, Lunge VR, et al. 2001. Detection of *Babesia equi* (Laveran, 1901) by nested polymerase chain reaction. Vet Parasitol, 101: 9–21.

Oladosu LA and Olufemi BE. 1992. Haematology of experimental babesiosis and ehrlichiosis in steroid immunosuppressed horses. Zentralblatt fur Veterinarmedizin.Reihe B, 39: 345–352.

Ueti MW, Palmer, GH, Scoles GA, et al. 2008. Persistently infected horses are reservoirs for intrastadial tick-borne transmission of the apicomplexan parasite *Babesia equi*. Infect Immun, 76: 3525–3529.

Ueti MW, Mealey RH, Kappmeyer LS, et al. 2012. Re-emergence of the apicomplexan *Theileria equi* in the United States: Elimination of persistent infection and transmission risk. PLoS ONE, 7(9): e44713.

Weiland G. 1986. Species-specific serodiagnosis of equine piroplasma infections by means of complement fixation test (CFT), immunofluorescence (IIF), and enzyme-linked immunosorbent assay (ELISA). Vet Parasitol, 20: 43–48.

World Organization of Animal Health. 2014 Equine piroplasmosis terrestrial manual. Available at: www.OIE.int Accessed November 15, 2014.

40

Assessment of Vaccination Status and Susceptibility to Infection

W. David Wilson

Department of Medicine and Epidemiology, School of Veterinary Medicine, University of California, California, USA

40.1 Introduction

Recovery from infection with microbial pathogens involves both innate and acquired immune responses, which are typically complex and generally involve a combination of humoral and cellular mechanisms. These responses can occur systemically, in which case pathogen-specific antibodies or effector T cells can be found in the bloodstream or locally, for instance on mucosal surfaces, in which case the antibodies and effector cells may be confined to the mucosa and will not be present in the bloodstream. In reality, the response to infection with most pathogens involves a combination of humoral and cell-mediated responses. The balance between humoral and cellular responses and between systemic and local responses is determined by the nature of the specific pathogen, the route of infection, the precise pathogenesis, the ability of the pathogen to evade or down regulate immune responses, and other factors. For each infectious disease, researchers and vaccine manufacturers have spent considerable time and effort attempting to characterize the key correlates for protection against a range of viral and bacterial pathogens following natural infection and vaccination. In some instances, levels of circulating antibody correlate well with protection, whereas for other infectious diseases the key correlates for protection may involve systemic or local cellular responses or local humoral responses that cannot be quantified readily, at least in the clinical setting.

Vaccines of various types have been developed to mimic infection and stimulate protective immune responses without causing disease. In general, the closer the response to vaccination mimics the response to natural infection, the more effective the vaccine will be. Replicating modified live virus (MLV) or vectored vaccines generally mimic natural infection well and induce an array of local and systemic immune responses similar to those induced by natural infection, whereas inactivated vaccines typically induce a more limited array of responses. Commercially available vaccines for horses include the following vaccine types: inactivated whole pathogen, inactivated subunit, inactivated toxoid, modified live (attenuated), chimera, and vectored viral. Most of these vaccines are administered by intramuscular injection, although a temperature sensitive modified live influenza vaccine, an inactivated influenza vaccine, and a modified live strangles vaccine are available for intranasal administration. Inactivated parenterally administered vaccines typically contain an adjuvant to enhance the immune response. In general, they are good inducers of systemic antibody responses but are generally less effective in inducing cellular and local responses. Attenuated parenterally administered live vaccines are generally effective at inducing both cellular and humoral responses, whereas intranasally administered vaccines may induce local mucosal responses without inducing significant increases in the level of circulating antibodies and effector T cells.

For pathogens such as influenza, equine herpes virus and *Streptococcus equi* ss. *equi* (*S. equi*) that infect the host via the respiratory tract, the major immune correlates for protection are the level of specific secretory antibody (typically of the IgA and IgG subclasses) and/or local effector T cells at the level of the respiratory mucosa and, in the case of *S. equi*, the local lymphoid tissues. For enteric pathogens such as rotavirus, mucosal immunity at the level of the enteric epithelium is important for protection against infection. If these specific mechanisms are in place, infection may be completely prevented (i.e., sterile immunity); otherwise, infection occurs, the pathogen gains systemic access, and clearance of the pathogen is then dependent on systemic humoral and/or cellular immune responses. Under these circumstances, high levels of circulating antibody and/or antigen-specific cytotoxic T lymphocytes may quickly clear the pathogen and significantly attenuate or prevent

Interpretation of Equine Laboratory Diagnostics, First Edition. Edited by Nicola Pusterla and Jill Higgins.
© 2018 John Wiley & Sons, Inc. Published 2018 by John Wiley & Sons, Inc.

development of clinical signs (i.e., provide clinical protection despite not inducing sterile immunity). Whereas parenterally administered vaccines may be sub-optimally effective in preventing infection with pathogens such as influenza that gain access to the body via mucosal routes, they are generally more effective in preventing infection and disease caused by pathogens that gain access to the body via systemic injection (e.g., tetanus toxin "injected" via puncture wounds, rabies via bites, and viral encephalitides via mosquito bites).

40.2 Duration of Immunity

In addition to understanding correlates for protection, it is important to understand that some pathogens are inherently more antigenic than others, which may result in a longer duration of protection. This is embraced in the concept of duration of immunity (DOI). For many respiratory and gastrointestinal pathogens, the DOI tends to be relatively short, even after recovery from natural infection. Because vaccines rarely induce the full array of immune responses induced by natural infection, it is not reasonable to expect that immunity following vaccination will be more complete or of longer duration than following natural infection. This is an important concept for veterinarians and horse owners to understand so that they do not place unrealistic expectations on the effectiveness of vaccines to prevent infections such as EHV-1 and EHV-4, for which immunity following natural infection is short-lived and incomplete. Similarly, it is important to understand that immunity is not absolute and that a level of immunity that will protect against low-level challenge may be overwhelmed by a higher challenge dose.

The minimum DOI is known for most commercially available vaccines, whereas the maximum DOI is rarely established during challenge studies that form an important part of the vaccine approval process. The USDA typically requires vaccination and challenge studies to be completed on relatively young, healthy, naïve horses that show no serologic evidence of previous infection or the presence of maternally derived antibodies. These horses tend to be at their peak regarding immune-competence and will show optimal immune responses. Additionally, challenge studies (if they are done as part of the approval process) are typically performed 3–6 weeks after completion of the primary vaccination series at a time when immunity and resistance to challenge infection are at their peak. Challenge studies are rarely done more than 6 or 12 months after vaccination; therefore, maximum DOI is not established and the revaccination interval of 6–12 months is typically approved and on the label, even though some vaccines undoubtedly induce protection of more than 12 months' duration. Additionally, because the approval process typically requires naïve horses, the duration of protection after subsequent booster doses, which one would expect to be more prolonged than after the primary vaccination series, is rarely established. Furthermore, there is no economic incentive for vaccine manufacturers to document a prolonged duration of protection beyond 1 year, even though more prolonged protection may have been documented for the same disease in other species such as dogs and humans.

The only definitive method to assess whether an animal is resistant to infection is through natural or experimental challenge. Clearly this is not a feasible or desirable approach to testing immunity in client-owned animals. Similarly, it is not practical or affordable to assess systemic cellular immunity or either local cellular or humoral protection at the mucosal level. The end result is that serologic testing for levels of circulating antibody becomes the only method available to the practitioner to assess levels of immunity to various pathogens. As noted previously, this approach is only reliable for those pathogens for which the key correlate for protection is measurable antibody in the circulation and for which published reports are available documenting the level of antibody that reliably correlates with protection against the disease in question, preferably in horses. If data is not available for the horse, extrapolation of information from other species, including humans, may be appropriate for some diseases. In many vaccination challenge studies, the circulating antibody titers in vaccinates and controls at the time of challenge are reported. This information gives some clue as to the level of antibody that may constitute a protective titer for those diseases for which circulating antibody titer is a good correlate for protection. Of relevance here is the type of serologic test used to determine vaccine responses. For example, the serum virus neutralization test detects the presence of antibody that will neutralize a virus in vitro. This test would therefore be likely to predict the ability of the antibodies to neutralize the pathogen *in vivo*, whereas others (e.g., tertiary tests such as a ELISA) may have less predictive value in terms of resistance to infection or disease. Additional important constraints on the use of serologic tests to predict the need to vaccinate are the limited commercial availability and cost of relevant serologic tests for many of the pathogens against which we vaccinate.

40.3 Rationale for Serologic Testing

For many years, the recommended "core" vaccines for all horses in North America were tetanus, eastern equine encephalomyelits (EEE), and western equine encephalomyelits (WEE). The introduction of West Nile virus (WNV) to North America 1991 and subsequent spread across the continent resulted in WNV being added to the AAEP-recommended core. Soon thereafter, the public health risk associated with rabies caused the AAEP to add annual rabies vaccination to list of core vaccinations. These changes, together with the tendency of organizers of equine competitions and events to require recent vaccination (and frequent revaccination) against the "risk-based" diseases, influenza and EHV-1 and EHV-4, has substantially increased the number of doses of vaccine that many horses receive annually in North America As a result, there is increased owner concern regarding the necessity for frequent administration of vaccines, particularly against diseases such as tetanus and rabies for which vaccines induce prolonged immunity in other species. This concern is heightened when individual horses experience an adverse reaction to a particular vaccine, prompting owners and veterinarians to ask whether it is possible to test the horse to determine if it is protected rather than simply administering a booster dose of vaccine that may not only be unnecessary but may also put the horse at risk for an adverse reaction. Conversely, there is a legitimate concern among equine practitioners that recommending a vaccination interval that is longer than the label recommendation, places the veterinarian at risk of legal action if the horse becomes ill with the disease in question. This dilemma is amplified by the following statement in the 2015 update to the AAEP equine vaccination guidelines:

> The use of antibody titers or other immunological measurements to determine if booster vaccination is warranted is not currently practiced in the horse as standardized tests and protective levels of immunity have not been defined for most diseases. A correlation between antibody levels and protective immunity under field conditions has not yet been identified.

It is this author's opinion that when the risk of an adverse reaction exceeds the risk from the disease in question, it is rational to attempt to predict immunity by serologic testing and extend the revaccination interval for as long as possible, rather than "blindly" vaccinating the horse. In the case of strangles, for which a high pre-vaccination titer of antibody against the M-protein appears to place a horse at increased risk for an adverse reaction, serologic testing is an aid to minimizing this risk rather than predicting disease susceptibility (Table 40.1 and 40.2). Additionally, serologic testing can prove helpful in assessing immunity in horses, such

Table 40.1 Antibody titers associated with protection, expected duration of protection and cautionary comments for various vaccine-associated equine pathogens and toxins.

Equine pathogen or toxin	Titer associated with protection	Expected duration of protection following revaccination of primed horses	Cautionary comments
Tetanus toxin	>0.01 IU/mL	2–8 years	Tetanus documented in vaccinated horses
Rabies virus	≥0.5 IU/mL	2–3 years	Protective titer only available for humans
EEE and EEW virus	>1:100	1 year	Rabies reported in vaccinated horses
West Nile virus	1:5	1 year	Protective titer only available for hamsters
EIV	SRH levels >140 mm^2	<1 year	Antibody titer not a measure of protection for modified live intranasal vaccine
EHV-1, EHV-4	Not reported	Not reported	Antibody titers don't predict susceptibility or resistance to infection
EAV	Not reported	Not reported	Documentation of sero-negative status prior to export or prior to vaccination
Streptococcus equi ss. *equi*	Not reported	Not reported	Titer-specific interpretations regarding risk associated with vaccination (see chapter on serology for *S. equi* ss. *equi*)
Clostridium botulinum type B toxoid	Not reported	Not reported	Vaccine as an aid in prevention of the shaker foal syndrome
Neorickettsia risticii	Not reported	Not reported	Antibody levels do not provide useful information regarding susceptibility to infection or the need for vaccination
Equine rotavirus	Not reported	Not reported	Antibody levels do not provide useful information regarding susceptibility to infection or the need for vaccination
Equine rhinitis A and B virus	Not reported	Not reported	No need for serologic testing to predict resistance to infection or need for vaccination

Table 40.2 Laboratories offering routine antibody testing for various equine vaccine pathogens or toxins.

Equine pathogen or toxin	Laboratory
Tetanus toxin	Animal Health Diagnostic Center, Cornell University
Rabies virus	Kansas State Veterinary Diagnostic Laboratory
EEE and WEE virus	National Veterinary Services Laboratory in Ames, Iowa
West Nile Virus	National Veterinary Services Laboratory in Ames, Iowa
EIV	OIE Reference Lab, Gluck Center, Lexington, Kentucky
	National Veterinary Services Laboratory in Ames, Iowa
EAV	National Veterinary Services Laboratory in Ames, Iowa
Streptococcus equi ss *equi*	IDEXX Laboratories
	Equine Diagnostic Solutions, Lexington, Kentucky
Clostridium botulinum type B toxoid	Unavailable
Neorickettsia risticii	National Veterinary Services Laboratory in Ames, Iowa
Equine rotavirus	Unavailable
Equine rhinitis A and B virus	Animal Health Diagnostic Center, Cornell University

those with pars intermedia dysfunction or those with combined variable immunodeficiency, that might be suspected to be "poor responders."

40.4 Tetanus

Levels of circulating tetanus toxin binding (To-Bi) antibody appear to correlate well with protection in horses (Lohrer and Radvila, 1970). To-Bi titers of 0.02 IU/mL or higher (i.e., >0.01 IU/mL) are considered to be protective (Lohrer and Radvila, 1970, Heldens et al., 2010, Kendall et al., 2015). Whereas the duration of persistence of vaccine-induced antibody levels above the 0.01 IU/mL threshold for protection varies somewhat depending on the adjuvant system used, the age and maternal antibody status of the horse at the time of primary vaccination and the vaccination schedule, tetanus toxoid is considered to be a potent antigen that induces a robust serologic response in immune-competent horses. For horses that receive the two-dose primary series of tetanus toxoid after 6 months of age, protective antibody levels persist for at least 12 months. A third dose of toxoid administered more than 2 months and up to 17 months after the second dose in the primary series has been shown to induce antibody titers that persist above the threshold for protection for periods ranging from 2 years to more than 10 years (Kendall et al., 2015, Heldens et al., 2010, Liefman, 1981, Jansen and Knoetze, 1979, Holmes et al., 2006), (Recknagel et al., 2015b, Ramon and Lemetayer, 1939). It is likely that subsequent doses of toxoid could protect for even longer, as is the case in people; however, duration of protection has not been confirmed in

challenge studies in horses vaccinated with products licensed in North America. A challenge study conducted in Europe almost 50 years ago found that three doses of tetanus toxoid induced protection lasting for at least 8 years, and perhaps for life, even when antibodies could no longer be detected (Lohrer and Radvila, 1970). These results suggest that, for a horse that reacts adversely to tetanus toxoid but has previously been properly vaccinated using a two- or three-dose primary vaccination series followed by at least one subsequent booster dose, the re-vaccination interval could be extended for as long as To-Bi antibody levels remain above 0.01 IU/mL. This period could be one year to more than 8 years and should be confirmed by monitoring of To-Bi titers at least once annually, depending on the magnitude of the measured titer (the higher the titer, the longer it will take to decline to levels of 0.01 IU/mL or less). A word of caution is warranted, however, based on the finding that tetanus has been documented in vaccinated horses in North America, although survival was strongly associated with previous vaccination (Green et al., 1994).

In earlier studies, antibody levels were measured using the expensive and time-consuming tetanus toxin-antitoxin neutralization assay in mice (Lohrer and Radvila, 1970, Liefman, 1980, 1981). More recent studies have employed a toxin-binding enzyme-linked immunosorbent (ELISA) assay (Heldens et al., 2010, Kendall et al., 2015, Wilson et al., 2001), or a microsphere bead assay (Davis et al., 2015). A "stall side" immunochromatographic dipstick test (Fassisi TetaCheck) that can be used on whole blood or serum is commercially available in Germany and was recently shown to be robust and reliable for assessing tetanus immunity in horses, yielding results that correlated well with those generated using ELISA (Recknagel et al., 2015a, Recknagel et al., 2015b, Thein et al., 2013). Unfortunately, none of these tests are yet available commercially in North America, although testing using the microsphere bead assay in a multiplex format will likely be offered soon (Davis E., personal communication).

40.5 Rabies

Research in several species indicates that the primary correlate of protection against rabies is the presence of rabies virus neutralizing antibodies (RVNA) in serum. (Hooper et al., 1998) The quantitative end-point Rapid Fluorescence Focus Inhibition Test (RFFIT) is currently the gold standard and reference technique used to measure the titer of RVNA induced by vaccination (Kostense et al., 2012, Moore and Hanlon, 2010, World Health Organization, 2013). The RFFIT is assay is available commercially through the Kansas State Veterinary Diagnostic Lab, Kansas State University, Manhattan, KS (ksvdl.org). An RVNA level of ≥0.5 IU/mL is considered by the World Health Organization (WHO) to be the threshold of seroconversion, and a predictor of protection, for humans (World Health Organization, 2013). A RVNA level of ≥0.5 IU/mL (as measured using the semi-quantitative Fluorescent Antibody Virus Neutralization (FAVN) Test or the RFFIT) is also the level recognized by regulatory authorities from most rabies-free areas as evidence of an adequate response to vaccination for importation of cats and dogs (Moore and Hanlon, 2010). It should be noted, however, that post-vaccination serologic test results in dogs were not found to be completely predictive of resistance to challenge exposure during tests performed with certain inactivated vaccines (Tizard and Ni, 1998).

The level of RVNA needed to confer protection in equids is not known at this time; however, it seems reasonable to extrapolate information from studies in humans and other species and use an RVNA level of ≥0.5 IU/mL as a guideline correlate for protection, pending challenge studies to better define the relationship between antibody levels and protection. One rabies challenge infection study in horses revealed that whereas clinical signs of rabies still occurred in some of the vaccinated horses after a challenge, none of the affected horses had RVNA levels above 0.5 IU/mL (Hudson et al., 1996). The test vaccine used in this study was not specified. Similarly, rabies was reported in vaccinated horses in one retrospective case study, although RVNA levels and accurate vaccine history were unavailable for affected horses (Green et al., 1992).

The AAEP vaccination guidelines designate rabies as a core vaccine for all horses in North America and recommend annual revaccination after completion of a two-dose primary series. This recommendation reflects the federal requirement for documentation of a 12-month minimum duration of immunity in challenge studies for licensing. Primary vaccination involves administration of one dose of an inactivated vaccine to horses age 3 months or older followed by a second dose of vaccine 1 year later. With the exception of foals of rabies-vaccinated mares, most horses show a detectable but short-lived serologic response after administration of the first dose of vaccine and almost all show a robust and durable response following the second dose. Maternally-derived antibodies significantly inhibit the response of foals to rabies vaccines until they are 6 months of age or older, leading to the recommendation that if foals from vaccinated mares are vaccinated at less than one year of age, they should receive two doses 4 weeks apart, followed by a third dose 6- to 12-months later to complete the primary series.

The response of horses to inactivated rabies vaccines is of similar magnitude and duration to that seen in people and small animals for which revaccination intervals of 3 or more years are now standard practice for most rabies vaccines. Revaccination of previously primed horses reliably resulted in a rapid and robust increase in RVNA antibody levels that persisted above the 0.5 IU/mL threshold for at least 36 months (Harvey et al., 2016). Considering that horses are significantly less likely to pose a public health risk from the standpoint of rabies transmission than are small domestic animals (Dyer et al., 2014), it is, therefore, reasonable to extend the revaccination interval beyond the recommended one year for horses that react adversely to rabies vaccine, provided that they have previously received at least two (and preferably at least three) doses of rabies vaccine after reaching 6 months of age and have circulating RVNA antibody levels of at least 0.5 IU/mL. The retesting interval will be dependent on the magnitude of the RVNA titer but should not exceed 2 years, pending further research.

40.6 Eastern and Western Equine Encephalomyelits (EEE, WEE)

Correlates for protection against EEE and WEE are not well established; however, circulating virus neutralizing antibodies likely play a prominent role because infection is acquired by vascular injection (mosquito bites) and current inactivated vaccines appear to be efficacious if administered sufficiently frequently (Barber et al., 1978, Hays, 1969). Considering the high morbidity and mortality rates associated with EEE infection and the documented need for frequent revaccination (twice or three times annually) to prevent this highly fatal disease in areas such as the southeastern US with year-round risk, it would not be prudent to attempt to extend the revaccination interval based on measurement of circulating antibody titers in EEE-endemic areas, unless the predicted risk of an adverse reaction is high. Whereas horses residing in the Western USA are at very low risk for EEE, they are at risk for infection with WEE and should be revaccinated annually. Because the available encephalomyelitis vaccines are bivalent (EEE plus WEE) or trivalent (EEE plus WEE plus VEE), it is inevitable that many horses will receive "unnecessary" antigens against diseases to which they are unlikely to be exposed.

The main indications for serologic testing for EEE or WEE are diagnosis of recent infection or documentation of prior exposure to these pathogens, either through natural infection or vaccination. Demonstration of specific IgM antibody (at a 1:400 dilution) in serum using the IgM antibody-capture ELISA test (MAC-ELISA) is a highly specific and sensitive method for diagnosis of active or recent infection with either EEE or WEE (Sahu et al., 1994). IgM antibody levels rise rapidly during acute infection and then decline quickly, persisting for about 6 weeks. In contrast, MAC-ELISA titers rarely increase following vaccination. A four-fold increase in titer of virus neutralizing antibody, typically determined using the plaque reduction neutralization test (PRNT), in acute and convalescent samples collected 3–4 weeks apart from horses that survive, also provides evidence of recent infection and confirms whether EEE or WEE was the pathogen involved with the disease. There is no cross reaction between EEE and WEE in either the PRNT test or MAC-ELISA tests.

A positive PRNT titer against EEE or WEE in serum provides evidence of previous infection or vaccination. Although the magnitude of the titer does not reliably predict protection, the degree of susceptibility can be inferred. Horses with PRNT titers of <1:10 are likely to be susceptible and should be revaccinated if conditions of risk exist, whereas those with titers of >1:100 are unlikely to be susceptible (Long, M., personal communication). Horses with PRNT titers between 1:10 and 1:100 are likely of intermediate susceptibility. Revaccination of horses in this category should be recommended; however, the decision to do so will depend on the risk of infection, the interval since the last vaccination, the titer level and trend (up or down) compared to the previous titer measurement, balanced against the predicted risk of an adverse event resulting from vaccination.

The MAC-ELISA and PRNT tests are available through the National Veterinary Services Laboratory in Ames, Iowa. A multiplex microsphere bead assay that detects IgG antibodies was recently described to assess the antigen-specific responses of foals to vaccination with a multivalent vaccine containing tetanus, EEE, WEE, West Nile Virus (WNV), equine influenza (EI), Equine herpesvirus-1 (EHV-1), and EHV-4 antigens (Davis et al., 2015). This test may be offered commercially in the near future (Davis, E., personal communication).

40.7 Venezuelan Equine Encephalomyelitis (VEE)

Venezuelan Equine Encephalomyelitis has not been diagnosed in North America or Central America for many years; therefore, there is no need to vaccinate against VEE except as mandated for importation into countries where the disease is endemic. Consequently, veterinarians are unlikely to be asked to submit samples for serologic testing for VEE.

40.8 West Nile Virus (WNV)

Comments regarding immune correlates for protection against infection with equine alphaviruses (EEE, WEE, VEE), as well as the serologic tests available to document recent infection or prior exposure through natural infection or vaccination, also apply to WNV. Of the various serologic assays used for detection of WNV-specific antibodies in serum, only the plaque reduction neutralization test (PRNT) is specific for WNV because other flaviviruses such as St. Louis encephalitis can cross-react in other assays (Balasuriya et al., 2006). Neither the PRNT nor a more recently developed highly sensitive and specific fluorescent microsphere immunoassay (MIA) incorporating recombinant WNV envelop protein (rE), can differentiate infected from vaccinated horses (Balasuriya et al., 2006). The most commonly used neutralizing antibody test formats are classic plaque reduction neutralization test (PRNT), more recently developed in a microwell format, available through the National Veterinary Services Laboratory (NVSL) in Ames, Iowa.

Research in hamsters predicted a minimal protective neutralizing titer (PRNT) for WNV of 1:5. Based on this finding, the NVSL runs the PRNT at serum dilutions of 1:10 and 1:100 and reports results as <1:10, 1:10 to 1:100 and >1:100 (Long, M., personal communication). Use of PRNT titers to assess disease susceptibility follows the same general principles as described above for EEE and WEE. WNV is endemic in almost all states and provinces in North America, whereas EEE and WEE have a more restricted geographic distribution. In contrast, the clinical attack rate and mortality rate in infected horses are much higher for EEE than for WNV. Because many WNV infections are subclinical, serological evidence of exposure is widespread, even in non-vaccinated horses (Gardner et al., 2007). Although currently available inactivated and recombinant WNV vaccines are highly effective in preventing clinical WNV when used according to label directions, vaccinated horses may become infected and experience a "boost" in immunity (Gardner et al., 2007). This explains why some previously vaccinated horses show an increase in circulating antibody levels despite not having been revaccinated. For these reasons, it is likely that extending the revaccination interval for WNV based on measured PRNT levels carries less risk of resulting in clinical disease and death than is the case for EEE.

40.9 Influenza

Correlates for protection against equine influenza are dependent on whether the immune response is triggered by natural infection or by vaccination and also influenced by the type of vaccine (modified live, recombinant or inactivated), the adjuvant system used and route of administration (intranasal or intramuscular). Infection with equine influenza A-2 (H3N8) virus generates a broad range of adaptive humoral and cellular immune responses in both the systemic and mucosal compartments and provides immunity to the same (homologous) strain that persists for a year or more (Soboll et al., 2003). These adaptive responses include induction of large amounts of virus-specific neutralizing IgG and secretory IgA antibody in nasal secretions, high levels of circulating IgG antibodies of isotypes a and b (IgGa and IgGb), and genetically restricted antigen-specific cytotoxic T-lymphocytes (CTLs) that kill infected cells (Nelson et al., 1998, Hannant et al., 1989, Hannant and Mumford, 1989, Soboll et al., 2003, van Maanen and Cullinane, 2002). Memory CTLs can be detected in peripheral blood for at least 6 months after infection, and solid immunity persists even when circulating antibody titers have declined to low or unndetectable levels (Hannant et al., 1989, 1994, Hannant and Mumford, 1989, Daly et al., 2004). Similarly, protection induced by the licensed modified live intranasal influenza vaccine (Flu-Avert™ I.N., Merck Animal Health) is presumably mediated through induction of local immune responses in the respiratory tract, because this vaccine does not typically induce high levels of circulating antibody (Chambers et al., 2001, Townsend et al., 2001). With the exception of ISCOM vaccines, inactivated vaccines administered by IM injection have limited potential to induce CTL or nasal secretory IgA responses, and induce only low levels of neutralizing antibody in nasal secretions (Crouch et al., 2004, Daly et al., 2004, Paillot and Prowse, 2012, Nelson et al., 1998).

Whereas the level of circulating antibody is the only portion of the immune response to influenza infection that can be easily quantified in the clinical setting, measurement of circulating antibodies is of limited value in predicting susceptibility to influenza infection in horses vaccinated with the intranasal vaccine or those that may have previously experienced natural infection. Under these circumstances, low antibody titers do not necessarily mean that the horse is susceptible to infection, whereas high titers likely correlate with protection. In contrast, the degree of protection induced by inactivated influenza vaccines is highly correlated with post-vaccination titers of circulating antibody, predominantly of the IgGa and IgGb sub-isotypes, as measured by the hemagglutination inhibition (HI) or single radial hemolysis (SRH) tests (Morley et al., 2000, Mumford and Wood, 1992, Townsend et al., 1999, Wood et al., 1983). SRH levels $\geq 100\,mm^2$ are considered to be at least partially protective; however, levels $>140\,mm^2$ are required for successful prevention of disease (Mumford and Wood, 1992). The partial protection induced by inactivated vaccines is of limited duration (up to about 7 months, depending on the vaccine) and is manifested as a reduction in clinical signs and attenuation of viral shedding in horses exposed to infection (Nelson et al., 1998, Wilson, 1993).

Circulating antibody has been measured using a variety of methods including conventional hemagglutination inhibition (HI), single radial hemolysis (SRH), virus neutralization (VN) and ELISA. Of these, SRH and ELISA tests have the highest sensitivity, and SRH results appear to be the best predictor of protection following vaccination. Recent work suggest that SRH results correlate closely with IgGb ELISA results (Landolt et al., 2014). Although HI testing on paired samples is considered by many to be the gold standard for serologic diagnosis of equine influenza infection, its main shortcoming is interlaboratory variation in results (Landolt et al., 2014, Wood et al., 1994). SRH tests have been shown to be more reproducible than HI tests (Wood et al., 1994), and since the level of SRH antibody after systemic vaccination correlates well with the level of protection, SRH may also be used to predict level of antibody-mediated immunity and determine the need for vaccination (Mumford et al., 1988, 1983, Newton et al., 2000, Mumford, 1990).

Influenza viruses of all species mutate in response to immune selection pressure, resulting in progressive changes in the antigenicity of the surface-exposed hemagglutinin (H) and neuraminidase (N) antigens, a process termed antigenic drift. As noted previously, horses appear to be solidly immune to reinfection with a homologues strain of influenza virus for a year or more after recovery from natural infection. Duration of resistance to infection with heterologs (drifted) strains is shortened, roughly proportional to the degree of antigenic relatedness of the strains. Considering that currently available vaccines contain strains of virus that were isolated more than a decade ago and that none of the available vaccines invokes the full range of immune responses induced by natural infection, the maximum duration of protection induced by currently available vaccines is less than 1 year. This finding is the basis for the recommendation that horses that are at risk for exposure to infected horses should be revaccinated at a 6-month or shorter interval.

The cold-adapted intranasal vaccine does not induce circulating antibodies; therefore, resistance to infection cannot be predicted by titers of antibody measured post-vaccination, no matter which serologic test is used. Another limiting factor is that the SRH and ELISA tests are not currently commercially available in the USA. Although readily available through NVSL, the HI test is not reliable for predicting resistance to influenza. As yet, it is not known how titers measured using the microsphere bead assay correlate with protection (Davis et al., 2015).

Considering that immunity following natural infection does not persist for much more than one year and that vaccine-induced immunity is more short-lived, particularly with inactivated vaccine administered by injection, it does not seem reasonable or advisable to extend the vaccination interval beyond one year, regardless of the serologic test results, particularly considering that the test that best correlates with protection, the SRH test, is not commercially available in the USA.

40.10 Equine Herpesvirus-1 (EHV-1) and EHV-4

Equine herpesvirus-1 (EHV-1) and EHV-4 are endemic in horse populations worldwide. Because innate and acquired immune responses are not completely effective in clearing virus after infection, many horses become latent carriers of one or both viruses. Infection of horses with EHV-1 and EHV-4 occurs via the respiratory tract; therefore, it is not surprising that an effective immune response requires a combination of mucosal, local (lymphoid) and systemic cellular and humoral immune responses (Slater, 2014, Patel et al., 2003, Edens et al., 1996). Systemic humoral immune responses alone are not sufficient to protect horses against EHV-1 infection; cytotoxic T-lymphocyte (CTL) responses are not only central to recovery, but the frequency of EHV-1 specific MHC class 1-restricted CTL precursors also provides a correlate for protective immunity against EHV infection (Kydd et al., 2003, O'Neill et al., 1999, Allen et al., 1995, Wilks, 1977). Infection with EHV-1 induces a strong humoral response but sterile immunity and protection from reinfection are short-lived (3–6 months) and are not achieved until the horse has experienced multiple infections with homotypic virus (Slater, 2007, 2014).

No clear relationship exists between protection from EHV-1 or EHV-4 infection and concentrations of circulating antibody induced by vaccination or infection; however, clinical manifestations of disease and the duration and amount of virus shedding from the nasopharynx are reduced in animals with high levels of circulating neutralizing antibody (Slater, 2014, Lunn et al., 2011, Goehring et al., 2010, Heldens et al., 2001, Burrows et al., 1984, Moore and Koonse, 1978). Currently available vaccines, which include inactivated and MLV vaccines administered by IM injection, induce some but not all of the desired immune responses and do not, therefore, induce persistent sterile immunity or complete protection from clinical disease. Their main role is to reduce contagion by reducing the duration and titer of virus shedding (Slater, 2014).

Serologic tests for antibodies to EHV-1 and EHV-4 include complement fixation (CF), virus neutralization (VN), ELISA and a recently described microsphere bead assay (Slater, 2014, Davis et al., 2015). Neither the CF nor VN tests distinguish between EHV-1 and EHV-4 infection, whereas the ELISA and microsphere bead assays do (Davis et al., 2015). The complement fixation (CF) test detects the IgM-mediated early humoral response to infection and is therefore useful for diagnosis but not for sero-surveillance or prediction of immune status. The VN test detects the more persistent IgG response that is likely more relevant from the standpoint of resistance to infection or attenuation of clinical signs resulting from vaccination. ELISA distinguishes between infection with EHV-1 and EHV-4 by measuring type-specific antibodies directed against glycoproteins D (gD) and G (gG) (Foote et al., 2002, 2006). The CF and VN tests are commercially available through NVSL and the type-specific ELISA is marketed by Boehringer Ingelheim Svanova in Sweden and is available through some State Diagnostic Laboratories. The laboratory that runs the microsphere bead assay will likely offer the test commercially in the near future (Davidson E., personal communication).

Given the complex and short-lived nature of the immune response to EHV and the fact that infection and induction of severe clinical signs such as abortion or myeloencephalopathy occur regularly in horses with measurable (high) levels of circulating VN antibody, the use of VN, ELISA or microsphere bead assays to predict susceptibility or resistance to infection and the need for vaccination cannot be recommended at this time.

40.11 Equine Viral Arteritis (EVA)

The virus neutralization (VN) assay available in microwell format at the NVSL is a sensitive and specific test for neutralizing antibodies to EAV and therefore remains the gold standard for assessing previous exposure or response to vaccination. The modified live virus EVA vaccine available for use in North America induces a persistent serologic response that cannot be distinguished from that resulting from natural infection using the VN assay (Timoney and McCollum, 1993, Timoney et al., 1988). From a regulatory standpoint, seropositive horses (particularly stallions) are considered to be persistently infected and potentially chronic shedders of the virus unless there is documented evidence that the horse was seronegative prior to vaccination and evidence of vaccination can be confirmed (Timoney and McCollum, 1993). Regardless, sero-positivity precludes export of positive horses to many countries and can also complicate interstate transfer; therefore, the indications for vaccination are limited.

Rather than being used to predict resistance to infection, the main indications for serologic testing for EVA are documentation of sero-negative status prior to export or prior to vaccination, and identification of stallions that are persistently infected and potentially shedding the virus in semen.

40.12 Strangles (*Streptococcus equi* subsp. *equi* Infection)

Most horses develop a solid immunity during recovery from strangles, which persists in more than 75% of animals for 5 years or longer (Hamlen et al., 1994). The cell wall M-protein of *S. equi* (Se-M) is recognized in the acquired immune response to *S. equi* infection, a response that involves both production of local antibodies in the nasopharynx and circulating opsonophagocytic antibodies (Flock et al., 2004, Sheoran et al., 1997, Timoney, 1993, Timoney and Eggers, 1985). The predominant opsonophagocytic antibodies are of the IgGb sub-isotype but also include IgGa and IgA, whereas IgGb and later mucosal IgA predominate in nasopharyngeal secretions (Sheoran et al., 1997, 2000b).

The finding that recovered horses rapidly clear intranasally inoculated *S. equi* despite not making circulating antibody to its surface proteins indicates that to be highly effective a strangles vaccine must stimulate local nasopharyngeal tonsillar immune clearance responses and that serum antibody is of lesser importance (Timoney et al., 2007). This conclusion is further supported by the finding that ponies with high levels of circulating antibody to multiple unique surface-exposed and secreted proteins after systemic vaccination remained susceptible to challenge with *S. equi* (Timoney et al., 2007). None of the available strangles vaccines, which include inactivated subunit vaccines administered by IM injection or modified live vaccines administered intranasally or mucosally, appear to be highly efficacious in preventing strangles the field setting, although they may offer some benefit by reducing the attack rate and severity of clinical signs if used on a herd-wide basis to enhance herd immunity (Staempfli et al., 1991, Rief et al., 1981, Hoffman et al., 1991). The most reactive and best studied of the 15 exposed or secreted proteins that stimulate a neutralizing response is the M protein (SeM).

Proprietary ELISA's for measuring antibodies to SeM are available from Idexx Laboratories (www.idexx.com) and Equine Diagnostic Solutions (EDS; www.edslabky.com) in the USA and the Animal Health Trust in England (AHT; www.aht.org.uk). These tests have been used diagnostically to confirm past infection with *S. equi* or vaccination and have increasingly been used in an attempt to reduce the risk of inducing untoward adverse effects such as purpura hemorrhagica following vaccination. An ELISA titer of 1:3200 or higher is considered a high positive and is found in horses 4–12 weeks after infection or vaccination. A horse with a titer of this magnitude is thought to be at increased risk for developing purpura hemorrhagica and should not be vaccinated (Sweeney et al., 2005, 2014). This conclusion is based on the belief that horses at risk for purpura hemorrhagica may be hyper-responders to SeM. Except in horses that have been exposed to *S. equi* within the past 2 weeks, a negative SeM titer is interpreted as no previous exposure to the bacterium or vaccine, while a weak positive (1:200 to 1:400) is equivocal and likely represents residual antibody from exposure to *S. equi* or vaccine in the remote past (Sweeney et al., 2014). Vaccination of horses in these two categories may be considered if warranted by the risk of exposure to *S. equi*. An intermediate positive titer (1:800 to 1:1600) titer may occur in horses exposed 2–3 weeks previously or in those infected 6 months to 2 years previously. If horses in this category have no history of strangles vaccination, it is assumed that presence of antibodies represent previous exposure and there is a high likelihood that these horses will be protected upon re-exposure to *S. equi*. For horses that have been vaccinated in the past, particularly if they have no history of previous infection, it is assumed that antibodies represent the response to vaccination and it is uncertain whether these horses are protected (Sweeney et al., 2014). In this case, two options are available; either retest in 3–6 months or go ahead with revaccination if warranted by risk of exposure.

40.13 Botulism

Protection against botulism appears to be antibody-mediated; therefore, measurement of antibody levels would be useful for predicting protection and the need for vaccination if serologic tests were readily available and affordable. The only available vaccine is a *C. botulinum* type B toxoid (BotVax®-B, Neogen Corporation, Tampa, FL) that is marketed primarily as an aid in prevention of the Shaker Foal Syndrome. Protection of the foal is accomplished via colostral transfer of antibodies induced by vaccination of the mare. For primary vaccination, mares should be given a series of three doses administered 4 weeks apart during gestation, scheduled so that the last dose will be administered 4–6 weeks before foaling (i.e., months 8, 9, and 10 of gestation). This regime is designed to maximize concentrations of type B-specific immunoglobulin in colostrum. Subsequently, mares should be revaccinated annually with a single dose 4–6 weeks prior to foaling.

The high and persistent antibody titers induced by administration of the three-dose primary series of the *C. botulinum* type B toxoid to naïve horses, or administration of a booster dose to previously vaccinated horses, is thought to be almost 100% protective in adult horses (Whitlock and Buckley, 1997, Crane et al., 1991). Foals born to vaccinated dams can occasionally present with botulism, suggesting that reliance on passive transfer of maternal antibody to protect foals may not be universally effective in endemic areas (Wilkins and Palmer, 2003). These failures could result from failure of the dam to mount an adequate serologic response, partial, or complete failure of passive transfer of maternal antibody to the foal, waning of maternal antibody so that older foals are no longer protected or exposure to a very high dose of toxin that overwhelms what would otherwise be protective levels of antibody (Wilkins, 2014).

Doubts regarding the adequacy of the vaccination program could be resolved by testing for specific antibodies to Type B toxin in either the mare pre-foaling or the foal at 24–72h after birth, or both, in addition to confirming the overall adequacy of passive transfer of IgG (>800 mg/dL) by testing post-nursing foal samples using one of the many available test kits. The mouse neutralization assay has been the gold standard for testing for antibodies against *C. botulinum* type B toxin for many years. A much less expensive ELISA test was developed at the University of Pennsylvania and was used in the original studies to asses responses to vaccination (Crane et al., 1991). Unfortunately, this test is no longer offered at the University of Pennsylvania and this author has been unable to identify an alternative. Because the levels of antibody necessary for protection have not been clearly defined, this test would likely have limited application, even if it were available.

40.14 Equine Neorickettsiosis (Potomac Horse Fever)

Recovery after natural infection with *Neorickettsia risticii* induces a strong antibody response and durable protection from reinfection lasting 20 months or longer. However, the presence of antibodies does not necessarily correlate with protection, and cell-mediated responses likely play a crucial role (Palmer, 1993). Although challenge studies conducted approximately 4 weeks after completion of a two-dose primary series with an inactivated vaccine (no longer marketed) documented protection against all clinical signs of disease except fever in 78% of horses, the results of epidemiological investigations involving a large number of horses failed to demonstrate any clinical or economic benefit from annual vaccination with currently available vaccines in New York State (Atwill and Mohammed, 1996a, 1996b). Failure of a substantial number of individual horses to mount an immune response to inactivated *N. risticii* vaccines, heterogeneity of *N. risticii* isolates, the presence of only one *N. risticii* strain in vaccines, and much more rapid waning of immunity after vaccination than after natural infection, likely account for the observed failure of vaccines to provide protection against field infection (Palmer, 1993, Dutta et al., 1998). Only one inactivated *N. risticii* vaccine for IM administration (Equine Potomavac®, Merial) is licensed and available for use in horses as an aid in prevention of equine neorickettsiosis (EN). Many practitioners who work in EN endemic areas believe that severity of disease is attenuated and mortality is reduced in vaccinated horses when vaccines are administered at a 4- to 6-month interval. An IFA test for antibodies to *N. risticii* is available through NVSL and has been used on paired samples for diagnostic purposes. However, the test appears to yield a high percentage of false positive results, as compared to ELISA and Western Blot (Madigan et al., 1995). Considering the above limitations and the perceived need for frequent revaccination to prevent PHF in the field, there is no rationale for serologic testing of horses to assess protection against EN or the need for revaccination.

40.15 Equine Rotavirus

Equine rotavirus is one of the most important causes of infectious diarrhea in foals during the first few weeks of life and often causes outbreaks involving the majority of the foal crop on individual farms (Browning et al., 1991, 1992, Dwyer, 1993). Older foals and adult horses are more resistant to infection. Although the most important correlate for protection against rotavirus infection is specific mucosal IgA in the intestinal tract, most of the immunological approaches to prevent the disease have been directed at maximizing the level of antibodies in colostrum and milk of the mare in the hope that the foal will gain at least some passive protection. An inactivated rotavirus A vaccine (Equine Rotavirus Vaccine, Zoetis) is conditionally licensed in the USA and is indicated for administration to pregnant mares as an aid to prevention of diarrhea in their foals caused by infection with RVs of serogroup A. The recommended three-dose series is administered to mares during each pregnancy at 8, 9 and 10 months of gestation. This protocol has been shown to induce significant increases in serum concentrations of neutralizing antibody in vaccinated mares and in the concentrations of antibodies of the IgG, but not IgA, subclass in the colostrum and milk (Powell et al., 1997, Sheoran et al., 2000a). It is essential that the newborn foal receive an adequate amount of good quality colostrum so that it absorbs sufficient anti-RV antibodies. A field study provided circumstantial evidence of at least partial efficacy by showing an approximately two-fold higher incidence of rotaviral diarrhea in foals from non-vaccinated mares compared to those from vaccinated mares, although this difference did not prove to be statistically significant (Powell et al., 1997). Rotavirus antibody tests on serum would not provide useful predictive information regarding susceptibility to infection or the need for vaccination.

40.16 Equine Rhinitis A (ERAV) and Equine Rhinitis B, types 1 and 2 (ERBV1 and ERBV2)

Although the role of these picornaviruses in causing clinically apparent disease remains a topic of debate, serological surveys using the VN test show them to be common and widely distributed in equine populations worldwide (Diaz-Mendez et al., 2010, Black et al., 2007, Kriegshauser et al., 2005, Dynon et al., 2007, Sugiura et al., 1987). It has been shown that the rate of seropositivity to ERBV1 and ERVB2 is already high when Thoroughbreds enter training as 2-year-olds and that the rate of seropositivity to ERAV increases substantially during the first year of training (Black et al., 2007), suggesting that there may be a place for vaccination of horses with the conditionally licensed inactivated ERAV vaccine before they enter training as 2-year-olds. Because immune correlates for protection of horses against ERAV, as well as the disease syndromes it causes, are poorly defined, there does not currently appear to be a need for serologic testing to predict resistance to infection or the need for vaccination.

References

Allen G, Yeargan M, Costa LR, and Cross R. 1995. Major histocompatibility complex class I-restricted cytotoxic T-lymphocyte responses in horses infected with equine herpesvirus 1. J Virol, 69: 606–612.

Atwill ER and Mohammed HO. 1996a. Benefit-cost analysis of vaccination of horses as a strategy to control equine monocytic ehrlichiosis. J Am Vet Med Assoc, 208: 1295–1299.

Atwill ER and Mohammed HO. 1996b. Evaluation of vaccination of horses as a strategy to control equine monocytic ehrlichiosis. J Am Vet Med Assoc, 208: 1290–1294.

Balasuriya UB, Shi PY, Wong SJ, Demarest VL, Gardner IA, Hullinger PJ, et al. 2006. Detection of antibodies to West Nile virus in equine sera using microsphere immunoassay. J Vet Diagn Invest, 18: 392–395.

Barber TL, Walton TE, and Lewis KJ. 1978. Efficacy of trivalent inactivated encephalomyelitis virus vaccine in horses. Am J Vet Res, 39: 621–5.

Black WD, Wilcox RS, Stevenson RA, Hartley CA, Ficorilli NP, Gilkerson JR, and Studdert, M. J. 2007. Prevalence of serum neutralising antibody to equine rhinitis A virus (ERAV), equine rhinitis B virus 1 (ERBV1) and ERBV2. Vet Microbiol, 119: 65–71.

Browning GF, Chalmers RM, Snodgrass DR, Batt RM, Hart CA, Ormarod SE, et al. 1991. The prevalence of enteric pathogens in diarrhoeic Thoroughbred foals in Britain and Ireland. Eq Vet J, 23: 405–409.

Browning GF, Sykes JE, Huntington PJ, Hollywell CA, and Begg AP. 1992. Rotavirus infections in Australian foals. Aust Eq Vet, 10: 123–126.

Burrows R, Goodridge D, and Denyer MS. 1984. Trials of an inactivated equid herpesvirus 1 vaccine: challenge with a subtype 1 virus. Vet Rec, 114: 369–374.

Chambers TM, Holland RE, Tudor LR, Townsend HG, Cook A, Bogdan J, et al. 2001. A new modified live equine influenza virus vaccine: phenotypic stability, restricted spread and efficacy against heterologous virus challenge. Equine Vet J, 33: 630–636.

Crane SA, Whitlock RH, and Buckley C. 1991. Vaccination of adult horses with a Clostridium botulinum type B toxoid: a comparison of vaccination intervals. AAEP Report, 37: 611.

Crouch CF, Daly J, Hannant D, Wilkins J, and Francis MJ. 2004. Immune responses and protective efficacy in ponies immunised with an equine influenza ISCOM vaccine containing an "American lineage" H3N8 virus. Vaccine, 23: 418–425.

Daly JM, Newton JR, and Mumford JA. 2004. Current perspectives on control of equine influenza. Vet Res, 35: 411–423.

Davis EG, Bello NM, Bryan AJ, Hankins K, and Wilkerson M. 2015. Characterisation of immune responses in healthy foals when a multivalent vaccine protocol was initiated at age 90 or 180 days. Equine Vet J, 47: 667–674.

Diaz-Mendez A, Viel L, Hewson J, Doig P, Carman S, Chambers T, et al. 2010. Surveillance of equine respiratory viruses in Ontario. Can J Vet Res, 74: 271–278.

Dutta SK, Vemulapalli R, and Biswas B. 1998. Association of deficiency in antibody response to vaccine and heterogeneity of *Ehrlichia risticii* strains with Potomac horse fever vaccine failure in horses. J Clin Microbiol, 36: 506–512.

Dwyer RM. 1993. Rotaviral diarrhea. Vet Clin N Am-Equine, 9: 311–319.

Dyer JL, Yager P, Orciari L, Greenberg L, Wallace R, Hanlon CA, and Blanton JD. 2014. Rabies surveillance in the United States during 2013. J Am Vet Med Assoc, 245: 1111–1123.

Dynon K, Black WD, Ficorilli N, Hartley CA, and Studdert MJ. 2007. Detection of viruses in nasal swab samples from horses with acute, febrile, respiratory disease using virus isolation, polymerase chain reaction and serology. Aust Vet J, 85: 46–50.

Edens LM, Crisman MV, Toth TE, Ahmed SA, and Murray MJ. 1996. In vitro cytotoxic activity of equine lymphocytes on equine herpesvirus-1 infected allogenic fibroblasts. Vet Immunol Immunopathol, 52: 175–189.

Flock M, Jacobsson K, Frykberg L, Hirst TR, Franklin A, Guss B, and Flock JI. 2004. Recombinant *Streptococcus equi* proteins protect mice in challenge experiments and induce immune response in horses. Infect Immun, 72: 3228–3236.

Foote CE, Love DN, Gilkerson JR, Wellington JE, and Whalley JM. 2006. EHV-1 and EHV-4 infection in vaccinated mares and their foals. Vet Immunol Immunopathol, 111: 41–6.

Foote CE, Love DN, Gilkerson JR, and Whalley JM. 2002. Serological responses of mares and weanlings following vaccination with an inactivated whole virus equine herpesvirus 1 and equine herpesvirus 4 vaccine. Vet Microbiol, 88: 13–25.

Gardner IA, Wong SJ, Ferraro GL, Balasuriya UB, Hullinger PJ, Wilson WD, et al 2007. Incidence and effects of West Nile virus infection in vaccinated and unvaccinated horses in California. Vet Res, 38: 109–116.

Goehring LS, Wagner B, Bigbie R, Hussey SB, Rao S, Morley PS, and Lunn DP. 2010. Control of EHV-1 viremia and nasal shedding by commercial vaccines. Vaccine, 28: 5203–5211.

Green SL, Little CB, Baird JD, Tremblay RR, and Smith-Maxie LL. 1994. Tetanus in the horse: a review of 20 cases (1970 to 1990). J Vet Intern Med, 8: 128–132.

Green SL, Smith LL, Vernau W, and Beacock SM. 1992. Rabies in horses: 21 cases (1970–1990). J Am Vet Med Assoc, 200: 1133–1137.

Hamlen HJ, Timoney JF, and Bell RJ. 1994. Epidemiologic and immunologic characteristics of *Streptococcus equi* infection in foals. J Am Vet Med Assoc, 204: 768–775.

Hannant D, Jessett DM, O'-Neill T, Livesay J, and Mumford JA. 1994. Cellular immune responses stimulated by inactivated virus vaccines and infection with equine influenza virus (H3N8). Equine infectious diseases VII: Proceedings of the Seventh International Conference, Tokyo, Japan 8th 11th June 1994. 169 174, 1994. Newmarket UK: R and W Publications (Newmarket) Ltd.

Hannant D, Jessett DM, O'Neill, T, and Mumford JA. 1989. Antibody isotype responses in the serum and respiratory tract to primary and secondary infections with equine influenza virus (H3N8). Vet Microbiol, 19: 293–303.

Hannant D and Mumford JA. 1989. Cell mediated immune responses in ponies following infection with equine influenza virus (H3N8): the influence of induction culture conditions on the properties of cytotoxic effector cells. Vet Immunol Immunopathol, 21: 327–337.

Harvey AM, Watson JL, Brault SA, Edman JE, Moore SM, Kass PH, and Wilson WD. 2016. Duration of serum antibody responses to rabies vaccination in horses. J Am Vet Med Assoc, 249(4): 411–418.

Hays MB. 1969. Definitive efficacy and safety testing for equine encephalomyelitis vaccine. J Am Vet Med Assoc, 155: 374–376.

Heldens JG, Hannant D, Cullinane AA, Prendergast MJ, Mumford JA, Nelly M, et al. 2001. Clinical and virological evaluation of the efficacy of an inactivated EHV1 and EHV4 whole virus vaccine (Duvaxyn EHV1,4). Vaccination/challenge experiments in foals and pregnant mares. Vaccine, 19: 4307–4317.

Heldens JG, Pouwels HG, Derks CG, Van De Zande SM, and Hoeijmakers MJ. 2010. Duration of immunity induced by an equine influenza and tetanus combination vaccine formulation adjuvanted with ISCOM-Matrix. Vaccine, 28: 6989–6996.

Hoffman AM, Staempfli HR, Prescott JF, and Viel L. 1991. Field evaluation of a commercial M-protein vaccine against Streptococcus equi infection in foals. Am J Vet Res, 52: 589–592.

Holmes MA, Townsend HG, Kohler AK, Hussey S, Breathnach C, Barnett C, et al. 2006. Immune responses to commercial equine vaccines against equine herpesvirus-1, equine influenza virus, eastern equine encephalomyelitis, and tetanus. Vet Immunol Immunopathol 111(1–2): 67–68.

Hooper DC, Morimoto K, Bette M, Weihe E, Koprowski H, and Dietzschold B. 1998. Collaboration of antibody and inflammation in clearance of rabies virus from the central nervous system. J Virol, 72: 3711–3719.

Hudson LC, Weinstock D, Jordan T, and Bold-Fletcher NO. 1996. Clinical presentation of experimentally induced rabies in horses. Zentralbl Veterinarmed B, 43: 277–285.

Jansen BC and Knoetze PC. 1979. The immune response of horses to tetanus toxoid. Onderstepoort J Vet Res, 46: 211–216.

Kendall A, Anagrius K, Ganheim A, Rosanowski SM, and Bergstrom K. 2015. Duration of tetanus immunoglobulin G titres following basic immunisation of horses. Equine Vet J 8(6): 710–771.

Kostense S, Moore S, Companjen A, Bakker AB, Marissen WE, Von Eyben R, et al. 2012. Validation of the rapid fluorescent focus inhibition test for rabies virus-neutralizing antibodies in clinical samples. Antimicrob Agents Chemother, 56: 3524–3530.

Kriegshauser G, Deutz A, Kuechler E, Skern T, Lussy H, and Nowotny N. 2005. Prevalence of neutralizing antibodies to Equine rhinitis A and B virus in horses and man. Vet Microbiol, 106: 293–296.

Kydd JH, Wattrang E, and Hannant D. 2003. Pre-infection frequencies of equine herpesvirus-1 specific, cytotoxic T lymphocytes correlate with protection against abortion following experimental infection of pregnant mares. Vet Immunol Immunopathol, 96: 207–217.

Landolt GA, Townsend HGG, and Lunn DP. 2014. Equine influenza infection. In DC Sellon and MT Long (eds), *Equine Infectious Diseases*. 2nd edn. St. Louis: Elsevier.

Liefman CE. 1980. Combined active-passive immunisation of horses against tetanus. Aust Vet J, 56: 119–122.

Liefman CE. 1981. Active immunisation of horses against tetanus including the booster dose and its application. Aust Vet J, 57: 57–60.

Lohrer J and Radvila P. 1970. Active tetanus protection in the horses and the duration of immunity. Schwei Arch Tierheikd, 112: 307–314.

Lunn DP, Sellers AD, Goehring LS, Townsend HGG, Hussey SB, Tuttle J, and Stenbom RM. Protection against EHv-1 challenge by inactivated vaccines. 57th Annual Convention of the American Association of Equine Practitioners, 2011 San Antonio, Texas, p. 322.

Madigan JE, Rikihisa Y, Palmer JE, Derock E, and Mott J. 1995. Evidence for a high rate of false-positive results with the indirect fluorescent antibody test for *Ehrlichia risticii* antibody in horses. J Am Vet Med Assoc, 207: 1448–1453.

Moore BO and Koonse HJ. 1978. Inactivated equine herpesvirus 1 vaccine - Pneumabort-K®. In FJ Milne (ed.), *24th Annual Convention of the American Association of Equine Practitioners*, St. Louis, MO, pp. 75–79.

Moore SM and Hanlon CA. 2010. Rabies-specific antibodies: measuring surrogates of protection against a fatal disease. PLoS Negl Trop Dis, 4: e595.

Morley PS, Townsend HG, Bogdan JR, and Haines DM. 2000. Risk factors for disease associated with influenza virus infections during three epidemics in horses. J Am Vet Med Assoc, 216: 545–550.

Mumford J, Wood JM, Scott AM, Folkers C, and Schild GC. 1983. Studies with inactivated equine influenza vaccine. 2. Protection against experimental infection with influenza virus A/equine/Newmarket/79 (H3N8). J Hyg (Lond), 90: 385–395.

Mumford JA. 1990. The diagnosis and control of equine influenza. 36th Annu Conv Am Assoc Equine Pract, pp. 377–385.

Mumford JA and Wood J. 1992. Establishing an acceptability threshold for equine influenza vaccines. Dev Biol Stand, 79: 137–146.

Mumford JA, Wood JM, Folkers C, and Schild GC. 1988. Protection against experimental infection with influenza virus A/equine/Miami/63 (H3N8) provided by inactivated whole virus vaccines containing homologous virus. Epidemiol Infect, 100: 501–510.

Nelson KM, Schram BR, McGregor MW, Sheoran AS, Olsen CW, and Lunn DP. 1998. Local and systemic isotype-specific antibody responses to equine influenza virus infection versus conventional vaccination. Vaccine, 16: 1306–1313.

Newton JR, Townsend HG, Wood JL, Sinclair R, Hannant D, and Mumford JA. 2000. Immunity to equine influenza: relationship of vaccine-induced antibody in young Thoroughbred racehorses to protection against field infection with influenza A/equine-2 viruses (H3N8). Equine Veterinary Journal, 32: 65–74.

O'Neill T, Kydd JH, Allen GP, Wattrang E, Mumford JA, and Hannant D. 1999. Determination of equid herpesvirus 1-specific, CD8+, cytotoxic T lymphocyte precursor frequencies in ponies. Vet Immunol Immunopathol, 70: 43–54.

Paillot R and Prowse L. 2012. ISCOM-matrix-based equine influenza (EIV) vaccine stimulates cell-mediated immunity in the horse. Vet Immunol Immunopathol, 145: 516–521.

Palmer JE. 1993. Potomac horse fever. Vet Clin N Amer: Equine Pract, 9: 399–410.

Patel JR, Bateman H, Williams J, and Didlick S. 2003. Derivation and characterisation of a live equid herpes virus-1 (EHV-1) vaccine to protect against abortion and respiratory disease due to EHV-1. Vet Microbiol, 91: 23–39.

Powell DG, Dwyer RM, Traub-Dargatz JL, Fulker RH, Whalen JW, Jr, Srinivasappa J, et al. 1997. Field study of the safety, immunogenicity, and efficacy of an inactivated equine rotavirus vaccine. J Am Vet Med Assoc, 211: 193–198.

Ramon G and Lemetayer E. 1939. The duration of the immunity conferred by tetanus anatoxin. Compte Rendu de l'Academie des Sciences, 209: 704–707.

Recknagel S, Snyder A, Blanke A, Uhlig A, Bruser B, and Schusser GF. 2015a. [Evaluation of an immunochromatographic dipstick test for the assessment of tetanus immunity in horses]. Berl Munch Tierarztl Wochenschr, 128: 376–383.

Recknagel S, Snyder A, Bruser B, and Schusser GF. 2015b. Immunization strategies and seroprotection against tetanus in horses in central Germany. Pferdeheilkunde, 31.

Rief JS, George JL, and Shideler RK. 1981. Recent developments in strangles research: observations on the carrier state and evaluation of a new vaccine. 27th Annu Conv Am Assoc Equine Pract, pp. 33–40.

Sahu SP, Alstad AD, Pedersen DD, and Pearson JE. 1994. Diagnosis of eastern equine encephalomyelitis virus infection in horses by immunoglobulin M and G capture enzyme-linked immunosorbent assay. J Vet Diagn Invest, 6: 34–38.

Sheoran AS, Karzenski SS, Whalen JW, Crisman MV, Powell, DG, and Timoney JF. 2000a. Prepartum equine rotavirus vaccination inducing strong specific IgG in mammary secretions. Veterinary Record, 146: 672–673.

Sheoran AS, Sponseller BT, Holmes MA, and Timoney JF. 1997. Serum and mucosal antibody isotype responses to M-like protein (SeM) of *Streptococcus equi* in convalescent and vaccinated horses. Vet Immunol Immunopathol, 59: 239–251.

Sheoran AS, Timoney JF, Holmes MA, Karzenski SS, and Crisman MV. 2000b. Immunoglobulin isotypes in sera and nasal Mucosal secretions and their neonatal transfer and distribution in horses. Am J Vet Res, 61: 1099–1105.

Slater J. 2007. Equine herpesviruses. In DC Sellon and MT Long (eds), *Equine Infectious Diseases*. 1st edn. St. Louis: Elsevier.

Slater J. 2014. Equine Herpesviruses. In: In DC Sellon and MT Long (eds), *Equine Infectious Diseases*. 2nd edn. St. Louis: Elsevier.

Soboll G, Horohov DW, Aldridge BM, Olsen CW, McGregor MW, Drape RJ., et al. 2003. Regional antibody and cellular immune responses to equine influenza virus infection, and particle mediated DNA vaccination. Vet Immunol Immunopathol, 94: 47–62.

Staempfli HR, Hoffman AM, Prescott JF, and Viel L. 1991. Clinical evaluation of a commercial M-protein vaccine in naturally infected foals. 37th Annu Conv Am Assoc Equine Pract, pp. 259–262.

Sugiura T, Matsumura T, Fukunaga Y, and Hirasawa K. 1987. Sero-epizootiological study of racehorses with pyrexia in the training centers of the Japan Racing Association. Nihon Juigaku Zasshi, 49: 1087–1096.

Sweeney CR, Timoney JF, Newton JR, and Hines MT. 2005. *Streptococcus equi* infections in horses: guidelines for treatment, control, and prevention of strangles. J Vet Intern Med, 19: 123–134.

Sweeney CR, Timoney JF, Newton JR, and Hines MT. 2014. *Streptococcus equi Subsp. equi. In: In DC Sellon and MT Long (eds), Equine Infectious Diseases*. 2nd edn. St. Louis: Elsevier.

Thein P, Rohm A, Jr., and Voss J. 2013. Experimental investigations to the immune response of foals and adult horses to tetanus toxoid using the Fassisi TetaCheckReg. Pferdeheilkunde, 29: 686–699.

Timoney JF. 1993. Strangles. Vet Clin North Am Equine Pract, 9: 365–374.

Timoney JF and Eggers D. 1985. Serum bactericidal responses to *Streptococcus equi* of horses following infection or vaccination. Equine Vet J, 17: 306–310.

Timoney JF, Qin A, Muthupalani S, and Artiushin S. 2007. *Vaccine potential of novel surface exposed and secreted proteins of Streptococcus equi*. Vaccine.

Timoney PJ and McCollum WH. 1993. Equine viral arteritis. Vet Clin North Am: Equine Pract, 9: 295–309.

Timoney PJ, Umphenour NW, and McCollum WH. 1988. *Safety evaluation of a commercial modified live equine arteritis virus vaccine for use in stallions*, Lexington, Kentucky: The University Press of Kentucky.

Tizard I and Ni Y. 1998. Use of serologic testing to assess immune status of companion animals. J Am Vet Med Assoc, 213: 54–60.

Townsend HG, Penner SJ, Watts TC, Cook A, Bogdan J, Haines DM, et al. 2001. Efficacy of a cold-adapted, intranasal, equine influenza vaccine: challenge trials. Equine Vet J, 33: 637–643.

Townsend HGG, Morley PS, Newton JR, Wood JLN, Haines DM, and Mumford JA. 1999. Measuring serum antibody as a method of predicting infection and disease in horses during outbreaks of influenza. In U Wernery, JF Wade, JA Mumford, and OR Kaaden (eds), *Equine Infectious Diseases VIII: Proceedings of the Eighth International Conference*. Newmarket, UK: R and W Publications (Newmarket Ltd).

Van Maanen C and Cullinane A. 2002. Equine influenza virus infections: an update. Vet Q, 24: 79–94.

Whitlock RH and Buckley C. 1997. Botulism. Vet Clin North Am: Equine Pract, 13: 107–128.

Wilkins PA. 2014. Botulism. In DC Sellon and MT Long (eds), *Equine Infectious Diseases*. 2nd edn. St. Louis: Elsevier.

Wilkins PA and Palmer JE. 2003. Botulism in foals less than 6 months of age: 30 cases (1989–2002). J Vet Intern Med, 17: 702–707.

Wilks CR. 1977. In vitro cytotoxicity of serum and peripheral blood leukocytes for equine herpesvirus type 1-infected target cells. Am J Vet Res, 38: 117–121.

Wilson WD. 1993. Equine Influenza. Vet Clin N Am-Eq. Prac, 9: 257–282.

Wilson WD, Mihalyi JE, Hussey S, and Lunn DP. 2001. Passive transfer of maternal immunoglobulin isotype antibodies against tetanus and influenza and their effect on the response of foals to vaccination. (Special Issue: Immunology). Eq Vet J, 33: 644–650.

Wood JM, Gaines-Das RE, Taylor J, and Chakraverty P. 1994. Comparison of influenza serological techniques by international collaborative study. Vaccine, 12: 167–174.

Wood JM, Mumford J, Folkers C, Scott AM, and Schild GC. 1983. Studies with inactivated equine influenza vaccine. 1. Serological responses of ponies to graded doses of vaccine. J Hyg (Lond), 90: 371–384.

World Health Organization 2013. WHO Expert Consulation on Rabies, Second Report. World Health Organization technical report series, 1.

41

Immune-Mediated Hemolytic Anemia

Julia B. Felippe

Cornell University, College of Veterinary Medicine, New York, USA

41.1   Clinical Background

Immune-mediated hemolytic anemia (IMHA) is caused by an antibody binding to antigens on red blood cells, and subsequent hemolysis. This condition in known as auto-immune hemolytic anemia (AIHA) when it involves a hypersensitivity reaction type II with production by the patient of auto-antibodies against red blood cell surface self-molecules. These antibodies (alone or along with a complement) bind to red blood cells, and promote their rapid removal or destruction; when destruction is greater than production, the resulting clinical anemia can be life-threatening.

Auto-immune hemolytic anemias can be classified as warm, cold, combined warm and cold (paroxysmal), and drug-induced (Michel, 2011, Chaudhary and Das, 2014). In addition, classification includes primary (idiopathic) or secondary (often to lymphoproliferative disorders, e.g., lymphoma; infections, e.g., equine infectious anemia, *Streptococcus* ssp., *Clostridium* spp.; drug administration, e.g., penicillin, cephalosporin, trimethoprim-sulfa, quinidine) (Reef et al., 1984, Sockett et al., 1987, Mair et al., 1990, Messer and Arnold, 1991, McConnico et al., 1992, Robbins et al., 1993, Thomas et al., 1998, Weiss et al., 2003, McGovern et al., 2011). In drug-induced hemolytic anemia, antibodies recognize directly red blood cell antigens or drugs bound to red blood cells (Gehrs and Friedberg, 2002). In acute hemolytic transfusion reaction that occurs within 24h, pre-existing antibodies in the recipient bind to incompatible red blood cells of the donor and cause hemolysis; in delayed hemolytic transfusion reaction that occurs in more than 24h, the incompatible red blood cells of the donor induce primary or secondary (anamnestic) antibody production by the recipient.

When complement is activated along with antibody (IgG or IgM) binding, hemolysis is fast and happens intravascularly, resulting in discolored serum and urine (hemoglobinuria). In extravascular hemolysis, the latter clinical signs are not obvious because the antibody (often IgG)-bound red blood cells are removed via phagocytosis when the antibody binds to the Fc receptor on phagocytes (Salama, 2009).

In the case of warm AIHA, IgG binds to red blood cells at >37 °C (but show decreased affinity at lower temperatures), and cause their destruction more frequently via their removal by the mononuclear phagocyte or reticuloendothelial system (also known as extravascular hemolysis), or more infrequently via complement activation (intravascular hemolysis). In human patients, it has been shown that some subclasses of IgG are less likely to activate complement and may induce milder hemolysis (Issitt et al., 1978).

In the case of cold AIHA, IgM binds to red blood cells at low body temperatures in the peripheral circulation (decreased affinity at physiologic temperature), efficiently facilitates complement binding and cell lysis (intravascular hemolysis), and subsequently dissociates as blood circulate to warmer areas; in this case, DAT may be positive for complement only, unless the assay is run at a cold temperature (0–4°C), which prevents dissociation of IgM. In horses, IgG appears to be the most common primary antibody associated with AIHA, although IgM may be involved in some cases (Wilkerson et al., 2000). Mixed warm and cold AIHA have been described in human patients (Shulman et al., 1985).

Clinical signs include depression and weakness; tachycardia and tachypnea; icterus; progressive decrease in red blood cell count, hematocrit, and hemoglobulin; increased mean corpuscular volume (MCV) and red cell distribution width (RDW); reticulocytosis can be detected with certain automated hematology analyzers; indirect hyperbilirubinemia; and hemoglobinuria (when there is intravascular hemolysis) (Figure 41.1).

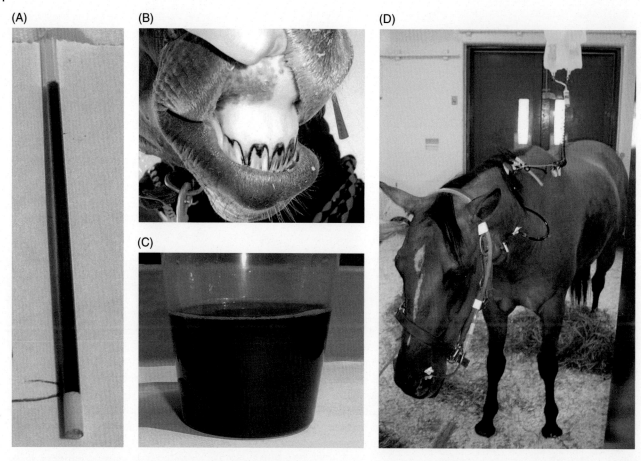

(A) **(B)** **(D)**

(C)

Figure 41.1 Clinical signs of a horse with immune-mediated hemolytic anemia. Pale mucous membranes (B) and depression (D) are signs of severe anemia; discolored serum (A, hemoglobulinemia) and urine (C, hemoglobinuria) indicate intravascular hemolysis.

41.2 Tests Available

Diagnosis of IMHA is based on the demonstration of antibodies and/or complement bound to red blood cells along with clinical evidence of anemia. Diagnostic tests for IMHA help determining prognosis, severity of disease, and type and duration of therapy by offering information about the antibody isotype(s) involved, antigenic-specificity, concentration, thermal amplitude, ability to fix complement, and ability to bind to Fc receptors on mononuclear phagocytes.

41.3 Sample Collection and Submission

Tests that detect the presence of red blood cells coated with antibody require whole blood samples carefully collected into tubes with ethylenediaminetetraacetic acid (EDTA) anti-coagulant, preferably, because it prevents complement fixation to red cells *in vitro*. Tubes with neutral gel separators have been associated with false positive results and should not be used.

For blood typing, whole blood is also preserved in EDTA. For crossmatch in the case of blood transfusion, blood is collected into a serum separator or clot tube without hemolysis.

41.4 Direct Antiglobulin Test (Direct Coombs Test)

The direct antiglobulin test (DAT) evaluates for the presence of red blood cells coated with antibodies and/or complement (Zantek et al., 2012) (Figure 41.2). This test is used to investigate immune-mediated AIHA, drug-induced AIHA, neonatal isoerythrolysis, and alloimmune reactions to a recent blood transfusion. In human patients, IgG-bound red blood cells are detected in about one quarter of AIHA cases; complement-bound red cells in one quarter of cases; and IgG and complement together in about half of cases (Chaudhary and Das, 2014). DAT detects a minimum level of 100–500 IgG molecules or 400–1100 complement molecules attached to red blood cells; therefore, clinical IMHA with negative DAT results

Direct Antiglobulin Test
(Direct Coombs Test)

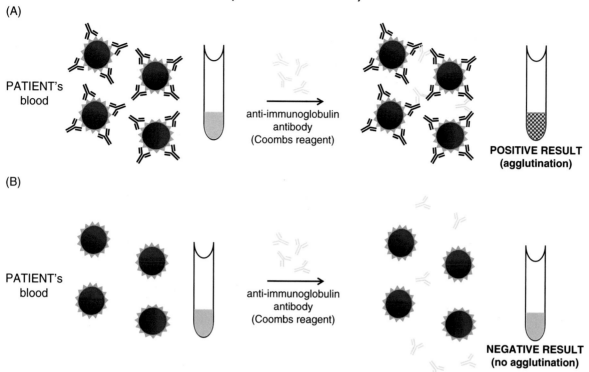

Figure 41.2 Direct antiglobulin test (direct Coombs test). DAT tests for the presence of antibody-coated red blood cells in the patient's blood. Washed red blood cells from the patient are incubated with anti-horse immunoglobulin (antibody reagent). (A) When the red blood cells are coated with immunoglobulin, antibody reagent binding promotes links between red blood cells and, consequently, agglutination (positive test). (B) In the absence of antibody-coated red blood cells, the antibody reagent cannot promote agglutination (negative test). False-positive and false-negative tests are possible, as discussed in the text.

(or DAT-negative IMHA) should be further investigated with more sensitive tests including flow cytometry or enzyme-linked DAT (Thedsawad et al., 2011).

The assay follows the following procedure (AABB Technical Manual, 2008):

1) The testing whole blood sample is washed with normal saline to remove unbound antibody and complement;
2) An aliquot of diluted washed red cells is mixed with polyspecific anti-IgG plus anti-IgM reagent, or monospecific anti-IgG or anti-IgM reagent for the species in a conventional test tube (gel matrix and solid phase methods are also available for human samples);
3) A negative control sample adds 6% bovine serum albumin (BSA) solution instead of antibody reagents to an aliquot of the testing washed blood sample;
4) A positive control sample uses IgG-coated or IgM-coated red blood cells instead of the patient's red cells plus monospecific anti-IgG or anti-IgM reagent, respectively;
5) When the reagent is available for the species (i.e., anti-C3), the presence of complement-coated red

blood cells is also tested using initially polyspecific reagents (anti-IgG, anti-IgM, and anti-C3 complement combined); and include the respective positive and negative controls. A positive result using polyspecific reagent should be followed by monospecific reagents;
6) The samples are centrifuged and the pellet dislodged by gentle tapping of the tube; agglutination is observed macroscopically and microscopically, and graded in a scale of 0 (no agglutination) to 4 (strong agglutination).

41.5 Indirect Antiglobulin Test (Indirect Coombs Test)

Determination of the presence or absence of antibodies against red blood cell surface molecules in the serum of a patient with hemolytic anemia by indirect antiglobulin test (IAT) and titration of the particular antibody for a semi-quantitative analysis offers information about the severity of disease: the greater the number of circulating

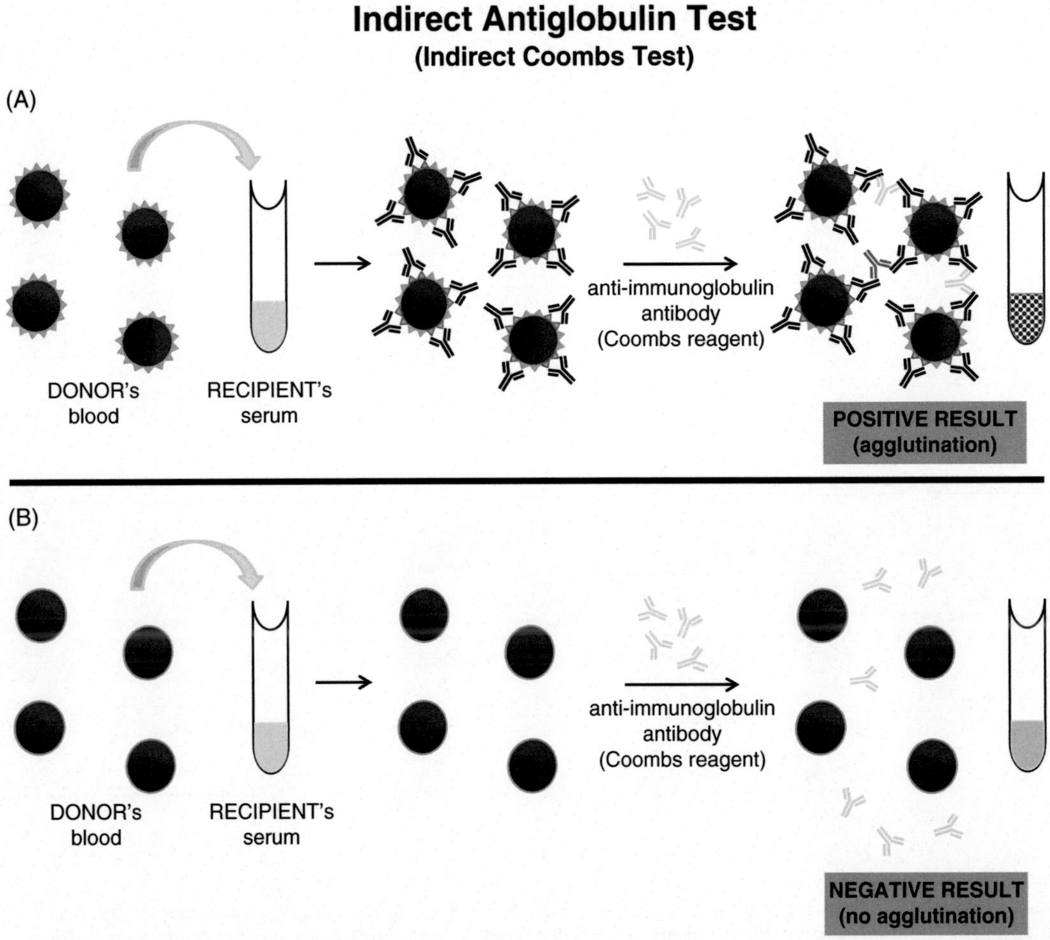

Indirect Antiglobulin Test
(Indirect Coombs Test)

Figure 41.3 Indirect antiglobulin test (indirect Coombs test). IAT tests for the presence of antibodies against red blood cell surface molecules in the serum of the patient with hemolysis or a patient in need of a blood transfusion. Dilutions of the patient/recipient serum is mixed with washed red blood cells of known antigenic expression or washed red blood cells from a blood donor. (A) When antibodies against red blood cell antigens are present in the recipient's serum, antibody-red blood cell complexes are formed, and subsequently detected by agglutination with the addition of antibody reagent (anti-horse immunoglobulin) (positive test). (B) In the absence of antibodies against red cell blood antigens in the serum of the patient/recipient, red blood cell link is not formed, and no agglutination is observed (negative test).

antibodies, the more efficient the complement activation and/or removal by the mononuclear phagocyte system, the more severe the anemia (Figure 41.3). Nevertheless, the presence of auto-antibodies against red blood cell molecules in serum alone does not imply their association with the cause of hemolysis. IAT is also used to measure the presence of antibodies against red blood cell surface molecules in the serum of a recipient of blood transfusion, in order to avoid transfusion reactions.

41.6 Possible Results and Interpretation

In the presence of clinical anemia and supporting clinical history, a positive result shows agglutination of red blood cells macroscopically and/or microscopically, and suggests an immune-dependent process for the destruction of red blood cells. A negative result does not show agglutination microscopically, and suggests the absence of an immune process in the destruction of red blood cells. However, the possibility of false-positive and false-negative results should be considered, and assay controls and clinical history used for thorough interpretation of results.

Comparably to human medicine, the sensitivity of DAT in veterinary medicine has been calculated at 58%, taken the high number of false-negative results; in contrast, specificity is 100% and a positive result, therefore, has a high association with IMHA (Wilkerson et al., 2000, Wang et al., 2001). The positive and negative predictive values have been calculated as 100 and 62%, respectively.

False-positive results (in the absence of hemolysis and anemia) are possible, and have been reported in a small percentage of human patients with spontaneous red blood cell agglutination, background disease (e.g., sickle-cell disease, renal disease, multiple myeloma, systemic lupus erythematosus), and in 1 per 10,000 healthy donors (Gorst et al., 1980, Bareford et al., 1985).

False-negative results (in the presence of clinical hemolysis and anemia) are possible when low-affinity IgG antibodies are removed from the red blood cell surface during washing; presence of low quantities of red blood cells coated with IgG or IgM; a different immunoglobulin isotype is not tested for (e.g., IgA, in rare cases); the assay is not run in cold conditions, and does not test for coating with complement (i.e., cold IMHA) (Segel and Lichtman, 2014). A negative result, therefore, does not rule out the diagnosis of IMHA.

For test validation, a negative result in the BSA control sample confirms a positive result in the testing tube containing anti-IgG reagent. A positive result in the BSA control sample indicates agglutination of red blood cells not due to antibody coating. Positive controls using IgG-coated (or complement-coated) red blood cells should show agglutination to validate the assay, in which a negative result invalidates the assay.

Clinical history and clinical signs are essential for the interpretation of diagnostics. Bone marrow cytology often reveals regenerative erythropoiesis, unless molecules on the red blood cell precursors are the target antigens for antibody production. When there is no evidence of a regenerative process with increased mean corpuscular volume (MCV) and red blood cell distribution width (RDW), impaired bone marrow production of red blood cells is possible, and bone marrow biopsy and cytology are indicated.

41.7 Direct Immunofluorescence Flow Cytometry

The presence of antibody-bound red blood cells in IMHA can be determined with high sensitivity using direct immunofluorescence flow cytometry (DIFC) (Roback et al., 2004, Alzate et al., 2015). The assay consists of incubating washed red blood cells from the patient with fluorescence-conjugated monospecific antibody against immunoglobulins of different isotypes (e.g. IgG, IgM, or IgA), and measuring positive fluorescence (i.e., antibody-coated red blood cell) using a flow cytometer. Background levels of antibody binding are measured using washed red blood cells from a control healthy animal; for some reagents, F(ab')2 fragment of the antibody reagent (e.g., anti-IgG) needs to be used to prevent readings of unspecific binding to red blood cells, perhaps the major challenging when stablishing an assay protocol. When compared to DAT, DIFC showed a sensitivity of 100% and a specificity of 87.5%, with positive

and negative predictive values of 92 and 100%, respectively, using dogs and horse samples (Wilkerson et al., 2000). The DIFC has also been shown to detect low number (<30%) of positive cells. Another advantage is the possibility to measure different immunoglobulin isotypes (i.e., IgG, IgM, and IgA), and reevaluate DAT-negative IMHA samples (Chaudhary et al., 2006).

The use of flow cytometry to detect the percentage of antibody-coated red blood cells has been successfully applied for the diagnosis of equine neonatal isoerythrolysis, penicillin-induced IMHA, and IMHA secondary to clostridial septicemia; DIFC has also been used to monitor response to therapy by measuring the percent of antibody-coated red blood cells through time (Davis et al., 2002).

41.8 Enzyme-Linked Antiglobulin Test

Although not widely used in veterinary medicine, enzyme-linked antiglobulin test (ELAT) has a high sensitivity for the detection of small amounts of IgG or IgM-coated red blood cells, and may be used in cases of clinical IMHA with negative DAT results (Sokol et al., 1985, Wang et al., 2001). Likewise flow cytometry, ELAT can detect IgA and, more importantly, the combination of antibody isotypes (IgG, IgM, and IgA), which can act synergistically in small amounts to cause hemolysis. This test has also shown high specificity based on negative results in patients without hemolysis, and with hemolysis of not immune origin. ELAT shows a high-agreement with DIFC when testing for antibody-coated red blood cells (Wang et al., 2001).

This method uses the principles of an enzyme-linked immunosorbent assay (ELISA): enzyme-conjugated monospecific anti-IgG, anti-IgM, anti-IgA, or anti-complement (when available for the species) react with a patient's washed red blood cell solution at 37°C; the substrate is added, and the absorbance of color developed during a positive result measured with a plate reader.

41.9 Clinical Case

A 10-year-old Thoroughbred mare presented with a history of fever (104.1°F) and icterus. Blood work revealed severe anemia (hematocrit 19%, hemoglobin 6.8g/dL), mature neutrophilia (9500 cells/μL), and elevated indirect bilirubin (6.3mg/dL). Total protein was normal at 7.0g/dL. Lactate was mildly elevated at 2.71mmol/L. On the blood smear, moderate anisocytosis, moderate macrocytes, few spherocytes, and agglutination were noted. A direct antiglobulin test was positive, indicating the presence of antibody-coated red blood cells.

Additional tests to investigate for a potential infectious inciting cause of the immune-mediated anemia included *Streptococcus equi* subspecies *equi* (guttural pouch culture negative; SeM protein titers low at 1:400), *Anaplasma phagocytophilum* (negative), *Theileria equi* (negative 1:5), *Babesia caballi* (negative 1:5), and equine infectious anemia (Coggin's test negative).

For precaution in case of deteriorating anemia, a blood donor was tested for compatibility with the patient. Major cross-match test of patient's serum and donor red blood cells revealed no agglutination and no hemolysis (compatible). Minor cross-match test of recipient red blood cells and donor serum revealed grade 3+ agglutination and no hemolysis (incompatible). A blood transfusion was not needed because hematocrit slowly improved in the subsequent days, and was never below 18%. Neutrophilia and indirect bilirubinemia also resolved.

The mare was treated with doxycycline for 10 days, and dexamethasone, azathioprine, and omeprazole for a total of 30 days, with the dexamethasone doses tapered gradually by 20% after every fourth dose. The mare made a full recovery.

References

American Association of Blood Banks (AABB) 2008. Standards for Blood Banks and Transfusion Services. 26th Edn, 2009. AABB Technical Manual, 16th Edn.

Alzate MA, Manrique LG, Bolaños NI, Duarte M, Coral-Alvarado P, and González JM. 2015. Simultaneous detection of IgG, IgM, IgA complexes and C3d attached to erythrocytes by flow cytometry. Int J Hematol, 37: 382–389.

Bareford D, Gilks G, Longster L, and Tovey LA. 1985. Follow-up of normal individuals with a positive antiglobulin test. Scand Journal J Haematol, 35: 348–353.

Chaudhary RK and Das SS. 2014. Autoimmune hemolytic anemia: From lab to bedside. Asian J Transf Sci, 8: 5–12.

Chaudhary R, Das SS, Gupta R, and Khetan D. 2006. Application of flow cytometry in detection of red-cell-bound IgG in Coombs-negative AIHA. An automatable format for accurate immunohematology testing by flow cytometry. Hematol, 11: 295–300.

Davis EG, Wilkerson MJ, and Rush BR. 2002. Flow cytometry: clinical applications in equine medicine. J Vet Int Med, 16: 404–410.

Gehrs BC and Friedberg RC. 2002. Autoimmune hemolytic anemia. AM J Hematol, 69: 258–271.

Gorst DW, Rawlinson VI, Merry AH, and Stratton F, 1980. Positive direct antiglobulin test in normal individuals. Vox Sangiunis, 38: 99–105.

Issitt PD and Pavone BG. 1978. Critical re-examination of the specificity of auto-anti-Rh antibodies in patients with a positive direct antiglobulin test. Brit J Haematol, 38: 63–74.

Mair TS, Taylor FG, and Hillyer MH. 1990. Autoimmune haemolytic anaemia in eight horses. Vet Rec, 126: 51.

McConnico RS, Roberts MC, and Tompkins M. 1992. Penicillin-induced immune-mediated hemolytic anemia in a horse. J Am Vet Med Assoc, 201: 1402–1403.

McGovern KF, Lascola KM, Davis E, Fredrickson RL, and Tan R. 2011. T-cell lymphoma with immune-mediated anemia and thrombocytopenia in a horse. J Vet Int Med, 25: 1181–1185.

Messer NT and Arnold K, 1991. Immune-mediated hemolytic anemia in a horse. J Am Vet Med Assoc, 198: 1415–1416.

Michel M, 2011. Classification and therapeutic approaches in autoimmune hemolytic anemia: an update. Exp Rev Hematol, 4: 607–618.

Reef VB, Dyson SS, and Beech J. 1984. Lymphosarcoma and associated immune-mediated hemolytic anemia and thrombocytopenia in horses. J Am Vet Med Assoc, 184: 313–317.

Roback JD, Barclay S, and Hillyer CD. 2004. Improved method for fluorescence cytometric immunohematology testing. Transfusion, 44: 187–196.

Robbins RL, Wallace SS, Brunner CJ, Gardner TR, DiFranco BJ, and Speirs VC. 1993. Immune-mediated haemolytic disease after penicillin therapy in a horse. Eq Vet J, 25: 462–465.

Salama A. 2009. Drug-induced immune hemolytic anemia. Exp Opin Drug Safety, 8: 73–79.

Segel GB and Lichtman MA. 2014. Direct antiglobulin ("Coombs") test-negative autoimmune hemolytic anemia: a review. Blood Cells, Mol, Disease, 52: 152–60.

Shulman IA, Branch DR, Nelson JM, Thompson JC, Saxena S, and Petz LD. 1985. Autoimmune hemolytic anemia with both cold and warm autoantibodies. J Am M Association, 253: 1746–1748.

Sockett DC, Traub-Dargatz J, and Weiser MG. 1987. Immune-mediated hemolytic anemia and thrombocytopenia in a foal. J Am Vet Med Assoc, 190: 308–310.

Sokol RJ, Hewitt S, Booker DJ, and Stamps R. 1985. Enzyme linked direct antiglobulin tests in patients with autoimmune haemolysis. J Clin Pathol, 38: 912–914.

Thedsawad A, Taka O, and Wanachiwanawin W, 2001. Development of flow cytometry for detection and quantitation of red cell bound immunoglobulin G in autoimmune hemolytic anemia with negative direct Coombs test. Asian Pacific J Allergy and Immunol, 29: 364–367.

Thomas HL and Livesey MA. 1998. Immune-mediated hemolytic anemia associated with trimethoprim-sulphamethoxazole administration in a horse. Can Vet J, 39: 171–173.

Wang Z, Shi J, Zhou Y, and Ruan C. 2001. Detection of red blood cell-bound immunoglobulin G by flow cytometry and its application in the diagnosis of autoimmune hemolytic anemia. Int J Hematol, 73: 188–193.

Weiss DJ and Moritz A. 2003. Equine immune-mediated hemolytic anemia associated with *Clostridium perfringens* infection. Vet Clin Pathol, 32: 22–26.

Wilkerson MJ, Davis E, Shuman W, Harkin K, Cox J, and Rush B, 2000. Isotype-specific antibodies in horses and dogs with immune-mediated hemolytic anemia. J Vet Int Med, 4: 190–196.

Zantek ND, Koepsell SA, Tharp DR Jr, and Cohn CS. 2012. The direct antiglobulin test: a critical step in the evaluation of hemolysis. Am J Hematol, 87: 707–709.

42

Equine Neonatal Isoerythrolysis

Julia B. Felippe

Cornell University, College of Veterinary Medicine, New York, USA

42.1 Clinical Background

Neonatal isoerythrolysis (NI) is an acquired form of immune-mediated hemolytic anemia in the foal that develops within hours to a few days of life, and involves the absorption from colostrum of maternally-derived alloantibodies against cell surface molecules expressed on the red blood cells of the foal. The absorbed anti-erythrocyte antibodies cause red blood cell agglutination, extravascular hemolysis, and, potentially, intravascular hemolysis (Becht, 1983, Becht et al., 1983).

This condition is more common in foals born to multiparous mares and in mules, and only manifests after the ingestion of colostrum for there is no transfer of antibodies during gestation in the mare; NI may happen even where there is partial transfer of antibodies through colostrum (i.e., foal serum IgG less than 800 mg/dL) (Scott and Jeffcott, 1978, Traub-Dargatz et al., 1995, Boyle et al., 2005).

Clinical signs vary depending on the severity of hemolysis, likely associated with the amount of red blood cell-specific antibodies absorbed; the closer to the first ingestion of colostrum the clinical signs are detected (e.g., 12 h of life), the more severe tends to be the hemolysis, which also progresses with time (i.e., within the initial 5–7 days of life) (Polkes et al., 2008). The most common clinical signs include depression, weakness, lethargy, lack of nursing, tachycardia, tachypnea, icteric or pale mucous membranes, anemia with normal total protein, metabolic acidosis due to poor tissue oxygenation, hyperbilirubinemia, hemoglobulinemia, and hemoglobinuria. In severe cases, pigmentary nephropathy, azotemia, tissue inflammation due to hypoxia (central nervous system, gastro-intestinal tract, liver), fever, seizures, and death occur. In addition, kernicterus or bilirubin encephalopathy may lead to severe depression, opisthotonus, rigidity, convulsions and death due to the deposition of unconjugated bilirubin (higher risk when blood unconjugated bilirubin concentration greater than 20 mg/dl), and necrosis of cerebral gray matter (Loynachan et al., 2007). Rarely, NI and alloimmune neutropenia may happen in the same patient (Wong et al., 2012).

The mule inherits the red blood cell factor (donkey factor) from the sire, which is incompatible with the mare's in 100% of pregnancies (Traub-Dargatz et al., 1995, Boyle et al., 2005). Nevertheless, the incidence of clinical NI is estimated as 10%, yet a higher incident of subclinical NI is possible; this incidence is still higher than the one in horse foals (1–2%) (Saint-Martin, 1952, McClure et al., 1994). Alloimmune thrombocytopenia may accompany NI, particularly in mules, when antibodies against platelet antigens are also transferred through colostrum, and signs include petechiae and echymoses, hematomas, hemorrhage, hemoarthroses, and hemoperitoneum.

Proteins expressed of the surface of red blood cells define blood groups, and function as antigens for the production of antibodies when the recipient's red blood cells lack that antigen. Alloantibodies are produced by the dam during gestation under specific conditions:

1) a gestation in which the fetus inherited antigenic red blood cell surface molecules from the sire that are incompatible to the dam's (i.e., incompatibility between the mare's and the sire's/foal's blood type) (Figure 42.1);
2) the mare is exposed to the fetus blood (perhaps in the case of placentitis or during parturition), which provides the antigenic stimulation for the antibody production against these factors;
3) these antibodies may not reach colostral levels in time to be absorbed and cause a clinical effect in the inciting foal; however, in the following pregnancies, the mare may transfer through the colostrum high levels of antibodies against that blood factor;

Interpretation of Equine Laboratory Diagnostics, First Edition. Edited by Nicola Pusterla and Jill Higgins.

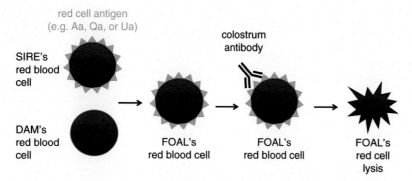

Figure 42.1 Incompatible blood types between the mare and the stallion predisposes to neonatal isoerythrolysis. When the sire's red blood cells express surface proteins that are not shared by the dam, the foal has a chance to inherit these proteins on their red blood cells. During gestation, the dam develops antibodies against the foal antigens, and transfers them to the colostrum. When that foal or a subsequent gestation foal (more likely) expressing the same incompatible antigen absorbs the antibodies in the colostrum, red blood cells become coated by these antibodies and hemolysis occurs.

4) a foal from a subsequent gestation is at risk of NI when it expresses the blood factor inherited from the sire with the same incompatibility with the blood type to the mare, and absorbs adequate amount of colostrum containing these maternal antibodies;

5) an exception to this sequence of events, and the possibility of neonatal isoerythrolysis in the immediate pregnancy happens when the mare received in the past blood transfusion of an incompatible blood type that is the same of the foal.

42.2 Diagnosis and Prevention of NI

Diagnosis of NI is based on demonstration of maternally-derived alloantibodies attached to the foal's red blood cells, often using direct antiglobulin test plus the presence of anti-erythrocyte antibodies in the mare's serum (and colostrum when available) using a hemolytic assay. Importantly, NI can be predicted and prevented when testing for incompatibility of blood factors expressed on the dam's and sire's red blood cells, and the presence of anti-erythrocyte antibodies in the mare's serum and colostrum using a hemolytic assay or a cross-match test, in the last month of pregnancy; if performed more than once during this period, a rising titer (e.g., from 1:4 serum dilution to 1:16 or greater) indicates an increase in the risk of NI.

42.3 Tests Available

There are two major groups of tests to detect antibodies against red blood cell antigens in serum or colostrum, and antibody-coated red blood cells: complement-mediated hemolytic tests and agglutination tests.

42.4 Sample Collection and Submission

Clinical diagnosis of NI starts with a supporting history of previous cases involving the same mare, clinical signs of anemia and a complete blood cell count of the foal. In most cases, a complete blood cell count and peripheral smear using blood samples preserved in ethylenediaminetetracetic acid (EDTA) anti-coagulant may indicate moderate to marked anemia (e.g., hematocrit < 25%, possibly < 15%). Clinical signs in the foal may not be apparent until the anemia is severe.

For blood factor assays (blood typing), a whole blood sample (e.g., mare, sire, blood donor) is collected in EDTA and shipped to a specialized laboratory; blood samples collected in anticoagulant citrate dextrose (ACD) solution can be processed within a week.

For screening anti-erythrocyte antibodies in the mare using a hemolytic assay, a serum sample (minimum 2 ml) is required.

The cross-match test can be run between the dam's serum and foal whole blood collected in EDTA or ACD, or between the dam's serum and the sire's whole blood. In addition, a blood donor can be cross-matched with the foal.

The jaundice foal agglutination test requires foal whole blood preserved in EDTA, and serial two-fold dilutions of mare's colostrum or serum.

A direct antiglobulin test requires foal whole blood sample preserved in EDTA.

All samples should be shipped overnight with an ice pack inside of an insulated box.

42.5 Blood Factor Assays (Blood Typing)

Blood groups are defined by inherited proteins on the surface of the red blood cells, and can function as antigens when exposed to an individual negative for that protein during a blood transfusion or pregnancy. There are seven distinct blood groups (cell surface antigens A, C, D, K, P, Q, and U) in the horse, and each blood group has additional antigenic molecules (defined 34 blood factors). The antigens Aa and Qa are responsible for more than 90% of the neonatal isoerythrolysis in horses (MacLeay, 2001). Other antigens associated with less frequent cases of NI include Ab, Ac, Da, Dc, Df, Dg, Ka, Pa, Pb, Qa, Qb, Qc, and Ua (Zaruby et al., 1992, MacLeay, 2001, Boyle, 2005). Therefore, all breeds can be affected but with different levels of incidence of disease (about 20% of Thoroughbred and Standardbred mares are negative for Aa; Qa is rare in Quarter Horses and Standardbreds; the risk of NI is high in Friesians) (Bailey, 1982, Bailey et al., 1988).

Blood factor assays test for the presence or absence of incompatible factors on the red blood cells of the dam and sire any time before breeding. Blood typing of mare and sire (stallion or jack) can be useful to prevent NI and plan breeding. Currently, blood factor tests include the following antigens: A (a,b,c), Ca, Ka, P (a,b), Q (a,b,c), and Ua.

Mares that are negative for Aa, Qa or a blood factor for which the stallion is positive for can transfer antibodies against these factors to the foal through colostrum. Subsequent breeding with the same sire, or sires with the same blood type of the inciting factor increases the chances of NI in the offspring. Therefore, mares with a history of offspring with NI should be tested and managed to prevent future cases. If a mare is negative for blood factors, a stallion also with negative antigen expression can be matched for the breeding. Sera from mares with mule pregnancies present hemolytic activity against donkey and mule red blood cells (McClure et al., 1994).

If the dam is positive for one of the blood groups, there is no risk for that specific blood group. If the sire is negative for these blood groups, there is no risk for the disease.

42.6 Complement-Mediated Hemolytic Assay

Hemolytic assay (Figure 42.2) is the preferred method to test for the presence of antibodies in the mare's serum against the blood factors, and assess the risk and support the diagnosis of NI because it offers objective analysis and better performance in samples with low levels of antibodies.

For the prevention of NI, the test should be run at 30 days and 15 days before the due date. The test can also be used to support the diagnosis of NI.

Different dilutions of the serum from the mare are mixed with red blood cells expressing different antigens (e.g., Aa or Qa, or other factors available in the

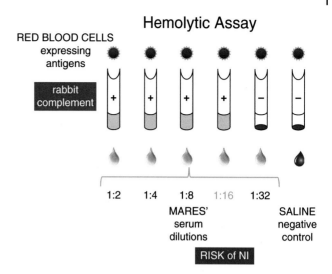

Figure 42.2 Hemolytic assay to detect serum antibodies against red blood cell surface proteins. Different two-fold dilutions (1:2 to 1:32) of the serum from the mare are mixed with red blood cells expressing different antigens (e.g., Aa or Qa). If antibodies are present in the mare's serum, they bind to the red blood cells and, after adding exogenous complement, red blood cell lysis is induced. A negative control uses saline instead of mare's serum. Serum dilutions above 1:16 for Aa and Qa that cause hemolysis *in vitro* may produce NI; therefore, withholding of the colostrum is recommended. Antibodies to Aa and Qa factors detected at 1:2 serum dilution require retest before foaling.

laboratory). If antibodies are present in the mare's serum, they bind to the red blood cells and, after adding exogenous complement, red blood cell lysis is induced. Cell lysis intensity is determined from 0–4, and the last dilution of serum that promoted cell lysis is identified. Serum dilutions above 1:16 for Aa and Qa that cause hemolysis *in vitro* may produce NI; therefore, withholding of the colostrum is recommended. Antibodies to Aa and Qa factors detected at 1:2 serum dilution require retest before foaling.

42.7 Cross-Match

A cross-match test can also be used to investigate an NI condition. A cross-match can detect a blood group incompatibility that is not used routinely in the screening panel. In addition, the mare' serum can be cross-matched with the sire's red blood cells: a negative reaction indicates no risk for the foal; a positive reaction indicates a 50% risk of NI, and a cross-match test should be done at foaling or colostrum withheld.

In the need of blood transfusion, the foal can be treated with the dam's washed red blood cells, or blood from a donor negative for the antigens causing the hemolysis (e.g., Aa and Qa negative, which are the most common involved blood factors). The cross-match test measures compatibility of red blood cells between the recipient and the donor beyond standard blood typing, with the goal to prevent post-transfusion red blood cell lysis and reactions. A major cross-match, the most relevant in blood transfusion, measures the presence of antibodies in the serum or plasma of the recipient's using the red blood cells of the donor. A minor cross-match measures the presence of antibodies in the serum or plasma of the donor's using the red blood cells of the recipient. A minor cross-match at the time of foaling can also test for the presence of dam's colostrum or serum antibodies against the foal red blood cells.

A positive test is considered when hemolysis occurs and indicates the presence of antibodies in the serum against red blood cell surface molecules. A scale of hemolysis is used for assessment: 1+ slight; 2+ moderate; 3+ severe hemolysis. If performed more than once before foaling, a rising titer (e.g., from 1:4 serum dilution to 1:16 or greater) indicates an increase in the risk of NI; consequently, colostrum should not be accessible to the foal and an alternate source of antibodies should be provided. A positive hemolytic test can also help diagnosing NI when a direct anti-globulin test is falsely negative (Boyle et al., 2005). False-negative results of direct antiglobulin tests occur when bound serum anti-erythrocyte antibody concentration is too low to cause enough cross-linking for agglutination to occur, or in excess of antigenic molecules on red blood cells, preventing obvious agglutination.

A negative test without hemolysis suggests the absence of antibodies in the serum against red blood cell surface molecules. False-negative tests may occur when the levels of antibodies are too low to cause hemolysis; therefore, a sample collected from the mare timely close to parturition offers the best assessment.

Cross-match can also be performed for agglutination, and a scale is used for assessment: 1+ weak or transient agglutination of red blood cells; 2+ microscopic small agglutinins; 3+ microscopic large agglutinin; and 4+ gross agglutination.

42.8   Direct Antiglobulin Test

Direct antiglobulin test (DAT, or direct Coombs' test) measures the presence of antibody- and/or complement-coated red blood cells. Washed red blood cells from the foal are incubated with a polyvalent antibody reagent (anti-IgG, anti-IgM, and anti-complement) at 37 °C. A positive agglutination does not specify the target (blood factor) for the antibody on red blood cells and, therefore, is not specific for the diagnosis of immune-mediated hemolytic anemia. A positive result should be interpreted along with the clinical history.

42.9   Jaundice Foal Agglutination Test

The jaundice foal agglutination test (Figure 42.3) is a crude method for the detection of antibodies in the colostrum against the foal's red blood cells, and should be run at parturition, before the ingestion of colostrum. In this test, two-fold dilutions of the dam's colostrum with saline (1 ml of 1:2 to 1:32 dilutions) are mixed with 1 drop of the foal's whole blood. A 1 ml saline is used as a negative control, and the mare's blood may be tested in the same conditions as another negative control. The presence of agglutination of the red blood cells may be observed after centrifugation for 2–3 min at a medium speed and inversion of the tubes. This test has also been performed on a glass slide when a centrifuge is not available.

Agglutination present at 1:16 or higher dilutions is considered positive and the foal should not ingest the colostrum from his dam. Caution should be taken with the interpretation of the results when using this test because of its simplicity (i.e., skipping the washing step of the testing red blood cells to remove serum proteins) and low sensitivity and specificity of agglutination tests. Agglutination tests may present dubious analysis (e.g., in the case of rouleaux formation) and are more dependent

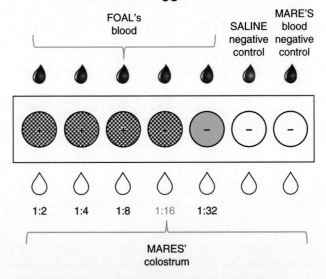

Figure 42.3 Jaundice foal agglutination test. This detects antibodies in the colostrum against the foal's red blood cells, and should be run at parturition, before the ingestion of colostrum. In this test, two-fold dilutions of the dam's colostrum with saline (1 ml of 1:2 to 1:32 dilutions) are mixed with one drop of the foal's whole blood. A 1 ml saline is used as a negative control, and the mare's blood may be tested under the same conditions as another negative control. The test can be performed in tubes for centrifugation or on a glass slide.

on an equivalent concentration of antibodies (in the mare's serum) and antigens (expressed on the red blood cells of the foal) for accuracy.

42.10 Clinical Case

A 7-day-old Warmblood colt presented with icterus, tachycardia, tachypnea, lethargy, and a mild systolic heart murmur. He nursed well and blood IgG concentration was greater than 800 mg/dL, indicating adequate passive transfer of antibodies through the colostrum. Blood hematocrit was measured at 9%, along with markedly decreased hemoglobin 5.0 g/dL, normal total protein 5.9. mg/dL, mildly elevated indirect bilirubin 3.8 mg/dL, and markedly elevated lactate 8.13 mmol/L. Age, clinical signs and blood work were suggestive of neonatal isoerythrolysis; a direct antiglobulin test was not performed.

Blood transfusion was indicated based on the low hematocrit and high lactate. Major cross-match test of patient's serum and donor#1 red blood cells revealed no agglutination and no hemolysis (compatible). Minor cross-match test of recipient red blood cells and donor#1 serum revealed grade 3+ agglutination and no hemolysis (incompatible). Because the major cross-match was compatible, washed red blood cells of the donor could still be used for transfusion to the patient. Nevertheless, two other donors were cross-matched with the patient, and result for donor#2 for major cross-match was no agglutination and no hemolysis (compatible) and for minor cross-match 1+ agglutination and no hemolysis (inconclusive); and for donor#3 major cross-match 1+ agglutination and no hemolysis (inconclusive), and minor cross match 3+ agglutination and no hemolysis (incompatible).

Blood transfusion was performed with blood from donor#2, which improved the hematocrit to 14% after 1 l, and to 19% after the second l. He was also treated with broad spectrum antibiotic therapy for 5 days. Lactate levels decreased gradually to 4.82, 2.42, and 1.64 mmol/l within 16 h post-transfusion. On the following day, hematocrit was 22% and lactate normal at 1.22 mmol/l; 3 days later hematocrit was 26% and indirect bilirubin still mildly elevated at 5.0 mg/dl. The foal had a complete recovery of the anemia in the subsequent days.

References

Bailey E. 1982. Prevalence of anti-red blood cell antibodies in the serum and colostrum of mares and its relationship to neonatal isoerythrolysis. Am J Vet Res, 43: 1917–1921.

Bailey E, Albright DG, and Henney PJ. 1988. Equine neonatal isoerythrolysis: Evidence for prevention by maternal antibodies to the Ca blood group antigen. Am J Vet Res, 49: 1218–1222.

Becht JL. 1983. Neonatal isoerythrolysis in the foal, Part I. Background, blood group antigens, and pathogenesis. Comp Cont Ed, 5: S5591.

Becht JL, Page EH, Morter RL, Boon GD, and Thacker HL. 1983. Evaluation of a series of testing procedures to predict neonatal isoerythrolysis in the foal. Cornell Vet, 73: 390–402.

Boyle AG, Magdesian KG, and Ruby RE. 2005. Neonatal isoerythrolysis in horse foals and a mule foal: 18 cases (1988–2003). J Am Vet Med Assoc, 227: 1276–1283.

Loynachan AT, Williams NM, and Freestone JF. 2007. Kernicterus in a neonatal foal. J Vet Diagn Invest, 19: 209–212.

MacLeay JM 2001. Neonatal isoerythrolysis involving the Qc and Db antigens in a foal. J Am Vet Med Assoc, 219: 79–81.

McClure JJ, Koch C, and Traub-Dargatz J. 1994. Characterization of a red blood cell antigen in donkeys and mules associated with neonatal isoerythrolysis. Anim. Genet. 25: 119–120.

Polkes AC, Giguère S, Lester GD, and Bain FT. 2008. Factors associated with outcome in foals with neonatal isoerythrolysis (72 cases, 1988–2003). J Vet Int Med, 22: 1216–1222.

Saint-Martin A. 1952. Prophylaxie et traitement de l'ictere dur nuleton. Revue de Médecine Vétérinaire, 103: 263–268.

Scott AM and Jeffcott LB. 1978. Haemolytic disease of the newborn foal. Vet Rec, 103: 71–74.

Traub-Dargatz JL, McClure JJ, Koch C, and Schlipf JW. 1995. Neonatal isoerythrolysis in mule foals. J Am Vet Med Assoc, 206: 67–70.

Wong DM, Alcott CJ, Clark SK, Jones DE, Fisher PG, and Sponseller BA. 2012. Alloimmune neonatal neutropenia and neonatal isoerythrolysis in a Thoroughbred colt. J Vet Diagn Invest, 24: 219–226.

Zaruby JF, Hearn P, and Colling D. 1992. Neonatal isoerythrolysis in a foal involving anti-Pa alloantibody. Eq Vet J, 24: 71–73.

43

Immune-Mediated Thrombocytopenia

Julia B. Felippe

Cornell University, College of Veterinary Medicine, New York, USA

43.1 Clinical Background

Immune-mediated thrombocytopenia (IMT) results from the production and binding of antibodies to platelet or megakaryocyte surface antigens, or from the binding of immunocomplexes (antibodies against microorganisms, or a drug hapten) to the Fc receptors on platelets. When the antibodies are produced by the patient due to hypersensitivity reaction type II, the condition is known as auto-immune thrombocytopenia (AIT). These antibodies (alone or along with complement) bind to platelets, and promote their rapid removal and/or destruction by the mononuclear phagocyte (reticuloendothelial) system, involving macrophages in the spleen and liver that phagocytose the platelets via their Fc and complement receptors. When destruction is greater than production, or when antibodies bind platelet precursors, the resulting clinical thrombocytopenia can be life-threatening. The mechanism for autoantibody production may involve autoreactive B cell clones that are stimulated during an immune response to infectious organisms, dysfunction in CD4+ T cell regulation of B cell response, antigenic mimicry, or altered anti-idiotypic regulation of antibody production.

Clinical signs include hemorrhagic diathesis characterized by epistaxis, prolonged bleeding from injection sites, mucosal petechiae and ecchymosis, hematomas, occult blood in urine and feces, melena, hemoarthritis, hyphema, and intracavitary hemorrhage.

Immune-mediated thrombocytopenia is classified as primary (idiopathic) or secondary to other disorders, including infectious agents (e.g., equine infectious anemia, *Clostridium* spp.); drug-induced (e.g., penicillin, sulfonamides, erythromycin, heparin, quinidine, thiazides, digoxin), or neoplasia (e.g., lymphosarcoma) (Byears and Greene, 1982, Larson et al., 1983, Reef et al.,

1984, Sockett et al., 1987, Clabough et al., 1991, Cohen et al., 1991, McGovern et al., 2011, Dunkel, 2013, Väänänen et al., 2013). Rarely, immune-mediated thrombocytopenia and anemia may happen in the same patient, a condition known as Evan's syndrome (Väänänen et al., 2013).

Differential diagnoses include non-immune-mediated causes of thrombocytopenia, for example, decreased megakaryopoiesis in malignancy, toxicity or infections; increased peripheral platelet consumption observed in hemorrhage, vasculitis and disseminated intravascular coagulopathy; platelet sequestration in splenomegaly; and dilution with administration of large amounts of fluids.

Two conditions studied in human medicine but not well reported in horses include heparin-induced thrombocytopenia (HIT) and post-transfusion purpura (PTP). HIT has been observed in 0.5–5% of patients 5–10 days after receiving therapeutic unfractionated or low-molecular weight heparin; in this condition, IgG auto-antibodies that recognize complexes of platelet-factor 4 bound to heparin engage platelet Fc receptors, and promote strong platelet activation and destruction (Warkentin, 2011). In PTP, clinical signs develop 5–14 days after platelet transfusion in patients who have received previous blood or platelet-enriched plasma transfusions, or in patients who had a previous pregnancy with a fetus of incompatible platelet type (Taaning et al., 1999).

Major and minor antigens are expressed on the surface of platelets. These glycoproteins are encoded by polymorphic genes and serve as alloantigens when there is incompatibility among individuals during blood transfusion or pregnancy. In equids, there is limited knowledge about platelet membrane alloantigens, and gene sequences with their respective predicted amino acid have been studied for platelet membrane glycoproteins Ia (integrin subunit a2),

Interpretation of Equine Laboratory Diagnostics, First Edition. Edited by Nicola Pusterla and Jill Higgins.
© 2018 John Wiley & Sons, Inc. Published 2018 by John Wiley & Sons, Inc.

Iba, IIb, and IIIa (integrin subunits aIIb and b3) in Holsteiner-Oldenburg cross, Quarter Horse, and Thoroughbred breeds, donkey, and zebra (Boudreaux and Humphries, 2013). Differences in amino acid sequences in these samples were identified, and they support the involvement of platelet alloantigens in transfusion reactions and neonatal alloimmune thrombocytopenia; however, larger sets of individuals in a species and breed are needed to better understand population polymorphism and frequency of platelet alloantigens, development of diagnostics, and calculation of clinical risks of disease.

43.2   Tests Available

Diagnosis of IMT is based on the demonstration of antibodies and/or complement bound to platelets along with clinical evidence of thrombocytopenia. Diagnostic tests for IMT help with determining prognosis, severity of disease, and duration of treatment. The fact that platelets express Fc receptors that can bind to antibodies nonspecifically challenges the specificity of tests that use antibody reagents.

43.3   Sample Collection and Submission

In most cases, a complete blood count and smear using peripheral blood samples preserved in ethylenediaminetetracetic acid (EDTA) anti-coagulant may indicate thrombocytopenia. The result should be confirmed with an automated and manual platelet count using a sample preserved in citrate anticoagulant in order to rule out pseudothrombocytopenia.

A coagulation panel should also be run to investigate for potential causes of nonimmune-mediated peripheral consumption of platelets; a blood sample collected directly into a citrate tube can be centrifuged for 15 min, and the plasma transferred to a clean plastic tube for shipping overnight on ice to a specialized veterinary laboratory.

For the possibility of equine infectious anemia, in which intermittent thrombocytopenia occurs concomitantly to viremic states, a Coggin's test is run using a serum sample from the patient (Crawford et al., 1996).

Direct immunofluorescence flow cytometry that test for the presence of antibody-bound platelet requires whole blood samples collected in EDTA, and shipped within 24 h.

Laboratorial diagnosis of drug-induced thrombocytopenia (DIT) in horses is available for penicillin, and requires a serum sample. In human medicine, these laboratorial tests are challenged by low sensitivity and the lack of standardization and validation across a range of assays (flow cytometry, platelet suspension immunofluorescence test, enzyme immunoassays, radiolabeled antiglobulin-based assays) and drugs. The desired test should provide sensitivity (i.e., patient's serum plus test drug or metabolite produce a measurable effect on test platelets) and specificity (i.e., neither non-implicated drugs nor serum from non-thrombocytopenic controls produce the effect to detect the presence of antibodies in the patient's serum) (Arnold et al., 2013).

Platelet glycoproteins can be potentially determined in individuals using molecular assays, gene sequencing, and amino acid determination in research laboratories; however, further characterization of these proteins in equid populations is required for development of assays relevant to prevention and diagnostics in clinical cases.

43.4   Possible Results and Interpretation

In general, clinical signs of thrombocytopenia are not detectable until platelet counts are <40,000/μL, and spontaneous bleeding may occur when counts are <10,000/μL.

Megakaryocytic hyperplasia is an expected response to the platelet destruction in the periphery, and the presence of immature platelets in the circulation as an indicator of bone marrow platelet production to thrombocytopenia can be assessed by a blood smear. Flow cytometric analysis of platelet mRNA content in whole blood using thiazole orange can also asses thrombocytopoiesis, as young platelets have greater mRNA content than older cells; although this assay has acceptable sensitivity and specificity, the current guidelines in human medicine do not consider it essential to evaluate bone marrow thrombocytopoiesis (Neunert et al., 2011, Jiménez et al., 2006). The absence of megakaryocytic hyperplasia and/or immature platelets may indicate immune-mediated destruction of megakaryocytes or myelophthisic disease. Nevertheless, bone marrow evaluation is not a required component of the initial diagnostics when other hematologic abnormalities are not present (e.g., pancytopenia, leukemia) (Neunert et al., 2011).

In immune-mediated thrombocytopenia, a coagulation profile often reveals prolonged bleeding time, abnormal clot retraction, slightly prolonged activated coagulation, elevated fibrinogen degradation products (FDP), normal prothrombin time (PT), and normal activated partial thromboplastin time (APTT).

43.5 Direct Immunofluorescence Flow Cytometry

Flow cytometric analysis has been used to identify the presence of IgG-, IgM-, and IgA-coated platelets in immune-mediated thrombocytopenia of human and horse patients (Nunez et al., 2001, Davis et al., 2002, McGurrin et al., 2004, Tomer, 2006). The test consists of first washing platelets to remove unbound-antibodies present in the blood, adding a fluorescence-conjugated anti-IgG, anti-IgM, or anti-IgA, and reading the sample in a flow cytometer that measures positive and negative control cells. Approximately 10,000 platelets are screened, and results indicate the percentage of fluorescent positive (antibody-bound) platelets; in general, percent-positive cells detected in clinical patients are around 8–10%, whereas < 4% of platelets are positive in healthy controls. Human medicine guidelines do not recommend to exclusively measure platelet-associated antibody using flow cytometry because of the low specificity of the test, that is, inability to differentiate pathologic from non-pathologic platelet-associated antibodies (Neunert et al., 2011). The use of flow cytometry to determine epitope specific (e.g., CD41a and CD42 glycoproteins) anti-platelet antibodies has been used with superior sensitivity and specificity in human medicine (Tomer, 2006); these assays are not currently available for horses.

In flow cytometric tests, false-positive results are obtained when fluorescence-conjugated antibody-reagents (e.g., anti-horse IgG) bind directly but non-specifically to Fc receptors normally expressed on platelets; also, the antibody reagents can bind to a large number of non-specific bound antibodies, with a potential overlap with the actual anti-platelet antibodies (Figure 43.1). In addition, platelet alpha-granules contain, among other active proteins, IgG. Consequently, not every detected platelet-associated antibody is anti-platelet antibody and, because platelets acquire IgG by fluid phase endocytosis from plasma, total platelet IgG is consistently increased in patients with high blood IgG concentrations (George, 1991, Harrison and Cramer, 1993). Although the concentration of platelet-surface IgG is greatly increased in patients with AIT, modest elevations of platelet-surface IgG are also found in patients with non-immune mediated thrombocytopenia. False negative results may result when there are low numbers of antibody-coated platelets in the sample, or *in vivo* bound-antibodies are removed from platelets during the washing process.

43.6 Clinical Case

An 18-month-old Standardbred filly presented with fever (103.9 °F), moderately enlarged mandibular lymph nodes, thrombocytopenia, petechiae on the mucous membranes (gum, nasal mucosa and vulva), bilateral epistaxis, and mild grade (1–2) ataxia. Blood work revealed severe thrombocytopenia at 22,000 platelets/μL (confirmed 25,000 platelets/μL in manual count using a citrate sample), mature neutrophilia 10,100 cells/μL, and hyperfibrinogenemia 500 mg/dL. Coagulation test revealed slightly decreased APTT (35.4 seconds, reference interval 45–66 seconds), and PT (12.7, reference interval 16–20 s), and elevated D-dimer (2277 ng/mL, reference interval 0–1000 ng/mL), characterizing a hypercoagulable state.

A diagnosis of immune-mediated thrombocytopenia was suspected based on blood work and clinical signs, and the filly was treated with immunosuppressive therapy (azathioprine and dexamethasone), and gastric protectant (omeprazole).

Further diagnostic tests to investigate for a potential infectious inciting cause of the immune-mediated thrombocytopenia included polymerase chain reaction for *Anaplasma phagocytophilum* (negative), equine infectious anemia (Coggin's test negative), *Streptococcus equi* subspecies *equi* (SeM titer 1:800 moderate positive, suggesting infection in the past 2–3 weeks). A biopsy sample was collected from the mandibular lymph node, and histology revealed lymphoid hyperplasia, with numerous secondary follicles. Direct fluorescence flow cytometry detected the presence of a higher percentage of antibody-bound platelets in the patient's blood (IgG-bound 26%, IgM-bound 10%, IgA-bound 2%) than control samples (less than 4%), supporting the diagnosis of immune-mediated thrombocytopenia.

Over the subsequent days, the mucosal petechiae, fever and ataxia improved, along with the platelet count (164,000 cells/μL), neutrophilia (7200 cells/μL), and fibrinogen (100 mg/dL). The azathioprine and dexamethasone treatments were continued for a total of 30 days, with the dexamethasone doses tapered gradually by 20% after every fourth dose.

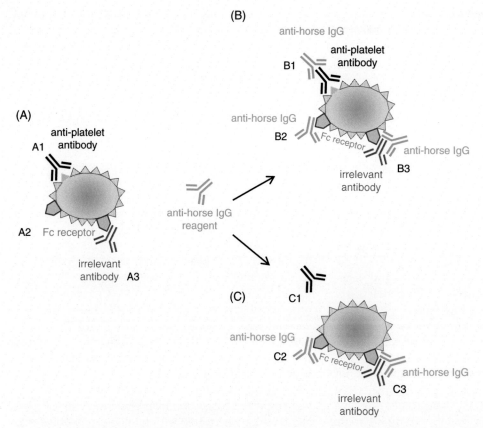

Figure 43.1 Direct immunofluorescence flow cytometry to detect antibody-coated platelets. Flow cytometric analysis identifies the presence of IgG-, IgM-, and IgA-coated platelets. Platelets from the patient are washed to remove unbound-antibodies present in the blood, and a fluorescence-conjugated anti-IgG, anti-IgM, or anti-IgA is added for subsequent reading using a flow cytometer. (A) Platelets from the patient may be coated by (A1) auto-immune antibodies that recognize a self cell-surface molecule or (A3) irrelevant antibodies may bind non-specifically to Fc receptors on the surface of platelets; in addition, (A2) Fc receptors may be *free* of antibodies. When fluorescence-conjugated anti-horse immunoglobulin is added to the platelet solution, (B) the reagent may (B1) bind specifically to an autoantibody recognizing a self-antigen (true positive results), (B2) bind non-specifically to a Fc receptor (false-negative), or (B3) bind to an antibody linked non-specifically to a Fc receptor (false-positive). (C) In addition, in a true-negative sample, there is no (C1) auto-antibody bound to a platelet self-antigen; yet, positive fluorescence is obtained with antibody reagent binding to (C2) an empty Fc receptor or (C3) an non-specific antibody bound to a Fc receptor. Consequently, not all detected platelet-associated antibody is anti-platelet antibody.

References

Arnold DM, Kukaswadia S, Nazi I, Esmail A, Dewar L, and Smith JW, et al. 2013. A systematic evaluation of laboratory testing for drug-induced immune thrombocytopenia. J Thrombo Haemost, 11: 169–176.

Boudreaux MK and Humphries DM. 2013. Identification of potential platelet alloantigens in the Equidae family by comparison of gene sequences encoding major platelet membrane glycoproteins. Vet Clin Pathol, 42: 437–442.

Byears TD and Greene CE. 1982. Idiopathic thrombocytopenic purpura in the horse. J Am Vet Med Assoc, 180: 1422–1424.

Clabough DL, Gebhard D, Flaherty MT, Whetter LE, Perry ST, Coggins L, and Fuller FJ. 1991. Immune-mediated thrombocytopenia in horses infected with equine infectious anemia virus. J Virol, 65: 6242–6251.

Cohen ND and Carter GK. 1991. Persistent thrombocytopenia in a case of equine infectious anemia. J Am Vet Med Assoc, 199: 750–752.

Crawford TB, Wardrop KJ, Tornquist SJ, Reilich E, Meyers KM, and McGuire TC. 1996. A primary production deficit in the thrombocytopenia of equine infectious anemia. J Virol, 70: 7842–7850.

Davis EG, Wilkerson MJ, and Rush BR. 2002. Flow cytometry: clinical applications in equine medicine. J Vet Int Med, 16: 404–410.

Dunkel B. 2013. Platelet transfusion in thrombocytopenic horses. Eq Vet Ed, 25(7): 359–362.

George JN 1991. Platelet IgG: measurement, interpretation, and clinical significance. Prog Hemost Thrombo, 10: 97–126.

Harrison P and Cramer EM. 1993. Platelet alpha-granules. Blood Rev, 7: 52–62.

Jiménez MM, Guedán MJ, Martín LM, Campos JA, Martínez IR, and Vilella CT. 2006. Measurement of reticulated platelets by simple flow cytometry: An indirect thrombocytopoietic marker. Eur J Int Med, 17: 541–544.

Larson VL, Perman V, and Stevens JB. 1983. Idiopathic thrombocytopenic purpura in two horses. J Am Vet Med Assoc, 183: 328–330.

McGovern KF, Lascola KM, Davis E, Fredrickson RL, and Tan R. 2011. T-cell lymphoma with immune-mediated anemia and thrombocytopenia in a horse. J Vet Int Med, 25: 1181–1185.

McGurrin MK, Arroyo LG, and Bienzle D. 2004. Flow cytometric detection of platelet-bound antibody in three horses with immune-mediated thrombocytopenia. J Am Vet Med Assoc, 224: 83–87.

Neunert C, Lim W, Crowther M, Cohen A, Solberg Jr. L, and Crowther MA. 2011. The American Society of Hematology 2011 evidence-based practice guideline for immune thrombocytopenia. Blood, 117: 4190–4207.

Nunez R, Gomes-Keller MA, Schwarzwald C, and Feige K. 2011. Assessment of Equine Autoimmune Thrombocytopenia (EAT) by flow cytometry. BioMed Cent Blood Disord, 1: 1.

Reef VB, Dyson SS, and Beech J. 1984. Lymphosarcoma and associated immune-mediated hemolytic anemia and thrombocytopenia in horses. J Am Vet Med Assoc, 184: 313–317.

Sockett DC, Traub-Dargatz J, and Weiser MG. 1987. Immune-mediated hemolytic anemia and thrombocytopenia in a foal. J Am Vet Med Assoc, 190: 308–310.

Taaning E and Tonnesen F. 1999. Pan-reactive platelet antibodies in post-transfusion purpura. Vox Sanguinis, 76: 120–123.

Tomer A. 2006. Autoimmune thrombocytopenia: determination of platelet-specific autoantibodies by flow cytometry. Ped Blood and Cancer, 47: 697–700.

Väänänen L, Sihvo HK, and Hewetson M. 2013. Cerebral haemorrhage in a pregnant Standardbred mare with Evan's syndrome. Eq Vet Ed, 25: 353–358.

Warkentin TE 2011. How I diagnose and manage HIT. Hematol Am Soc Hematol Ed Prog, 2011: 143–149.

44

Neonatal Alloimmune Thrombocytopenia
Julia B. Felippe

Cornell University, College of Veterinary Medicine, New York, USA

44.1 Clinical Background

Neonatal alloimmune thrombocytopenia (NAIT) is a condition that involves alloantibodies absorbed through the colostrum produced by the mare against paternally inherited, incompatible surface molecules expressed on the foal's platelets. The condition happens when the dam is negative for the antigens expressed on the sire's platelets that are inherited by the foal. The alloantibodies, alone or along with complement, bind to platelets of the foal, and accelerate their removal and/or destruction. Thrombocytopenia develops despite platelet production by the foal because the binding of maternally-derived antibodies decreases platelet survival time to a few hours. This disease only manifests after the ingestion of colostrum for there is no transfer of antibodies during gestation in the mare. Theoretically, this condition should be more common in mules but it is likely underdiagnosed. In human medicine, severe alloimmune thrombocytopenia happens in a first pregnancy history in 50% of the cases, and risk of disease increases in subsequent pregnancies, but such data is not available for horses (Roberts and Murray, 2008).

NAIT is a transient but potentially life-threatening passive disease in an otherwise healthy newborn. Clinical signs manifest in the first week of life and include petechiations, extensive bleeding from injection sites, hematomas, hemoarthrosis, and hyphema. In human infants, intracranial hemorrhage with long-term neurodevelopmental sequelae happens in 15% of untreated newborns (Ghevaert et al., 2007). Differential diagnoses include sepsis, disseminated intravascular hemolysis, drug-induced thrombocytopenia, and myelophthisic disease. The risk for bleeding alleviates as colostral antibody levels drop, antibody-bound platelets are removed from circulation, and platelet numbers return to normal (Arnold et al., 2008).

In horses, NAIT has been described in a Quarter Horse foal with profound thrombocytopenia, which recovered after platelet-rich plasma and supportive therapy. Confirmation of the presence of platelet-bound immunoglobulins in the foal's blood and platelet-bindable antibodies in the mare's plasma and milk was accomplished using direct and indirect immunoradiometric assays (Buechner-Maxwell et al., 1997). In another report, transient ulcerative dermatitis, severe thrombocytopenia, and mild neutropenia were diagnosed in six newborn foals from four mares.

Flow cytometric platelet-bound immunoglobulin test was negative in a blood sample from one tested foal (Perkins et al., 2005). All foals improved after supportive treatment; the two mares with two affected foals each had subsequent healthy foals when an alternate source of colostrum was given. Experimentally-induced neonatal alloimmune thrombocytopenia in mule pregnancies was accomplished by immunization of dams during the last trimester of pregnancy with whole acid-citrate-dextrose-anticoagulated donkey blood; a non-immunized control group was used for comparison and mules did not develop thrombocytopenia after ingestion of colostrum (Ramirez et al., 1999). An indirect enzyme-linked immunosorbent assay demonstrated significantly higher concentration of platelet-bindable immunoglobulin G in serum from thrombocytopenic mule foals, compared with nonthrombocytopenic mule foals.

44.2 Tests Available

The diagnosis of NAIT is based on a markedly low platelet count in the newborn foal, laboratory tests that indicate foal-dam incompatibility for platelet-associated antigens (platelet typing), and the presence of antibodies in the plasma or serum of the dam (and foal after ingestion of colostrum) reactive against the foal and sire platelet antigens but not the dam's. A history of NAIT in previous pregnancies is supportive of the diagnosis.

44.3 Sample Collection and Submission

In most cases, a complete blood count and peripheral smear using blood samples preserved in ethylenediaminetetracetic acid (EDTA) anti-coagulant may indicate thrombocytopenia. The result should be confirmed with an automated and manual platelet count using a sample preserved in citrate anticoagulant in order to rule out pseudothrombocytopenia.

A coagulation panel investigates for potential causes of non-immune thrombocytopenia due to peripheral consumption of platelets; a blood sample collected directly into a citrate tube should be centrifuged for 15 min, and the plasma transferred to a clean plastic tube for shipping overnight on ice to a specialized veterinary laboratory.

Laboratory diagnosis of NAIT can be attempted by demonstrating the presence of antibody-bound platelets in the foal blood using flow cytometry, taking into consideration the limitations of the test.

44.4 Diagnosis and Prevention of NAIT

In contrast to neonatal isoerythrolysis, there is no routine screening test available to plan mare and sire breeding in order to prevent or anticipate the possibility of NAIT (Bussel and Sola-Visner, 2009). Platelet genotyping and phenotyping that determine the antigen expressed on platelets of the mare, sire, and foal are not available commercially for horses.

Ideally, a screening test would investigate platelet antigen incompatibility between dam and foal (typing), and the presence of antibodies in the mother's plasma or serum against a platelet-specific antigen (platelet-bindable antibody) expressed on the sire's platelets, and inherited by the foal (Kaplan, 2006). In human medicine, platelet-bindable antibodies are usually detected with antigen capture enzyme-linked immunosorbent assay (ELISA), and platelet phenotype and genotype of both parents and infant are accomplished with molecular techniques using an experienced reference laboratory, with appropriate controls (Kiefel et al., 1987, Kroll et al., 1998). Molecular assays also allow pre-natal tests of mother and father to predict the chances of alloimmune thrombocytopenia in the upcoming pregnancy.

Accordingly, NAIT is almost always identified in a newborn foal with signs of bleeding or incidentally when complete blood cell count is performed for other reasons (e.g., infection or sepsis). In mules or in foals with a history of NAIT in their siblings, platelet count may be proactively performed in the first week of life to verify for the condition. Any difficulties in confirming the diagnosis should not delay therapy when thrombocytopenia is life-threatening.

44.5 Possible Results and Interpretation

The diagnosis of NAIT is often made based on clinical history and signs of bleeding in the first 2 weeks of life, with the diagnostic exclusion on non-immune causes of thrombocytopenia. In general, clinical signs of thrombocytopenia are not detectable until platelet counts are <40,000/μL, and spontaneous bleeding may occur when counts are <10,000/μL.

In immune-mediated thrombocytopenia, a coagulation profile often reveals prolonged bleeding time, abnormal clot retraction, slightly prolonged activated coagulation, elevated fibrinogen degradation products (FDP), normal prothrombin time (PT), and normal activated partial thromboplastin time (APTT).

In addition, confirmation of diagnosis can be attempted by platelet aggregation and immunoradiometric assays using staphylococcal protein A to test for platelet-bindable antibody. The latter technique may reveal the absence of antibodies on the maternal platelets, circulating antibodies in the maternal plasma that bind foal and sire platelets, allotypic differences between dam and foal platelets, and/or the presence of antibodies in the dam's serum and colostrum against the foal and sire platelets.

Flow cytometric analysis has been used to identify the presence of IgG-, IgM-, and IgA-coated platelets in immune-mediated thrombocytopenia of human and horse patients (Nunez et al., 2001, Davis et al., 2002, Tomer 2006). The test consists of first washing platelets to remove unbound-antibodies present in the blood, adding a fluorescence-conjugated anti-IgG, anti-IgM or anti-IgA, and reading the sample in a flow cytometer. Approximately 10,000 platelets are screened, and results indicate the percentage of fluorescent positive (antibody-bound) platelets; in general, percentage-positive cells detected in patients are around 8–10%, whereas < 4% of platelets are positive in healthy controls. Human medicine guidelines do not recommend to exclusively measuring platelet-associated IgG because of the low specificity of the test, that is, to differentiate pathologic from non-pathologic platelet-associated antibody (Neunert et al., 2011).

The knowledge of platelet surface glycoproteins in the horse would help developing assays of greater specificity with antibody reagents that recognize these molecules.

In human medicine, the monoclonal antibody-specific immobilization of platelet antigens (MAIPA) tests for and quantifies serum platelet-bindable antibody in plasma against the patient platelets or a panel of platelets of known antigens, and in the presence of monoclonal antibodies (made in mice) against the most common glycoproteins expressed on human platelets; the test platelets are then solubilized and attached to microtiter plates coated with anti-murine IgG, and an ELISA procedure follows (Kiefel et al., 1987). The MAIPA test detects a trimolecular complex formed by the glycoprotein expressed on the platelet, the murine monoclonal antibody that recognizes this antigen, and the anti-platelet antibody present in the testing serum against the same antigen. When using a platelet panel with known alloantigens, test sera with multiple platelet reactive antibodies can be accurately characterized in a single test run. Platelet-bindable antibody levels in the mothers' plasma measured via MAIPA at delivery correlate inversely with the neonatal platelet count, with a clinical sensitivity and specificity of 93 and 63%, respectively, for risk of disease.

44.6 Clinical Case

A reported case in the literature describes a one-day-old Quarter Horse foal presented to a veterinary medical center with severe depression, inability to nurse, moderate dehydration, and diffusely swollen hind limbs (Buechner-Maxwell et al., 1997). An automated complete blood cell count revealed severe thrombocytopenia (13,000 platelets/uL), which was confirmed by manual count (9,000 platelets/uL). Prothrombin time and activated partial thromboplastin time were within normal reference ranges and comparable to an aged-matched healthy foal. The affected foal presented prolonged bleeding from venipuncture sites but did not show petechiae or swollen joints. Supportive therapy was provided with intravenous fluids and antibiotic. Three liters of platelet-rich plasma from a blood donor identified based on minor crossmatch compatibility initially improved the platelet count to 33,000 cells/uL, eliminated prolonged bleeding at venipuncture sites, and improved attitude, strength and nursing. Platelet counts varied from 14,000 to 188,000 in the 10 days post-transfusion. The foal recovered completely.

In this report, antibodies in the mare's plasma and milk were documented to bind to the foal's platelets using immunoradiometric assays. For the direct assessment of platelet-bound immunoglobulin, platelets harvested from blood samples preserved in citrate anticoagulant from the test and a control foal were washed with saline buffered solutions and incubated with radiolabeled staphylococcal protein A (SPA); after removing the excess, not-bound SPA with washes, the platelet-bound radioactivity (which correlates with platelet-bound antibody) was measured using a gamma counter. Using similar approach, an indirect assay detected high levels antibodies in the mare's plasma and milk that bound to the foal's platelets (i.e., platelet-bindable antibodies) but not normal control platelets, with 43 and 34 times greater levels in comparison to control plasma and milk, respectively. Platelet-bindable antibodies were also detected in the mare's plasma when using platelets of a full sibling foal born the year before. Nowadays, these tests are performed using fluorescence-conjugated reagents rather than radioisotopes.

References

Arnold DM, Smith JW, and Kelton JG. 2008. Diagnosis and management of neonatal alloimmune thrombocytopenia. Transfusion Med Rev, 22: 255–267.

Buechner-Maxwell V, Scott MA, Godber L, and Kristensen A. 1997. Neonatal alloimmune thrombocytopenia in a quarter horse foal. J Vet Intern Med, 11: 304–308.

Bussel JB and Sola-Visner M. 2009. Current approaches to the evaluation and management of the fetus and neonate with immune thrombocytopenia. Semin Perinatol, 33: 35–42.

Davis EG, Wilkerson MJ, and Rush BR. 2002. Flow cytometry: clinical applications in equine medicine. J Vet Intern Med, 16: 404–410.

Ghevaert C, Campbell K, Walton J, Smith GA, Allen D, Williamson LM, et al. 2007. Management and outcome of 200 cases of fetomaternal alloimmune thrombocytopenia. Transfusion, 47: 901–910.

Kaplan C. 2006. Foetal and neonatal alloimmune thrombocytopenia. Orphanet J Rare Dis, 1: 39.

Kiefel V, Santoso S, Weisheit M, and Mueller-Eckhardt C. 1987. Monoclonal antibody-specific immobilization of platelet antigens (MAIPA): A new tool for the identification of platelet-reactive antibodies. Blood, 70: 1722–1726.

Kroll H, Kiefel V, and Santoso S. 1998. Clinical aspects and typing of platelet alloantigens. Vox Sanguinis, 74: 345–354.

Neunert C, Lim W, Crowther M, Cohen A, Solberg L Jr, and Crowther MA. 2011. American Society of Hematology. The American Society of Hematology 2011 evidence-based practice guideline for immune thrombocytopenia. Blood. 117: 4190–4207.

Nunez R, Gomes-Keller MA, Schwarzwald C. and Feige K. 2001. Assessment of Equine Autoimmune Thrombocytopenia (EAT) by flow cytometry. BMC Blood Disord. 1:1.

Perkins GA, Miller WH, Divers TJ, Clark CK, Belgrave RL, and Sellon DC. 2005. Ulcerative dermatitis, thrombocytopenia, and neutropenia in neonatal foals. J Vet Intern Med, 19: 211–216.

Ramirez S, Gaunt SD, McClure JJ, and Oliver J. 1999. Detection and effects on platelet function of anti-platelet antibody in mule foals with experimentally induced neonatal alloimmune thrombocytopenia. J Vet Intern Med, 13: 534–539.

Roberts I and Murray NA. 2008. Neonatal thrombocytopenia. Semin Fetal and Neonatal Med, 13: 256–264.

Tomer A. 2002. Antiphospholipid antibody syndrome: rapid, sensitive, and specific flow cytometric assay for determination of anti-platelet phospholipid autoantibodies. J Lab Clin Med. 139: 147–154.

45

Cellular Immunity

Julia B. Felippe

Cornell University, College of Veterinary Medicine, New York, USA

45.1   Clinical Background

Immunodeficiency is a rare disorder of the immune system that results in failure to build protection against pathogens and, consequently, in the predisposition to recurrent or fatal infections.

The presence of infections and fevers is essential for the diagnosis of immunodeficiency, and recurrent episodes are supportive; in general, clinical signs are similar (fever, inflammatory blood work, system-related inflammatory signs), independent of the cause of the immunodeficiency. Every effort should be in place to identify the pathogen causing recurrent disease because the type of organism (i.e., bacterium, virus, fungus; encapsulated bacterium; opportunistic or highly virulent; intracellular versus extracellular) may suggest the impaired area of the immune system. Intracellular organisms take advantage of impaired cellular immunity to establish infection.

In equine neonates and weanlings, the clinical recognition of underlying primary cellular immunodeficiency may not be obvious because of the common presentation of infections at this age, the high frequency of failure of transfer of immunoglobulins through colostrum, and the physiologic, gradual development of the immune system (i.e., immune population expansion) that creates windows of susceptibility to infections.

45.2   Tests Available

Cellular immunodeficiencies are more difficult to diagnose and, therefore, apparently less prevalent in the horse. Testing immunologic parameters in a growing foal (i.e., less than 12 months of life) requires comparison with samples from an age-matched healthy foal, in order to account for physiologic and developmental parameters.

Peripheral blood lymphocyte absolute counts and subpopulation distributions reflect lymphoid tissue activity, as lymphocytes constantly circulate throughout the body. Cellular immune disorders more commonly affect CD4+ T cells, with implications to cytotoxic and/or humoral functions, depending on the underlying mechanism. Therefore, determining the distribution of CD4+ T cells, CD8+ T cells, and B cells in peripheral blood using immunophenotyping and flow cytometry may reflect unbalanced activity in the lymphoid tissues. In addition, the expression of major histocompatibility class II in lymphocytes can be used as a developmental marker, and this molecule has an age-dependent expression in the foal (Lunn et al., 1993).

Cytokines are soluble protein mediators secreted by cells involved in immunity and cell development (e.g., epithelial cells, stromal cells, immune cells). Cytokines modulate cell differentiation, activation or suppression, and their collective profile characterizes and defines an immune response at the site of inflammation. In inflammatory responses and autoimmunity, blood cytokines have been studied as biomarkers for disease severity and as target for therapy (O'Shea et al., 2002). Thus far, serum cytokine concentrations have limited applications for the diagnosis of immunodeficiencies.

Lymphocyte proliferation assays in response to mitogens or cell signaling stimulants (e.g., phytohemagglutinin, PHA; pokeweed, PWM; concanavalin A, ConA; phorbol 12-myristate 13-acetate plus ionomycin, PMAi) have been used to determine response to stimuli in vitro using carboxyfluorescein succinimidyl ester (CSFE) staining decay and flow cytometry. Results that would suggest impairment of cell proliferation are rarely observed in clinically immunodeficient patients (Flaminio et al., 2000, Felippe, personal observation). Therefore, the value

Interpretation of Equine Laboratory Diagnostics, First Edition. Edited by Nicola Pusterla and Jill Higgins.
© 2018 John Wiley & Sons, Inc. Published 2018 by John Wiley & Sons, Inc.

of proliferation assays is to induce and measure peak response of cytokines (e.g., interferon-gamma) or co-stimulatory molecules (e.g., CD40 ligand, CD28, MHC class II) upon stimulation in order to better understand potential mechanisms of cell dysfunction.

Cellular dysfunction may also be induced by upstream events of immunity, through impaired antigen presentation and signaling, and consequent failure to activate T lymphocytes. Assessment of antigen presenting cell competency requires sophisticated and laborious *in vitro* systems, which are currently suitable for developmental research and vaccinology but not clinical diagnostics (Flaminio et al., 2007, Cavatorta et al., 2009).

In addition, the expression of a variety of receptors, ligands and activation of signaling pathways could be involved, making the choice of test complex.

45.3 Sample Collection and Submission

Immunologic testing requires fresh samples maintained cooled at all times with an ice pack or in the refrigerator and shipped overnight to specialized laboratories in order to preserve their integrity and cellular function. Prolonged storage can affect cell viability and profile.

A complete blood count and peripheral smear using blood samples preserved in ethylenediaminetetracetic acid (EDTA) anti-coagulant shows the distribution of lymphocytes in the developing foal and adult horse.

For evaluation of the distribution of lymphocyte subpopulations (CD4+ T cells, CD8+ T cells, and B cells), whole blood samples preserved in EDTA or heparin can be submitted to specialized laboratories for immunophenotyping.

For proliferation and cytokine activation tests, whole blood samples preserved in EDTA or heparin can be submitted to specialized laboratories.

Quantification of cytokines in cells and tissues can be performed using real-time reverse-transcriptase polymerase chain reactions (RT-PCR), flow cytometry, and multiplex assays, often used in research. Secreted cytokine concentrations in fluids can be determined using bioassays, enzyme-linked immunosorbent assay (ELISA), and microsphere multiplex assays (Luminex®), which are more practical for clinical applications (de Jager et al., 2003, Wagner and Freer, 2009). Microsphere multiplex assays allow simultaneous detection of cytokines (IL-4, IL-10, IL-17, IFN-gamma, IFN-alpha) in small amounts of samples. Serum samples are more routinely tested for systemic measurements, whereas body fluids (e.g., synovial fluid, cerebrospinal fluid shipped in tubes without anti-coagulants) can be submitted in tubes without anticoagulants for assessment of local inflammatory mediators.

Phagocytosis and oxidative burst activity can be tested via flow cytometry using opsonized inactivated fluorescence-conjugated bacteria (e.g., *Staphylococcus aureus*, *E. coli*) and an indicator of production of reactive oxygen species (e.g., oxidation of 123 dihydrorhodamine into fluorescent 123 rhodamine) (Flaminio et al., 2002). These assays require whole blood samples preserved in heparin.

The definitive diagnosis of severe combined immunodeficiency syndrome (SCID) in an affected foal, and the identification of heterozygous carriers can be done by DNA test using whole blood or cheek swab samples (Shin et al., 1997). The defective B and T cell development is caused by a frame-shift mutation in the gene encoding DNA-dependent protein kinase catalytic subunit (DNA-PKc), which results in faulty V(D)J recombination for B and T cell receptor formation (Wiler et al., 1995, Shin et al., 1997). The mutation has been detected in Arabian and Arabian-cross horses. Carrier horses are heterozygous for the defective gene, and are immunocompetent; yet, the breeding of two carriers will produce an affected foal in 25% of the offsprings (McGuire and Poppie, 1973, Perryman and McGuire, 1980).

Necropsy and histopathology provide useful postmortem diagnostics. Lymphoid tissues can be evaluated for lymphoid hypoplasia and abnormal architecture. In addition, immunohistochemistry can test for the presence and distribution of immune cells, including lymphocyte subpopulations. In SCID, lymphoid tissues are hypoplastic for both B and T cells, and lack germinal centers; the thymus has a paucity of lymphocytes and prevalence of adipose tissue (Wyatt, 1987). Necropsy and histopathology can also detect and characterize lymphosarcoma, the most important differential diagnosis of cellular immunodeficiencies, although lymphoid neoplasias may accompany immunodeficiencies.

45.4 Possible Results and Interpretation: Immune Disorders of the Young Horse

The initial development and structural organization of primary and secondary lymphoid tissues happens during fetal life in the absence of foreign antigens; consequently, peripheral blood lymphocyte counts

(1000–2000 cells/uL) in healthy equine neonates are somewhat comparable to adult horses (Perryman et al., 1980, Becht and Semrad, 1985, Tallmadge et al., 2009). In the case of prematurity/immaturity and perinatal infection, lymphopenia may be present and persist for a few or several days.

The progressive exposure to an abundant and diverse population of pathogens in early life induces a massive expansion of antigen-specific lymphocyte populations in the naïve foal. Therefore, an increase in peripheral blood absolute lymphocyte count of at least 2.5–3 times is expected in the foal by the third month of life, and blood counts may reach 6000–8000 cells/μL by 6 months of life (Banks et al., 1999, Flaminio et al., 2000). Failure to expand lymphocyte populations is an indication of delayed immunologic development or primary cellular immunodeficiency (e.g., severe combined immunodeficiency syndrome).

Consequently, there is also an age-dependent increase in the distribution of lymphocyte subpopulations in peripheral blood within the first 3–5 months of life (Flaminio et al., 1998, 1999, 2000, Smith et al., 2002). The increase in circulating lymphocytes likely reflects the intense lymphocyte priming and population expansion in the secondary lymphoid tissues in response to antigens/pathogens. Individual variability in the distribution of the different lymphocyte subpopulations should be expected, and some foals may take longer to reach normal values than others; a prolonged delay predisposes to recurrent infections.

Infections with opportunistic organisms (e.g., *Pneumocystis joroveci, Cryptosporidium parvum*, adenovirus) are also suggestive of primary or transient/delayed cellular immunodeficiency in foals, and some of these organisms may require combination of immune mechanisms for protection (e.g., humoral and cellular immunity). These cases often present decreased peripheral blood CD4+ T cell distribution (<50%) and, consequently, decreased CD4:CD8 ratio (<2.0) (Felippe, personal observation, Tanaka, 1994, Flaminio et al., 1998, 1999). This finding is often accompanied by a decrease in the proportion of lymphocytes expressing the MHC class II molecules, or failure to timely show an increase in its expression when compared to age-matched control healthy foals. The actual implications of the lack of MHC class II expression on lymphocytes in the young foal are unknown; yet, this molecule serves as a marker for maturation of lymphocytes. This condition may also be accompanied by transient hypogammaglobulinemia, but it is uncertain if both conditions (i.e., transient CD4+ T cell lymphopenia and delayed hypogammaglobulinemia) involve the same disorder

background because they can also present independently (Felippe, personal observation).

Immunologic testing based on lymphocyte immunophenotyping (CD4+ and CD8+ T cells, B cells, MHC class II expression) along with serum IgG and IgM concentrations every 2–3 months can be used to determine progress in immunologic competence, and guidance for the need of antibiotic therapy (i.e., when immunologic parameters reach reference intervals for the age, antibiotic therapy may be discontinued).

SCID foals present severe peripheral blood lymphopenia (<1000 cells/μL), with absence of T and B cells; immunoglobulin production is totally impaired, and serum IgM concentration undetectable; when present, serum IgG concentration reflects colostrum-derived antibodies.

45.5 Possible Results and Interpretation: Immune Disorders of the Adult Horse

In the adult horse, infections with intracellular organisms (e.g., *Rhodococcus equi, Pneumocystis jiroveci, Candida albicans, Aspergillus* spp., *Bipolaris* spp.) are suggestive of faulty cellular immune mechanisms.

Persistent absolute lymphopenia could reflect lymphoid tissue hypoplasia, which also contributes to decreased circulating lymphocyte subpopulation distributions; alternatively, disease and stress often cause lymphopenia that resolves or improves with clinical recovery.

Results for distribution of lymphocyte subpopulations should be compared to reference or confidence intervals determined by the laboratory. In general, for adult horses, median CD4+ T cell distribution is 64.4% with a confidence interval (CI) 4.7; median CD8+ T cell 18.3% with CI 2.6; median B cell 9.0 with CI 2.0; and median MHC class II 95.0% with CI 4.1. Changes in CD4:CD8 ratio suggest immune imbalance; the cause could be an underlying immunodeficiency or secondary to an existing infection process, and values improve in the latter once the infection is resolved. In any case, decreased CD4:CD8 ratio (less than 2.5) in peripheral blood is associated with susceptibility to infections with intracellular organisms. Failure of lymphocytes to respond to stimuli with proliferation and/or adequate cytokine and co-stimulatory molecule expression indicate intrinsic cellular dysfunction.

Cytokine concentration in supernatant after *in vitro* lymphocyte stimulation may be compared with assay negative control (non-stimulated cells) and positive control (stimulated cells from a healthy horse), which allow analysis of adequate or impaired relative responses. On the other hand, systemic (serum) cytokine concentration for the diagnosis of immuno-deficiencies can be difficult to interpret because of the wide normal reference ranges or confidence intervals, particularly with low concentrations. Serum cytokine concentrations may be more revealing of and applica-ble to the monitoring of inflammatory conditions and autoimmunity, when values are markedly increased. The sensitivity of cytokine detection by multiplex assays is much increased when compared to other methods; however, due to need of sample dilutions for analysis, the sensitivity of the test is low for sam-ples with low concentrations (e.g., IL-4). In addition, dilutions also overestimate cytokine concentrations when they promote dissociation of cytokines from soluble receptors or binding proteins, which are natural mechanisms that control their function *in vivo* (i.e., blocking of their biological activity) (de Jager et al., 2009). Interpretation of results should also take in consideration a diurnal rhythm of cytokine secretion because of its neuroendocrine control under cortisol, melatonin, and progesterone (Petrovsky and Harrison, 1998).

45.6 Possible Results and Interpretation for Phagocyte Dysfunction

Inherited forms of neutrophil dysfunction have not been described in the horse but should be suspected in cases of recurrent infection (dermatitis, cutaneous, or intra-cavitary abscesses, cellulitis, periodontal diseases) not associated with humoral immunodeficiency, and caused by *Staphylococcus, Pseudomonas, Serratia, Klebsiella*, or fungi (*Aspergillus, Candida*).

In the neonate foal, transient neutrophil dysfunction has been reported during sepsis. Although healthy foals are born with competent neutrophil function, septic foals demonstrate a decrease in phagocytosis and oxidative burst activity that improves during the hospitalization period (Flaminio et al., 2002, Gardner et al., 2007).

45.7 Clinical Case

An 8-month-old Quarter Horse filly presented with non-respiratory *Rhodococcus equi* abscess, endodontic abscess (no organism identified), and tibial tarsal effusion with lameness (no signs of osteomyelitis

Table 45.1 Peripheral blood immunophenotyping and serum immunoglobulin concentrations in a filly with delayed cellular immune development.

Age	CD4+ T cells %	CD8+ T cells %	CD4/ CD8 Ratio	B cells %	MHC class II %	IgM mg/dL	IgG mg/dL
10 mo	54.2	21.9	2.5	14.5	37.9	1232	80
13 mo	45.1	24.7	1.8	19.8	40.0	1407	116
15 mo	50.7	35.7	1.4	18.7	43.9	1358	93

radiographically. Peripheral blood lymphocyte pheno-typing at 10 months of life revealed mildly decreased CD4+ T cell distribution (54.2%), and decreased percent positive MHC class II lymphocytes (37.9%), perhaps expected for the age, and CD4/CD8 ratio at the low end of normal reference interval (2.5) (Table 45.1). Absolute lymphocyte count was appropriate for the age at 3,770 cells/μL. Serum IgG and IgM concentrations were nor-mal at 1232 and 80 mg/dL, respectively, indicating nor-mal humoral development.

The filly was treated with antibiotic therapy for a month, and response was favorable. Three weeks after the antibiotics were discontinued, she developed a cough, nasal discharge and enlarged submandibular lymph nodes. Subsequent immunologic testing at 13 and 15 months of life indicated persistence of decreased CD4+ T cell distribution (45.1 and 50.7%, respectively), low percentage of lymphocytes express-ing MHC class II molecules (40 and 43.9%, respec-tively), and low CD4/CD8 ratio (1.8 and 1.4, respectively). Lymphocyte stimulation *in vitro* with mitogen (phyto-hemagglutinin, PHA) induced robust proliferation of cells, and upregulation of expression of MHC class molecule (Figure 45.1). Based on these results, sus-tained inability to promote the maturation of lympho-cytes and overcome infections does not seem to be intrinsic to lymphocyte dysfunction but secondary to a lack of appropriate stimulus *in vivo* (e.g., activation from antigen presenting cells or adequate levels of cytokines).

This case reflects the need to monitor through time immunologic parameters of foals with intermittent signs of infection, particularly when antibiotics are discon-tinued. This case shows delayed development of the cellular immunity without apparent consequences to the humoral function. Antibiotic treatment can be tailored to the patient according to the immunologic develop-ment, with the potential for resolution.

Figure 45.1 Peripheral blood lymphocyte subpopulation distribution and serum immunoglobulin concentrations in a filly with delayed cellular immunity development. An 8-month-old Quarter Horse filly presented for veterinary care with recurrent fevers and infections, including a non-respiratory *Rhodococcus equi* abscess. Infection with a facultative intracellular bacterium at this age suggests impaired cellular immunity. Peripheral blood lymphocyte immunophenotyping performed every 2 months revealed CD4+ T cell lymphopenia, low CD4/CD8 ratio, and low percentage of lymphocytes expression the MHC class II molecule. When stimulated *in vitro* with a mitogen (PHA, phytohemagglutinin), the lymphocytes proliferated robustly, and flow cytometric analysis measured an increase in the percentage of lymphocytes expressing the MHC class II molecule, in comparison to freshly isolated lymphocytes and non-stimulated lymphocytes. In this case, intrinsic lymphocyte dysfunction was not documented, and delayed cellular immunity development due to lack of appropriate stimulus *in vivo* is likely.

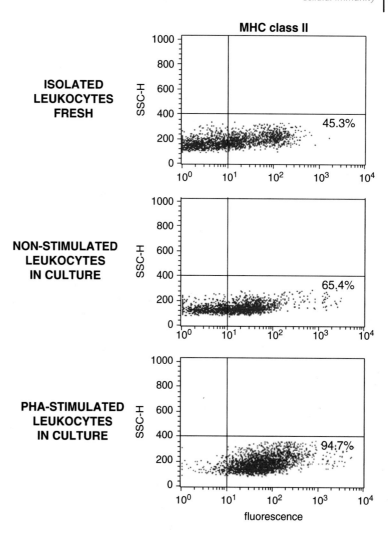

References

Banks EM, Kyriakidou M, Little S, and Hamblin AS. 1999. Epithelial lymphocyte and macrophage distribution in the adult and fetal equine lung. J Comp Pathol, 120: 1–13.

Becht JL and Semrad SD. 1985. Hematology, blood typing, and immunology of the neonatal foal. Vet Clin North Am Equine Pract, 1: 91–116.

Cavatorta, DJ, Erb HN, and Flaminio MJ. 2009. Ex vivo generation of mature equine monocyte-derived dendritic cells. Vet Immunol Immunopath, 131: 259–267.

de Jager W, Te Velthuis H, Prakken BJ, Kuis W, and Rijkers GT. 2003. Simultaneous detection of 15 human cytokines in a single sample of stimulated peripheral blood mononuclear cells. Clin Diagn Lab Immunol, 10: 133–139.

de Jager W, Bourcier K, Rijkers GT, Prakken BJ, and Seyfert-Margolis V. 2009. Prerequisites for cytokine measurements in clinical trials with multiplex immunoassays. BioMed Cent Immunol, 10: 52.

Flaminio MJ, Rush BR, Cox JH, and Moore WE. 1998. CD4+ and CD8+ T-lymphocytopenia in a filly with *Pneumocystis carinii* pneumonia. Aust Vet J, 76: 399–402.

Flaminio MJ, Rush BR, and Shuman W. 1999. Peripheral blood lymphocyte subpopulations and immunoglobulin concentrations in healthy foals and foals with *Rhodococcus equi* pneumonia. J Vet Intern Med, 13: 206–212.

Flaminio MJ, Rush BR, and Shuman W. 2000. Characterization of peripheral blood and pulmonary leukocyte function in healthy foals. Vet Immunol Immunopath, 73: 267–285.

Flaminio MJ, Rush BR, Davis EG, Hennessy K, Shuman W, and Wilkerson MJ. 2002. Simultaneous flow cytometric analysis of phagocytosis and oxidative burst activity in equine leukocytes. Vet Res Commun, 26: 85–92.

Flaminio MJ, Borges AS, Nydam DV, Horohov DW, Hecker R, and Matychak MB. 2007. The effect of CpG-ODN on antigen presenting cells of the foal. J Immune Based Therapy Vacc, 25(5): 1.

Gardner RB, Nydam DV, Luna JA, Bicalho ML, Matychak MB, and Flaminio MJ, 2007. Serum opsonization capacity, phagocytosis, and oxidative burst activity in neonatal foals in the intensive care unit. J Vet Intern Med, 21: 797–805.

Lunn D, Holmes M, and Duffus W. 1993. Equine T-lymphocyte MHC II expression: variation with age and subset. Vet Immunol Immunopath, 35: 225–238.

McGuire TC and Poppie MJ. 1973. Hypogammaglobulinemia and thymic hypoplasia in horses: a primary combined immunodeficiency disorder. Infection and Immunity, 8: 272–277.

O'Shea JJ, Ma A, and Lipsky P, 2002. Cytokines and autoimmunity. Nat Rev Immunol, 2: 37–45.

Perryman LE and McGuire TC. 1980. Evaluation for immune system failures in horses and ponies. J Am Vet Med Assoc, 176: 1374–1377.

Perryman LE, McGuire TC, and Torbeck RL. 1980. Ontogeny of lymphocyte function in the equine fetus. Am J Vet Res, 41: 1197–1200.

Petrovsky N and Harrison LC 1998. The chronobiology of human cytokine production. Intern Rev Immunol, 16: 635–649.

Shin EK, Perryman LE, and Meek K. 1997. Evaluation of a test for identification of Arabian horses heterozygous for the severe combined immunodeficiency trait. J Am Vet Med Assoc, 211: 1268–1270.

Smith R 3rd, Chaffin MK, Cohen ND, and Martens RJ. 2002. Age-related changes in lymphocyte subsets of quarter horse foals. Am J Vet Res, 63: 531–537.

Tallmadge RL, McLaughlin K, Secor E, Ruano D, Matychak MB, and Flaminio MJ. 2009. Expression of essential B cell genes and immunoglobulin isotypes suggests active development and gene recombination during equine gestation. Dev Comp Immunol, 33: 1027–1038.

Tanaka S, Kaji Y Taniyama H, Matsukawa K, Ochiai K, and Itakura C. 1994. *Pneumocystis carinii* pneumonia in a thoroughbred foal. J Vet Med Sci, 56: 135–137.

Wagner B and Freer H. 2009. Development of a bead-based multiplex assay for simultaneous quantification of cytokines in horses. Vet Immunol Immunopath, 127: 242–248.

Wiler R, Leber R, Moore BB, VanDyk LF, Perryman LE, and Meek K. 1995. Equine severe combined immunodeficiency: a defect in V(D)J recombination and DNA-dependent protein kinase activity. Proc National Acad Sci USA, 92: 11485–11489.

Wyatt CR, Magnuson NS, and Perryman LE. 1987. Defective thymocyte maturation in horses with severe combined immunodeficiency. J Immunol, 139: 4072–4076.

46

Immunoglobulins
Julia B. Felippe

Cornell University, College of Veterinary Medicine, New York, USA

46.1 Clinical Background

Hypogammaglobulinemia is the most common and more readily diagnosed type of immunodeficiency in horses. The condition may manifest in early age (e.g., failure in the passive transfer of immunoglobulins to the foal, transitory hypogammaglobulinemia of the young, X-linked agammaglobulinemia, foal immunodeficiency syndrome, severe combined immunodeficiency syndrome), or later in life (e.g., common variable immunodeficiency). In general, hypo- or agammaglobulinemia is caused by intrinsic failure of B cell development or function; or dysfunction of CD4+ helper T cells that provide survival signals to B cells.

In the horse, the immunoglobulin repertoire includes IgM, IgA, IgE, IgD, and seven different IgG isotypes (IgG$_{1 \text{ to } 7}$) defined by different amino acid sequences in the heavy chain constant region; IgGT comprises two isotypes named IgG$_3$ and IgG$_5$, and IgGb includes the IgG$_4$ and IgG$_7$, which share 96% nucleotide sequence homology. The equine immunoglobulin isotypes IgD, IgG$_2$ and IgG$_6$ have no identified function to date (Wagner, 2006a) (Table 46.1).

The inadequate production of immunoglobulins may affect one (selective) or more isotypes (e.g., IgG, IgM, IgA, and/or IgE). Each immunoglobulin isotype offers distinct functions for neutralization (e.g., IgG, IgA, IgM), opsonization (IgG and IgA), complement fixation (e.g., IgM and IgG), mast cell degranulation (e.g., IgE), natural killer cell-mediated cytotoxicity (e.g., IgG), and mucosal protection (e.g., IgA, IgG). Therefore, the combination of isotypes provides a functional strategy for removal of pathogens, and lack of specific isotypes may facilitate certain pathogen establishment and disease. Nevertheless, IgG hypogammaglobulinemia is the most significant humoral deficiency because its broader role in mechanisms of protection and greater concentration in the circulation in comparison to other isotypes; other selective-isotype

deficiencies (e.g., selective IgM deficiency or selective IgA deficiency, with normal IgG) may be asymptomatic. The lack of IgG leads to susceptibility to bacterial infections, particularly encapsulate bacteria (e.g., *Streptococcus* spp., *Staphylococcus* spp., *Klebsiella* spp.), since these organisms require both antibody and complement for effective opsonization and phagocytosis. Therefore, recurrent respiratory clinical signs are the most common, followed by sinusitis, sepsis, meningitis, osteomyelitis, hepato- or splenomegaly, dermatitis, oral candidiasis, and failure to grow.

As a general practice, blood IgG concentration is measured in the newborn foal between 12 and 24h after birth to evaluate for adequate passive transfer of immunoglobulins through colostrum. Blood IgG concentration is rarely measured in different times of the horse's life unless there are clinical signs of recurrent infections and fevers, and persistent hypoglobulinemia detected in blood biochemistry. Importantly, when evaluating for humoral competency, age-dependent developmental changes in the immune system should be taken into consideration, as they may confound a definitive diagnosis of immunodeficiency in the growing horse.

In contrast, marked hyperglobulinemia can be further characterized using protein electrophoresis to investigate for monoclonal gammopathy. In some cases, monoclonal gammopathies may create susceptibility to certain infections when there is suppression of polyclonal immunoglobulin production.

46.2 Tests Available

Humoral function can be readily and precisely assessed by measuring serum IgG concentrations, as antibodies are the final products of humoral immunity.

In foals less than 3–4 months old, serum IgG concentration interpretation should take into account circulating

Interpretation of Equine Laboratory Diagnostics, First Edition. Edited by Nicola Pusterla and Jill Higgins.
© 2018 John Wiley & Sons, Inc. Published 2018 by John Wiley & Sons, Inc.

Table 46.1 Immunoglobulin isotypes of the horse.

Immunoglobulin isotypes of the horse	Previous nomenclature
IgG_1	IgGa
IgG_2	none
$IgG_{3/5}$	IgGT
$IgG_{4/7}$	IgGb
IgG_6	IgGc
IgM	IgM
IgA	IgA
IgE	IgE
IgD	IgD

levels of colostrum-derived antibodies, which vary individually depending on the initial amount of absorption (colostral IgG half-life is estimated at 28–32 days) (Lavoie et al., 1989). Therefore, serum IgM concentration is more specific for B cell function in foals, as IgM production occurs already *in utero*, and the low transferred amounts of colostrum-derived IgM has a short half-life of 5–16 days.

Measuring antigen-specific antibody titers in response to vaccination (e.g., tetanus toxoid) is a useful strategy to evaluate *in vivo* immunoglobulin production. In general, if patients have been vaccinated before with a tetanus toxoid, a 15–21-day interval between the pre-vaccination and post-vaccination samples is recommended. When using enzyme-linked immunosorbant assay (ELISA) to measure antibody concentrations, it is important that pre-vaccination and post-vaccination serum samples are run in the same test because variable magnitude of results is often obtained between assays. This approach may not be useful in young foals without optimal vaccines for the age, and during the period of development of their immune system (i.e., <8 months of life) that requires many boosters to achieve protection.

Evaluation of peripheral blood B cell distribution adds information about faulty humoral immunity, and can be processed using immunophenotying and flow cytometry. Humoral immunity disorders can also be secondary to cellular deficiencies, with low levels or dysfunctional CD4+ T cells that cannot co-stimulate and support B cell differentiation and survival.

In Foal Immunodeficiency Syndrome (FIS), a mutation in the gene SLC5A3 on chromosome ECA26 has been associated with the disease, although the mechanistic implications of this mutation in the impaired red blood cell and B cell productions have not been fully resolved (Fox-Clipsham et al., 2011a, 2011b). Pedigree analysis of the Fell Pony breed suggests that FIS may have an autosomal recessive inheritance, with normal carriers

(Butler et al., 2006). A DNA-based test has been developed and offers powerful herd management planning to avoid the mating of two carriers with the genetic defect.

Monoclonal gammopathies can be diagnosed using protein electrophoresis, which separates blood proteins into albumin, alphaglobulins, betaglobulins, and gammaglobulins when exposed to an electric current.

Necropsy and histopathology provide useful postmortem diagnostics. Lymphoid tissues can be evaluated for lymphoid hypoplasia and abnormal architecture, particularly lack of germinal centers, in which B cell development occurs. In addition, immunohistochemistry can test for the presence and distribution of immune cells, including lymphocyte subpopulations. Necropsy and histopathology can also detect and characterize lymphosarcoma, the most important differential diagnosis of cellular immunodeficiencies, although lymphoid neoplasias may accompany immunodeficiencies.

46.3 Sample Collection and Submission

For immunoglobulin quantitation, blood should be collected in red top blood tubes and serum transferred to fresh tubes for shipping or storage; some tests offer the option of whole blood samples (e.g., samples collected in ethylenediaminetetraacetic acid, EDTA) or plasma.

Antigen-specific antibody titers in response to vaccination require serum pre- and post-vaccination samples collected 15–21 days apart.

Peripheral blood immunophenotyping requires blood samples collected in tubes with anticoagulant (i.e., heparin or EDTA), and shipped overnight with an ice pack.

For protein electrophoresis, blood should be collected in red top blood tubes and serum transferred to fresh tubes for shipping or storage.

46.4 Serum Immunoglobulin Concentrations

Serum, plasma or whole blood IgG concentration in horses has been measured by glutaraldehyde agglutination test, zinc sulfate turbidity test, latex agglutination test, radial immunodiffusion (RID) test, enzyme immunoassays, turbidimetric immunoassays, quantitative colorimetric assay, and infrared spectroscopy (Rumbaugh et al., 1978, Beetson et al., 1985, Kent and Blackmore, 1985, Bauer and Brooks, 1990, LeBlanc et al., 1990, Erhard et al., 2001, Pusterla et al., 2002, Davis and Giguère, 2005, Metzger et al., 2006, Wong et al., 2013). Serum total protein has also been used to indirectly assess circulating IgG values in the newborn after ingestion of colostrum.

Radial immunodiffusion has been considered the gold-standard quantitative test for determining serum IgG or IgM concentration, although there are no publications supporting the reference standards and test performance; in addition, RID kits from different companies have wide limits of agreement, particularly when values are greater than 800 mg/dL (Buening et al., 1977, Flaminio et al, 1999, Davis and Giguère, 2005). In this test, species-specific antibody-reagent that binds to a certain immunoglobulin isotype is diffusely distributed in a gel slide. The testing sample (serum) is placed in a punched hole, and diffuses radially in the gel, forming precipitations when the amount of antibody-reagent and serum antibody is equivalent. The diameter of the precipitation reaction corresponds to a certain concentration obtained from measurements of a standard curve (i.e., known antibody concentrations of standard solutions versus their diameter of diffusion and precipitation). This test requires dilutions of testing samples when concentrations are above the standard values, and does not provide an actual result when below the standard values; in addition, it may take 24–48 h to obtain the results, accordingly. Therefore, due to its limited commercial availability and practicability for the diagnosis of failure of passive transfer of immunoglobulins, RID has been slowly replaced by tests with a faster turnaround in results. A RID test for IgA concentrations is not commercially available at the moment.

Turbidimetric immunoassay measures loss of intensity of light transmitted through a solution with antibody-antigen complexes (i.e., species-specific antibody-reagent bound to an immunoglobulin in serum or plasma). When compared to RID, this test offers accurate results particularly for the detection of low IgG concentrations (i.e., less than 400 mg/dL) (Kent and Blackmore, 1985, Bauer and Brooks, 1990, McCue, 2007, Wong et al., 2013). To date, there is no turbidimetric test commercially available for serum IgM or IgA concentration in horses.

A stall-side equine semi-quantitative commercially available enzyme immunoassay (SNAP® Test, Idexx Laboratories, Inc.) measures serum, plasma or whole blood IgG concentration in a scale of less than 400 mg/dL, 400–800 mg/dL, and greater than 800 mg/dL. The test uses the same principles of an enzyme-linked immunosorbent assay (ELISA). The sample and an enzyme-conjugated antibody reagent are first mixed into a solution, and form a complex. The complex binds to capture antibodies in the device matrix during the snap activation phase. A wash solution is applied to remove unbound elements and reagents. The enzyme activity changes the reporting color into blue, and the color intensity of the sample spot is compared to calibrator spots for quantitation. This test has been widely used for the timely diagnosis of failure of passive transfer of immunoglobulins in foals. Other ELISAs applicable to research have also been shown to provide accurate quantitative results of serum immunoglobulin concentrations, including total IgG, individual IgG subtypes, IgM, IgA and IgE (Erhard et al., 2001, Wagner et al., 2006b, Tallmadge et al., 2009).

Early semi-quantitative tests used to measure serum IgG concentration for the diagnosis of failure of passive transfer of immunoglobulins in foals, including zinc sulfate turbidity test, glutaraldehyde coagulation test, and latex agglutination test were considered adequate and inexpensive when compared to RID, with sensitivity values of approximately 85% and specificity values of approximately 60–70% for IgG values less than 800 mg/dL; however, these tests have also been slowly replaced throughout the years with most recent commercially available devices (Kent and Blackmore, 1985, Beetson et al., 1985, Clabough et al., 1989, Saikku et al., 1989, Davis and Giguere, 2005). In contrast, sodium sulfite precipitation reactions were reported with low sensitivity and specificity (Rumbaugh et al., 1978).

Infrared spectroscopy, in conjunction with classification or quantification algorithms, has been proposed as an inexpensive candidate methodology for the diagnosis of failure of passive transfer in foals taken its comparable or superior sensitivity, specificity, and predictive positive and negative values in comparison to RID, but requires further studies for its clinical application (Riley et al., 2007, Hou et al., 2014).

Serum IgA concentration can be measure by ELISA but tests are not widely available; in general, serum IgA concentration is not reflective of mucosal concentrations, although deficiencies could be diagnosed based on serum results.

Serum IgG subtype concentrations (IgG_1, $IgG_{4/7}$, $IgG_{3/5}$) can be determined by ELISA and multiplex fluorescent bead-based assay, and they have been used in studies addressing developmental immunology and vaccinology; their value in the context of immunodeficiencies is uncertain and, to date, not validated (Keggan et al., 2013).

46.5 Failure of Passive Transfer of Immunoglobulins in Foals

Total or partial failure of passive transfer of immunoglobulins through the colostrum increases the foal's susceptibility to infection by environmental pathogens. Immunoglobulin production is possible during gestation, and the equine neonate is born with trace levels of circulating IgG (around 0.2 to 17 mg/dL) and IgM (around 25 mg/dL) (Perryman and McGuire, 1980,

Tallmadge et al., 2009). Serum or whole blood IgG concentrations in the foal after ingestion of colostrum during the first 24 hours of life less than 400 mg/dL indicate total failure of passive transfer of antibodies, values of 400–800 mg/dL indicate partial failure, and values greater than 800 mg/dL are considered adequate. In general, good quality colostrum and timely nursing provides transfer of antibodies to levels often greater than 2000 mg/dL (Flaminio et al., 2002). Therefore, the measurement of IgG concentration in the foal's blood after nursing colostrum determines the need for clinical intervention with administration of immunoglobulins and other prophylactic measures.

In general, the assays routinely used for the diagnosis of failure of passive transfer of immunoglobulins in foals have high sensitivity (with high negative predicted value), and moderate to low specificity. Therefore, the tests are useful for the detection of the majority of foals in need of supplementary IgG but may overdiagnose that need when using a cut-off value of 800 mg/dL. In any case, sensitivity, specificity, positive and negative predicted values should be consulted for each (commercially) available test in order to determine limitations in the interpretation of results.

The sensitivity of the SNAP® test to detect serum IgG concentration has been compared to RID as a reference method and calculated at 89–90% for values less than 400 mg/dL, and 81–95% for values less than 800 mg/dL; and the specificity at 79–96% for values less than 400 mg/dL, and 52–95% for values less than 800 mg/dL (Pusterla et al., 2002, Davis et al., 2005, Metzger et al., 2006). The DVM Stat (VDx Inc.) quantitative colorimetric assay has shown a sensitivity of 100 and 97.6%, and specificity of 96 to 82.8% for values below 400 and 800 mg/dL, respectively (Davis and Giguere, 2005).

In comparison to RID, a turbidimetric assay for values below 400 mg/dL has shown 92.3% sensitivity, 99.1% specificity, 98.1% positive predicted value, and 96.4% negative predicted value. For values greater than 400 mg/dL, turbidimetric immunoassays may underestimate concentrations, with a consequent drop in the specificity and positive predicted value to 70.5 and 71.5%, respectively. In another study, a statistically significant linear relationship was measured between serum IgG concentrations between the turbidimetric and RID tests, with slightly lower sensitivity and specificity values (Davis et al., 2005).

Serum total protein concentration less than 4.5 g/dL is suggestive of failure of passive transfer of immunoglobulins in foals (i.e., IgG values less than 400 mg/dL), and values greater than 6.0 g/dL suggest adequate transfer of immunoglobulins (i.e., IgG values greater than 800 mg/dL) (Davis and Giguère, 2005, Hurcombe et al., 2012). Nevertheless, the sensitivity and specificity of serum

total protein in predicting passive transfer of immunoglobulins were low at an intermediate interval (between 4.5 and 6.0 g/dL), which altogether discourage its use as a screening test (Rumbaugh et al., 1978, Davis and Giguère, 2005, Metzger et al., 2006).

When confirming definitive hypogammaglobulinemia in a patient, the next step is to measure peripheral blood lymphocyte distribution via immunophenotyping in order to evaluate for the distribution of B cells and CD4+ helper T cells. In addition, vaccination response tests can also be performed to further evaluate humoral response *in vivo*. In this case, paired pre- and post-vaccination (e.g., tetanus toxoid) serum samples can be used for comparison of antibody titers; in normal humoral response, an increase in titer is expected; one caution about this test is the fact that amplitude of response is quite variable among healthy horses, and this approach may not be useful in young foals for they require many boosters to achieve protection.

46.6. Immunodeficiencies of the Young Horse

It is not common practice to measure serum IgG and IgM concentrations in foals beyond the time of ingestion of colostrum. Colostral IgG concentrations decrease with a half-life of 28–32 days in the healthy foal, and total serum IgG concentration in the foal may drop to levels below 500 mg/dL around 8 weeks of life (Lavoie et al., 1989). Meanwhile, endogenous antibody production that reaches protective levels (i.e., greater than 500 mg/dL) happens by 8–12 weeks of life, and values greater than 800 mg/dL are usually measured beyond 6 to 8 months of life. Consequently, serum immunoglobulin concentrations in foals should be compared to age-matched control foals of the same breed, preferably of the same heard, in order to assess normal humoral response.

Relative decay of total colostral antibody is proportional to the initial amount of immunoglobulin absorbed at birth taken the IgG half-life. To some extent, larger transfer of IgG through colostrum (i.e., foal serum IgG concentration greater than 2000 mg/dL after ingestion of colostrum) will maintain adequate levels for a longer period of time, beyond the time the foal's endogenous production reaches protective levels. On the other hand, low initial colostral IgG concentrations (i.e., values not much higher than 800 mg/dL) may not persist until endogenous production reaches protective levels in some foals; in this case, transient susceptibility to infection may occur around the first and second months of life. The knowledge of the actual concentration (i.e., rather than a value greater than 800 mg/dL) of serum IgG in the foal after the ingestion of colostrum provides prospective assessment of antibody protection during the transition phase between the decay of colostrum-derived antibodies and the endogenous production. In other words, while minimum serum IgG values of 800 mg/dL are important at birth for protection during the first and second weeks of life, values greater than 1200 mg/dL would more likely protect the foal beyond that period until endogenous production reaches protective levels.

When colostrum-derived IgG are still present in high concentrations (i.e., in foals less than 2 months of life), serum IgM concentrations more clearly reflect endogenous humoral competency because colostrum has low levels of IgM, and colostrum-derived IgM has a short half-life (around 10–15 days). Serum IgM concentrations greater than 25 mg/dL after ingestion of colostrum and 50 mg/dL in the first month of life and thereafter (100 mg/dL) are expected in the developing healthy foal.

In foals older than 3–5 months of life and with delayed antibody production, serum IgG concentration is below protective levels (less than 500 mg/dL), and IgM levels are often decreased (less than 25 mg/dL). If IgG and IgM production is recovered in the subsequent months, the condition is known as transient hypogammaglobulinemia of the young, which often resolves around 8 months of life but could persist up to 18–24 months (Felippe, personal observation). Although a progressive increase in serum IgG and IgM concentrations may be measured in some foals during the recovery phase, others show little or no improvement in immunologic parameters for months until suddenly they start showing evidence of sustained antibody production (Felippe, personal observation). Foals often need intermittent treatment with antibiotics during this period due to recurrent respiratory infections and fevers; periodic measurement of serum IgG and IgM concentrations allows treatment planning and follow-up of the transient condition.

When IgG and IgM production do not resume during this period, B cell impaired development (B cell lymphopenia) or dysfunction may characterize a permanent condition as observed in X-linked agammaglobulinemia or early manifestation of common variable immunodeficiency (CVID) (Banks et al., 1976, McGuire et al., 1976, Perryman et al., 1977, 1983). In foals of Arab breed with concomitant B and T cell depletion and recurrent infections with opportunistic organisms, SCID can be confirmed with genetic tests and necropsy findings (McGuire and Poppie, 1973, Shin et al., 1997). In foals of Fell Pony and Dales breeds with persistent infection, progressive anemia and B cell lymphopenia, serum IgM concentration of less than 25 mg/dL are found in FIS, which can be confirmed by genetic test or necropsy findings (Scholes et al., 1998, Richards et al., 2000, Gardner et al., 2006, Tallmadge et al., 2012). In SCID- and FIS-affected foals, serum IgG concentrations reflect colostrum-derived

antibodies, and can be within normal reference values for the age. All these conditions are fatal in the horse.

Selective IgM deficiency has been reported in foals with chronic infections when serum IgM concentrations are more than two standard deviations below the normal mean (nowadays serum IgM concentration less than 25 mgdL), and IgG and IgA were within normal reference range for the age group, along with normal B and T cell distribution in the blood (Perryman et al., 1977). In the foal, it is uncertain if selective IgM deficiency is an independent condition or reflects transient hypogammaglobulinemia of the young, as most of the reported foals recovered IgM and IgG productions as yearlings (Perryman and McGuire, 1980).

Small amounts of IgE are transferred to foals through colostrum, and IgE is found either bound to peripheral blood leukocyte membranes or soluble in serum for a period of 2 and 4 months of life, respectively (Wagner et al., 2006b). In the foal, there is a long delay in endogenous IgE production, and serum IgE values are detectable around 9 months of life (Marti et al., 2009). Studies on passive transfer of antibodies against *Streptococcus equi* subspecies *equi* through colostrum in the foal revealed the presence of colostral polymeric IgA on the nasopharyngeal mucosa, with peak levels at 2 days of life (Galan et al., 1986, Sheoran et al., 2000). Endogenous IgA concentrations become measurable beyond 28 days of life, reaching levels comparable to adult horses by 42 days. The onset of production of different IgG subtypes has been described in the foal but offers limited use for evaluation of humoral competency because of confounding developmental and antigenic exposure factors (Holznagel et al. 2003).

46.7 Immunodeficiencies of the Adult Horse

The presence of infections and fevers is essential for the suspicion of immunodeficiency, and recurrent episodes are supportive. Therefore, significance of serum immunoglobulin concentrations is determined based on the clinical history and signs.

Serum immunoglobulin concentrations should be interpreted using reference intervals and confidence intervals determined by the laboratory performing the test, ideally beyond the reference intervals supplied by the manufacturer of the testing device. Nevertheless, an example of reference interval for adult horses of different breeds is enclosed for serum IgG concentration 1159–2667 (mean 1913) mg/dL; serum IgM concentration 98–108 (mean 103) mg/dL; and serum IgA concentration 85–365 (mean 225) mg/dL (Tallmadge et al., 2009, de Camargo et al., 2009).

Common variable immunodeficiency (CVID) in the horse is a rare late-onset (average age of diagnosis 10 years, range 2–23 years) fatal humoral disorder. B cell lymphopenia or depletion due to impaired production in the bone marrow leads to hypogammaglobulinemia that predisposes to recurrent infections and fevers, particularly encapsulated bacteria (Freestone et al., 1987, MacLeay et al., 1997, Flaminio et al., 2002, 2009). Serum IgG (less than 800 mg/dL, with fluctuations) and IgM (less than 25 mg/dL) concentrations are markedly reduced. Peripheral blood lymphocyte immunophenotyping reveals persistent, severe B cell lymphopenia (less than 2% of the total lymphocyte population). To date, there is no ante-mortem definitive diagnostic test; the disease involves gene silencing of essential transcription factors for B cell development in the bone marrow (Tallmadge et al., 2015). Necropsy, histopathologic, and immunohistochemical findings confirm the immunologic impairment by the lack of B cells and plasma cells in tissues, and abnormal structure of lymphoid tissues due to the lack of germinal centers.

Selective IgM deficiency has been reported in adult horses of both genders and different breeds with and without association with susceptibility to infections. In these reports, serum IgM concentrations were more than two standard deviations below the mean normal value of age-matched controls, along with normal serum concentrations for IgG and IgA, and normal B and T cell lymphocyte distribution. This condition is poorly defined and distinct from the condition described in foals. Conditions that affect antibody production in adult horses may be secondary to lymphosarcoma, prolonged immunosuppressive therapy or stress. Caution should be used when interpreting low serum IgM concentrations: persistent serum IgM concentrations less than 25 mg/dL better define deficiency (Perkins et al., 2003). The positive predicted value of serum IgM concentration of less than 25 mg/dL for the diagnosis of lymphoma or lymphosarcoma is not reliable, and these conditions should be investigated using more effective and definitive diagnostic tests (e.g., lymph node biopsy, cytology, and histology). Selective IgA deficiency has not been systematically studied in the horse.

46.8 Monoclonal Gammopathies

Serum protein electrophoresis separates blood proteins based on their net charge (positive or negative), and physical properties (size and shape). The gamma region comprises mostly of immunoglobulins, primarily IgG. Nevertheless, immunoglobulins can be found throughout the electrophoretic spectrum (Figure 46.1).

In agammaglobulinemia or hypogammaglobulinemia, the gamma region is decreased. Nevertheless, serum immunoglobulin concentration should be measured for its specificity and subsequent monitoring.

In clinical infections and monoclonal gammopathies, the gamma region is increased. In the case of infections, the pattern of proteins is broad, formed by diverse immunoglobulin heavy and light chains. In the case of monoclonal gammopathy (multiple myeloma, B cell neoplasm), the pattern shows a homogeneous spike-like peak, secondary to the secretion of a single heavy and a single light chain immunoglobulin by clonal neoplastic plasma cells or B cells. Taken the high specificity of monoclonal immunoglobulins, the lack of immunoglobulin diversity and their decreased production may predispose the patient to infections.

Protein Electrophoresis

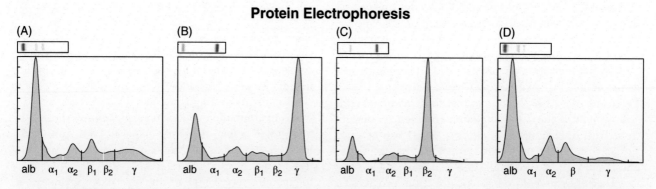

Figure 46.1 Serum protein electrophoresis pattern. Protein electrophoresis separates blood proteins based on their net charge (positive or negative), and physical properties (size and shape) when exposed to an electric current: albumin, alphaglobulins, betaglobulins, and gammaglobulins. The gamma region comprises mostly of immunoglobulins, primarily IgG. Nevertheless, immunoglobulins can be found throughout the electrophoretic spectrum. (A) normal electrophoretic pattern; (B) electrophoretic pattern showing a monoclonal spike in the gamma region in a horse with B cell leukemia; note the low albumin levels; (C) electrophoretic pattern showing a monoclonal spike in the beta2 region in a horse with B cell leukemia; note the low albumin and gammaglobulin levels; (D) electrophoretic pattern showing increased alpha and beta inflammatory proteins, and decreased gammaglobulins in a horse with common variable immunodeficiency.

46.9 Clinical Case

An 8-month-old Warmblood filly was evaluated by a veterinarian for pneumonia at weaning. The filly displayed hyperfibrinogenemia, scattered comet tails and a small area of consolidation in the cranioventral lung field observed by ultrasound examination; transtracheal wash culture yielded growth of *Streptococcus equi* subspecies *zooepidemicus*. The filly was treated with intramuscular antibiotics with favorable response but showed intermittent fevers when switched to oral antibiotics. At 10 months of life, she presented with acute onset of fever (103 °F) and respiratory distress; thoracic ultrasound and radiographs were normal, and a second transtracheal wash culture yielded no bacterial growth. She was treated again with broad-spectrum antibiotics. Transient hypogammaglobulinemia of the young was suspected based on the lower than expected for age serum IgM (less than 50 mg/dL) and serum IgG concentrations (less than 1000 mg/dL) as well as the history of chronic infections (Figure 46.2). In the subsequent months, her rectal temperature fluctuated from 100–101.8 °F, and blood work showed marked mature neutrophilia and hyperfibrinogenemia. The filly was kept on intermittent antibiotic

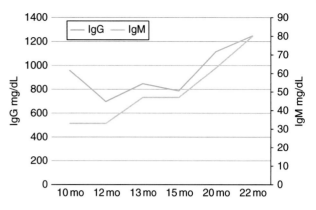

Figure 46.2 Transient hypogammaglobulinemia of the young. Serum IgG (left *y*-axis) and IgM (right *y*-axis) concentrations through time in a filly with history of recurrent fevers, hyperfibrinogenemia and pneumonia.

therapy, and serum IgG and IgM concentrations monitored through time. The filly failed to increase serum IgG concentrations linearly until around 20 months of life, when both IgM and IgG hypogammaglobulinemia gradually resolved. At that time, antibiotic therapy was discontinued, and the filly maintained normal temperature and lack of respiratory signs of infection.

References

Banks KL, McGuire TC, and Jerrells TR. 1976. Absence of B lymphocytes in a horse with primary agammaglobulinemia. Clin Immunol, 5: 282–290.

Bauer JE and Brooks TP 1990. Immunoturbidimetric quantification of serum immunoglobulin G concentration in foals. Am J Vet Res, 51: 1211–1214.

Beetson SA, Hilbert BJ, and Mills JN. 1985. The use of the glutaraldehyde coagulation test for detection of hypogammaglobulinaemia in neonatal foals. Aust Vet J, 62: 279–281.

Buening GM, Perryman LE, and McGuire TC. 1977. Practical methods of determining serum immunoglobulin M and immunoglobulin G concentrations in foals. J Am Vet Med Assoc, 171: 455–458.

Butler CM, Westermann CM, Koeman JP, and Sloet van Oldruitenborgh-Oosterbaan MM. 2006. The Fell pony immunodeficiency syndrome also occurs in the Netherlands: a review and six cases. Tijdschr Diergeneeskd, 131: 114–118.

de Camargo MM, Kuribayashi JS, Bombardieri CR, and Hoge A, 2009. Normal distribution of immunoglobulin isotypes in adult horses. Vet J, 182: 359–361.

Clabough DL, Conboy HS, and Roberts MC. 1989. Comparison of four screening techniques for the diagnosis of equine neonatal hypoglobulinemia. J Am Vet Med Assoc, 194: 1717–1720.

Davis R and Giguère S. 2005. Evaluation of five commercially available assays and measurement of serum total protein concentration via refractometry for the diagnosis of failure of passive transfer of immunity in foals. J Am Vet Med Assoc, 227: 1640–1645.

Davis DG, Schaefer DM, Hinchcliff KW, Wellman ML, Willet VE, and Fletcher JM. 2005. Measurement of serum IgG in foals by radial immunodiffusion and automated turbidimetric immunoassay. J Vet Intern Med, 19: 93–96.

Erhard MH,C Luft C, Remler HP, and Stangassinger M. 2001. Assessment of colostral transfer and systemic availability of immunoglobulin G in newborn foals using a newly developed enzyme-linked immunosorbent assay (ELISA) system. J Animal Physiol Nutr, 85: 164–173.

Flaminio MJ, LaCombe V, Kohn CW, and Antczak DF. 2002. Common variable immunodeficiency in a horse. J Am Vet Med Assoc, 221: 1296–1302, 1267.

Flaminio MJ, Rush BR, and Shuman W. 1999. Peripheral blood lymphocyte subpopulations and immunoglobulin concentrations in healthy foals and foals with *Rhodococcus equi* pneumonia. J Vet Intern Med, 13: 206–212.

Flaminio MJBF, Tallmadge R, Salles-Gomes CM, and Matychak MB. 2009. Common variable immunodeficiency in horses is characterized by B cell depletion in primary and secondary lymphoid tissues. J Clin Immunol, 29: 107–116.

Fox-Clipsham LY, Brown EE, Carter SD, and Swinburne JE. 2011a. Identification of a mutation associated with fatal foal immunodeficiency syndrome in the Fell and Dales Pony. PLoS Genetics, 7: e1002133.

Fox-Clipsham LY, Carter SD, Goodhead I, Hall N, Knottenbelt DC, May PDF, Ollier WE, and Swinburne JE. 2011b. Population screening of endangered horse breeds for the foal immunodeficiency syndrome mutation. Vet Rec, 169: 655–658.

Freestone JF, Hietala S, Moulton J, and Vivrette S. 1987. Acquired immunodeficiency in a seven-year-old horse. J Am Vet Med Assoc, 190: 689–691.

Galan JE, Timoney JF, and Lengemann FW. 1986. Passive transfer of mucosal antibody to *Streptococcus equi* in the foal. Infect Immun, 54: 202–206.

Gardner RB, Hart KA, Stokol T, Divers TJ, and Flaminio MJ. 2006. Fell Pony syndrome in a pony in North America. J Vet Intern Med, 20: 198–203.

Holznagel DL, Hussey S, Mihalyi JE, Wilson WD, and Lunn DP. 2003. Onset of immunoglobulin production in foals. Eq Vet J, 35: 620–622.

Hou S, McClure JT, Shaw RA, and Riley CB. 2014. Immunoglobulin G measurement in blood plasma using infrared spectroscopy. App Spectr, 68: 466–474.

Hurcombe SD, Matthews AL, Scott VH, Williams JM, Kohn CW, and Toribio RE. 2012. Serum protein concentrations as predictors of serum immunoglobulin G concentration in neonatal foals. J Vet Emerg Crit Care (San Antonio), 22: 573–579.

Keggan A, Freer H, Rollins A, and Wagner B. 2013. Production of seven monoclonal equine immunoglobulins isotyped by multiplex analysis. Vet Immunol Immunopathol, 153: 187–193.

Kent JE and Blackmore DJ 1985. Measurement of IgG in equine blood by immunoturbidimetry and latex agglutination. Eq Vet J, 17: 125–129.

Lavoie JP, Spensley MS, Smith BP, and Mihalyi J. 1989. Absorption of bovine colostral immunoglobulins G and M in newborn foals. Am J Vet Res, 50: 1598–1603.

LeBlanc MM, Hurtgen JP, and Lyle S. 1990. A modified zinc sulfate turbidity test for the detection of immune status in newly born foals. J Eq Vet Sci, 10: 36–39.

MacLeay JM, Ames TR, Hayden DW, and Tumas DB. 1997. Acquired B lymphocyte deficiency and chronic enterocolitis in a 3-year-old quarter horse. Vet Immunol Immunopathol, 57: 49–57.

Marti E, Ehrensperger F, Burger D, Ousey J, Day MJ, and Wilson AD. 2009. Maternal transfer of IgE and subsequent development of IgE responses in the horse (*Equus callabus*). Vet Immunol Immunopathol, 127: 203–211.

McCue PM. 2007. Evaluation of a turbidimetric immunoassay for measurement of plasma IgG concentration in foals. Am J Vet Res, 68: 1005–1009.

McGuire TC and Poppie MJ. 1973. Hypogammaglobulinemia and thymic hypoplasia in horses: a primary combined immunodeficiency disorder. Infect Immun, 8: 272–277.

McGuire TC, Banks KL, and Davis WC. 1976. Alterations of the thymus and other lymphoid tissue in young horses with combined immunodeficiency. Am J Pathol, 84: 39–54.

Metzger N, Hinchcliff KW, Hardy J, Schwarzwald CC, and Wittum T. 2006. Usefulness of a commercial equine IgG test and serum protein concentration as indicators of failure of transfer of passive immunity to hospitalized foals. J Vet Intern Med, 20: 382–387.

Perkins GA, Nydam DV, Flaminio MJBF, and Ainsworth DM. 2003. Serum IgM concentrations in normal, fit horses and horses with lymphoma or other medical conditions. J Vet Intern Med, 17: 337–342.

Perryman LE, McGuire TC, and Hilbert BJ. 1977. Selective immunoglobulin M deficiency in foals. J Am Vet Med Assoc, 170: 212–215.

Perryman LE and McGuire TC. 1980. Evaluation for immune system failures in horses and ponies. J Am Vet Med Assoc, 176: 1374–1377.

Perryman LE, McGuire TC, and Banks KL. 1983. Animal model of human disease. Infantile X-linked agammaglobulinemia. Agammaglobulinemia in horses. Am J Pathol, 111: 125–127.

Pusterla N, Pusterla JB, Spier SJ, Puget B, and Watson JL. 2002. Evaluation of the SNAP foal IgG test for the semiquantitative measurement of immunoglobulin G in foals. Vet Rec, 151: 258–260.

Richards AJ, Kelly DF, Knottenbelt DC, Cheeseman MT, and Dixon JB. 2000. Anaemia, diarrhoea and opportunistic infections in Fell ponies. Eq Vet J, 32: 386–391.

Riley CB, McClure JT, Low-Ying S, and Shaw RA. 2007. Use of Fourier-transform infrared spectroscopy for the diagnosis of failure of transfer of passive immunity and measurement of immunoglobulin concentrations in horses. J Vet Intern Med, 21: 828–834.

Rumbaugh GE, Ardans AA, Ginno D, and Trommershausen-Smith A. 1978. Measurement of neonatal equine immunoglobulins for assessment of colostral immunoglobulin transfer: comparison of single radial immunodiffusion with the zinc sulfate turbidity test, serum electrophoresis, refractometry for total serum protein, and the sodium sulfite precipitation test. J Am Vet Med Assoc, 172: 321–325.

Saikku A, Koskinen E, and Sandholm M. 1989. Detection of hypogammaglobulinaemia in neonatal foals using the glutaraldehyde coagulation test. Zentralblatt für Veterinärmedizin Reihe B, 36: 168–174.

Scholes SF, Holliman A, May PD, and Holmes MA. 1998. A syndrome of anaemia, immunodeficiency and peripheral ganglionopathy in Fell pony foals. Vet Rec, 42: 128–134.

Sheoran, AS, Timoney JF, Holmes MA, Karzenski SS, and Crisman MV. 2000. Immunoglobulin isotypes in sera and nasal mucosal secretions and their neonatal transfer and distribution in horses. Am J Vet Res, 61: 1099–1105.

Shin EK, Perryman LE, and Meek K. 1997. Evaluation of a test for identification of Arabian horses heterozygous for the severe combined immunodeficiency trait. J Am Vet Med Assoc, 211: 1268–1270.

Tallmadge RL, McLaughlin K, Secor E, Ruano D, Matychak MB, and Flaminio MJ. 2009. Expression of essential B cell genes and immunoglobulin isotypes suggests active development and gene recombination during equine gestation. Dev Comp Immunol, 33: 1027–1038.

Tallmadge RL, Stokol T, Gould-Earley MJ, Earley E, Secor EJ, Matychak MB, and Felippe MJ. 2012. Fell Pony syndrome: characterization of developmental hematopoiesis failure and associated gene expression profiles. Clinical and Vaccine Immunology, 19: 1054–1064.

Tallmadge RL, Shen L, Tseng CT, Miller SC, Barry J, and Felippe MJ. 2015. Bone marrow transcriptome and epigenome profiles of equine common variable immunodeficiency patients unveil block of B lymphocyte differentiation. Clin Immunol, 160: 261–276.

Wagner B 2006a. Immunoglobulins and immunoglobulin genes of the horse. Dev Comp Immunol, 30: 155–164.

Wagner B, Flaminio BJ, Hillegas J, Leibold W, Erb HN, and Antczak DF. 2006b. Occurrence of IgE in foals: evidence for transfer of maternal IgE by the colostrum and late onset of endogenous IgE production in the horse. Vet Immunol Immunopathol, 110: 269–278.

Wong DM, Giguère S, and Wendel MA. 2013. Evaluation of a point-of-care portable analyzer for measurement of plasma immunoglobulin G, total protein, and albumin concentrations in ill neonatal foals. J Am Vet Med Assoc, 242: 812–819.

47

Equine Blood Groups and Factors

K. Gary Magdesian

Department of Medicine and Epidemiology, School of Veterinary Medicine, University of California, California, USA

47.1 Clinical Background

Surface molecules (proteins, glycoproteins) on erythrocytes can be homogenous, or uniform across individuals within a species; they can also be heterogeneous, meaning they vary in structure due to genetic polymorphisms within the population. These polymorphisms can be variable enough in make up to be immunologically antigenic to individuals who lack them, stimulating an immune response and the development of antibodies directed against the erythrocytes with those specific glycoproteins.

Previously, blood typing was used for parentage verification and pedigree analysis, but this has now been replaced by DNA genotyping. Now blood typing is primarily done to minimize immune sensitization to incompatible blood types. Blood typing is based on erythrocyte surface antigens, termed groups and factors, because these antigens are responsible for blood transfusion reactions, as well as neonatal isoerythrolysis (NI). The most common factors associated with NI in horses include Aa and Qa, however, several additional factors, including Ab, Qrs, Qb, Qc, Dc, Da, Db, Dg, Ka, Pa, Pb, and Ua, have been associated with NI (Boyle et al., 2005). Aa is also responsible for many blood transfusion reactions in horses, as are Qa and Ca.

In summary, blood typing is performed in horses to minimize blood transfusion reactions and to prevent NI.

47.2 Tests Available

1) Blood typing is useful for ensuring that blood transfusions are as compatible as possible. With more than 30 factors and 7–8 systems, there are over 400,000 possible red cell phenotypes in horses. While completely compatible blood transfusions are not possible, the major or most antigenic factors can be evaluated for and ensured to be compatible. Blood typing also has a place in NI screening, in that blood typing of the mare and stallion can evaluate for potential incompatibilities. For mares that have a history of having foals that developed NI, the blood typing of mare and a number of potential sires can allow for selection of a sire without the offending blood factor. For example, if the mare is Aa negative, and has antibodies against Aa factor, then a stallion with Aa factor should be avoided. Only Aa negative stallions should be used to breed this mare.

Blood typing is currently done by evaluating for lytic (with added complement) or agglutinating reactions when mixing the horse's red blood cells and specific anti-erythrocyte antibodies directed against known factors. Sera with antibodies that are monospecific to factors within the seven major blood systems are used. For example, if a positive reaction occurs when combining anti-Aa antibody with the patient's red blood cells, then the patient is known to have Aa factor on its red blood cell surface. Most of these genetic markers are expressed semi-dominantly, so that alleles on both chromosomes are usually expressed phenotypically.

A rapid (15 min), emergency blood typing protocol has been described to detect the presence or absence of Aa and Ca on patient erythrocytes in order to aid in blood donor selection (Owens et al., 2008). This also uses equine derived specific antibodies against Aa and Ca.

2) Anti-erythrocyte antibody screening has two clinical applications. The first is in selection of blood donors, who would ideally not have any anti-erythrocyte antibodies in their serum. The second is in prevention or diagnosis of NI. The mare should be tested for anti-erythrocyte antibodies 1–2 weeks prior to foaling due date. The test is performed with the mare's serum using a panel of red cells from 11 horses with known blood types and one donkey. If the sire's blood is

Interpretation of Equine Laboratory Diagnostics, First Edition. Edited by Nicola Pusterla and Jill Higgins.
© 2018 John Wiley & Sons, Inc. Published 2018 by John Wiley & Sons, Inc.

available, his red blood cells can be added to the panel as well. A positive result is agglutination or hemolysis of one or more of the panel horse's red blood cells. If the antibody screen is positive for antibodies, particularly against those of the sire's factors, then NI is highly likely. Colostrum can also be tested for anti-erythrocyte antibodies (Johnson, 2015).

47.3 Sample Collection and Submission

1) For blood typing, 5 mL EDTA or ACD tubes are required. Samples should be shipped overnight and kept cool. EDTA samples should be shipped within 24 h of collection, whereas ACD tubes are more stable and can be shipped within one week of the collection. The overnight shipment should be with an ice pack; however, the samples should not be allowed to have direct contact with the ice pack (Equine Blood Typing, UC Davis, 2016).

2) For anti-erythrocyte antibody screening, as is done for potential blood donors or for screening mares for NI within 2 weeks prior to foaling, 2 mL of serum is required. The blood from a 5- or 10-mL red top tube should be allowed to clot for 30–60 min, and then the sample should be spun with removal of serum into another tube (Equine Blood Typing, UC Davis, 2016).

47.4 Possible Results

Horses have seven different red blood cell "Groups," also called "Systems," which correspond to a specific gene encoding for that antigen. Within each of these genes, two or more different alleles exist (Table 47.1). These alleles code for "Factors," which are antigenic sites on the surface of the red blood cells. So far, over 30 factors have been identified in horses (Table 47.1).

The blood type result for an individual horse is a list of the genetic markers that have been identified for that individual.

47.5 Interpretation

Each blood group or system is denoted by an uppercase letter, including A, C, D, K, P, Q, and U which are the seven blood groups or systems recognized by the International Society for Animal Blood Group Research (Bowling and Clark, 1985). Additionally, specific laboratories recognize additional blood groups or systems in horses, including Group T.

The factors, representing different alleles within each blood group gene, are recognized by lower case letters. Factors are the antigenic sites on the surface molecules, making the red blood cells antigenic to horses that lack those factors. The number of different alleles within each blood group varies from 2, as is the case for the C, K, and U blood groups, up to 27 for the D system (Table 47.1). Examples of factors include lower case letters of the alphabet, ranging from a-i and k-r, which can exist in combinations. For example, As, Dadl, Qbc, and Ua represent alleles within their respective groups. Groups of factors on a single allele, for example, "adl" or "abc" are termed "phenogroups".

47.6 Case Example

A 20-year-old Warmblood mare was presented with a maxillary sinus cyst associated with a chronic sinusitis caused by *Streptococcus equi* ss *zooepidemicus*. In anticipation of sinus flap surgery, a blood donor was selected based on the mare's blood type. The mare's blood type results were: Aabf, Ca, Dk, K-, Pb, Qabc, U-. In addition, the mare had no anti-erythrocyte antibodies, either lysins or agglutinins.

Table 47.1 Equine blood groups and factors.

Group or system	Factors	Examples of varying alleles
A	a,b,c,d,e,f,g	Aa, Aabf, Aadf, Adg, Aabdf, Aabdg, Ab, Abc, Abce, Abe, Ac, Ace, Ae, A-
C	a	Ca, C-
D	a,b,c,d,e,f,g,h,I,k,l,m,n,o,p,q,r	Dad, Dadl, Dadlr, Dadlnr, Dbc, Dbcmq, Dcg, Dcegi, Ddk, Dd, Dcefg, Ddfk, Dcfgk, Ddef, Dde, Ddh, Ddeo, Ddn, Dcg, Ddgh, Dadn, Dcg, D-
K	a	Ka, K-
P	a,b,c,d	Pa, Pac, Pacd, Pad, Pb, Pbd, Pd, P-
Q	a,b,c	Qa, Qab, Qabc, Qac, Qb, Qbc, Qc, Q-
U	a	Ua, U-

Source: Adapted from Bowling and Clark (1985) and Rodriguez-Gallardo et al. (1992).

In this case, an appropriate donor would be relatively easy to find because the mare is positive for the most antigenic factors, Aa, Qa, and Ca. Therefore, the donor could have these same factors as this mare, and the mare would not develop antibodies against them. In addition, the donor would not have antibodies against these factors since they have them on their red cell surface as well. Ideally the donor would lack Ua, Ka, Pa, Qrs, and Dabcg factors, because the mare lacks these factors on her red cell surface and could become sensitized to them; while they are far less antigenic and less likely to cause

significant transfusion reactions than Aa, Qa, or Ca, they have been reported to cause NI and therefore would be ideal to avoid, especially if the mare may be bred in the future. It would be difficult to nearly impossible to find a donor that lacks all of these secondary factors, but one that is free of as many as possible would be the top choice. The factors previously associated with NI include: Aa, Qa, Ab, Qrs, Qb, Qc, Dc, Da, Db, Dg, Ka, Pa, Pb, and Ua (Boyle et al., 2005). A donor that is Aa, Qa or Ca negative can also be used for this mare, as long as it is tested negative for antibodies against these factors.

References

Bowling AT and Clark RS. 1985. Blood group and protein polymorphism gene frequencies for seven breeds of horses in the United States. Animal Blood Groups and Biochem Genet, 16: 93–108.

Boyle AG, Magdesian KG, and Ruby RE. 2005. Neonatal isoerythrolysis in horse foals and a mule foal: 18 cases (1988–2003). J Am Vet Med Assoc, 227: 1276–1283.

Equine blood typing. 2016. UC Davis Veterinary Medicine; Veterinary Medical Teaching Hospital Clinical Diagnostic Laboratories. www.vetmed.ucdavis.edu/vmth/lab_services/clinical_labs.

Johnson JR. 2015. Diseases caused by allogeneic incompatibilities (Horses and ruminants). In BP Smith (ed.),

Large Animal Internal Medicine, Mosby, St Louis: Elsevier, pp. 1564–1567.

Owens SD, Snipes J, Magdesian KG, and Christopher MM. 2008. Evaluation of a rapid agglutination method for detection of equine red cell surface antigens (Ca and Aa) as part of pretransfusion testing. Vet Clin Pathol, 37: 49–56.

Rodriguez-Gallardo PP, Aguilar Sanchez P, Vega Pla JL, and de Anndres Cara DF. 1992. Blood group and protein polymorphism gene frequencies for the Andalusian horse breed. A comparison with four American horse breeds. Arch Zootec, 41(extra): 433–442.

48

Bacteriology and Mycology Testing

Joshua B. Daniels[1] and Barbara A. Byrne[2]

[1] Department of Microbiology, Immunology and Pathology, College of Veterinary Medicine & Biomedical Sciences, Colorado State University, Colorado, USA
[2] Department of Pathology, Microbiology and Immunology, School of Veterinary Medicine, University of California, California, USA

48.1 Introduction

Culture for diagnosis of bacterial and fungal-associated disease is unique among laboratory techniques for diagnosis of infectious diseases. The majority of the microbiota that cause disease are opportunists and may variably colonize and/or contaminate different body sites of healthy patients and sick patients alike. Additionally, successful cultivation of microorganisms requires appropriate sampling and transport to optimize recovery and detection of the agent(s) of interest (Miller, 1999). Therefore, it is critical to always consider the following when interpreting bacteriology or mycology results: (1) sterility or degree of normal microbiota content of the anatomic site, (2) appropriateness of transport media and timely conveyance to the laboratory, and (3) most importantly, clinical signs, history, and differential diagnosis.

48.2 Preanalytical Variables

Interpretation of culture results is most straightforward when the anatomic site sampled is sterile in nature (Table 48.1). As long as the site and/or sample were not inadvertently contaminated during the sampling process, the results will usually be meaningful. Parallel cytological evaluation of samples from sterile sites is also informative; results of cytology are often the impetus for ordering cultures.

However, negative results from sterile sites do not necessarily indicate that the site(s) in question are free of infection. Confidence in negative results is increased by submitting reasonable amounts of specimen. Sending a single culturette swab (which usually holds approximately 50 μl of fluid) can lead to false negative results, especially if the infection is paucibacillary. The small-specimen size problem is compounded when one culturette or an otherwise miniscule sample is used for multiple cultures (e.g., aerobic culture, anaerobic culture, and mycology). Whenever possible, one is advised to send large amounts of sample material.

When interpreting culture results from non-sterile sites, clinical history and differential diagnosis are extremely important. This history and clinical signs may direct the laboratory to use specialized media for bacterial cultivation to enhance the ability to isolate key bacteriological differential diagnosis organisms.

Because the microbiology laboratory must have viable organisms to cultivate, selection of transport media (Table 48.2) and management of time and ambient temperature are key factors to optimizing recovery of microbiota in culture. When possible, tissue is preferred over swabs because tissue essentially acts as a transport medium, as microbiota are relatively stable in the tissue where they are putatively propagating to cause infection. However, very small volumes of tissue may desiccate in transport, therefore for tissue volumes less than $1\,cm^3$, it is advisable to make a small "nest" for the tissue using sterile gauze moistened with sterile non-bacteriostatic physiologic saline, in a sterile specimen container such as a sealed sterile urine collection cup. Aseptically acquired biopsy specimens are ideal, however for necropsy, larger "chunky" specimens that may be seared to decrease surface contaminants are invariably preferred.

When tissue cannot be sampled directly, and the sample is not a fluid, specialized transport media are required. A clinic should be reasonably stocked with transport media or at worst, have a working relationship with a human healthcare facility nearby that may provide materials on short notice. It is also important

Interpretation of Equine Laboratory Diagnostics, First Edition. Edited by Nicola Pusterla and Jill Higgins.

Table 48.1 Sterile anatomical sites.

Sterile Anatomic Sites	
Site/sample	Comment
CSF	
Joint space/synovial structure	
Lower respiratory tract	Usually sterile below trachea
Thoracic cavity	
Peritoneal cavity	
Blood culture	

Table 48.2 Media used for specimen transport.

Transport Media	
Microorganisms	Media
Non-fastidious aerobic or facultatively anaerobic bacteria, or fungi	Amies medium in culturette with foam sponge at the bottom
Anaerobic bacteria	Amies or Cary-Blair medium in pre-reduced agar
Taylorella equigenitalis	Amies medium with charcoal
Mycoplasma spp.	Amies medium or "CVM" medium (Chlamydia, Virus, Mycoplasma)

for veterinary clinic staff to be mindful of expiration dates of transport media as part of a quality control program.

Samples bound for the laboratory should be kept cold (approximately 4 °C), but not frozen. While freezing samples will minimize bacterial overgrowth (which could obscure the ability to detect at pathogen of interest in a specimen sourced from a non-sterile site), freezing samples with very low numbers of organisms may completely obscure the ability to cultivate the organism(s) of interest because the freeze-thaw cycle will impact overall viability of microbiota. Differences in cryotolerance among microbial species are not completely understood; therefore, it is reasonable to avoid freezing altogether (Walker et al., 2006). Importantly, if virus isolation is desired from the same sample, freezing would adversely affect the ability to isolate most viruses.

Some bacteria and all fungi require specialized media and/or culture conditions for isolation (Box 48.1). If any of these bacteria are suspected in a disease process, this should be made clear to the microbiology laboratory so that samples are processed and incubated appropriately.

Box 48.1 Bacteria and fungi that require specialized media or growth conditions that should be specifically requested.

Anaerobes including clostridial organisms
Mycobacterium paratuberculosis, other mycobacteria
Mycoplasma
Campylobacter
Leptospira
Listeria (cold enrichment for neural tissues)
Salmonella (selection/enrichment)
Fungi

48.3 Interpretation of the Gram Stain

Most laboratories supply Gram stain results of the initial sample that can be used to guide empirical therapy. The Gram stain is useful to delineate the presence of bacteria or fungi, the Gram reaction of any bacteria observed, and their morphology. Occasionally the genus of the bacteria present can be inferred by the Gram stain appearance. For example, the presence of Gram-positive cocci in chains or cultures is suggestive of *Streptococcus* spp. or *Staphylococcus* spp., respectively. Filamentous Gram-positive beaded rods may be consistent with *Actinomyces* or *Nocardia* whereas pleomorphic Gram-positive coccobacilli can indicate *Rhodococcus equi* or *Corynebacterium pseudotuberculosis*. Gram-negative rods might be enterics, non-enteric bacteria (e.g., *Pseudomonas* spp.), or anaerobic Gram negative rods. The presence of inflammatory cells is more difficult to determine based on the Gram stain as it does not adequately illuminate the cellular features that differentiate the cell types. Therefore, for sites where demonstration of inflammatory cells is important for interpretation of positive culture results, a Wright-Giemsa stain of the sample is also warranted.

48.4 Upper Respiratory Infections

The nasal cavity, nasopharynx, and guttural pouches are not sterile sites. Given that these sites are heavily colonized with microflora in healthy patients, culture is only useful in specific clinical situations.

Streptococcus equi ssp. *equi* (SEE) is the predominant cause of guttural pouch empyema, thus culturing samples from animals with abnormal endoscopic findings for this agent is useful. The guttural pouches are also regarded as the predominant carriage site for SEE in non-clinical horses and culture of a sample from this site is also useful as a screening tool in SEE surveillance. Because SEE is a high-consequence pathogen in populations of horses, it is critical to maximize sensitivity of detection. The presence of competing flora in culture could obscure the ability to detect it, and as with all culture based methods, the volume and viability of the specimen also affect sensitivity. Therefore, in recent years, multiple studies have shown that PCR-based methods offer superior sensitivity to culture (Sweeney et al., 2005, Lindahl et al., 2013).

Suspicion of guttural pouch mycosis is the other primary reason to culture this anatomic site. Culture is also performed on the basis of abnormal endoscopic findings. Frequently the diagnosis is made upon the endoscopic examination due to the presence of grossly-visible mats of fungal mycelia in the pouches, but speciation of the fungal agent is made upon culture. The most frequent fungal pathogens of horses are *Aspergillus* spp. Often with mycosis due to *Aspergillus* spp., the etiologic diagnosis is attainable upon cytology because of the large amount of intact visible fruiting structures and conidia (Figure 48.1). One case series found that histopathology was more sensitive than culture for diagnosis of pouch mycosis (Ludwig et al., 2005).

The clinical significance of isolation of other microorganisms from the guttural pouch is questionable, therefore, the general approach of associating culture results with cytology or histopathology is necessary for ascribing associations of individual agents with disease states.

48.5 Bronchopneumonia and Pleuropneumonia

Acquisition of material for culture from the lower respiratory tract is best accomplished by transtracheal wash. This method, when performed carefully, will avoid oropharyngeal contaminating flora. It is also superior to

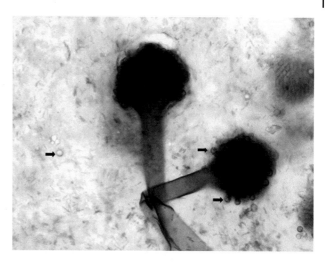

Figure 48.1 Fruiting structure of *Aspergillus* spp. including conidia (arrows) observed in a cytological sample collected from an equine guttural pouch.

bronchoalveolar lavage for culture, in that bronchoscopes pass through the oropharynx and become contaminated by oral flora. If performing both techniques is indicated, such as with animals that may have chronic disease due to suspected underlying recurrent airway obstruction, performance of the transtracheal wash for culture should precede the BAL.

Many organisms may be associated with bronchopneumonia and pleuropneumonia (Table 48.3) (Reuss and Giguere, 2015). Both aerobic and anaerobic culture is advised in cases of pleuropneumonia, as approximately one-third of cases involve anaerobes (Sweeney et al., 1991). Ideally, in cases of pleuropneumonia, both pleural fluid and tracheal fluid are submitted for culture. However, as inflammation usually precedes the invasion

Table 48.3 Possible causative organisms in cases of bronchopneumonia or pleuropneumonia.

Possible causative organisms in cases of bronchopneumonia or pleuropneumonia			
Non-Enteric Gram-Negative Bacteria	*Enteric Gram-Negative Bacteria*	*Gram-Positive Aerobes*	*Anaerobes*
Pasteurella spp.	*Klebsiella* spp.	β-Hemolytic streptococci[a]	*Bacteroides* spp.
Actinobacillus spp.	*Escherichia coli*	*Staphylococcus* spp.	*Clostridium* spp.
Bordetella spp.	*Enterobacter* spp.	*Rhodococcus equi*[b]	*Peptostreptococcus* spp.
Pseudomonas spp.[c]	*Salmonella enterica*	*Streptococcus pneumoniae*[d]	*Fusobacterium* spp.
			Prevotella spp.

a) *Streptococcus equi* subsp. *zooepidemicus* most commonly.
b) Rare in immunocompetent adults.
c) Rarely a primary cause of pneumonia and more commonly due to sampling equipment contamination.
d) Common pathogen of humans and has been correlated with disease in young Thoroughbred racehorses in the United Kingdom but rarely isolated from horses in the United States.
Source: Reuss and Giguere (2015). Reproduced with permission of Elsevier.

of bacteria into the pleural space, a tracheal aspirate will have a greater diagnostic yield (i.e., is more likely to be positive) if only able to obtain and submit one of the two samples for culture (Sweeney et al., 1991).

Transtracheal aspirates can occasionally be contaminated with oropharyngeal flora should the horse cough during the procedure leading to introduction of the tube used for aspiration into the upper respiratory tract or if there is laryngeal dysfunction leading to aspiration of material. While many lower respiratory tract pathogens are opportunistic arising from the oropharynx, the presence of numerous bacterial species in low numbers may be consistent with contamination. Isolation of alpha-hemolytic streptococci, *Corynebacterium* spp. (other than *C. pseudotuberculosis*), or certain non-enteric bacteria such as *Neisseria* or *Moraxella* spp. are suggestive of oropharyngeal contamination.

Common agents of bacterial pneumonia include *S. equi* ssp *zooepidemicus*, *Actinobacillus equuli* ssp *hemolyticus*, *E. coli*, *Rhodococcus equi* (foals), and *Klebsiella pneumoniae*. *Mycoplasma felis* is an unusual cause of pleuritic and/or pericarditis in horses. Since *Mycoplasma* spp. require specialized media for isolation, a special request for *Mycoplasma* culture should be made if this condition is suspected.

48.6 Peritonitis

Septic peritonitis is classified as primary (idiopathic or spontaneous) or secondary. Primary peritonitis has no obvious direct cause, and occurs most often in foals (Davis, 2003). Secondary peritonitis is usually associated with a primary GI event, such as a ruptured GI viscous or due to bacterial translocation across a devitalized segment of intestine.

Primary peritonitis is usually associated with a sole agent: *Streptococcus equi* spp. *zooepidemicus.*, *Rhodococcus equi*, or *Actinobacillus* spp. (Davis, 2003).

Secondary peritonitis is frequently polymicrobial, because of the heterogeneous nature of GI microbiota. Bacteria recovered usually include enteric Gram-negative bacilli (especially *E. coli*), as well as *Staphylococcus* spp., *Enterococcus* spp., and anaerobic bacteria including anaerobic Gram-negative organisms such as *Bacterioides* spp. and *Prevotella* spp. that are frequently penicillin-resistant (Davis, 2003).

Individual infectious agents have not been meaningfully associated with survival; rather the strongest association that has been established with mortality to date is any association of peritonitis development following abdominal surgery (Hawkins et al., 1993, Nogradi et al., 2011). Notably, clinicians are frequently concerned about *Enterococcus* spp., because they are intrinsically resistant to several classes of antimicrobial agents, and targeted antimicrobial therapy may not be possible in a horse (Murray, 1990). The significance of the presence of *Enterococcus* spp. is controversial, and there are no data in horses that establish their clinical importance in septic peritonitis. The importance of isolation of enterococci is also controversial in human peritonitis (Harbarth and Uckay, 2004).

48.7 Enterocolitis

Differential diagnoses of bacterial enterocolitis include salmonellosis, *Clostridium difficile*, *Clostridium perfringens*, and *Lawsonia intracellularis*. Other agents that may cause diarrhea include *Clostridium piliforme* and *Rhodococcus equi* that are both foal pathogens. *Salmonella* spp., which may be recovered from a low proportion of asymptomatic carriers, is of particular concern because of its potential to spread among horses, especially in clinical settings. In horses with gastrointestinal signs, *Salmonella* has been detected in up to 13% of the animals; in the general US horse population, the overall prevalence has been estimated at 0.8% (Ernst et al., 2004, Traub-Dargatz et al., 1990). When using fecal culture to establish *Salmonella* negative status for biosurveillance, or as a rule-out test in a symptomatic animal, it is important to evaluate multiple serially-collected fecal samples of adequate volume and cultured using an enrichment technique before confidently concluding that an animal is negative (Burgess and Morley, 2014). Because *Salmonella* tends to be unevenly distributed in feces, it is recommended that feces are homogenized before submitting at least 1 g to the laboratory for culture (Burgess and Morley, 2014). When submitting serial samples from asymptomatic animals for surveillance, it is often more cost effective to send several samples in bulk to the laboratory. Fortunately, freezing does not seem to significantly affect viability of *Salmonella* from feces up to 14 days (O'Carroll et al., 1999).

A *Salmonella*-positive culture result from horse is always significant given the importance of this agent in nosocomial spread. However, just because *Salmonella* is detected does not mean that this agent is causing clinical signs of gastrointestinal disease. Interpretation should be made in light of the clinical picture including clinical signs of gastroenteritis and the presence of an inflammatory leukogram perhaps with neutropenia. Appropriate testing for additional agents such as *C. difficile* may help to identify alternative diagnoses. However, given the low frequency of isolation of this agent from normal horses, detection of *Salmonella* in horses with compatible clinical signs is likely significant.

Culture for *C. difficile* is not always useful in making a clinical diagnosis, because nontoxigenic and toxigenic strains alike may be shed by both healthy and diarrheic horses; moreover, viability declines rapidly after sampling and is best attempted when the sample is transported in anaerobic transport media and processed by the laboratory within 24 h of collection (Weese et al., 2000). Foal carrier rates range from 0–3%, and adult carrier rates range from 0–10% (Diab et al., 2013). Presence of toxin in feces has a higher positive predictive value than culture. Toxin (*TcdA* and/or *TcdB*) may be detected via enzyme immunoassay, or by cytotoxicity assay.

While culture is not as useful as toxin detection in establishing *Clostridium difficile* as the cause of diarrhea, isolation in culture is necessary for determining antimicrobial susceptibility (Magdesian et al., 2006). Isolation in culture is also necessary for molecular epidemiologic studies.

Similarly, as an antemortem diagnostic culture, detection of *Clostridium perfringens* is of very limited utility because it is found in a high percentage of normal horses. Toxin typing of *C. perfringens* isolates by PCR is helpful in establishing a diagnosis. Toxin type "A" strains (production of α toxin only) are very common in both healthy adult horses and foals. Establishing a role for type "A" *C. perfringens* in enterocolitis requires parallel histopathologic studies and is therefore more useful post-mortem. However, some *C. perfringens* type A strains produce β_2 toxin, which is believed to increase their virulence. Recovery of such strains from compatible antemortem cases increases the index of suspicion for their role in disease; however, histopathologic evaluation is necessary for a definitive diagnosis. The presence of *C. perfringens* type "C" (α and β toxins) has also been correlated with severe disease in foals.

There are also an ELISA-based tests available that can detect the presence of *C. perfringens* toxins. Detection of enterotoxin is of doubtful significance as there has been no evidence that this toxin is active on equine tissues. Detection of beta, epsilon, or iota toxins in gastrointestinal contents by ELISA can be beneficial in establishing *C. perfringens* as a causative agent of gastrointestinal disease (Diab et al., 2012).

48.8 Urogenital

48.8.1 Cystitis

Diagnosis of cystitis requires collection of urine via catheter or by midstream free-catch. Because the urethra is not a sterile body site, quantitative culture is critical in establishing the significance of bacteria that are present. A mixed culture result with low numbers of bacteria is suggestive of contamination. Suggested reference ranges for healthy adult horses are (1) midstream free-catch <20,000 cfu/ml and (2) catheterized <500 cfu/ml with males having fewer bacteria isolated (MacLeay and Kohn, 1998). Some of the bacteria isolated from normal horses are normal inhabitants of the equine lower urogenital tract and include streptococci, Gram-positive diptheroids, *Bacillus*, enterococci, and enterics. The most common uropathogens include *Streptococcus equi* ssp. *zooepidemicus* and Gram–negative enteric bacilli, including *E. coli* and *Klebsiella* spp. Staphylococci and *Corynebacterium* spp. are also occasionally isolated as pathogens from equine urine (Saulez et al., 2005).

48.8.2 Metritis

Bacterial culture with accompanying endometrial cytology of the uterus is most often performed as a pre-breeding screen, or as a rule-out test in mares that have not been successfully bred, ideally in conjunction with uterine biopsy. Among microbiota that are associated with metritis, *Taylorella equigenitalis* is of greatest concern due to its highly contagious nature. Culture for *T. equigenitalis* must be ordered specifically from the laboratory because specialized media and conditions are necessary for its cultivation. It also requires specialized transport media for specimens for results to be recognized by regulatory agencies (OIE, 2012).

While bacterial endometritis has been associated with organisms including *E. coli*, *Klebsiella* spp., *Enterobacter* spp., *Pseudomonas aeruginosa*, and *Streptococcus equi* subsp. *zooepidemicus*, the clinical utility of screening for these and other common opportunistic pathogens in the absence of accompanying cytology or histopathology to substantiate the presence of inflammation prior to breeding in healthy mares has not been demonstrated. Collection of uterine samples either via guarded swab or via uterine lavage may result in contamination with vaginal flora; thus, it is important to examine samples cytologically for the presence of neutrophils with or without bacteria to interpret a positive culture result as significant. Pre- and post-breeding swab cultures of the stallion urethra and prepuce have also been recommended to assess for the presence and potential venereal transfer of such opportunistic pathogens. While such transmission has been documented (Samper and Tibary, 2006), appropriate clinical studies assessing factors such as successful breeding and occurrence of metritis have not been performed to assess any benefit that the results of these cultures might provide.

Fungal endometritis has been associated with a variety of organisms including *Candida* spp. and *Aspergillus* spp.

among others. As with bacterial endometritis, concurrent cytopathologic and/or histopathologic evaluation are necessary to attribute endometritis to these agents.

48.9 Septicemia

Neonatal foals are the most likely patients to require blood culture. Up to 45% of neonatal mortality is due to sepsis (Gayle et al., 1998). One of the most common indications for blood culture is failure of passive transfer or suspicion thereof.

There are two methods of blood culture, each of which requires a special transport container. The method that a given end user employs in practice is usually a function of the preference of their laboratory, as there are distinctly different workflows for each during laboratory processing.

1) *Enrichment culture*: Blood is inoculated directly into a collection bottle that contains a nutrient broth, which may or may not also contain a resin to adsorb previously administered aminoglycoside antimicrobial agents. Theoretically the resin will increase the likelihood of obtaining viable bacteria and an *in vitro* study has supported this (Lorenzo-Figueras et al., 2006). Typically, the collection bottles are incubated for up to one week and subcultured to semi-solid media at 24 h, 48 h, and at 5–7 days. Semi-solid media is subsequently incubated and observed for colonial growth for several days. One advantage of this system is that it can be more sensitive than non-enrichment techniques in that small numbers of bacteria will amplify in the enrichment broth. However, bacterial contaminants introduced into the collection bottle will also multiply, confounding interpretation in some cases.
2) *Lysis centrifugation*: Blood is inoculated into a collection tube that contains a mild detergent that does not adversely affect bacterial viability. The detergent lyses blood cells including leukocytes that contain phagocytosed bacteria. The lysate is plated onto semi-solid media that is incubated and observed daily for colonial growth. Isolated bacterial colonies may be obtained up to 24 h earlier than via enrichment culture. Also, because there is no enrichment step, the likelihood of obtaining false positive culture due to contamination is lower.

It is recommended that up to four blood samples collected from different anatomical sites over 24-h period of time be used to adequately detect bacteremia in animals and humans. Examination of multiple cultures allows the clinician and microbiologist to interpret the findings and identify potential contaminants.

A wide variety of bacteria are associated with neonatal sepsis, including Gram-negative enteric bacilli (especially *Actinobacillus equuli* ssp. *equuli* and *E. coli*), enterococci, staphylococci, and streptococci (Marsh and Palmer 2001). However, it is notable that while the blood is considered a sterile body site, healthy foals may manifest transient bacteremia (Hackett et al., 2015). Isolation of skin flora such as coagulase-negative staphylococci from only one time point is suggestive of contamination. Whereas isolation of the same bacterial species from multiple time points or sites is more consistent with actual sepsis.

48.10 Bacterial Meningitis

Infection of the central nervous system is a rare event in horses fortunately. The most likely patients to have bacteria isolated from the CSF are foals where *E. coli* is the most commonly isolated bacterium (Viu et al., 2012). The interpretation of a positive bacterial isolation from equine patients should always be correlated with clinicopathological findings of the CSF. Pleocytosis, increased protein, and the presence of bacteria are all highly supportive of a bacterial infection (Viu et al., 2012). The presence of common skin flora such as coagulase negative staphylococci without compatible cytological findings is more consistent with contamination. Some of the more common bacteria isolated from the CSF of horses include *S. equi* ssp *zooepidemicus*, SEE, and *E. coli*. More unusual isolates could include *Klebsiella pneumoniae*, *Corynebacterium pseudotuberculosis*, and *Listeria monocytogenes* (Toth et al., 2012). Many cases of bacterial meningitis have infections affecting other body systems and spread to the central nervous system occurs hematogenously (Toth et al., 2012). Thus, culture of samples from these other sites can aid identification of infectious agents in cases with compatible CSF cytological findings where CSF culture fails to yield bacterial growth.

Agents that cause neurologic disease but are not found in the central nervous system include the causative agents of tetanus and botulism, *Clostridium tetani* and *C. botulinum*, respectively. It can be very difficult to isolate and identify *C. tetani* from wound infections; hence a culture negative for this agent does not rule out this disease. Although isolation of *C. botulinum* is less problematic most horses are ingesting botulinum toxin resulting in disease rather than an infection per se (foals with toxicoinfectious botulism are the exception). Consequently, isolation of this organism is generally not indicated. Rather, detection of botulinum toxin in feed or water is a more useful diagnostic test. Furthermore *C. botulinum* can be ubiquitous in feces and the environment and isolation would be of unknown significance.

48.11 Musculoskeletal Infections

Bone, muscle, joints, and other synovial structures are sterile sites; consequently, isolation of bacteria from them is almost always significant. However, contamination during sampling may result in inadvertent isolation of bacteria. This is particularly true with wounds. In these cases, superficial swabs of the area are inadequate to determine the primary agent(s) and frequently have substantial contamination including enterococci and *Staphylococcus* spp. It is best to disinfect the superficial aspect of the wound and collect a deep culture, preferably a tissue sample for bacterial isolation.

Common aerobic bacteria isolated from musculoskeletal infections include *Escherichia coli,* coagulase-negative staphylococci, *Staphylococcus aureus, Streptococcus equi* subspecies *zooepidemicus, Actinobacillus* spp., *Enterococcus* spp., and *Pseudomonas* spp. (Byrne unpublished observations). Another important agent includes *Brucella abortus* that can infect the atlantal or supraspinus bursa. Detection of coagulase-negative staphylococci and enterococci should be interpreted cautiously as these are frequent skin contaminants. Obligate anaerobic bacteria include *Clostridium* spp. and *Fusobacterium* spp. may often be found in many musculoskeletal infections. In foals, any agent associated with septicemia may result in joint or epiphyseal infection.

Cytological evaluation of synovial fluid can assist with interpretation of positive culture findings. Isolation of bacteria from synovial structures can be often be frustratingly difficult; the results of clinicopathological analysis is essential for determining sepsis in these cases. Some laboratories and clinics inoculate blood culture enrichment broths to increase the likelihood of detecting bacteria. However, this practice can also lead to detection of contaminants (Dumoulin et al., 2010).

48.12 Dermatological and Subcutaneous Infections

Equine patients are less likely to suffer from bacterial pyoderma that is common in small animal patients. If a superficial bacterial skin infection is suspected, a skin biopsy may be warranted. The skin should be disinfected prior to collection of the biopsy as there are a number of bacteria that are considered normal flora of equine skin including staphylococci, *Corynebacterium,* and occasionally enterococci. Superficial disinfection allows removal of normal flora and more accurate identification of the causative agent.

Unfortunately, normal bacterial flora is most frequently the causative agents of dermatological infections making differentiation between contamination and a true infection difficult for example, *Staphylococcus aureus.* Most frequently agents found in moderate to large numbers in pure or nearly pure growth are likely to be significant.

Some of the bacterial agents that are associated with dermatological manifestations that are not part of the normal flora include *Dermatophilus congolensis, Rhodococcus equi* (cutaneous and subcutaneous abscesses), *Burkholderia mallei* (subcutaneous with cutaneous ulceration), and *Corynebacterium pseudotuberculosis.*

Dermatophytosis is a more common skin infection in horses than bacteria. Cultures of hair and/or crusts from suspected lesions on suitable media, such as dermatophyte test media, along with histopathologic examination are excellent ways to detect these fungi. It is important that mold that grows on dermatophyte test medium be identified microscopically or molecularly as a number of non-pathogenic saprophytic fungi are capable of growing on this media and may even result in the characteristic red color change usually associated with dermatophyte growth. Fortunately, a culture result that identifies a dermatophyte is always significant as these fungi are not part of the normal flora of skin. Some of the common dermatophytes in horses include *Trichophyton equinum, T. mantagrophytes,* and *Microsporum equinum.*

Pythium insidiosum is an aquatic oomycete often confused with a fungus that causes severe subcutaneous pyogranulomatous inflammation and ulceration. Isolation of this agent can be difficult and requires specialized media (Grooters et al., 2002). Thus, if this organism is suspected, it is important to notify the laboratory so that appropriate media and culture conditions can be utilized.

Cellulitis is often a rapidly progressive condition accompanied by fever, severe pain, and swelling. Antimicrobial therapy must be initiated early in the infection prior to the availability of culture and susceptibility results. Regardless, collection of samples prior to administration of antimicrobial agents is important to guide definitive therapy or a change in therapy if empirical treatment is insufficient. As for other infections, collection of an appropriate sample is critical for interpretation of a positive culture. Cellulitis in horses can be primary or secondary associated with surgical or traumatic wounds. Common agents of cellulitis include coagulase positive *Staphylococcus, S. equi* ssp *zooepidemicus,* and *Clostridium* spp. (Adam and Southwood, 2007) Less common agents include *Rhodococcus equi, Corynebacterium pseudotuberculosis, Actinobacillus ligneresii,* and *Actinobacillus equuli* (Perdrizet and Scott, 1987, Carmalt et al., 1999, Castagnetti et al., 2008).

48.13 Lymph Node/Lymphatic Infections

The frequency of equine lymphatic infections varies across the world but there are only a few agents that cause primary lymphangitis including the bacteria *Corynebacterium pseudotuberculosis* and *Burholderia mallei* and the fungi *Histoplasma farcinimosum* and *Sporothrix schenkii*. Isolation of these agents from the lymph node or lymphatics is a significant finding. Lymph node infections are more common in horses and the agents most commonly associated with this organ, particularly the mandibular lymph nodes include *Streptococcus equi* ssp *equi* (strangles) and *Actinomyces* spp. (Albini et al. 2008, Fielding et al. 2008).

48.14 Ocular Infections

The conjunctiva of the eye contains a variety of Gram-positive and Gram-negative bacteria including streptococci, staphylococci, micrococci, and non-enterics.

In the event of ocular trauma that results in corneal ulceration any of these opportunistic organisms may colonize the disrupted surface. A more serious infection may result from a fungal organism; most commonly *Aspergillus* spp. in horses. Care should be taken to only sample the ulcer itself when collecting a specimen for culture as touching the eyelid or conjunctiva may result in isolation of this normal flora confounding interpretation. Most cultures of corneal ulcers yield only one or two primary pathogen(s). A highly mixed population of bacteria is more consistent with contamination.

Interpretation of bacterial or fungal culture results is largely dependent on the anatomical site sampled, methodology of sample collection, and the microbial flora at the sampling site. Proper collection of samples for microbial isolation is essential for obtaining meaningful and interpretable results. Communication with the laboratory can be quite helpful in determining sample type and meaning of results. The number of bacteria isolated, whether in mixed or pure culture, and the specific genus and species can guide determination of the significance of any particular isolate (Figure 48.2).

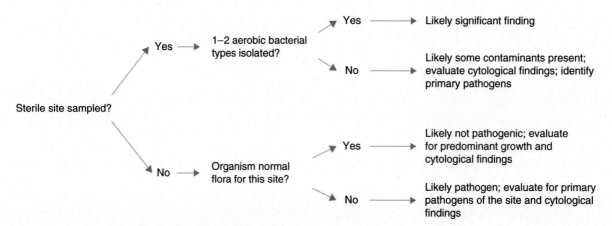

Figure 48.2 General algorithm for interpretation of aerobic bacterial culture results.

References

Adam EN and Southwood LL. 2007. Primary and secondary limb cellulitis in horses: 44 cases (2000–2006). J Am Vet Med Assoc, 231(11): 1696–1703.

Albini S, Korczak BM, Abril C, et al. 2008. Mandibular lymphadenopathy caused by *Actinomyces denticolens* mimicking strangles in three horses. Vet Rec, 162(5): 158–159.

Burgess BA and Morley PS. 2014. Managing *Salmonella* in equine populations. Vet Clin N Am-Eq, 30(3): 623–640.

Carmalt JL, Baptiste KE, and Chirino-Trejo JM. 1999. *Actinobacillus lignieresii* infection in two horses. J Am Vet Med Assoc, 215(6): 826–828.

Castagnetti C, Rossi M, Parmeggiani F, et al. 2008. Facial cellulitis due to *Actinobacillus equuli* infection in a neonatal foal. Vet Rec, 162(11): 347–329.

Davis JL. 2003. Treatment of peritonitis. Vet Clin N Am-Eq, 19(3): 765–778.

Diab SS, Kinde H, Moore J, et al. 2012. Pathology of *Clostridium perfringens* type C in horses. Vet Pathol, 49(2): 225–263.

Diab SS, Songer G, and Uzal FA. 2013. *Clostridium difficile* infections in horses. Vet Microbiol, 167(1–2): 42–49.

Dumoulin M, Pille F, van den Abeele AM, et al. 2010. Use of blood culture medium enrichment for synovial fluid culture in horses: a comparison of different culture methods. Eq Vet J, 42(6): 541–546.

Ernst NS, Hernandez JA, MacKay RJ, et al. 2004. Risk factors associated with fecal *Salmonella* shedding among hospitalized horses with gastrointestinal disease. J Am Vet Med Assoc, 225(2): 275–281.

Fielding CL, Magdesian KG, Morgan RA, et al. 2008. *Actinomyces* species as a cause of abscesses in nine horses. Vet Rec, 162(1): 18–20.

Gayle JM, Cohen ND, and Chaffin MK, 1998. Factors associated with survival of septicemic foals: 65 cases (1988–1995). J Vet Intern Med, 12(3): 140–146.

Grooters AM, Whittington A, Lopez MK, et al. 2002. Evaluation of microbial culture techniques for the isolation of *Pythium insidiosum* from equine tissues. J Vet Diagn Invest, 14(4): 288–294.

Hackett ES, Lunn DP, Ferris RA, et al. 2015. Detection of bacteraemia and host response in healthy neonatal foals. Eq Vet J, 47(4): 405–409.

Harbarth S and Uckay I. 2004. Are there patients with peritonitis who require empiric therapy for *Enterococcus*? Eur J Clin Microbiol Infect Diseases, 23(2): 73–77.

Hawkins JF, Bowman KF, Roberts MC, et al. 1993. Peritonitis in horses: 67 cases (1985–1990). J Am Vet Med Assoc, 203(2): 284–288.

Lindahl S, Baverud V, Engenvall A, et al. 2013. Comparison of sampling sites and laboratory diagnostic tests for *Streptococcus equi* subsp *equi* in horses from confirmed strangles outbreaks. J Vet Intern Med, 27(3): 542–547.

Lorenzo-Figueras M, Pusterla N, Byrne BA, et al. 2006. *In vitro* evaluation of three bacterial culture systems for the recovery of *Escherichia coli* from equine blood. Am J Vet Res, 67(12): 2025–2029.

Ludwig A, Gatineau S, Reynaud MC, et al. 2005. Fungal isolation and identification in 21 cases of guttural pouch mycosis in horses (1998–2002). Vet J, 169(3): 457–461.

MacLeay JM and Kohn CW. 1998. Results of quantitative cultures of urine by free catch and catheterization in healthy adult horses. J Vet Intern Med, 12(2): 76–78.

Magdesian KG, Dujowich M, Madigan JE, et al. 2006. Molecular characterization of *Clostridium difficile* isolates from horses in an intensive care unit and association of disease severity with strain type. J Am Vet Med Assoc, 228(5): 751–755.

Marsh PS and Palmer JE. 2001. Bacterial isolates from blood and their susceptibility patterns in critically ill foals: 543 cases (1991–1998). J Am Vet Med Assoc, 218(10): 1608–1610.

Murray BE. 1990. The life and times of the *Enterococcus*. Clin Microbiol Rev, 3(1): 46–65.

Miller JM. 1999. *A Guide to Specimen Management in Clinical Microbiology*. Washington, D.C.: ASM Press.

Nogradi N, Toth B, and MacGillivray KC. 2011. Peritonitis in horses: 55 cases (2004–2007). Acta Veterinaria Hungarica. 59(2): 181–193.

O'Carroll JM, Davies PR, Correa MT, et al. 1999. Effects of sample storage and delayed secondary enrichment on detection of *Salmonella* spp. in swine feces. Am J Vet Res, 60(3): 359–362.

OIE. 2012. Contagious Equine Metritis. *Manual of Diagnostic Tests and Vaccines for Terrestrial Animals*. World Organization for Animal Health. Chapter 2.5.2. pages 1–7. www.oie.int/international-standard-setting/terrestrial-manual/access-online/. Accessed Dec. 4, 2015.

Perdrizet JA and Scott DW. 1987. Cellulitis and subcutaneous abscesses caused by *Rhodococcus equi* infection in a foal. J Am Vet Med Assoc, 190(12): 1559–1561.

Reuss SM and Giguere S. 2015. Update on bacterial pneumonia and pleuropneumonia in the adult horse. Vet Clin N Am-Eq, 31(1): 105–120.

Samper JC and Tibary A. 2006. Disease transmission in horses. Theriogenology, 66(3): 551–559.

Saulez MN, Cebra CK, Heidel JR, et al. 2005. Encrusted cystitits secondary to *Corynebacterium matruochotii* infection in a horse. J Am Vet Med Assoc, 226(2): 246–248.

Sweeney CR, Holocombe SJ, Bamington SC, et al. 1991. Aerobic and anaerobic bacterial isolates from horses with pneumonia or pleuropneumonia and antimicrobial susceptibility patterns of the aerobes. J Am Vet Med Assoc, 198(5): 839–842.

Sweeney CR, Timoney JF, Newton JR, et al. 2005. *Streptococcus equi* infection: guidelines for treatment, control, and prevention of strangles. J Vet Intern Med, 19(1): 123–134.

Traub-Dargatz JL, Salman MD, and Jones RL. 1990. Epidemiologic study of salmonellae shedding in the feces of horses and potential risk factors for development of infection in hospitalized horses. J Am Vet Med Assoc, 196(10): 1617–1622.

Toth B, Aleman M. Nogradi N, et al. 2012. Meningitis and meningoencephalomyelitis in horses: 28 cases (1985–2010). J Am Vet Med Assoc, 240(5): 580–587.

Viu J, Monreal L, Jose-Cunilleras E, et al. 2012. Clinical findings in 10 foals with bacterial meningoencephalitis. Eq Vet J, Supplement. Feb(41): 100–104.

Walker VK, Palmer GR, and Voordow G. 2006. Freeze-thaw tolerance and clues to winter survival of a soil community. Appl Env Microbiol, 72(3): 1784–1792.

Weese JS, Staempfli HR, and Prescott JF. 2000. Survival of *Clostridium difficile* and its toxin in equine feces: Implications for diagnostic test selection and interpretation. J Vet Diagn Invest, 12(4): 332–336.

49

Antimicrobial Susceptibility Testing

K. Gary Magdesian

Department of Medicine and Epidemiology, School of Veterinary Medicine, University of California, California, USA

49.1 Clinical Background

Antimicrobial susceptibility testing evaluates the concentrations of antimicrobials which inhibit (minimum inhibitory concentration; MIC) or kill (minimum bactericidal concentration; MBC) bacterial agents *in vitro*, as a means of predicting the ability of the specific antimicrobial to be effective *in vivo*. The MIC is reported most commonly. There are established susceptibility (S) and resistance (R) breakpoints, which are concentrations of the antimicrobial determined by the Clinical and Laboratory Standards Institute (CLSI), which are physiologically achievable in animals and are therefore consistent with efficacy *in vivo*. However, the number of antimicrobials for which CLSI has guidelines for in veterinary species is limited; many of the S and R breakpoints used in veterinary medicine are from human recommendations.

The S and R breakpoints relate the MIC of the microbe to what is attainable in plasma following administration of safe doses of the antimicrobial to the patient species. Because many of these breakpoints have been determined by pharmacokinetics and plasma concentrations in humans, they are not always relatable to veterinary species, especially for oral drugs where differences in bioavailability may be present. This is particularly true for adult horses, where the bioavailability of many orally administered drugs is markedly lower than that in humans. For example, doxycycline has a susceptibility breakpoint of 2–4 μg/mL for many human infections. However, because of relatively poor oral bioavailability in adult horses, this concentration is not achievable in equine plasma or tissues at the recommended dose of 10 mg/kg PO, q 12 h. A pathogen isolated from a horse with a MIC of 2 μg/mL would be reported as "susceptible" by the microbiology lab, even though these concentrations are not achievable *in vivo*. Based on published pharmacokinetic studies in horses, the recommended S

breakpoint should be ≤ 0.25 μg/mL (Bryant et al., 2000, Davis et al., 2006).

49.2 Test(s) Available

49.2.1 Disk Diffusion (Kirby-Bauer)

The disk diffusion is a qualitative test. There is no MIC value reported, rather simply "susceptible" or "resistant" based on a zone of inhibition of bacterial growth on agar by the antimicrobial contained in a paper disk. The disc is impregnated with a single concentration of the antibiotic. The discs are then placed on the surface of an agar plate previously inoculated with the test bacteria. The antimicrobial diffuses outward concentrically from the disc into the agar, thereby creating a concentration gradient. After incubation for 18–24 h, the zone of inhibition of bacterial growth around the disc is measured. Based on the zone diameter, the bacteria are determined to be susceptible, intermediate or resistant. One of the disadvantages is that only once concentration is used for testing per disk, and the relative susceptibility is not determined as it would with broth microdilution.

49.2.2 Broth Microdilution

Broth microdilution has the advantage of providing quantitative results. Knowing the actual MIC is helpful in determining relative efficacy of antimicrobials, and knowing which can be achieved *in vivo* after dosing. With this technique, the cultured bacteria are inoculated into tubes or wells containing serial dilutions of the antimicrobial to be tested. For example, the wells may contain 8, 4, 2, 1, 0.5, and 0.25 μg/mL for ceftiofur. After 18–24 h of incubation, the plates are examined with an analytical instrument for bacterial growth. The MIC is read out as the lowest concentration of antibiotic

Interpretation of Equine Laboratory Diagnostics, First Edition. Edited by Nicola Pusterla and Jill Higgins.

(most dilute), which still inhibits bacterial growth. For example, if growth is present in the wells containing 0.25, 0.5, and 1 µg/mL of ceftiofur, but not in those with 2 µg/mL or above, then the MIC of that microbe is 2 µg/mL.

49.2.3   E-Test

The E-test method has features of both techniques described previously. It uses a strip which has the antimicrobial impregnated on one side, at varying concentrations. The strip is then placed on the agar plate that contains the bacteria of question. The result (MIC) is read as the point on the strip where the zone of inhibition of growth intersects the lowest concentration of drug on the strip. This is the MIC, and in this manner the E-test is quantitative.

The Clinical and Laboratory Standards Institute provides standards from which good laboratory practices are described for laboratories providing antimicrobial susceptibility testing. For example, they provide standards for the medium to be used, inoculum density, incubation time, and optimal testing conditions for MIC determination.

49.3   Sample Collection and Submission

The sample type to be cultured will vary with each disease process. These can include transtracheal wash, blood cultures, urine, uterine, cerebrospinal fluid or biopsy tissue cultures, or third space effusions (e.g., peritoneal fluid), among others. The samples are submitted to a clinical microbiology lab for culture and susceptibility testing. If the samples are to be sent out, then a commercial culturette with transport medium should be used, as well as anaerobic transport media when anaerobic culture is desired. Urine samples should be submitted unaltered in sterile specimen cups. The original sample, stored in a sterile, uncoated container or tube, should be submitted along with the culturette. Blood cultures are submitted in blood culture vials, with specific vials for aerobic and anaerobic culture. Blood cultures should be kept at room temperature rather than refrigeration and sent to the lab as soon as possible.

49.4   Possible Results

The interpretation of antimicrobial susceptibility testing is largely under the guidance of two major international bodies, the Clinical and Laboratory Standards Institute (CLSI) and the European Committee on Antimicrobial Susceptibility Testing (EUCAST). The EUCAST focuses on setting breakpoints for human pathogens, whereas the CLSI has separate standing committees to consider antimicrobials in human and veterinary medicine.

Possible results of antimicrobial susceptibility testing include susceptible (S), intermediate (I), and resistant (R).

49.5   Interpretation

1) Susceptible: A microbe is defined as susceptible (S) when it is inhibited by a level of antimicrobial activity that is readily achievable in serum (serum concentration) after safe dosing of the antimicrobial in the targeted animal species, in this case horses. The antimicrobial would therefore be expected to have a high likelihood of therapeutic success.
2) Intermediate: A microbe is defined as intermediate (I) when it is inhibited by antimicrobial activity that may or may not be achievable in serum (serum concentration) after recommended dosing in the targeted animal species. Therefore, the therapeutic effect is uncertain. The antimicrobial may be effective in body sites where the drug is concentrated, or when a higher dose of the drug can be used.
3) Resistant: A microbe is defined as resistant (R) when the concentration of antimicrobial required for inhibition of growth is higher than achievable serum concentrations after recommended dosing protocols. The isolate is not inhibited by the usual achievable concentrations of the antimicrobial with normal doses and dosing schedules for the target species. There is a high likelihood of therapeutic failure.

It is important to note that the MIC should be interpreted in light of the pharmacokinetic and pharmacodynamic data for the specific antimicrobial in horses. For example, some of the CLSI susceptibility breakpoints used for orally administered antimicrobials are extrapolated from humans, yet the same plasma concentrations cannot be achieved in horses as in humans because of differences in bioavailability. Because of this, the interpretation of a result of "S" for orally administered antimicrobials should be made with caution. Therefore, the MIC should be compared to results of pharmacokinetic studies for the specific antibiotic in horses whenever available. For example, the CLSI "S" breakpoint for doxycycline recommended for many common bacteria is ≤ 2–4 µg/mL and this is the breakpoint used by most commercial microbiology laboratories when reporting microbes as susceptible. However, the pharmacokinetic study of doxycycline in adult horses shows the steady state plasma concentrations to be far lower than in humans, making the clinical susceptibility breakpoint for oral doxycycline in adult horses ≤ 0.25 μg/mL (Bryant et al., 2000). Because achievable plasma concentrations of orally administered doxycycline are relatively low as compared to humans, bacteria with higher MICs (0.5–2 μg/mL) would not be expected to respond to oral doxycycline at commonly prescribed doses in horses, even though they would be considered susceptible for human infections. This same interpretation must be applied to other orally administered antimicrobials with variable absorption in adult horses, including chloramphenicol, enrofloxacin, trimethoprim-sulfamethoxazole, and minocycline. For these antimicrobials, differences in oral bioavailability make the achievable plasma concentrations in horses much lower than those in humans or small animals for which CLSI guidelines have been developed. For these antimicrobials, based on results of oral pharmacokinetic studies, the author regards the following values as the "S" breakpoints when administered orally to *adult* horses at recommended doses:

1) Chloramphenicol (≤1 μg/mL) (Magdesian, unpublished data 2016)
2) Enrofloxacin (oral route) (≤0.5 μg/mL) (Boeckh et al., 2001)
3) Trimethoprim-sulfamethoxazole or trimethoprim-sulfadiazine (≤0.5 for trimethoprim/9.5 for sulfonamide μg/mL) (Gustaffson et al., 1999)
4) Minocycline ≤0.25 μg/mL (Schnabel et al., 2012)
5) Doxycycline ≤0.25 μg/mL (Bryant et al., 2000, Davis et al., 2006)

Because of higher bioavailability of most oral drugs in foals, as well as differences in pharmacokinetic parameters in this age group, these values would be expected to be different for foals (higher "S" breakpoints).

In addition to these differences in achievable plasma concentrations, the MIC should also be interpreted as they relate to pharmacokinetic parameters depending on whether the antimicrobial is time- or concentration-dependent. Those antimicrobials which are time-dependent should be evaluated in terms of T > MIC, where T is time. For concentration-dependent antimicrobials, the AUC/MIC (e.g., for fluoroquinolones) or Cmax/MIC (e.g., for aminoglycosides and fluoroquinolones) ratios should be evaluated, where AUC is the area under the plasma concentration-time curve and Cmax is the maximal achievable plasma concentration. The Cmax/MIC for aminoglycosides and fluoroquinolones should be ≥8–10, in order to ensure maximal efficacy. The AUC/MIC for enrofloxacin ideally should be ≥100–125 for optimal efficacy.

49.6   Case Example

A 3-year-old Thoroughbred gelding was presented for an acute onset of cellulitis-lymphangitis of one hind leg. Culture of exudate from the limb revealed a *Staphylococcus aureus* isolate. The antimicrobial susceptibility pattern from broth microdilution was as follows:

PENICILLIN G	R	0.50
AMOXICILLIN/CLAV	S	≤4
OXACILLIN	S	≤1
CHLORAMPHENICOL	S	≤4
CEPHALOTHIN	S	≤0.5
CEFTIZOXIME	S	2
CEFTIOFUR	S	0.5
ENROFLOXACIN	S	≤0.25
AMIKACIN	S	2
GENTAMICIN	R	16
TETRACYCLINE	R	>16
TRIMETH/SULFA	S	≤0.25

Based on the MIC results, including susceptibility to oxacillin and other beta lactam antimicrobials, this isolate is *not* a methicillin resistant *Staph aureus* (MRSA). There are many choices for antimicrobial therapy in this case. The antimicrobials that are listed as "R" here have a MIC greater than the "S" breakpoint and include penicillin, gentamicin, and tetracycline and these would be expected to be ineffective. From the other choices, chloramphenicol is an unknown in terms of expected efficacy, even though it is listed as "S," because the lowest concentration tested by this lab includes 4 μg/mL. Based on recent pharmacokinetic studies, a serum concentration of 4 μg/mL would be unachievable in most adult horses for long enough (T > MIC), and it would therefore not be a good choice in this case unless the MIC was determined to be ≤1 μg/mL. In addition, chloramphenicol is a bacteriostatic drug, and with acute cellulitis use of a bactericidal drug is optimal.

Potential therapeutic choices in this case include cephalosporins (first and third generations are both effective, however, with a 0.5 μg/mL MIC for ceftiofur it would have to be administered at 2 mg/kg q 12h), enrofloxacin, amikacin, and trimethoprim sulfamethoxazole. Enrofloxacin and trimethoprim-sulfamethoxazole have the advantages of being both bactericidal and having good tissue penetration. If enrofloxacin is used, the clinical response should be monitored closely, as resistance can develop during treatment, however this is more common with MRSA.

References

Boeckh S, Buchanan C, Boeckh A, Wilkie S, Davis C, Buchanan T, and Boothe D. 2001. Pharmacokinetics of the bovine formulation of enrofloxacin (Baytril 100) in horses. Vet Ther, 2(2): 129–134.

Bryant JE, Brown MP, Gronwall RR, et al. 2000. Study of intragastric administration of doxycycline: pharmacokinetics including body fluid, endometrial and minimum inhibitory concentrations. Equine Vet J, 32: 233–238.

Clinical and Laboratory Standards Institute. 2015. Performance standards for antimicrobial susceptibility testing. *Twenty-fifth informational supplement (M100-S25)*. Clinical and Laboratory Standards Institute, Wayne, PA.

Davis JL, Salmon JH, and Papich MG. 2006. Pharmacokinetics and tissue distribution of doxycycline after oral administration of single and multiple doses in horses. AJVR, 67: 310–316.

Gustaffson A, Baverud V, Franklin A, Gunnarsson A, Ogren G, and Ingvast-Larsson C. 1999. Repeated administration of trimethoprim/sulfadiazine in the horse- pharmacokinetics, plasma protein binding and influence on the intestinal microflora. J Vet Pharmacol Therap, 22: 20–26.

Schnabel LV, Papich MG, Divers TJ, Altier C, Aprea MS, McCarrel TM, and Fortier LA. 2012. Pharmacokinetics and distribution of minocycline in mature horses after oral administration of multiple doses and comparison with minimum inhibitory concentrations. Eq Vet J, 44: 453–458.

50

Parasite Control Strategies

Wendy Vaala[1] and Robin Houston[2]

[1] Merck Animal Health, New York, USA
[2] William R. Pritchard Veterinary Medical Teaching Hospital, School of Veterinary Medicine, University of California, California, USA

50.1 Introduction

An effective parasite control program considers the susceptibility of the host to parasitic disease, the parasite(s) of interest and clinical significance, the impact of local environment and general husbandry practices, the history and frequency of anthelmintic use on the farm, and the chemical and non-chemical treatment options available. Designing and maintaining an effective deworming regimen requires an appreciation of how to use and interpret fecal egg counts (FEC) and fecal egg count reduction tests (FECRT), a knowledge of the basic life-cycles of equine parasites of clinical significance and an understanding of the mode of action, spectrum, and duration of activity of the three major classes of anthelmintics licensed for horses. The goals of a comprehensive parasite control program include minimizing the health risk of parasitic disease among individual animals, controlling parasite egg shedding and environmental contamination, and optimizing drug efficacy to combat development of anthelmintic resistance.

Small stronglyes (cyathostomins) and *Parascaris* spp. are considered the most important parasites of well-managed horses. Chemical control of these parasites has evolved around the use of three major drug classes, the benzimidazoles, tetrahydropyrimidines, and macrocyclic lactones. Not surprisingly, this heavy reliance on anthelmintic administration, frequently in the absence of any parasite surveillance program, has contributed to the appearance of multi-drug-resistant isolates among well-cared-for horse populations throughout the world. There are numerous reports of confirmed or suspected resistance in small strongyles to piperazine, benzimidazoles, pyrantel salts, and more recently, macrocyclic lactones (e.g., ivermectin, moxidectin). The fact that cyathostomins are not usually serious pathogens in healthy adult horses has allowed practitioners and horse owners to remain fairly complacent

that such resistance, although warranting caution, was manageable. That comfort level disappeared with reports of anthelmintic resistance among populations of *Parascaris* spp. in young horses. Anecdotal reports of anthelmintic lack of efficacy also exist for other less pathogenic parasites including pinworms and *Habronema* spp. There are a growing number of reports of cyathostomins and ascarids becoming resistant to more than one drug class. Interestingly there are no documented cases of drug resistance among large strongyle species including *Strongylus vulgaris.* An in-depth discussion of equine parasite biology and anthelmintic resistance is beyond the scope of this chapter, the reader is referred to other resources as well as the current and comprehensive set of guidelines for equine parasite control strategies available on the American Association of Equine Practitioners' website (Nielsen et al., 2013).

50.2 Useful Terminology and Concepts

Anthelmintic resistance is an inherited trait and is defined as the ability of worms to survive treatments that are considered effective against that species and stage of infection. In order for anthelmintic resistance to develop on a farm, the gene mutations that confer drug resistance must already be present within the resident worm population. Frequent drug therapy increases selection pressure on parasite populations and allows only resistant isolates to survive, reproduce, and pass on their resistance genes to future generations of parasites. Without routine surveillance measures, including fecal egg counts (FEC) using a sensitive assay and post-treatment drug monitoring, it is easy to understand how intensively managed horse operations, accustomed to following deworming strategies based on tradition rather than science, can become permissive breeding grounds for resistant parasite populations. The intensity of drug use on a farm influences how quickly resistance develops and which drugs are involved.

The *fecal egg count* (FEC) remains the only method currently available for evaluating drug efficacy and egg shedding status. The FEC also permits identification of the type of parasite eggs being shed. It is important to recognize the inherent short-comings of the fecal exam while trying to optimize results. The FEC should be viewed as an estimate of parasite eggs contained in a manure sample. Results from fecal samples collected from the same horse over the course of a day will vary, as will FECs performed by different individuals using the same assay technique and manure sample. Different assay techniques have different lower thresholds of egg detection. The lowest limit of detection, defined as the lowest positive FEC that can be detected by a given technique, can vary from 1 egg per gram (EPG) to greater than 50 EPG. The less sensitive assays are acceptable when screening horses to determine egg shedding status, but assays with the lowest detection limits should be used when performing a fecal egg count reduction test (FECRT) to evaluate drug efficacy. The FEC is not a direct reflection of the total parasite burden of an individual horse. Because the FEC only detects eggs shed by reproductively mature parasites, fecal exams do not detect or reflect burden size of immature or larval stages of large and small strongyles and *Parascaris* spp. or encysted stages of cyathostomins. Unless this concept is explained to owners, a fecal egg count of "0" EPG may be misinterpreted to mean that their horse is "parasite free." Additionally, no fecal assay alone can be used to diagnose between cyathotomin versus large strongyle infections as these nematode eggs are virtually morphologically indistinguishable from each other. Reported "strongyle ova" counts are more likely to be cyathostomins based on the fecundity of these worms, but the results do not rule out the occasional large strongyle infection. Finally, unless a centrifugation-enhanced flotation technique is used, most fecal exams tend to miss or underestimate cestode (e.g., *Anoplocephala perfoliata*) eggs. Collecting a fecal sample 18–24 h after administering a cestocide increases the likelihood of finding tapeworm eggs, if a patent infection is present and an appropriate fecal assay is used.

The accuracy of the FEC is affected by the quality of the sample submitted, whether it was collected during a season of high or low parasite transmission and when it was collected with respect to the last anthelmintic treatment administered. A fresh fecal sample should be collected and stored in an air-tight container and refrigerated until processing. Freezing will damage the sample. Exposing the sample to high ambient temperatures encourages parasite eggs contained in the sample to hatch resulting in misleadingly low egg counts.

The most common reasons to perform a FEC include:

- Determination of strongyle egg shedding potential of individual mature horses
- Detection of anthelmintic resistance using the FECRT
- Monitoring the duration of drug-induced suppression of egg shedding (e.g., egg reappearance period) for the various drug classes

The *fecal egg count reduction test* (FECRT) is the only method currently available to determine if anthelmintic resistance is developing. Originally designed to evaluate resistance among strongyle species, the FECRT has also been applied to ascarids, although results should be interpreted cautiously. To perform a FECRT a fecal sample is collected prior to deworming and another 10–14 days following treatment. The number of eggs per gram (EPG) in the pre-treatment and post-treatment samples is used to calculate the percent reduction in fecal egg count (FECR) using the following equation:

$$EPG\,(pre-treatment)-EPG\,(14\,days\,post-treatment)$$
$$\times 100 = FECR\,(\%)$$

$$EPG\,(pre)-EPG\,(14\,days)/EPG\,(pre)\times 100 = FECR\,(\%)$$

Only horses that are shedding significant numbers of eggs pre-treatment (e.g., FEC ≥ 100 EPG) should be used to calculate the FECRT. The FECR values obtained from those horses are used to infer drug efficacy for the resident farm population. Ideally horses being tested should not have received anthelmintic treatments for at least a time interval ≥ the egg reappearance period for the last drug administered. For example, if moxidectin was the last drug administered, it is preferable to wait at least 12 weeks before collecting a pre-treatment sample. The FECRT can also be used to screen newcomers to the farm. Only foals old enough to be shedding parasite eggs should be included in the screening. Shedding of (small) strongyle eggs typically does not commence until foals are at least 6 weeks of age or older and ascarid eggs usually do not appear in fecal exams until foals are at least 10–15 weeks of age. Guidelines for interpreting FECRT results are presented in Table 50.1.

Egg reappearance period (ERP) is defined as the time interval between the last effective deworming treatment and the resumption of significant egg shedding. Table 50.2 lists the ERP for commonly used equine dewormers. A shortening of the ERP suggests that deworming regimens have selected for parasite populations with shorter prepatent periods and is considered to be a precursor to the development of full resistance. Occasional monitoring of the ERP for a given drug class

Table 50.1 Interpretation of fecal egg count reduction (FECR) values used to determine anthelmintic efficacy.

Anthelmintic	Susceptible (no evidence of resistance) (%)	Suspected resistance (%)	Resistance present (%)
Benzamidazoles	>95	90–95	<90
Pyrantel	>90	85–90	<85
Ivermectin/Moxidectin	>98	95–98	<95

Source: Luksovsky (2013). Reproduced with permission of Elsevier.

Table 50.2 Cyathostomin egg reappearance periods (ERP) for commonly used equine anthelmintics.

Anthelmintic	Expected ERP when Drug is still effective (weeks)	ERP when drug was first introduced (weeks)
Benzimidazoles	4–5	6
Pyrantel	4–5	5–6
Ivermectin	6–8	9–13
Moxidectin	10–12	16–22

Source: Luksovsky (2013). Reproduced with permission of Elsevier.

on a farm is a reasonable way to determine if resistance is beginning to develop against drugs previously considered effective. When monitoring the ERP, it is only necessary to collect fecal samples from a subset of the resident equine population (e.g., adult horses classified as higher egg shedders and youngsters <2 years of age). For example, if ivermectin was last used, the expected ERP is 6–8 weeks. Performing fecal exams on a group of high shedders 4 weeks after ivermectin treatment will help determine if the drug is still suppressing strongyle egg counts as long as expected.

The *strongyle egg shedding potential* varies among adult horses older than 3 years of age and is considered an innate trait for that individual. Within groups or bands of adult horses strongyle egg counts are often concentrated in a small percentage of the herd leading to the commonly quoted statistic: "Twenty percent of adult horses shed approximately 80% of the eggs." Over-dispersion is the term used to describe this distribution of strongyle egg shedding within a group of horses. In some horse populations, high egg counts may be concentrated in as few as 5–15% of the herd. This egg shedding potential tends to remain stable for a healthy horse over time unless the original classification was based on an improperly collected or performed fecal exam or the horse's immune status has changed due to disease or other factors. Aging alone does not impact shedding status, but development of PPID has been associated with increased fecal egg counts in affected equine seniors.

Since there is little data available to scientifically establish the FEC thresholds used to classify horses as low, moderate, and high shedders, the author (WV) prefers not to use black and white cut-off values, but rather generate FEC data for a specific herd and environment and classify animals in relationship to each other as low and high shedders for that farm. The high and low FEC ranges can vary greatly between farms based on a variety of factors including innate parasite susceptibility of the individual, general husbandry practices, stocking density, presence of younger horses (<3 years of age) on the property, time spent on pasture, region of the country and recent weather patterns. High shedders are generally considered to be animals with FEC > 500 EPG. Horses with FEC < 200 EPG are usually classified as low shedders. Horses with low strongyle shedding potential often require an average of two anthelmintic treatments per year, while those individuals identified as high shedders may require at least 3–4 anthelmintic treatments per year. Suggested guidelines for classifying the contaminating potential are discussed in detail elsewhere. Since deworming recommendations for mature horses are influenced by shedding status, it is advisable to retest horses at least twice during a 12–24-month period to reconfirm the individual's shedding status.

A fecal exam used to determine shedding status should be done during seasons of optimal parasite exposure and transmission (e.g., not during cold, freezing winters or hot, dry summers). To ensure the FEC obtained reflects the horse's innate immunity to cyathostomin infection rather than the lingering effects of the last drug used, it is important to wait a suitable period of time following the last anthelmintic treatment, preferably well beyond the drug's egg reappearance period (ERP), before collecting a fresh fecal.

Refugia is represented by the population of parasites or stages of parasites that escape exposure to a drug treatment and remain susceptible to anthelmintics. On a farm, this susceptible sub-population includes free-living stages of parasite eggs and larvae on pasture, all stages of parasites in horses left untreated (e.g., the low shedders), and stages of parasites unaffected by the anthelmintic administered as in the case of encysted stages of cyathostomins whenever non-larvicidal treatments are given (e.g., ivermectin, pyrantel pamoate). A variety of climatic and management factors also affect pasture refugia. Heat (temperatures above 85 °F) and drought will kill infective L3 strongyle larvae on pasture. Cold temperatures below 45 °F will arrest development of infective strongyle larvae and disrupt successful horse to horse parasite transmission. However, cold does not kill strongyle larvae which will resume development once warm temperatures return. Unfortunately, ascarid eggs are far most resilient to both hot and cold temperatures and can survive on pastures for up to 10 years. Picking up and disposing manure on a bi-weekly basis effectively disrupts the transmission cycle since parasite eggs/larvae require a minimum of 7–10 days to become infective even under ideal conditions. The higher the proportion of worms in refugia, the more slowly resistance develops. Hopefully this pool of susceptible parasites dilutes out the numbers of more resistant worms. The concept of refugia can be applied when designing the frequency and timing of anthelmintic treatments. Ideally, the frequency of drug treatments should be kept to a minimum when pasture refugia is low (e.g., during temperature extremes of cold winters and hot summers and during droughts). Using fecal egg counts, only horses classified as moderate to high shedders need to be treated more frequently, leaving a large percentage of the herd identified as low shedders untreated.

50.3 Fecal Flotation Assays

Table 50.3 summarizes the more commonly used fecal diagnostic tests used in equine medicine. The two most popular fecal egg counting techniques are the Modified Wisconsin method and the McMasters technique, while the Centrifugal Fecal Flotation technique is employed when sensitivity is most crucial and quantitative results are not as essential. Other methods, such as the FLOTAC technique are versions of the McMaster procedure but with a higher sensitivity. A lab may choose a standard published FEC to run routinely based on multiple factors, for example the minimal amount (in grams) of feces and the amount of flotation solution required per assay, the need for a centrifuge and/or McMaster slide, and the time required to perform each test.

50.3.1 The Modified Wisconsin Method

The modified Wisconsin method uses Sheather's solution (sucrose solution at specific gravity of 1.27) as a flotation medium and involves centrifugation at 1000 rpm followed by gravitational flotation of the sample. This assay can detect egg counts as low as 1–5 EPG. The procedure is outlined next:

50.3.1.1 Equipment and Supplies
- Disposable cups, wooden tongue depressors, laboratory scale, cheesecloth or tea strainer, funnel, Sheather's sugar solution [454 g (i.e., 1 lb of table sugar added to 355 mL of hot water); stir to dissolve; cool and keep refrigerated to prevent mold growth; the solution should be periodically checked with a hydrometer to confirm a specific gravity of 1.27], 15-mL taper bottom centrifuge tubes, test tube racks, microscope slides and 22 × 22 mm cover slips, centrifuge with buckets to accommodate 15 mL tubes, and a microscope.

50.3.1.2 Procedure
- Line funnel with cheesecloth (or place tea strainer inside funnel). Place funnel tip in centrifuge tube supported by rack.
- Weigh 1 g of feces in a disposable cup.
- Add 10 mL of Sheather's sugar solution to the feces and mix well with a tongue depressor.
- Pour fecal-sugar solution mixture through funnel into tube. Use a tongue depressor to squeeze all additional liquid through cheesecloth/strainer into tube, leaving at least 1 mL of air space at the top.
- Balance tubes and centrifuge them for 7–10 min at 1000 rpm.
- Place tube in rack and top off with sugar solution until meniscus bulges over top of tube. Place cover slip on top of tube and allow to sit undisturbed for 10 min.
- Lift the cover slip straight off and place on slide. Scan entire cover slip methodically and count all eggs of each species observed. Number of eggs counted is the number of eggs per gram of feces (EPG), therefore the detection limit of this method is 1 EPG.

50.3.1.3 Advantages of Modified Wisconsin Method
- Other than a clinical grade, fixed-angle table top centrifuge, no specialized equipment is required.
- Procedure allows examination of a large number of samples in a short time period. Multiple samples can be centrifuged at one time and then slides prepared and read at one time. Once cover slips are placed on slides, the slides can be refrigerated inside a slightly humidified, airtight container (i.e., petri dish containing a moistened piece of filter paper) and read within the next several days.
- The low egg detection limit of this assay makes it the ideal method to use when performing a FECRT to evaluate drug efficacy.
- Centrifugation increases the likelihood of detecting cestode eggs.

Table 50.3 Fecal diagnostic tests summary.

Technique type	Published method	Quantitative	Sensitivity = detection limit (e.p.g.)	Counting chamber required	Feces required (g)	Flotation solution required (ml)	Centrifuge required
Centrifugal Fecal Flotation		No	<1, but results only reported as pos. or neg.	No	2–5	10–13	Yes
Modified Wisconsin Centrifugal Flotation	Zajac & Conboy (2012)	Yes	1	No	3	12	Yes
Modified Stoll's Centrifugal Flotation		Yes	5	No	2	13	Yes
McMaster	Henriksen & Aagaard (1976)	Yes	20	Yes	4	56	Yes
	Roepstorff & Nansen (1998)	Yes	20	Yes	4	56	Yes
	Zajicek (1978)	Yes	33	Yes	1	15	Yes
	Kassai (1999)	Yes	50	Yes	3	42	Yes
	Gronvold (1991)	Yes	50	Yes	4	56	No
	Wetzel (1951)	Yes	67	Yes	2	60	No

50.3.1.4 Limitation of the Modified Wisconsin Method

- Because the sample size (only 1 g) is small in comparison to the total volume of a typical bowel movement of a horse, the resulting FEC may result in false negative results for parasite stages in very low numbers. A qualitative fecal flotation test using a 5–10 g, well mixed fecal sample, should be performed to rule in/out parasite stages that may be suspected, but not found in a FEC (e.g., to detect *Habronema* spp. and/or cestode ova).

50.3.2 The McMasters Technique

The McMasters Technique uses a flotation medium containing either sodium chloride or sodium nitrate and requires a glass or plastic calibrated counting chamber, for instance, the "McMasters slide." Under the top portion of the slide are engraved (or printed) two grids each subdivided into six columns. Because the grid is in the same focal plane as the worm eggs that float up against it, the microscopist can keep track of what eggs fall within the grid, and those that don't get counted There are multiple variations of this technique used by various labs worldwide, each with varying levels of sensitivity and requirement of a centrifuge (see Table 50.3). The procedure described next is one of them, having a lower limit of sensitivity of 50 EPG and does not require the use of a centrifuge:

50.3.2.1 Equipment and Supplies

- Disposable cups, wooden tongue depressors, and disposable pipettes.
- Laboratory scale.
- Cheesecloth or tea strainer.
- McMasters slide.
- Flotation solution with specific gravity in the range of 1.18–1.25 (e.g., 37% zinc sulfate, saturated NaCl Sheather's sugar solution).
- Microscope.

50.3.2.2 Procedure

- Weigh out 4 g of feces in a disposable cup.
- Add 56 mL of flotation solution and mix vigorously using a tongue depressor.
- When mixing, pour suspension through cheesecloth or strainer into another disposable cup.
- Immediately aspirate a sample of suspension with the pipette and transfer liquid into one of the chambers of the McMasters slide. Fill the entire area under the grid and avoid forming any bubbles. Mix again and repeat the procedure to fill the other chamber.

- Wait 1–2 min to allow eggs to float to the bottom of the top portion of the chamber. Examine the slide under the 10× objective of the microscope and count all of the eggs seen within all six columns of each grid – keeping separate counts of each worm species. Multiply the total number of each type of parasite egg counted within both grids (e.g., strongyle, ascarid) by 50. This is the FEC and is reported as EPG; thus, the detection limit of this procedure is 50 EPG. Example: sevenstrongyle eggs and 10 ascarid eggs were counted under the left grid; five strongyle eggs and 11 ascarid eggs were counted under the right grid. Total strongyle egg count is 12. Total ascarid egg count is 21. Therefore, this horse has a FEC of $12 \times 50 = 600$ EPG strongyle ova and $21 \times 50 = 1050$ EPG *Parascaris* ova.

50.3.2.3 Sample Collection and Handling

The deworming guidelines available on the AAEP website (www.AAEP.org) provide an excellent overview of fecal collection, handling and processing as well as interpretation of fecal egg counts. It is recommended that only fresh fecal samples be collected and stored in airtight containers such as Ziploc plastic bags to reduce the likelihood of eggs hatching. Each sample should be labeled with the horse's identification and date of collection. Samples should be refrigerated (never frozen) soon after collection. If samples are shipped by mail they should be packed on cold packs and sent via next day delivery. Ideally all samples should be processed within 7 days after collection. Formed fecal samples are ideal since watery diarrheic feces are too dilute for accurate quantitative fecal egg counts.

50.4 Biology of Selected Equine Parasites of Concern

A comprehensive classification of the diverse array of internal parasites with the potential to affect horses is presented in Table 50.4 together with recommended diagnostic tests. While it is beyond the scope of this chapter to review the life-cycle of all of these parasites, it is important to be familiar with the biology of the most commonly encountered parasites with respect to their life-cycle, the stages (larval vs adult) associated with clinical disease, optimal diagnostic assays, and chemical and non-chemical control strategies. Clinicians with the desire to run their own fecal assays should invest in at least one good diagnostic parasitology reference manual to assist with identification of diagnostic stages; some of these manuals also include information on individual parasite life cycles.

Table 50.4 Equine parasites: classification and diagnostic assays.

Common name	Genus species	Classification	Sample	Diagnostic tests	Diagnostic stage(s)	Considerations
Tapeworms	*Anoplocephala* spp. *Paranoplocephala* spp.	Helminth • Cestoda • anoplocephalids	5–10 g fresh feces, refrigerated or shipped w/cool pack	QCF (s.g. >1.3), MWCF, MSCF, MMT, sedimentation	Ova, sometimes intact proglottids	Portions of the adult tapeworm may be found in fresh feces and themselves be diagnostic.
Threadworm	*Strongyloides westeri*	Helminth • Nematoda • rhabditoids	5–10 g fresh feces, refrigerated or shipped w/cool pack	QCF, MWCF, MSCF, MMT	Ova containing a larva	Larvae may be recovered w/Baermann if fecal sample is not fresh.
Eye worm	*Thelazia* spp.	Helminth • Nematoda • spirurids	Adult nematodes in 70% ethanol	Eye exam	Adult worms found under conjunctivae	Muscid flies serve as intermediate hosts.
Lungworm	*Dictyocaulus arnfieldi*	Helminth • Nematoda • trichostrongyles	5–10 g fresh feces, refrigerated or shipped w/cool pack	Baermann technique	Ova containing a larva; motile (hatched) larvae	Larvae and ova containing larvae may be found in fresh feces. More common in donkeys.
Roundworm	*Parascaris equorum*	Helminth • Nematoda • ascarids	5–10 g fresh feces, refrigerated or shipped w/cool pack	QCF (s.g. >1.3), MWCF, MSCF, MMT	Ova	More likely in young and very old horses.
Pinworm	*Oxyuris equi*	Helminth • Nematoda • oxyurids	Scotch tape preparation of perianal region	Scotch tape preparation	Ova w/unipolar plug	Ova also may occasionally be found on flotation.
Stomach worms	*Habronema* spp. & *Draschia megastoma*	Helminth • Nematoda • spirurids	5–10 g fresh feces, refrigerated or shipped w/cool pack	QCF, MWCF, MSCF, MMT	Ova containing a larva	Larvae in skin cause "summer sores" (see below).
Summer sores	*Habronema* spp.	Helminth • Nematoda • spirurids	Deep tissue biopsy	Histopathological examination of biopsy	Larvae	PCR has been used in diagnosis; not widely available.
Equine onchocerciasis	*Onchocerca cervicalis*	Helminth • Nematoda • filarids	Full skin thickness biopsy (≥6 mm)	Baermann technique to collect microfilariae	Microfilariae	*Culicoides* spp. ("biting midges") serve as intermediate hosts.
Large strongyles	*Strongylus vulgaris, S. edentatus & S. equinus*	Helminth • Nematoda • strongylids	5–10 g fresh feces, refrigerated or shipped w/cool pack	QCF, MWCF, MSCF, MMT, fecal culture	Ova, third-stage larvae	Ova cannot be morphologically differentiated from small strongyle ova.
Small strongyles	Various, mostly in subfamily Cyathostominae	Helminth • Nematoda • cyathostomes	5–10 g fresh feces, refrigerated or shipped w/cool pack	QCF, MWCF, MSCF, MMT	Ova, third-stage larvae	Ova cannot be morphologically differentiated from large strongyle ova.

(*Continued*)

Table 50.4 (Continued)

Common name	Genus species	Classification	Sample	Diagnostic tests	Diagnostic stage(s)	Considerations
Hairworm	*Trichostrongylus axei*	Helminth ● Nematoda ● trichostrongyles	5–10g fresh feces, refrigerated or shipped w/cool pack	QCF, MWCF, MSCF, MMT	Ova, third-stage larvae	Ova cannot be morphologically differentiated from strongyle ova.
EPM (equine protozoal myeloencephalitis)	*Sarcocystis neurona/ Neospora hughesi*	Protozoa ● Apicomplexa ● coccidia	Cerebral spinal fluid (CSF) and/or serum	Serology	Antibodies to schizonts & merozoites	Definitive diagnosis supported by serum/CSF antibody ratio.
Giardia	*Giardia* spp.	Protozoa ● Sarcomastigophora ● mucosoflagellates	5–10g fresh feces, refrigerated or shipped w/cool pack	QCF, DFA test	Cysts	Trophozoites may be recovered in direct smear, but flotation of cysts more reliable; potentially zoonotic.
Crypto	*Cryptosporidium* spp.	Protozoa ● Apicomplexa ● coccidia	5–10g fresh feces, refrigerated or shipped w/cool pack	Kinyoun's acid fast stain technique, DFA test	Oocysts	More common in foals; potentially zoonotic
Coccidia	*Eimeria leuckarti*	Protozoa ● Apicomplexa ● coccidia	5–10g fresh feces, refrigerated or shipped w/cool pack	QCF, MWCF, MSCF, MMT	Oocysts	More common in foals.
Equine piroplasmosis	*Babesia caballi/ Theileria equi*	Protozoa ● Apicomplexa ● Piroplasmida	Whole blood for hematological exam; serum/plasma for serological tests.	Stained blood smears, ELISA, IFA, PCR	Intra-erythrocytic piroplasms	Contact state or federal animal health officials for instructions. Organisms may be zoonotic.

50.4.1 Ascarids (*Parascaris equorum* and *Parascaris univalens*)

Parascaris equorum and *Parascaris univalens* are the only ascarid nematode of horses and infection is most common in foals and young horses less than 2 years of age. The two species are morphologically identical, and the only current method to differentiate them is through karyotyping primordial germ cells prior to their first cell division. Contrary to the general assumption, available evidence now suggests that *P. univalens* is the main equine ascarid, whereas *P. equorum* is rare (Nielsen et al., 2014). Immunity typically develops by 8–18 months of age and is believed to be age-related and exposure induced. Following ingestion of larvated eggs from pastures, paddocks, dry lots, or stalls, larvae emerge in the small intestinal lumen, penetrate through the intestinal mucosa, enter the lymphatics and are transported to the liver. After a period of hepatic migration lasting as long as one week, third-stage ascarid larvae (L3) are transported to the lungs via the posterior vena cava. Larvae erupt from pulmonary capillaries and enter the alveoli where they enjoy 2–3 weeks of pulmonary migration. Larvae are then coughed up and swallowed to continue their development through to egg-laying adults in the small intestinal lumen. The prepatent period of *Parascaris* spp. is approximately 10–15 weeks. Clinical signs associated with pulmonary migration include mucopurulent nasal discharge, cough, and low-grade fever. Large burdens of ascarid larvae and adults within the small intestine have been associated with poor growth or weight loss, unthrifty appearance, inappetance, and diarrhea. Small intestinal impaction, resulting in colic and occasionally bowel rupture, does occur and is often associated with recent deworming using a macrocyclic lactone or pyrimidine anthelmintic. If surgical intervention is required to relieve ascarid impactions, the outcome is often guarded due to post-operative complications related to refractory ileus, peritonitis, and systemic toxemia. Ascarid eggs (Figure 50.1) are covered by a thick capsule that renders them environmentally hardy and capable of withstanding extremes in temperatures resulting in pasture persistence for a minimum of 5–10 years. Therefore, it is easy to appreciate how breeding farm pastures can become heavily contaminated with ascarid eggs if there has not been vigilant monitoring of the deworming regimen for foals, weanlings and yearlings.

Drugs that can be used in young foals to treat ascarid infections include fenbendazole, oxibendazole, pyrantel, and ivermectin. As noted on the label, fenbendazole should be administered at 10 mg/kg (2× the label dose recommended for adult horses) for juveniles ≤18 months of age. Moxidectin is not labeled for use in young foals

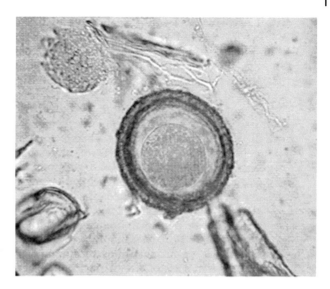

Figure 50.1 Ascarid eggs are surrounded by a thick proteinaceous capsule.

<6 months of age and must be dosed carefully and accurately in all horses. During the last 10 years there have been a growing number of reports from around the world of ascarids developing resistance to ivermectin. Recent research has shown that the larvicidal dose of fenbendazole (10 mg/kg orally q24 h for 5 days) is effective against all stages of ascarids, including migrating larvae and including isolates known to be resistant to ivermectin.

50.4.2 Large Strongyles (*Strongylus vulgaris*, *Strongylus edentatus*, *Strongylus equinus*)

Older foals and horses of all ages can be affected by both larval and adult stages of the three large strongyle species, *S. vulgaris*, *S. edentatus*, and *S. equinus*. The basic life cycle for large strongyles includes excretion of fertilized eggs in the manure followed by the emergence of a first stage larva (L_1). The first stage larva molts to L_2 in the feces. A second molt gives rise to the infective, free-living third stage larva (L_3) that retains its L_2 cuticle. Third stage larvae migrate away from the fecal pat and onto forage. Climatic conditions affect the three larval stages differently. Temperatures above 100 °F, especially if hot weather is accompanied by dry conditions, are detrimental to survival of all free-living larval stages. Development into infective stages is inhibited when temperatures fall below 45 °F and the likelihood of parasite transmission on pasture becomes minimal. Freezing temperatures kill developing L_1 and L_2, but L_3 can survive for cold winter weather for months. The optimal temperature range for development of eggs and larvae is 77–91 °F. Once ingested by an equine host, the infective third stage larva exsheathes and invades the mucosa of the large intestine.

Larval migration patterns and prepatent periods vary between the three large strongyle species. Following ingestion, third-stage *S. vulgaris* larvae invade the mucosa of the distal small intestine, cecum and colon and molt to L_4. Fourth stage larvae migrate and penetrate the intimal layer of the walls of small arterioles, ultimately ending their migration near the root of the cranial mesenteric artery approximately 2 weeks post-infection. A final molt to L_5 occurs while larvae are residing within arterial walls. Within 4 months of initial infection, fifth-stage larvae resume migration and return via the bloodstream to the submucosa of the ventral colon and cecum. Small, pea-size nodules form around the embedded L_5 stages. Adult worms emerge from the nodules and mature within the intestinal lumen. The prepatent period for *S. vulgaris* is estimated to be 5.5–7 months. Clinical signs ascribed to *S. vulgaris* infection include episodes of potentially fatal thromboembolic colic involving large colon and cecum.

Third stage *S. edentatus* larvae exsheathe in the small intestine, penetrate the bowel wall, travel via the portal system to the liver. Third stage larvae molt to L_4 within the hepatic parenchyma followed by migration through the liver and retroperitoneal space, including subperitoneal spaces of various abdominal organs. After an indeterminate migratory period, larvae undergo a final molt to L5 and return to the large intestinal walls. Nodules form and eventually rupture to release adults back into the intestinal lumen. The prepatent period ranges from 10–12 months. Liver pathology and mild peritonitis have been associated with *S. edendatus* migration.

After ingestion *S. equinus* third stage larvae invade the mucosa of the cecum and large colon. Larvae molt to L_4 followed by a migratory route that includes the liver and pancreas. The prepatent period of *S. equinus* is 8–9 months. This large strongyle species has become relatively rare based on necropsy findings.

Large strongyle infections are typically acquired by horses grazing on pasture or near manure piles. The incidence of large strongyle infections among well-managed horse populations is rare. Using larval cultures to identify strongyle species, the majority of strongyle-type eggs (Figure 50.2) observed in fecal samples are from cyathostomins and not large strongyles. The low prevalence of large strongyle infections is probably due mostly to the absence of anthelmintic resistance among large strongyle species. All three drug classes (e.g., benzimidazoles, tetrahydropyrimidines, and macrocyclic lactones) remain effective against adult stages of large strongyle species. Drugs effective against migrating larval stages include ivermectin, moxidectin, and a larvicidal dose of fenbendazole. Due to the long prepatent period for

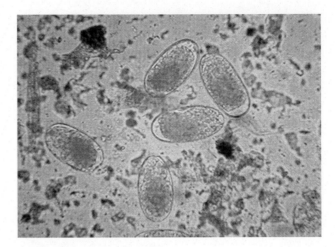

Figure 50.2 Strongyle eggs.

S. vulgaris, it is possible to eradicate potential *S. vulgaris* infection by deworming the resident horse population with a drug effective against *S. vulgaris* for a minimum of 18 months, or three deworming treatments. Selective drug therapy based on fecal egg counts and risk of parasite exposure has decreased the frequency of anthelmintic treatments on many premises. Interestingly, some farms have experienced a reappearance of *S. vulgaris*, confirmed by larval culture and/or PCR fecal testing, when routine drug treatments are administered at greater than 6–12 month intervals.

50.4.3 Small Strongyles (Cyathostomins)

Cyathostomins are the most common parasites observed in fecal samples from well-cared-for horses. All ages can be infected, but the young and the debilitated are more likely to exhibit clinical signs associated with heavy cyathostomin burdens. There are over 50 species of small strongyles comprising numerous genera with each species having its own predilection site within the horse's large intestines. Among domesticated horses there are approximately ten species that predominate which undoubtedly reflects selection pressure associated with routine deworming protocols. Similar to large strongyles, the cyathostomin life-cycle is direct. Eggs are passed in feces and develop into infective (L_3) larvae on pasture where they are susceptible to the same temperature extremes as described before for large strongyles. Following ingestion, infective L_3 invade and become encysted in the mucosa or submucosa of the cecum and ventral or dorsal colon. Cyathostomins invade the large intestines as early L_3 (EL_3). Once encysted, EL_3 are surrounded by a fibrous capsule produced by the host. Encysted larvae can range in numbers from several thousand to more than several million per horse and can remain dormant from weeks to several years or longer.

It is important to recognize that fecal egg counts do not reflect the numbers of encysted small strongyles. Once stimulated, EL_3 resume their progressive development within the cyst and undergo two successive molts to become late L_3 (LL_3) and then fourth stage larva (L_4). The cyst eventually ruptures to release L_4 into the intestinal lumen. Late L_4 (LL_4) mature into the final adult stage, the L_5.

Synchronous, mass emergence of fourth stage larvae can be devastating to the host. Clinical signs of cyathostominosis include colic, inflammatory enteritis, diarrhea, weight loss, ventral and limb edema, emaciation, and death. Laboratory findings include hypoproteinemia, hypoalbuminemia, hyperglobulinemia, and leukocytosis. The stimuli for excystment and emergence of L_4 are poorly understood. When pasture conditions are adverse for larval survival (e.g., during hot dry summers or cold winters) larger numbers of small strongyles remain encysted within the host. Anthelmintic treatment with a drug effective against only adult cyathostomins residing in the intestinal lumen may also trigger excystment of mucosal stages. This effect is thought to be due to feedback from luminal to mucosal worms, and when adult stages within the lumen have been eliminated by anthelmintic treatment, larval stages in arrested development are stimulated to excyst. Killing dormant, hibernating larvae is preferable to waiting for mass emergence and associated clinical disease to occur.

All three major drug classes report efficacy against adult cyathostomins. However, there are numerous reports of confirmed or suspected resistance among certain small strongyles species to benzimidazoles, pyrantel salts, and more recently, macrocyclic lactones (e.g., ivermectin, moxidectin). Resistance to any drug class should not be assumed, even within one region of the country. The FECRT should be utilized to determine efficacy. For example, one recent study examining the incidence of fenbendazole-resistant cyathostomins on four Texas ranches, demonstrated a wide difference in pre-treatment FECs on the four premises and a difference in drug efficacy. Fenbendazole resistance was detected on three ranches, while the fourth ranch showed no evidence of resistance. Unfortunately, mucosal larval stages are not fully susceptible to any anthelmintic. Only two anthelmintics have demonstrated efficacy against encysted larvae. Moxidectin has labeled efficacy against the LL_3 and a larvicidal dose of fenbendazole has a label claim of efficacy beginning with EL_3 stages.

Mature horses vary in their genetic susceptibility to cyathostomins with at least 80% of most horse populations being classified as low shedders. The risk of exposure and infection increases among horses on pasture compared to those that spend the majority of their time in stalls.

50.4.4 Tapeworms (*Anoplocephala perfoliata*)

Horses harbor only three cestode species and of those *Anoplocephala perfoliata* is the cestode species most commonly isolated from horses in North America. Older foals and horses of all ages can be affected. Eggs are shed intermittently in the feces and then ingested by free-living oribatid mites that are endemic on pastures throughout North America. Egg hatch occurs in the mite to release the cysticercoid stage. Horses ingest infected mites while grazing and cysticercoids are released and continue to develop into adult tapeworms. Scolex attachment occurs primarily in the cecum with a tendency for clustering along the cecal side of the ileocecal valve. *A. perfoliata* infections have been associated with colic, diarrhea, ileal impactions, and ileo-cecal intussusceptions.

Detection of cestode eggs (Figures 50.3 and 50.4) is challenging. Tapeworms are intermittent egg layers and eggs are unevenly distributing in feces as proglottids disintegrate. The sensitivity of most fecal assays is too low to make a reliable diagnosis. Tapeworm eggs are less likely to be observed using only flotation techniques like the McMasters assay, and more likely to be visualized using the Modified Wisconsin Method or qualitative fecal flotation that employs centrifugation using a larger fecal sample. Using a modification of the Stoll technique increases detection rate for cestode eggs. Collecting a fecal sample 18–24 h after administering a cestocide also increases the likelihood of observing cestode eggs. An ELISA method is available that detects antibodies against the 12/13 kDa excretory/secretory antigens of *A. perfoliata* for serodiagnosis of cestode exposure. This serological assay has been validated using horses whose tapeworm status was

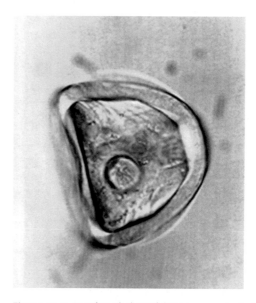

Figure 50.3 *Anoplocephala perfoliata* eggs are typically D-shaped.

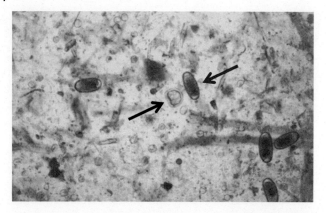

Figure 50.4 Strongyle (red arrow) and cestode (black arrow) eggs.

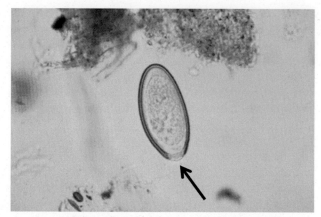

Figure 50.5 *Oxyuris* equi eggs contain an operculum (black arrow) at one end.

confirmed at necropsy. Antibody titers reflect exposure and not necessarily active infection, since some horses may remain antibody-positive for up to 5 months following cestocidal treatment.

The only two anthelmintic treatments effective against tapeworms are praziquantel and pyrantel pamoate (administered at a dose of 13.2 mg/kg).

50.4.5 Pinworms (*Oxyuris equi*)

Adult *Oxyuris equi* are found primarily in the small colon. The gravid female migrates down the colon and rectum and out the anus to cement her eggs in masses to the surrounding perianal skin. Adult females range in length from 5–8 cm and can be seen in fresh feces, protruding from the anus or coating a rectal sleeve following a rectal exam. Once laid the eggs become infective in 4–5 days. The egg masses flake off into the environment and adhere to a variety of surfaces including buckets, hay mangers and stable walls. Infective, larvated eggs are passed to other horses via ingestion. Following ingestion, third-stage larvae emerge to continue their development in the cecum and colon. The prepatent period is approximately 5 months. Signs of infection include tail rubbing and loss of tail hair. Younger horses are generally more susceptible. *Oxyuris* eggs are not typically found in feces due to the unique egg-laying behavior of the female. One of two methods commonly used to collect eggs involves applying a piece of cellophane tape to the perianal area and then transferring the tape to a microscope slide to scan for *Oxyuris* eggs (Figure 50.5). Another method is to coat a tongue depressor with a small amount of lubricant and gently perform a perianal scraping and then transfer collected material to a slide and examine for eggs. All three classes of dewormers have label efficacy against pinworms, although there are both anecdotal and confirmed reports of macrocyclic lactones failing to clear pinworm infections and variable reports regarding efficacy of pyrantel salts. Because of the unusual egg

laying behavior of *O. equi* females, accurate pre- and post-treatment fecal egg counts are not possible, thereby rendering the FECRT meaningless. Treatment failure is suspected when there is rapid reappearance of *O. equi* eggs following anthelmintic administration. If treatment failure is suspected, the hierarchy of expected drug efficacy against *O. equi* seems to be benzimidazoles, followed by pyrantel salts followed by macrocyclic lactones.

50.4.6 Threadworms (*Strongyloides westeri*)

Strongyloides westeri is the first nematode to mature in foals with a prepatent period of less than 2 weeks. Infective third-stage larvae can be transmitted to foals via their dam's milk for up to 40 days post-partum or acquired from the environment via oral or percutaneous routes. Following pulmonary migration, larvae return to the small intestines to complete their development. *Strongyloides westeri* eggs (Figure 50.6) pass in the feces and infective third stage larvae hatch out in the environment. *Strongyloides westeri* is usually considered benign unless present in large numbers. Clinical signs of strongyloidosis that include diarrhea, lethargy, and anorexia are usually observed in foals with high fecal egg counts (>2000 EPG). Historically, the incidence of patent *S. westeri* infections was much higher prior to the approval and widespread use on ivermectin in foals and horses. A recent study of foals in Kentucky, ranging in ages from 17–117 days of age, that had never been dewormed revealed a prevalence rate of 30% for patent *S. westeri* infections, which was substantially greater than reports from the same geographic area approximately 15 years earlier. It was hypothesized that this recent increase in *S. westeri* positive fecals was related to the diminished use of ivermectin in response to the increased prevalence of ML-resistant populations of *P. equorum*. This observation

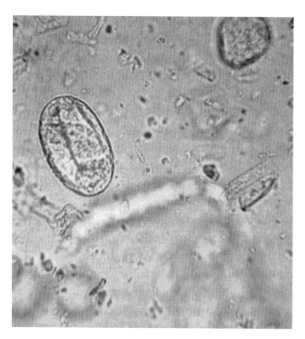

Figure 50.6 *Strongyloides westeri* eggs are small (50 × 40 μm), thin-shelled elliptical eggs that already contain a larva.

serves as a reminder that changing the use of a single drug class to address resistance among one parasite species may have consequences in terms of other parasitic infections. Due to age-related immunity patent *S. westeri* infections are rare in juveniles older than 5 months of age. Anthelmintics with labeled efficacy against *S. westeri* are ivermectin (0.2 mg/kg) and oxibendazole (15 mg/kg). Drudge and associates demonstrated that a single dose of fenbendazole administered at 50 mg/kg was highly effective against *S. westeri*. Strategic deworming of the mare may help alleviate the pervasive fear of *S. westeri* that still prompts some farms to routinely deworm foals beginning at 2–4 weeks of age.

50.5 Anthelmintic Mode of Action and Spectrum of Activity

50.5.1 Benzimidazoles

Fenbendazole and oxibendazole are members of this drug class. Their mode of action is to disrupt parasite energy metabolism at a cellular level. Mode of action is slower than that of other drug classes and drug half-life is relatively short. Bioavailability is improved if administered on an empty stomach. This family of anthelmintics provides broad spectrum of efficacy against large strongyles, cyathostomins, *Parascaris*, and *Oxyuris* infections. Oxibendazole is effective against *S. westeri* when administered at 15 mg/kg. When administered at an elevated dose of 10 mg/kg for 5 consecutive days, fenbendazole

exhibits larvicidal efficacy against migrating large strongyles, and susceptible populations of migrating and encysted small strongyles. Although not part of the label claim, the larvicidal dose of fenbendazole has demonstrated efficacy against migrating *Parascaris* spp. *larvae*, including ivermectin-resistant isolates. Benzimidazoles often remain the drug of choice to treat multi-drug resistant *Parascaris* spp. and *Oxyuris equi* infections. This drug class has an exceptionally wide safety index.

50.5.2 Tetrahydropyrimidines

First introduced more than four decades ago, pyrimidines are marketed for horses in North America as pyrantel pamoate, available in paste or suspension formulations and as pyrantel tartrate, available as a pelleted formulation designed to be used as a daily feed additive. The mode of action for these drugs is as selective acetylcholine agonists resulting in fast, spastic paralysis of susceptible worms that are then usually expelled by intestinal peristalsis. Since there is no intestinal absorption of the pyrimidine anthelmintics, their effect is confined to luminal stages of parasites and does not include migrating or encysted larval stages. Pyrimidines are considered to be broad spectrum with efficacy against cyathostomins, large strongyles, ascarids, and pin worms. In addition, pyrimidines have demonstrated good efficacy against the equine cestode, *Anoplocephala perfoliata*. The label dose of pyrantel pamoate (6.6 mg/kg) may provide at least 80% cestocidal efficacy and administration of twice that dose (13.2 mg/kg) affords greater than 95% efficacy against tapeworms. Confirmed and suspected cyathostomin resistance to pyrimidine dewormers has been reported. While the pyrimidines are usually considered effective against *Parascaris* spp. infections, there are a growing number of reports of pyrantel-resistant ascarid populations.

Daily administration of pyrantel tartrate (PT) at the label dose of 2.64 mg/kg has been promoted for use in both adult horses and youngsters as a means to control cyathostomin infections by killing ingested parasite larvae before they begin their tissue damaging migrations. Clinical trials with PT in mares, foals, and yearlings have produced controversial results. Potential benefits associated with daily PT administration to post-foaling mares was effective in reducing fecal egg counts with a subsequent decrease in pasture contamination with infective strongyle eggs and larvae, thus providing a safer grazing environment for foals. Foals of medicated mares maintained low strongyle and ascarid FECs until weaning, which allowed the first anthelmintic treatment to be delayed until after weaning. However, when those weanlings were dewormed with pyrantel pamoate for the first time, the drug had little effect on FEC reduction.

A separate study examined the effect of three different management and deworming strategies on foals. Two groups of foals were raised with mares on pasture with one group receiving daily PT and one group receiving no anthelmintic treatment. A third group of foals were raised under parasite-free conditions. After weaning, when foals in each group were challenged with large numbers of infective large and small strongyle larvae, those foals reared on pasture without benefit of anthelmintic treatment demonstrated evidence of protective resistance to the challenge, while the other two groups were more susceptible to clinical disease associated with larval challenge. This response suggested that daily PT prevented the development of acquired resistance to subsequent challenge.

Parasitologists continue to debate whether the use of daily pyrantel tartrate in North America has predisposed to the development of pyrantel resistant populations of cyathostominae and *Parascaris* spp. In response to reports of pyrantel pamoate resistance in horses receiving daily administration of pyrantel tartrate, farms should be monitored for pyrimidine-resistant cyathostomins prior to the use of pyrantel tartrate.

50.5.3 Macrocyclic Lactones (ML)

This drug class contains two subgroups, the avermectins and milbemycins. These drugs cause neuromuscular flaccid paralysis in susceptible parasites by interfering with the function of glutamate-gated chloride channels found only in neurons and myocytes of invertebrates. Affected parasites can no longer ingest nutrients and die of starvation or are expelled by intestinal peristalsis if they are residing within the gut lumen at the time of treatment. Similar to the pyrimidines, onset of action is rapid and occurs within 48 h following treatment. Both ivermectin and moxidectin have broad parasiticidal activities and are effective against luminal stages of nematodes as well as migrating larval stages of ascarids, large strongyles, and *Strongyloides*. In addition to nematodes, these drugs also exhibit efficacy against arthropods and are useful in the treatment of *Gastrophilus* larvae. Drugs in this class are also effective against *Onchocerca* larvae, *Habronema* and *Draschia*.

Moxidectin was introduced in the mid-1990s and differs from ivermectin in several ways. Moxidectin is more lipophilic, which accounts for its accumulation in fatty tissues, longer elimination half-life, and prolonged egg reappearance period. Unlike ivermectin, moxidectin demonstrates efficacy against encysted LL3 stage cyathostomin larvae. The efficacy of moxidectin parallels that of ivermectin in many areas, but safety profiles differ. Due to its lipophilic nature, moxidectin becomes highly concentrated in serum when administered to horses with very little body fat, such as foals or thin, debilitated individuals. The immature blood brain barrier of young foals renders them more susceptible to moxidectin toxicity. Signs associated with toxicity in juvenile equids include dyspnea, depression, weakness, ataxia, coma, and seizures. Consequently, moxidectin is not labeled for use in foals less than 6 months of age. When faced with multi-drug resistant cyathostomin populations, moxidectin remains one of the last drugs to demonstrate continued efficacy, despite increasing reports of reduced ERPs. Therefore, it is the recommendation of many parasitologists that this anthelmintic be used strategically for those horse populations at increased risk for parasite-associated disease due to cyathostominosis and for those farms where FECRTs have confirmed decreased efficacy for other drug classes.

Provided the ascarid population on a given farm is not ML-resistant, ivermectin exhibits efficacy against *Parascaris* spp. larval and adult stages. If ivermectin-resistant ascarids are identified in pre-weaning age foals, it is probable that moxidectin will be equally ineffective in clearing ascarid infections in older foals and yearlings. The macrocyclic lactones continue to demonstrate good efficacy against cyathostomins at 14 days post-treatment and large strongyles remain susceptible. However, there are reports of the strongyle ERPs becoming shorter after treatment with both compounds in this drug class. When first marketed, ivermectin and moxidectin suppressed strongyle egg-shedding for 8 weeks and >12–16 weeks, respectively. Recent reports have documented reduced ERPs of less than 5 weeks for both drugs. Additional studies have demonstrated that fourth-stage small strongyle larvae residing in the intestinal lumen are able to survive treatment with macrocyclic lactones.

50.6 Environmental Control Strategies

The goals of any deworming program include prevention of parasite-related disease in the individual animal as well as reduction of egg contamination of the environment. While strategic use of effective anthelmintics is usually the backbone of most parasite control programs, it is important to remember good general husbandry is vital to the success of any deworming regimen. An "open" breeding farm should have biosecurity protocols for new and returning mares and foals that include fecal exams and prophylactic therapy targeted against potentially drug-resistant cyathostomins and ascarids acquired during recent visits to other farms. New arrivals should be treated prior to gaining access to home pastures. Strategies to reduce parasite egg and larvae build-up in the environment include cross-grazing pastures with other ruminant species, preferably sheep, and keeping pastures mowed and/or resting pastures for at least several months during periods of warm ambient temperatures sustained above 85°F to optimize desiccation of vulnerable strongyle larvae. Harvesting a hay crop off pastures helps reduce parasite burdens. Regular manure removal from paddocks and pastures at least twice weekly, while labor intensive and unpopular, can greatly reduce mare and foal exposure to infective stages of strongyle and ascarid eggs and larvae. A testimony to the impact of a clean environment is the observation that most stallions, usually confined to individual, well-groomed paddocks and pastures, typically have low to negligible fecal egg counts. It is unlikely that all stallions are genetically more resistant to strongyle parasites and serves as a reminder that good husbandry practices are among the best parasite control measures. If pastures are harrowed, this procedure should only be done during hot, dry periods and pastures rested for 3–4 weeks or longer before re-introducing mares and foals. Young foals are the most susceptible age group and ideally should be turned out on the farm's "cleanest" pastures. Overcrowding and limited pastures often contribute to the accumulation of heavy parasite burdens by late spring which will be a challenge for any deworming program to control. Fresh manure should never be spread on active pastures. Properly composted manure can attain high enough temperatures to kill both strongyle larvae and ascarid eggs.

50.7 Risk Assessment: Age and General Husbandry

When designing an equine parasite control program there are at least two populations of horses to consider: mature adults, 3 years of age or older; and foals, weanlings, and juveniles 2 years of age and younger. Parasites of concern and risk of infection vary considerably between these two populations and necessitate different monitoring and control strategies.

50.8 Parasite Control Strategies for Mature Horses

Among well-managed adult horse populations *Strongylus vulgaris* infections are rare and cyathostomins are recognized as the major parasite of concern. Mature horses, including broodmares and breeding stallions, vary in their innate susceptibility to cyathostomin infection and their strongyle egg shedding potential. This is a heritable trait. Consequently, deworming regimens can be

individualized among adult horses (≥3 years of age) once their shedding status is determined using properly performed FECs. The majority of horses in a herd that are shedding low to moderate numbers of strongyle eggs can be managed with two to three anthelmintic treatments per year administered during periods of peak parasite exposure and transmission. Low shedders may only require a larvicidal treatment for encysted cyathostomins every other year. The small percentage of horses classified as high egg contaminators benefit from more frequent deworming with as many as four or more treatments annually. Herd size, pasture availability, general husbandry practices, history of past drug use on the farm, prevalence of other parasite species, and local climate also impact deworming recommendations and anthelmintic selection. The FECRT should be used on a farm-by-farm basis to determine which drug classes are still effective against cyathostomins and ascarids.

Specific treatments for other parasites of interest, including *Anoplocephala perfoliata*, *Oxyuris equi*, *Habronema* spp., *Strongyloides westeri*, and *Strongylus vulgaris* can be incorporated into the annual treatment plan. Two treatments a year are sufficient to prevent reappearance of large strongyles. All drug classes are still effective against adult stages of *S. vulgaris*, while ivermectin, moxidectin and larvicidal doses of fenbendazole are effective against larval stages of *S. vulgaris*. Ideally, anthelmintic treatments should be concentrated during seasons of parasite transmission, typically spring and fall in most regions, as well as during winter months in warmer climates and temperate summers in cooler regions. Consider including a treatment against encysted cyathostomins (e.g., larvicidal dose of fenbendazole or moxidectin) at a time when the mucosal burden is dormant and expected to be at its peak. This is typically at the end of the grazing season (i.e., late fall/early winter in northern climates and late spring/early summer in warmer climates). If tapeworms are a proven regional concern, incorporate a cestocidal treatment at least once a year, preferably at the end of the grazing seasons.

Broodmares that are low shedders typically receive a treatment in the fall and again in the spring prior to foaling or immediately post-partum. Ivermectin, with or without praziquantel, remains a popular post-delivery treatment. The incidence of clinical neonatal disease associated with *Strongyloides westeri*, a parasite that can be transferred to the foal via the milk, is extremely low on most well-managed farms. Therefore, the practice of routinely deworming young foals at 2–4 weeks of age to prevent *Strongyloides*-associated diarrhea is no longer warranted. Maintaining the broodmare on a good deworming regimen should continue to control this parasite. Even though some anthelmintics have a "safe in pregnant mare" claim and all commonly used drug classes have been administered throughout pregnancy, the author (WV) still prefers to minimize the administration of unnecessary drugs to the broodmare during the early period of fetal organogenesis.

Adult horses with limited pasture access or confined to individual paddocks with limited exposure to large numbers of other horses, usually can be properly managed with 2–3 anthelmintic treatments per year. Horses that spend a considerable amount of time in stalls are at reduced risk of exposure to cyathostomins, large strongyles, and cestodes since transmission of these parasites occurs more frequently on pasture. In addition, horse urine is toxic to developing strongyle larvae which may also explain why stalled horses are less likely to be exposed to large numbers of infective strongyle larvae. Daily stall cleaning also provides excellent parasite control by removing parasite eggs and larvae before infective stages are reached. Low to moderate shedders and horses in a well-groomed environment can receive on average one (or two treatments) in the spring and early summer and then one (or two) treatments again in the fall. A popular treatment at the end of the grazing season is a macrocyclic lactone (with or without praziquantel) to provide broad spectrum parasite control in addition to a boticide.

Stables with large numbers of horses, multiple owners and over-stocked pastures provide the greatest challenge. It may be too labor intensive and too difficult to achieve owner compliance in this setting to individualize horse deworming regimens. In this environment, a deworming program may be designed to minimize pasture worm burdens for the majority of horses. In some cases, it might be beneficial to pasture high shedders together to permit more targeted treatment of this population. The use of low-dose, daily pyrantel tartrate might also be helpful to reduce an individual's exposure to high pasture parasite burdens when other non-chemical strategies or changes in husbandry practices are unavailable or impractical. It should be remembered that pyrantel resistance can develop in the face of daily deworming and routine FECs should still be employed to monitor drug efficacy.

50.9 Parasite Control Strategies for Juvenile Horses

Foals and weanlings are susceptible to a wide range of parasites including ascarids, cyathostomins, large strongyles, tapeworms, pinworms, and threadworms. The most pathogenic of these parasites is *Parascaris* spp. Although acquired immunity develops in most horses by 8–18 months of age, effective larvicidal anthelmintics are often needed to ensure adequate control of all stages of ascarid infections in juvenile equids. Failure of ML anthelmintics to reduce *P. equorum* egg counts in foals on many stud farms has been reported. Many farms with documented ML resistant ascarids share several common management practices (Robert et al., 2015): (1) Foals often receive their first anthelmintic treatment prior of 60 days of age (often as early as 14–30 days of age), (2) Deworming intervals are often ≤ 30–60 days, (3) Ivermectin is used frequently, if not exclusively, and (4) Prior to the discovery of clinical disease due to ascarid infection, FEC monitoring had not been routinely performed.

During the first year of life foals typically receive a minimum of four to five anthelmintic treatments. The first treatment should be performed no earlier than 2 months of age, unless there is a documented medical indication to do treat at a younger age. A benzimidazole drug is recommended to ensure efficacy against ascarids. The label dose of fenbendazole for juvenile horses less than 18 months of age is 10 mg/kg. This is double the label dose for mature horses. The higher drug dose in young animals is critical to ensure efficacy against ascarids, the dose-limiting parasite for most equine anthelmintics. One or two additional treatments are recommended prior to weaning. Pyrantel is another drug class with good efficacy against ascarids. The average interval between these early anthelmintic treatments should range between 8–12 weeks with the goal of reducing the number of patent ascarid infections among the foal population while minimizing the drug selection pressure on resistant *Parascaris* spp. isolates.

On an annual basis, fecal egg count reduction tests should be performed on at least a subset of foals and weanlings on breeding farms in order to monitor drug efficacy against cyathostomins and ascarids. The cleanest pastures should be reserved for the youngest foals. Stepwise suggestions for implementing new control strategies for foals include the following principles:

- Unless medically indicated, delay the first anthelmintic treatment for foals until foals are at least 2–3 months of age. Reasons to consider therapy at an earlier age include treatment of symptomatic disease due to *Strongyloides westeri* infection or a strong index of suspicion that foals are harboring dangerously heavy burdens of migrating *Parascaris spp.* larvae. Ivermectin (0.2 mg/kg) or oxibendazole (15 mg/ kg) have been used successfully to treat *Strongyloides westeri* infection. Ivermectin (0.2 mg/kg) or a larvicidal treatment with fenbendazole (10 mg/kg orally once daily for 5 consecutive days) have demonstrated efficacy against migrating ascarid larvae. Due to widespread reports of macrocyclic lactone resistant ascarids, a FECRT should be performed on each breeding farm before relying on ivermectin to treat *Parascaris* spp. infections. If ivermectin resistant ascarids are confirmed, then fenbendazole (10 mg/kg) or pyrantel pamoate (6.6 mg/kg) are reasonable selections for the first anthelmintic treatment.

- Perform a FEC prior to deworming foals for the first time to address two issues of concern for young foals. Document the incidence of patent ascarids, and to a lesser degree cyathostomins, infections among that age group. The FECs will reflect the level and intensity of early parasite exposure for foals on that particular farm. If the majority of foals have negative or low eggs counts, delaying the first treatment until foals are slightly older can be discussed with farm management. Identify those foals with positive FECs (e.g., patent infections). Those are the only foals that require 14-day, post-treatment fecal collections that will be used to calculate the FECRT for the drug class about to be administered. On each farm, anthelmintics from the three major drug classes, pyrimidines, benzimidazoles, and macrocyclic lactones, should be evaluated for efficacy against ascarids in pre-weaning age foals. This can be accomplished over the courses of one or two foaling seasons.

- Determine the longest and safest deworming interval between drug treatments. Delay the second anthelmintic treatment for as long as possible while still reducing the risk of parasite-related clinical disease and minimizing fecal egg shedding to control pasture contamination with weather resistant ascarid eggs. A deworming interval of at least sixty days or longer is recommended to reduce drug selection pressure for resistance.

- On farms with a high stocking density and/or a high percentage of foals exhibiting positive FECs between treatments, the challenge becomes finding a treatment regimen that prevents rapid resumption of egg shedding without relying on frequent anthelmintic administration as the only solution. A 5-day, larvicidal dose of fenbendazole has been shown to eliminate juvenile and adult ascarid burdens, even macrocyclic lactone-resistant ascarids. Since larvicidal treatment removes both migrating and intraluminal larval stages as well as *Parascaris* spp. adult worms. A minimum of 8–10 weeks will be necessary before treated foals can acquire new infections that develop into egg-laying adults. If given close to weaning, such larvicidal therapy can eliminate existing ascarid burdens at a time when the foal's advancing age should help suppress new ascarid infections.

- At weaning, a FEC should be performed to determine whether foals are shedding primarily strongyles and/or ascarids. At least two additional treatments should be administered between weaning and 12 months of age. Unless ascarid infection remains a persistent problem, these later drug treatments should target cyathostomins. Ivermectin is often a viable option. A tapeworm treatment, using either a double dose of pyrantel (13.2 mg/kg) or a product containing praziquantel, should be included as one of these later treatments. Include a larvicidal treatment for encysted small strongyles at the end of the grazing season. The author (WV) prefers larvicidal fenbendazole for this purpose in older foals.

Figure 50.7 outlines a general approach to monitoring young horse populations based on risk of exposure and the parasite life cycle.

As yearlings and 2-year-olds, juvenile horses remain at increased risk for parasitic disease. Hopefully, age-related immunity will have decreased the incidence of patent ascarid infections among yearlings. On stud farms, a representative subset of this age group can be selected to monitor FECs at convenient times when youngsters are already being handled for vaccinations, foot care or other routine procedures. Control of cyathostomin and tapeworm infections becomes the more important focus of the deworming regimen for this age group unless ascarid infections are observed. If *Parascaris* spp. are detected, benzimidazoles and tetrahydropyrimidines remain the drugs of choice unless FECRT indicate otherwise. Yearlings and 2-year-olds benefit from larvicidal treatments against encysted small strongyles at least once a year. Moxidectin often remains the drug of choice, if FECRT reveals unacceptable results following larvicidal doses of fenbendazole, for treatment of encysted cyathostomins. It should be remembered that FECs are not reflective of the prepatent stages of any equine parasite, including encysted small strongyles.

50.10 Summary

Strategic deworming/restrained deworming regimens coupled with sound husbandry practices and a supplemental, targeted fecal surveillance program should be the hallmark of parasite control programs on all stud farms. Veterinarian consultation is critical to determine when and why to perform fecal exams as well as how to interpret and apply the results.

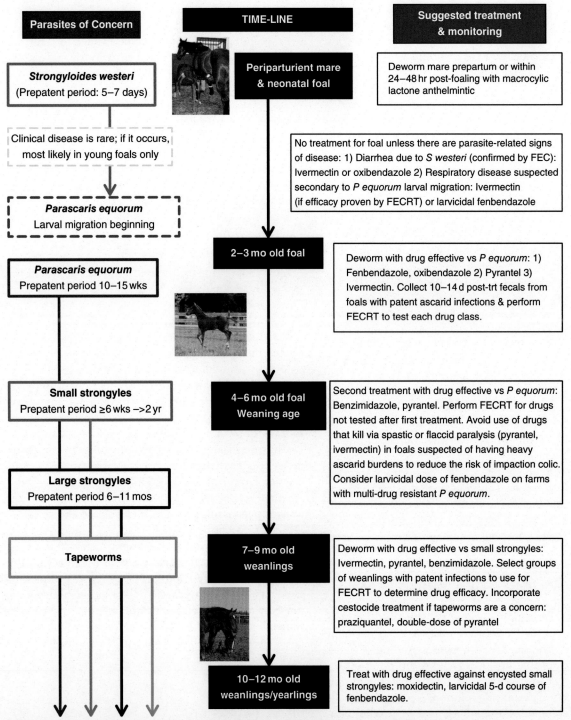

Parasites of Concern

Strongyloides westeri
(Prepatent period: 5–7 days)

Clinical disease is rare; if it occurs, most likely in young foals only

Parascaris equorum
Larval migration beginning

Parascaris equorum
Prepatent period 10–15 wks

Small strongyles
Prepatent period ≥6 wks –>2 yr

Large strongyles
Prepatent period 6–11 mos

Tapeworms

TIME-LINE

Periparturient mare & neonatal foal

2–3 mo old foal

4–6 mo old foal
Weaning age

7–9 mo old weanlings

10–12 mo old weanlings/yearlings

Suggested treatment & monitoring

Deworm mare prepartum or within 24–48 hr post-foaling with macrocylic lactone anthelmintic

No treatment for foal unless there are parasite-related signs of disease: 1) Diarrhea due to *S westeri* (confirmed by FEC): Ivermectin or oxibendazole 2) Respiratory disease suspected secondary to *P equorum* larval migration: Ivermectin (if efficacy proven by FECRT) or larvicidal fenbendazole

Deworm with drug effective vs *P equorum*: 1) Fenbendazole, oxibendazole 2) Pyrantel 3) Ivermectin. Collect 10–14 d post-trt fecals from foals with patent ascarid infections & perform FECRT to test each drug class.

Second treatment with drug effective vs *P equorum*: Benzimidazole, pyrantel. Perform FECRT for drugs not tested after first treatment. Avoid use of drugs that kill via spastic or flaccid paralysis (pyrantel, ivermectin) in foals suspected of having heavy ascarid burdens to reduce the risk of impaction colic. Consider larvicidal dose of fenbendazole on farms with multi-drug resistant *P equorum*.

Deworm with drug effective vs small strongyles: Ivermectin, pyrantel, benzimidazole. Select groups of weanlings with patent infections to use for FECRT to determine drug efficacy. Incorporate cestocide treatment if tapeworms are a concern: praziquantel, double-dose of pyrantel

Treat with drug effective against encysted small strongyles: moxidectin, larvicidal 5-d course of fenbendazole.

* Reprinted with permission from : Vaala WE, How to Design a Parasite Control Program for the First Year of Life: Focus on *Parascaris equorum*, accepted for publication in AAEP Proceedings 2016.

Figure 50.7 Chronological approach to parasite control for foals during the first 12 months of life.

References

Grønvold J. 1991. Laboratory diagnoses of helminths common routine methods used in Denmark. In P Nansen, J Grønvold, H Bjørn (eds), Seminars on Parasitic Problems in Farm Animals Related to Fodder Production and Management. Tartu, Estonia: The Estonian Academy of Sciences, pp. 47–48.

Henriksen SA and Aagaard KA. 1976. A simple flotation and McMaster method. Nord Vet Med, 28: 392–397.

Kassai T. 1999. Veterinary Helminthology. Oxford: Butterworth-Heinemann, pp. 260.

Luksovsky J, Craig TM, Bingham GM, et al. 2013. Determining treatment to control two multidrug-resistant parasites on a Texas horse farm. J of Equine Vet Sci, 33: 115–119.

Nielsen MK, Mittel L, Grice S, et al. 2013. AAEP Equine Parasite Control Guidelines. American Association of Equine Practitioners. www.aaep.org/custdocs/ParasiteControlGuidelines.pdf.

Nielsen, MK, Wang, J, Davis, R., et al. 2014. *Parascaris univalens* – a victim of large-scale misidentification. Parasitol Res, 113: 4485–4490.

Robert M, Hu W, Nielsen MK, et al. 2014. Attitudes towards implementation of surveillance-based parasite control on Kentucky Thoroughbred farms – Current strategies, awareness and willingness-to-pay. Equine Vet J, 47:6 94–700.

Roepstorff A and Nansen P. 1998. A Simple McMaster technique. Epidemiology, diagnosis and control of helminth parasites of swine. FAO. Animal Health Manual. Rome, Italy, pp. 47–56.

Wetzel E. 1951. Verbesserte McMaster-Kammer zum Auszählen von Wurmeiern. Tierärztl Umsch, 6: 209–210.

Zajac AM and Conboy, GA. 2012. Veterinary Clinical Parasitology, 8th Edn, John Wiley & Sons, Ltd, Chichester, UK.

Zajicek D. 1978. Comparison of the efficiency of two quantitative ovoskopic methods (article in Czech). Vet Med, 23: 275–280.

51

Molecular Diagnostics for Infectious Pathogens

Nicola Pusterla[1] and Christian M. Leutenegger[2]

[1] *Department of Medicine and Epidemiology, School of Veterinary Medicine, University of California, California, USA*
[2] *IDEXX Laboratories, Inc., California, USA*

51.1   Introduction

The ready availability of a correct etiologic diagnosis, particularly in contagious infections, enables the veterinarian to make early decisions regarding the patient's care and management, address appropriate treatment, and allow timely notification and discussion of management issues pertaining to the prevention of disease spread. The past two decades have seen a revolution in the understanding, management, diagnosis, control, and prevention of infectious diseases. This period has encompassed the discovery of emerging equine agents, antimicrobials, and vaccines, as well as a wealth of improved diagnostic tests and molecular methods for equine practitioners. Despite these advances, infectious diseases remain a leading cause of equine morbidity and mortality, with resurgence of certain infections, an increasing population of elderly, more susceptible horses, and growth of international equine commerce, expanding the geographic distribution of pathogens. The focus of rapid diagnosis of infectious diseases has also shifted during this time. The most obvious change has been the appearance and increasing importance of nucleic acid (NA) amplification-based techniques, primarily polymerase chain reaction (PCR), at the expense of traditional methods of clinical microbiology.

PCR has become an increasingly important tool in microbial diagnosis in recent years, mainly because of its rapidity, affordability, high sensitivity, and high specificity (Box 51.1). These superior characteristics have propelled the field of PCR-based molecular diagnostics into the arena of applied diagnostics for infectious agents. Because the number of published and offered PCR assays is steadily rising, there is a need for critical evaluation, comparison of performance, and eventually also standardization of methods to enable equine practitioners to select the optimal methodology.

51.2   Molecular Awareness and Panel Strategy

As more and more veterinarians are using PCR to diagnose infectious diseases, it is important for them to have a basic understanding of the processes involved. Further, indications to use PCR and interpretation of results are often confusing and require more education within the veterinary community. In addition, the differences in protocols used by laboratories add to the confusion and highlight the need for standardized protocols.

Parallel testing of multiple infectious agents in highly standardized platforms is a central component of molecular assays; it essentially allows several detections to happen simultaneously on a single sample for both DNA and RNA pathogen targets. This so-called panel strategy allows an efficient work-up of complex clinical syndromes with general symptomatology. These clinical situations do not allow easy diagnostic decision making for the veterinarian. In such organ-related complex problems with general or unspecific clinical signs, multiple infectious agents can be responsible for a clinical picture. Even though veterinarians tend to make a single pathogen diagnosis, it has become more evident in recent years that many syndromes are caused by co-infections. Panel testing on a large scale will uncover unknown dual or triple infections in animals that can diffuse the clinical picture. It has long been speculated that seemingly clinically irrelevant EHV-2 infections in horses may be the underlying cause to aggravate and cloud the clinical picture by setting up for secondary infections. More characteristic examples are known from companion animal respiratory infections, often times initiated by a subclinical viral infection leading the way to secondary infections.

Box 51.1 Key features for the adoption of molecular diagnostics for infectious agents.

- Superior sensitivity and specificity compared to most immunoassays
- Automated technology increasing accuracy and throughput
- Quantitative assessment of specific pathogens allowing a better interpretation of disease stage, infectious risk and response to treatment
- Fast turnaround time that speeds detection and reduces overall costs
- Simultaneous analysis of multiple pathogens (panel strategy)

51.3 Pre-Analytical Variables and Quality Controls

Diagnostic laboratories provide strict recommendations for sample type collection including shipping instructions (see Chapter 1 for more details). These instructions include specimen type, volume, anticoagulant, and specimen transport specifications, storage, and handling. The sample type(s) is largely influenced by the pathogenesis of the disease and plays a key role in the performance and interpretation of the test results. Veterinarians are advised to adhere to these recommendations as the quality of the result is directly correlated to the quality of the sample and preservation of the nucleic acid content (Box 51.2).

Veterinarians can use a variety of guidelines to select laboratories for molecular diagnostics. There are questions worth asking before samples are submitted to a molecular diagnostic laboratory. These questions should cover three areas. First, it is worthwhile to obtain information about the nature of the PCR testing platform (traditional PCR versus qPCR). Second, questions addressing the quality control and quality assurance system within a particular laboratory should be asked. In particular it is relevant to know whether whole processes are controlled or just single point controls are used and how contamination is avoided and confirmed to be absent within the laboratory. Third, turnaround time, pricing, and the level of guidance provided when interpreting results are additional questions worth asking before samples are submitted.

Biological samples received by diagnostic laboratories are generally processed the same day and PCR results are usually available within 24–72 h (including shipping) assuming all relevant standards are met. These standards should include internal sample quality controls (to confirm proper collection, storage, shipping, and NA extraction) and other associated quality controls, such as PCR positive and negative controls (to confirm PCR reagents were properly made and are contaminate free), internal positive control (to confirm absence of PCR inhibitors), and negative extraction control (to confirm absence of cross-contamination during the NA extraction process).

Interpretation of results obtained with molecular assays for infectious diseases requires understanding of the pathogenesis and biology of the target organism(s). Some challenges are unique to molecular tests and are different from considerations in interpreting other microbiological tests. Such differences are related to the distinction of viable versus nonviable organisms and the correlation of NA detection with presence of disease or disease association.

Box 51.2 Recommendations for sample collection and shipping for PCR testing of infectious pathogens.

- Specimen type should be compatible with the biology of the pathogen (blood for blood-borne pathogen, feces for enteric pathogens, respiratory secretions for respiratory pathogens).
- Whole blood samples should be collected aseptically into evacuated blood tubes containing EDTA.
- Body fluids (thoracic, abdominal, joint, cerebrospinal, tracheal wash, bronchoalveolar, nasopharyngeal, or guttural pouch lavage fluid) and tissues should be collected into serum tubes without additives.
- Nasal or nasopharyngeal secretions should be collected with rayon- or Dacron-tipped swabs and are best kept in a serum or conical tube with or without transport medium.
- Feces should be collected into small fecal cups and rectal swabs should be collected with 6″ rayon- or Dacron-tipped swabs and best kept in a serum tube.

- All samples must be sent cooled on ice by express mail overnight to the laboratory. Freezing of samples should be avoided due to the degradation of NA during the thawing process and prevention of inhibition due to hemolysis.
- Short-term storage for a period of 2–3 days before shipment (over a weekend) should be done in a refrigerated compartment.
- Label sample properly (date, sample identification with name of owner and patient) and fill out laboratory specific submission form (information pertaining to animal, owner, veterinarian, sample, and pathogen(s) to be tested).
- The laboratory should be notified in advance and inquiry should be made about the availability of the offered tests as well as the expected turnaround time and the associated costs.

Interpretation considerations for PCR results:

- Interpretation of a negative PCR result requires information about the sensitivity of the PCR test, limit of detection and the NA extraction efficiency as indicated by the use of quantitative internal sample controls. A false-negative PCR result may be caused by a degraded or unstable sample. Insufficient or inappropriate sample type, inadequate sampling procedures or transport problems are additional sources of false-negative results. Sample-specific internal positive controls targeting endogenous genes help to overcome this problem. In addition, inhibition phenomena originating from sample matrixes such as feces, urine or environmental samples contaminated with soil or surface water have to be controlled with internal positive controls to assess the inhibitory effects on the PCR process.
- The factors requiring consideration for the interpretation of PCR positive results include assay specificity and contamination issues. PCR or any other target amplification method is subjected to these considerations. Quantitative PCR (qPCR) using closed-tube detection procedures reduces the risk of PCR product carry-over as a source for false-positive results.
- In general, molecular assays do not provide information about the viability of an infectious agent. Exceptions to this are DNA viruses, bacteria, and parasites analyzed for the presence of RNA molecules such as rRNA and transcribed genes in form of messenger RNA instead of their genomic DNA equivalents.
- Detection of NA of a pathogen does not necessarily indicate the organism is the cause of the disease. However, using the quantitative information of a qPCR result may give further insight and provide a means to evaluate disease association. Primary examples are herpesvirus infections (EHV-1 and EHV-4) where the quantitative detection of DNA may indicate presence of lytic, non-replicating or latent virus. Laboratory specific cut-off values in EHV-4 and EHV-1 DNA load allow differentiation between lytic and non-replicating virus. In these particular cases, high viral loads are generally associated with the presence of clinical signs and the presence of viral RNA transcripts indicating virus replication. Therefore, qPCR can provide a means to obtain information about the disease association, a crucial criterion for the equine practitioner to obtain the correct diagnosis.

51.4   Blood-Borne Pathogens

See Table 51.1. Whole, uncoagulated blood is generally used for the detection of specific blood-borne pathogens. It is important to collect the blood in evacuated tubes containing ethylenediaminetetraacetic acid (EDTA) since other anti-coagulants, such as heparin, have been shown to have an inhibitory effect on the PCR. Further, severely hemolyzed blood should not be used for PCR analysis due to the presence of biological inhibitors such as hemin. Most commercially available nucleic acid purification systems have been found to be suitable extraction methods for eliminating inhibitors from samples with mild hemolysis. Therefore, blood should be properly handled and stored at 4°C prior to analyses and accidental freezing of blood samples should be avoided to minimize hemolysis of red blood cells.

- *Equine granulocytic anaplasmosis* (EGA) is caused by *Anaplasma phagocytophilum*, a rickettsial pathogen transmitted by *Ixodes* spp. ticks. Diagnosis is often based on awareness of the geographic area for infection, typical clinical signs, abnormal laboratory findings, and identifying characteristic pathogen inclusions in the cytoplasm of neutrophils and eosinophils in a peripheral blood smear. PCR has been used for many years to study several aspects of the epidemiology and pathophysiology of EGA. For clinical purposes, the material of choice is whole blood. PCR has been shown to be a very sensitive and specific tool, confirming the diagnosis especially during the early and late stage of the disease, at times when the number of organisms is too small to be detected via microscopy.
- *Equine herpesvirus-1* (EHV-1) is an important, ubiquitous equine viral pathogen that exerts its major impact by inducing respiratory disease, abortion in pregnant mares, early neonatal death in foals and myeloencephalopathy (also see EHV-1 under neurologic and abortogenic pathogens). Due to the lymphotropism of EHV-1, PCR detection should always be attempted from whole blood concurrently with other biological samples determined by the clinical presentation. Although EHV-1 is ubiquitous in horse populations and a high percentage of horses are estimated to be latently infected with the virus, it is uncommon to detect EHV-1 by qPCR in the blood and nasal secretions from healthy horses outside an outbreak. The random testing of clinically normal horses for EHV-1 by qPCR should be avoided, however, since practicing veterinarians and regulatory officials, on receipt of positive test results may be unaware of the complexities involved in test interpretation, leading to inappropriate decision-making in relation to the quarantine of equine facilities or the cancellation of competitions.
- *Neorickettsia risticii* is the agent of equine neorickettsiosis (formerly known as Potomac horse fever) and responsible for serious enterocolitis, laminitis, and occasionally abortion in horses. While nucleic acid of *N. risticii* can be detected in blood and feces of

Table 51.1 Testing considerations for selected blood-borne pathogens.

Pathogen	Sample type		Considerations
	Whole blood	Others	
Anaplasma Phagocytophilum	X	Cavitary effusion	Expect negative results if patient has been pre-treated with antimicrobials
Equine herpesvirus-1	X	Nasal secretions, cerebrospinal fluid	Combine with additional biological samples depending on the clinical presentation Avoid testing asymptomatic horses outside an outbreak
Neorickettsia risticii	X	Feces	PCR testing should be done on blood and feces Expect negative results if patient has been pre-treated with antimicrobials
West Nile virus	X	Cerebrospinal fluid	An ante-mortem diagnosis should rely on the serological detection of IgM in blood and/or cerebrospinal fluid
Babesia caballi, Theileria equi	X	Not applicable	Always combine PCR testing with serology to confirm the diagnosis in clinical cases and detect infection in unapparent chronic carriers of EP agents

naturally or experimentally infected horses, the detection period does not necessarily coincide between the two sample types. It is therefore recommended to analyze both biological samples from suspected horses in order to enhance the chance of molecular detection of *N. risticii*.

- *West Nile virus* (WNV) is a flavivirus transmitted by *Culex* spp. mosquitos and responsible for systemic and neurological abnormalities mainly in unvaccinated horses. The diagnosis of WNV infection is generally supported by clinical signs, whether the horse resides in an area in which WNV has been confirmed in the current calendar year in mosquitos, birds, humans, or other horses, absence of incomplete vaccination against WNV and detection of IgM antibodies against WNV that consistently occur in acutely infected horses but is rarely observed post-vaccine administration. Because of the short-lived viremia, PCR detection of WNV in blood should be avoided and the ante-mortem diagnosis should rely on serological testing.

- *Equine piroplasmosis* (EP) is a tick-borne protozoal disease of horses, mules and donkeys that is characterized by acute hemolytic anemia. There are two distinctive EP causative agents, *Babesia caballi* and *Theileria equi*. Clinical signs can alert the veterinarian to the possibility of EP. In cases having clinical signs consistent with EP, examination of blood smears can assist the diagnosis. As an alternative, molecular techniques for the detection of *T. equi* and *B. caballi* have been described based on species-specific PCR. Because the parasitemia can be very low in horses that have recovered from clinical disease, the examination of direct blood smears or PCR testing may not allow for

detection of the infection in chronic carriers. To confirm the diagnosis in clinical cases and detect infection in unapparent chronic carriers of EP agents, serological tests should be used.

51.5 Respiratory Pathogens

See Table 51.2. The sample of choice for the molecular detection of viruses associated with infectious respiratory tract disease is nasal secretions, which are generally collected from the nasal passages and/or the nasopharynx using rayon- or Dacron-tipped swabs. The use of viral transport medium for the transportation of respiratory swabs is not necessary for PCR detection, since NA-based assays do not rely on viability of the target pathogen. PCR assays testing for the presence of EIV, EHV-1, EHV-4, and *S. equi* subsp. *equi* have shown greater sensitivity than antigen-capture ELISAs and/or conventional culture systems. Another advantage of molecular assays is their ability to detect non-viable virus, a situation that may occur when nasal or nasopharyngeal samples are frozen or not adequately stored and/or shipped to a diagnostic laboratory. Further, novel PCR platforms allow quantitation of DNA or RNA content in a given sample. This is of interest in order to assess the kinetics of viral shedding, to determine the infectious nature of a clinically or subclinically infected horse and to assess the response to treatment.

- *Equine influenza virus* (EIV) is routinely detected from upper airway secretions collected from horses during the early febrile stage of the disease. Nasopharyngeal

Table 51.2 Testing considerations for selected respiratory pathogens.

Pathogen	Sample type		Considerations
	Respiratory secretions	Others	
Equine influenza virus	X	Not applicable	Nasopharyngeal swabs are superior in the detection of EIV when compared to nasal swabs Inability to discriminate between clade I and II Florida sublineage EIV
Equine herpesvirus-1	X	Whole blood	Discriminate between lytic and non-replicating virus using absolute quantitation and transcriptional activity of the target genes at the messenger RNA level
Equine herpesvirus-4	X	Not applicable	
Streptococcus equi subsp. *equi*	X	Aspirate from draining lymph node	Diagnostic sensitivity varies based on type and location of biological sample Inability to distinguish between viable and non-viable organisms and between vaccine-derived and wild-type organisms
Streptococcus equi subsp. *zooepidemicus*	X	Aspirate from draining lymph node	Upper respiratory secretions should not be tested due to the ubiquitous nature of the bacterial organism Strangles-like disease should be considered after detection of *S. zooepidemicus* from a draining lymph node and ruling out other respiratory pathogens
Equine rhinitis A virus	X	Urine	Very short detection period in nasal secretions Concurrent serological testing indicated to support infection
Equine rhinitis B virus	X	Not applicable	Always collect nasal secretions during the acute phase of the disease and possibly sample multiple affected animals
Equine arteritis virus	X	Blood, conjunctival swab, placenta, fetal tissues	Nasal/nasopharyngeal swabs or washes, conjunctival swabs and whole blood are appropriate biological specimens for horses with respiratory signs
Equine herpesvirus-2	X	Blood	Testing of upper airway secretions and blood from horses with respiratory signs is, at this time, not recommended due to the high prevalence of these viruses in horse populations Detection of EHV-5 in bronchoalveolar lavage and/or lung biopsy in a horse with atypical interstitial pneumonia is suggestive of EMPF
Equine herpesvirus-5	X	Blood Bronchoalveolar lavage	

swabs have been shown to be superior to nasal swabs in the detection of EIV, with increased frequency and amount of virus detected via nasopharyngeal swabs. Amplification of the single stranded RNA of EIV is performed by reverse transcription-PCR (RT-PCR) technology, in addition to qPCR. The haemagglutinin, nucleoprotein, and matrix gene are the commonly targeted genes for these molecular assays. Nucleotide and deduced amino-acid sequences of portions of the haemagglutinin gene are now routinely used for phylogenetic characterization of outbreak strains. Routine diagnostic testing for EIV does not allow differentiation between clade I and clade II viruses of the Florida sublineage.

- *Equine herpesvirus (EHV)-1 and EHV-4* are double-stranded DNA alphaherpesviruses that affect the equine respiratory tract and can establish life-long latent infection following exposure. The diagnostic sample of choice is a nasal or nasopharyngeal swab which should be taken early in the febrile phase of the

disease. Due to the lymphotropism of EHV-1, detection can also be attempted from whole blood. PCR assays used in the diagnostic field are based on the detection of viral genomic DNA and are therefore unable to distinguish between lytic, inactive, or latent virus. Alternative molecular approaches have recently been established using qPCR to allow discrimination between the different viral states in horses naturally infected with EHV. Discrimination between the different viral states is now possible by (1) targeting several genes (e.g., glycoprotein, latency-associated transcripts), (2) detecting viral genomic DNA and transcriptional activity of the target genes at the messenger RNA (mRNA) level, and (3) using absolute virus quantification. Quantitative thresholds are used in selected human infectious diseases (i.e., HIV, HCV, herpes simplex virus) to determine disease stage and response to antiviral therapy. A similar concept is used diagnostically for EHV-1 or EHV-4 infected horses in order to discriminate between lytic and non-replicating virus, to determine their infectious risk based on viral load in nasal secretions and to monitor their response to treatment.

- *Streptococcus equi* subsp. *equi (S. equi)* infection rarely is associated with detection difficulties when using conventional culture in clinically affected horses. Culture of nasal swabs, nasopharyngeal or guttural pouch washes or exudates aspirated from an abscess remains the gold standard for the detection of *S. equi*. Culture, however, may be unsuccessful during the incubation and early clinical phases of infection. Further, the presence of other beta-hemolytic streptococci, especially *S. equi* subsp. *zooepidemicus*, may complicate the interpretation of the culture. Available PCR assays are designed to detect the DNA sequence of the *S. equi* M protein (SeM) gene, the gene for the antiphagocytic M protein of *S. equi*. This gene offers sufficient nucleotide variability between the two *S. equi* subspecies, allowing full discrimination in clinical specimens. One of the pitfalls of PCR has been its inability to distinguish between viable and non-viable organisms, therefore, positive results have been considered presumptive in the past until confirmed by culture. Nowadays, the viability issue can be addressed by quantitation of the SeM gene or detection of transcriptional activity of the SeM gene at the RNA level. In several studies, PCR proved to be up to three times more sensitive than culture. Nasopharyngeal lavages analyzed by a combination of qPCR directly and after culture, or, alternatively, qPCR directly on a nasopharyngeal lavage and a nasal/nasopharyngeal swab can identify *S. equi* in over 90% of acute strangles cases. PCR accompanying culture on a nasal/nasopharyngeal swab or nasopharyngeal/guttural pouch lavage may be used in a control program to select possible carrier animals, because PCR is capable of detecting *S. equi* DNA in guttural pouch lavages for weeks after disappearance of live organisms. PCR should be considered to detect asymptomatic carriers, to establish the *S. equi* infection status of asymptomatic horses and to determine the success of elimination of *S. equi* from the guttural pouch. Unfortunately, diagnostic PCR assays are unable to differentiate between wild-type and the non-encapsulated, avirulent vaccine strains of *S. equi* (Pinnacle I.N., Pfizer Animal Health, Overland Parks, KS 66210). However, when needed for forensic reasons, differentiation can be done via the morphology of colonies, biochemical analysis, genotyping and restriction digest. Together, these assays allow differentiation between wild-type and vaccine/ancestor strains.
- *Streptococcus equi* subsp. *zooepidemicus (S. zooepidemicus)* is a commensal, opportunistic equine pathogen that is generally present in the upper respiratory tract and responsible for secondary bacterial bronchopneumonia in young and adult horses. The literature reports on a few outbreaks of upper respiratory disease associated with *S. zooepidemicus*. The clinical signs are indistinguishable from *S. equi* infection and include depression, anorexia, elevated rectal temperature, serous to purulent nasal discharge, coughing, and lymphadenopathy with abscessation. Single clones of *S. zooepidemicus*, as determined by sequencing of the szP gene and multilocus sequence typing have been associated with increased pathogenicity. From a diagnostic standpoint, one should not test for *S. zooepidemicus* in nasal secretions from horses with upper airway disease due to the ubiquitous nature of this bacterial organism. However, *S. zooepidemicus* should be considered as the etiological agent in respiratory cases when detected by culture or qPCR from a draining lymph node and other respiratory pathogens have been ruled out.
- *Equine rhinitis A (ERAV) and B (ERBV) viruses* have been given little attention by practitioners compared to other respiratory viruses, mainly because of the lack of diagnostic modalities. These viruses are common in horse populations, but knowledge of their epidemiology, pathogenesis and association with disease is poor. ERAV (*Aphthovirus*), formerly known as equine rhinovirus 1, and ERBV (*Erbovirus*), formerly known as equine rhinovirus 2, are capable of affecting both the lower and upper airways. In young performance horses ERAV has been associated with the development of inflammatory airway disease. Both natural and experimental infection of seronegative horses with ERAV has been associated with fever, anorexia, seromucoid nasal discharge, coughing, lymphadenopathy, and occasionally lower limb swelling. The diagnosis has remained a true challenge for ERVs until recently. The infection may be diagnosed by virus isolation, detection of viruses by qPCR, or demonstration of rising antibody titers to ERAV or ERBV through virus neutralization using an acute and convalescent serum sample. One of the diagnostic challenges with ERAV is that the shedding time is very short following the development of clinical signs. Further, prolonged excretion of ERAV in urine of racehorses appears to be common, particularly in 2- and 3-year-old animals and is probably an important source of infection for other susceptible horses.
- *Equine arteritis virus* (EAV) infection occurs throughout much of the world with the vast majority of infected horses being inapparently or subclinically infected. Sporadic cases as well as occasional outbreaks of EAV infection are characterized by upper-airway illness in adult horses, abortion in pregnant mares, and interstitial pneumonia in neonates. Depending on the disease presentation several

biological specimens should be collected for either virus isolation or PCR detection. Nasal/nasopharyngeal swabs or washings, conjunctival swabs, and whole blood are appropriate biological specimens for horses with respiratory signs. Placenta, fetal fluids, lung, spleen, and lymphoid tissues should be collected to confirm EAV-induced abortion. PCR has several advantages (greater sensitivity, shorter turnaround time) over viral culture, which is considered the OIE-approved gold standard for the detection of EAV in semen and is the prescribed test for international trade.

- *Equine herpesvirus* (EHV)-2 *and* EHV-5 are wide spread in horse populations, therefore, the detection of any of these viruses can occur in healthy but also in sick animals. These two viruses are optimally adapted to their host, which means that significant clinical expression of infection is rarely encountered. Experimental studies have shown that EHV-2 and EHV-5 contribute to various forms of clinical disease in young horses, including upper respiratory tract signs, fever, pharyngitis, and enlarged lymph nodes. Recent work has shown that different genetic variants of these viruses circulate amongst healthy horses, hypothesizing that viral re-infections or re-activations may be the origin of clinical disease and also explaining the sporadic occurrence of such cases. Another characteristic of the gammaherpesviruses is their ability to immunomodulate the immune system potentially increasing the susceptibility of horses to various infectious pathogens. A recently described atypical interstitial pneumonia named equine multinodular pulmonary fibrosis (EMPF) has been linked to the presence of EHV-5 in affected pulmonary tissue. The diagnosis of this disorder is based on clinical signs, radiographic abnormalities of the lungs, lower airway fluid cytology, histopathology of pulmonary tissue, and EHV-5 detection by qPCR in bronchoalveolar fluid and/or pulmonary tissue. Due to their high prevalence in the horse population, and in order to avoid dilemmas with the interpretation of PCR results, testing of EHV-2 and EHV-5 in horses with upper respiratory tract disease is not recommended at this time.

51.6 Neurologic Pathogens

See Table 51.3. Various PCR assays have been developed for the detection of viral, bacterial, and protozoal pathogens in the cerebrospinal fluid (CSF) of neurologic horses. Although highly sensitive and specific, these methods often are of limited value in the routine

Table 51.3 Testing considerations for selected neurologic pathogens.

| Pathogen | Sample type | | Considerations |
	Cerebrospinal fluid	Others	
Sarcocystis neurona	X	CNS tissue	An ante-mortem diagnosis should rely on the serological detection of IgG in blood and/or cerebrospinal fluid
Neospora hughesi	X	CNS tissue	PCR can be used to diagnose EPM on post-mortem examination using neurologic tissue
West Nile virus	X	Blood, CNS tissue	An ante-mortem diagnosis should rely on the serological detection of IgM in blood and/or cerebrospinal fluid PCR can be used to diagnose WNV on post-mortem examination using neurologic tissue
Borrelia burgdorferi	X	CNS tissue	An ante-mortem diagnosis should rely on the serological detection of specific antibodies in blood and/or cerebrospinal fluid PCR can be used to diagnose Lyme disease on post-mortem examination using neurologic tissue and determine infection in *Ixodes* ticks
Equine herpesvirus-1	X	Nasal secretions, blood, CNS tissue	Combine with additional biological samples such as nasal secretions and blood Discriminate between lytic and non-replicating virus using absolute quantitation and transcriptional activity of the target genes at the messenger RNA level SNP at position 2254 of the ORF 30 gene allows discrimination between neuropathogenic ($G_{2254}=D_{752}$) and non-neuropathogenic genotype ($A_{2254}=N_{752}$) PCR can be used to diagnose EHM on post-mortem examination using neurologic tissue

diagnosis because either the presence of the pathogen within the CSF is very short-lived or the pathogen has no affinity to the nucleated cells of the CSF. Consequently, pathogens are usually no longer molecularly detectable at the onset of systemic or neurologic signs.

- *Sarcocystis neurona* and *Neospora hughesi* are both apicomplexan protozoal organisms associated with equine protozoal myeloencephalitis (EPM). A diagnosis of EPM is generally considered when neurologic horses display progressive asymmetrical neurological deficits, other neurological disorders have been ruled out and specific antibodies to either *S. neurona* or *N. hughesi* are detected in serum and preferentially in CSF. Molecular antigen detection assays, such as qPCR, have been shown to be very specific but are lacking analytic sensitivity (too many false-negative results because the parasite is rarely found free or cell-bound in the CSF). PCR is used to document the presence of *S. neurona* and/or *N. hughesi* in neurological tissue to support the post-mortem diagnosis of EPM when direct detection of the apicomplexan protozoal organisms is unsuccessful via immunohistochemistry.
- *West Nile virus* is a flavivirus transmitted by *Culex* spp. mosquitos and responsible for systemic and neurological abnormalities mainly in unvaccinated horses (see also WNV under blood-borne pathogens). Horses are considered dead-end hosts, which imply that the viremia and disease course are generally short-lived. Although qPCR detection of WNV in blood and/or CSF is very specific it lacks sensitivity and should therefore not be used as an ante-mortem diagnostic tool. Rather, the diagnosis of WNV infection should depend on history, clinical signs, and serology. A definitive diagnosis of WNV infection is commonly based on the detection of the virus at necropsy either by viral culture, qPCR, or immunohistochemistry of neurological tissue.
- *Borrelia burgdorferi*, the causative agent of Lyme disease, is a helical-shaped, Gram-negative, unicellular spirochete transmitted by infected *Ixodes* ticks. In general, the diagnosis of Lyme disease in horses is made based on the geographic origin of the horse, ruling out other causes of clinical signs and a high antibody titer to *B. burgdorferi*. qPCR for *B. burgdorferi* in CSF has been shown to be very specific but the results are often negative due to the rare occurrence of the spirochetes in the CSF. However, PCR can be used to help document the presence of *B. burgdorferi* at post-mortem on neurological tissue or infected ticks.
- *Equine herpesvirus 1* (EHV-1) *myeloencephalopathy* (EHM), although a relatively uncommon manifestation of EHV-1 infection, can cause devastating losses on individual farms, boarding stables, veterinary hospitals, and show

and racing venues. In general, EHM is supported by historical and clinical findings, the presence of xanthochromia and elevated total protein concentration in CSF and laboratory detection of EHV-1 in blood and/or nasal secretions by qPCR. Because affected horses can shed the virus in nasal secretions, and thus represent a risk of infection for unaffected, in-contact horses, it is imperative to determine the risk of shedding in a suspected horse in order to initiate an appropriate infectious disease control protocol. The dilemma as to whether the virus is in a lytic, non-replicating or latent state can be addressed by using absolute quantitation or transcriptional activity of the target gene similar to the approach used for EHV-4. A recently identified single nucleotide polymorphism (SNP) at position 2254 in the DNA polymerase gene (ORF 30) correlates with neurological disease. This SNP is responsible for a single amino acid residue at position 752 of the DNA polymerase with EHV-1 strains associated with neurological outbreaks involving a D_{752} genotype (also referred as G_{2254}), whereas most non-neurological outbreaks involve a N_{752} genotype (also referred as A_{2254}). However, the genotyping of field isolates needs to be interpreted carefully as 14–24% of EHV-1 isolates from horses with EHM do not have this neuropathogenic marker. Strain characterization may be important given that the potential of EHM development is greater in horses infected with a neuropathogenic genotype (D_{752}). Furthermore, detection of a neurotropic EHV-1 strain may influence therapy, especially in the use of antiviral drugs such as valacyclovir, used to decrease viremia and prevent the development of neurological sequelae.

51.7 Enteric Pathogens

See Table 51.4. The detection of equine gastrointestinal pathogens using conventional or molecular tests can be very challenging because these pathogens are either difficult to grow in cell culture systems or can be present in pathogenic or non-pathogenic forms, making interpretation of positive results difficult. Furthermore, the use of fecal material for molecular diagnostics has been associated with false-negative results due to the presence of inhibitory substances in the feces that can interfere with NA extraction or amplification. However, development and use of specific extraction kits and a set of appropriate controls (internal positive control) have improved the yield and quality of NA from feces and expanded the usability of molecular methods. As with other biological sample types, it is important that sample quality and inhibition be monitored using internal or external controls.

- *Neorickettsia risticii*, agent of equine neorickettsiosis (EN) (formerly Potomac horse fever), causes serious

Table 51.4 Testing considerations for selected enteric pathogens.

Pathogen	Sample type		Considerations
	Feces/rectal swab	Others	
Neorickettsia risticii	X	Whole blood	PCR testing should be done on blood and feces Expect negative results if patient has been pre-treated with antimicrobials
Lawsonia intracellularis	X	Not applicable	Combine PCR testing with serology Expect negative results if patient has been pre-treated with antimicrobials
Salmonella enterica	X	Gastric reflux, colonic content, environmental swabs	Always perform testing following selective enrichment to increase sensitivity Culture is needed to determine serotype and antimicrobial susceptibility
Clostridium difficile	X	Gastric reflux, colonic content	Diagnosis relies on identification of toxin A and/or B and not on antigen detection Expect higher colonization rates with *C. difficile* in young horses and horses treated with antimicrobials
Clostridium perfringens	X	Gastric reflux, colonic content	Diagnosis relies on identification of virulence toxin genes (CPE, β2, netF) and not on antigen detection Expect higher colonization rates with *C. perfringens* in young horses
Equine coronavirus	X	Not applicable	PCR positive results are difficult to interpret in foals because healthy foals are known to shed ECoV PCR positive results are consistent with ECoV infection in adult horses
Equine rotavirus	X	Not applicable	Restricted to foal diarrhea

enterocolitis in horses of all ages. The diagnosis of EN is based on the detection of *N. risticii* from blood and/or feces of infected horses. Isolation of the agent in cell culture, although possible, is time-consuming and not routinely available in many diagnostic laboratories. The development of *N. risticii*-specific PCR assays has greatly facilitated the diagnosis of EN. These molecular assays have been the key in the investigation of the epidemiology of EN, allowing the discovery of helminthic vectors and intermediate and definitive helminthic hosts as well as determining the natural route of infection. While NA of *N. risticii* can be detected in the blood and feces of naturally or experimentally infected horses, the detection period does not necessarily coincide between the two sample types. It is therefore recommended to analyze both biological samples from suspected horses in order to enhance the chance of molecular detection of *N. risticii*.

- *Lawsonia intracellularis*, agent of equine proliferative enteropathy (EPE), is an emerging equine gastrointestinal pathogen of young horses. Because culture of *L. intracellularis* from feces is currently not possible, the ante-mortem diagnosis relies on serology and PCR. The combination of both tests will increase the chance

of diagnosing EPE. PCR has the advantage of being fast and can yield positive results in the early stage of disease, when antibodies are not yet measurable. Prior use of antimicrobials can negatively affect the molecular detection of *L. intracellularis* in feces. Therefore, in a suspected case, fecal collection for PCR testing should be performed prior to institution of any antimicrobial treatment.

- Infection with *Salmonella enterica* is an important cause of enteric disease and death in horses. However, *Salmonella* can also be associated with subclinical shedding, representing a source of infection for other animals. In recent years, PCR assays for the detection of *Salmonella* in fecal samples from horses admitted to veterinary hospitals have been evaluated. Collectively, these studies have shown an unquestioned higher analytical sensitivity for the detection of *Salmonella* by qPCR when compared to conventional microbiological culture. The higher detection rate of *Salmonella* by PCR has been attributed to the detection of non-viable organisms and of previously undescribed *Salmonella*-like bacterial organisms. The use of novel virulence target genes for the molecular detection of *Salmonella* has considerably improved the performance and accuracy of such assays. More and more veterinary hospitals across North America are switching from conventional microbiological culture to PCR for the testing of *Salmonella* as part of their infectious disease control program. In such instances, PCR is performed on fecal and environmental samples following a 24-h selective enrichment step. The use of PCR is very cost-effective and has the potential to reduce contamination risks and turnaround time, with results being available within 22–28 h from sample collection (18–24 h enrichment time, 4 h for DNA purification and amplification). Further, the use of absolute quantitation allows assessment of the infectious nature of hospitalized animals and may be an excellent alternative to conventional culture methods for surveillance and research studies. One must keep in mind, however, that a positive PCR result should be confirmed by culture so that serotyping of the *Salmonella* isolate and antimicrobial susceptibility can be determined.

- *Clostridium difficile* is a fastidious anaerobe considered an important cause of colitis, although, it can also be found in the intestinal tract of healthy horses. Whilst the dynamics of colonization are unknown, it is likely that horses can carry *C. difficile* for long periods without ever developing disease. Carrier status is generally higher in foals and in adult horses treated with antimicrobials. The diagnosis of *C. difficile* infection is generally based on the detection of toxin A or B or both in feces, gastric reflux or colonic content, ideally using a test that has been validated in horses. A variety of immunoassays are available, however, only one assay has been validated in horses (*Clostridium difficile* TOX A/B II ELISA, Techlab, Blacksburg, VA). This test, which detects toxin A and B has a reported sensitivity of 84% and specificity of 96% compared to the gold standard (cell cytotoxicity assay). qPCR targeting the toxin A and B genes of *C. difficile* has been shown to be highly sensitive with the advantage of a short turnaround time. However, the clinical specificity will depend on the overall background prevalence of *C. difficile* colonization in the population of horses tested. qPCR is considered an acceptable screening tool to rule in or rule out *C. difficile* infection, allowing proper management and isolation of qPCR positive patients.

- *Clostridium perfringens* type A and C are important causes of enteric disease in young foals. Disease induced by *C. perfringens*, especially type C, is associated with hemorrhagic diarrhea, abdominal distention and circulatory shock. The diagnosis of *C. perfringens* infection is challenging because the microbe can be cultured from the feces of healthy foals. Therefore, identification of toxins and ruling out other etiologies of diarrhea are key. For toxin assays, fresh feces should be submitted to a laboratory with immunoassays for *C. perfringens* toxins, including alpha, beta and epsilon toxins. Fecal assays for *C. perfringens* enterotoxin (CPE) are readily available but lack sensitivity because only minorities of equine isolates produce CPE. The alternative diagnostic avenue is to submit isolates cultured from feces for PCR analysis. The novel pore-forming necrotizing toxin (netF) of *C. perfringens* type A is an important advance in understanding the virulence of this pathogen and potentially improves the diagnostic field.

- Historically, the detection of *equine coronavirus* (ECoV) has relied on either electron microscopy, antigen-capture ELISA, or viral isolation from the feces. All of these detection modalities lack sensitivity, especially if viral particles are not present in sufficient numbers. qPCR for the detection of coronaviruses has supplanted many conventional virological assays, mainly due to its short turnaround time, high throughput capability and increased analytical sensitivity and specificity. The detection of ECoV by qPCR in the feces of foals with fever and diarrhea is difficult to interpret because ECoV has also been detected in the feces of healthy foals. Healthy foals have been found to be infected mostly by ECoV in a single infection without any other co-infecting agents, whereas ECoV was found exclusively in association with other co-infecting agents in sick foals. This is in sharp contrast to the detection of ECoV by qPCR in adult horses, where the virus has been shown to be responsible for a self-limiting disease characterized by depression, anorexia, fever, and less frequently, changes in fecal character and colic.

- *Equine rotavirus* poses a challenge each foaling season to farm managers and veterinarians in intensive horse breeding areas throughout the world. A quick and reliable diagnosis is essential in order to separate affected foals with diarrhea and reduce the spread of this virus. The diagnosis of rotavirus infection in the past has relied on direct virus detection using a rapid antigen-capture immunoassay or latex agglutination. Commercially available qPCR assays have shown high analytical sensitivity, specificity and accuracy in the diagnosis of equine rotavirus infection and will likely replace the less sensitive ELISA test in the near future.

51.8 Abortogenic Pathogens

See Table 51.5. Placentitis continues to represent a significant problem and common cause of equine abortions. These are generally sporadic cases but occasionally can be associated with abortion storms. Pathogens associated with placentitis and abortions are either primary or opportunistic microorganisms. A variety of biological

Table 51.5 Testing considerations for selected abortogenic pathogens.

Pathogen	Sample type		Considerations
	Placenta	Others	
Equine herpesvirus-1	X	Uterine swab, placenta, fetal tissue	For cost-effectiveness consider pooling various fetal tissues from the same aborted fetus In cases of sporadic abortions, nasal secretions and whole blood from the mare are generally PCR negative
Leptospira interrogans	X	Placenta, fetal tissue	Fetal kidneys and placenta are reliable samples for molecular testing
Fungi	X	Not applicable	Identification of genus or species is generally performed via sequencing of the PCR amplicons
Nocardioform actinomycetes	X	Not applicable	PCR testing for selected nocardioform actinomycetes is offered by various diagnostic laboratories

samples can be used to test for selected abortogenic pathogens, including placenta, fetal tissues, and uterine swabs. Applications of molecular diagnostics in this field would include the detection of contagious pathogens for which a rapid diagnosis is relevant from a husbandry standpoint, but also pathogens that are difficult to grow or present in small numbers, often missed via conventional methods (culture and/or histology).

- *Equine herpesvirus 1* (EHV-1) can cause late-term abortions and premature delivery of foals that die soon after birth. Mares infected with EHV-1 can appear healthy and abort two weeks to several months after infection or reactivation of the virus. Abortion usually occurs in the last trimester of pregnancy without warning and the placenta is expelled together with the fetus, which has died from asphyxia or dies shortly after birth. Sporadic abortions in individual mares are most common, but EHV-1 outbreaks with high attack rates have been reported and depend on herd management, immune status, and viral factors. The ideal biological samples for molecular detection of EHV-1 are fetal tissues, uterine swabs, and placenta. Amongst fetal tissues, no definitive conclusion has been made as to the best possible biological samples. Several studies have evaluated the detection of EHV-1 in various fetal tissues and shown that lungs, spleen, thymus, and liver represent adequate sample types for the molecular detection of EHV-1. From a practical standpoint, the various tissue samples can be pooled for the detection of EHV-1. Recent work has shown an increased prevalence of neuropathogenic (D_{752}) strains of EHV-1 in equine abortions from 1951 to 2006. This is of concern, knowing that D_{752} strains of EHV-1 are overall more virulent than N_{752} strains.
- There are more than 250 serovars of *Leptospira* spp., but equine leptospirosis has been attributed primarily

to *L. interrogans* serovar Pomona type Kennewicki in North America and serovars Bratislava, Grippotyphosa, Copenhageni, Autumnalis, Hebdomadis, Arborea, and Icterohaemorrhagiae in other parts of the world. Infection of pregnant mares can result in placentitis, abortion, or still birth. Definitive diagnosis of leptospiral infections has, in the past, relied on culture, histology, fluorescence antibody test (FAT), and serology. Many of these diagnostic assays are difficult to perform in diagnostic laboratories or lack sensitivity. A recent study evaluated the diagnostic performance of qPCR, FAT, and microscopic agglutination test (MAT) on 21 confirmed leptospiral abortions. qPCR detected all 21 leptospiral abortions using fetal kidneys or placenta, while the use of FAT and MAT supported the diagnosis of leptospiral infection in 18/21 and 19/21 of the abortions, respectively.

- Fungi, especially *Candida* spp., *Aspergillus* spp., and *Mucor* spp. are important causes of endometritis and placentitis. Most fungi induce a chronic focally extensive placentitis, most often observed in the late gestational period and arising from ascending infections. Currently, the standard for detection of fungal infections is mycological culture and direct microscopic evaluation of cytologic or biopsy specimens, placenta, or fetal tissues. Microscopy often lacks specificity (inability to positively identify an organism), whereas diagnosis by mycological culture often requires a substantial period to allow the growth phase of mycotic organisms and requires considerable laboratory expertise for accurate identification. Amplification of fungal DNA by qPCR has been used in recent years to provide a rapid diagnosis of mycological infections of equids. Most of the qPCR assays diagnostically available target the conserved 28S ribosomal gene of various fungi. Fungal identification of the genus or species is determined via sequence analysis of the PCR

Table 51.6 Interpretation of common qPCR results for selected equine pathogens.

Clinical scenario	Biological sample	Pathogen tested	qPCR	Interpretation
Acute onset of fever, mucosal bleeding, icterus, limb edema	Whole blood	*A. phagocytophilum*	Positive	Confirmation of EGA
			Negative	Absence of *A. phagocytophilum*, consider quality of sample and previous use of antimicrobials
Acute onset of fever, depression, mucoid nasal discharge, occasional cough, mandibular lymphadenopathy	Nasal/nasopharyngeal swab or wash, guttural pouch lavage	EIV, EHV-1, EHV-4, ERAV, ERBV, EAV, *S. equi* subsp. *equi*	Positive	Shedding of EIV, EHV-1, EHV-4, EAV & *S. equi* subsp. *equi* consistent with etiological agent
			Negative	No shedding of selected respiratory pathogens, consider quality of sample and timing of collection
Acute onset of upper respiratory catarrh, fever and drainage of mandibular lymph node	Nasal/nasopharyngeal swab or wash, guttural pouch lavage, swab of draining abscess	*S. equi* subsp. *equi*, *S. equi* subsp. *zooepidemicus*	Positive	Any positive sample for *S. equi* subsp. *equi* is consistent with strangles, *S. equi* subsp. *zooepidemicus* in upper airway secretions to be expected, positive pus from abscess consistent with etiological pathogens for both microorganisms
			Negative	No shedding of microorganisms, consider quality of sample and timing of collection
Adult horse with chronic lower airway signs, coughing, occasional nasal discharge	Nasal/nasopharyngeal swab, tracheal wash, bronchoalveolar lavage	EHV-2, EHV-5	Positive	Expect positive results due to ubiquitous nature of EHV-2/-5 in upper airway secretions BAL positive for EHV-5 may support EMPF
			Negative	Absence of EHV-2/-5, consider quality of sample
Fever, acute onset of spinal cord deficits, urinary incontinence	Whole blood and nasal/nasopharyngeal swab	EHV-1	Positive	Laboratory confirmation of EHM
			Negative	No viremia and shedding of EHV-1, consider quality of sample and timing of collection
Progressive hind limb ataxia, asymmetrical muscle wasting	Cerebrospinal fluid	EHV-1, WNV, *S. neurona*, *N. hughesi*, *B. burgdorferi*	Positive	Intrathecal presence of any of the selected pathogens is supportive of infection
			Negative	To be expected for WNV, *S. neurona*, *N. hughesi* and *B. burgdorferi* because rarely found free or cell-bound in the CSF
Weanling foal with fever, peripheral edema, weight loss, diarrhea	Feces/fecal swab	*N. risticii*, *L. intracellularis*, *Salmonella enterica*, *C. difficile* toxin A/B, ECoV	Positive	Supportive diagnosis for *N. risticii*, *L. intracellularis* and *S. enterica*, high prevalence of *C. difficile* and ECoV to be expected in this age group
			Negative	Consider quality of sample, timing of sample collection and previous use of antimicrobials (*L. intracellularis*, *N. risticii*), add serology testing for *L. intracellularis* and whole blood PCR for *N. risticii*
Adult horse with acute onset of fever, depression, anorexia, cow-pie feces	Feces/fecal swab	*N. risticii*, *L. intracellularis*, *Salmonella enterica*, *C. difficile* toxin A/B, ECoV	Positive	Supportive diagnosis for any of the selected pathogens
			Negative	Consider quality of sample, timing of sample collection and previous use of antimicrobials (*L. intracellularis*, *N. risticii*)
Multiparous mare with abortion in last trimester of gestation	Placenta, fetal tissues	EHV-1, EAV, *Amycolatopsis* spp., *Crosiella equi*	Positive	Supportive diagnosis for any of the selected pathogens
			Negative	No evidence for involvement in disease process for any of the selected pathogens, consider quality of sample

amplicons. qPCR may prove to be clinically useful as an adjunct to microbial culture and histological examination of tissue samples for identification of fungal organisms in a timely manner and allow for early development and implementation of a treatment plan.

- *Nocardioform placentitis* is caused by various groups of filamentous, branching bacteria including *Nocardia* spp., *Amycolatopsis* spp., *Crosiella equi*, and *Cellulosimicrobium cellulans*. These pathogens induce chronic placentitis that results in late-term abortion, stillbirth, or birth of term weak foals. Due to the difficulty in culturing these pathogens, several diagnostic laboratories offer the qPCR testing for selected nocardioform actinomycetes.

The diagnosis of botulism is often based on history and clinical presentation since the laboratory detection of *C. botulinum* neurotoxin is difficult, requiring an expensive, time-consuming, and poorly sensitive mouse bioassay. To improve sensitivity, culture enrichment is recommended. The likely presence of *C. botulinum* spores in clinical samples coupled with the need for a rapid and cost-effective assay has prompted the development of qPCR assays targeting the various *C. botulinum* neurotoxins. qPCR assays targeting the various *C. botulinum* neurotoxins using culture-enriched samples (feces, gastrointestinal content, feed, wounds, and carrions) have shown greater sensitivity and specificity than the mouse bioassay.

51.9   Miscellaneous Pathogens

- *Corynebacterium pseudotuberculosis* is a common cause of external and internal abscesses in horses from arid regions of North America. The epidemiology has recently been investigated with the help of PCR and flies have been identified as mechanical vectors. *Corynebacterium pseudotuberculosis* is easy to grow on culture and the indication to use PCR is restricted to specific situations (e.g., culture-negative aspirates or body fluids).
- Botulism is a neuromuscular disease of horses and other mammals caused by neurotoxins of *Clostridium botulinum*. Amongst the eight serotypes of *C. botulinum*, only types A, B, and C have been reported in the USA, while types C and D are most common in Europe.

51.10   Interpretation of qPCR Results for Common Pathogens

See Table 51.6. The diagnostic market for qPCR testing of infectious equine pathogens will continue to grow with improved robotic extraction platforms and new generations of NA amplification assays. This technology, however, needs to be used judiciously and one must keep in mind the biology of the suspected pathogen(s) to be detected, the disease stage of the animal and the adequacy of the biological specimen to be collected. PCR results should always be interpreted within the clinical context. Table 51.6 illustrates common qPCR results for selected equine pathogens and their interpretation in association with clinical scenarios.

Further Reading

Desmettre P. 1999. Diagnosis and prevention of equine infectious diseases: present status, potential, and challenges for the future. Adv Vet Med, 41: 359–377.

Frederick J, Giguère S, and Sanchez LC. 2009. Infectious agents detected in the feces of diarrheic foals: a retrospective study of 233 cases (2003–2008). J Vet Intern Med 23, 1254–1260.

Holland PM, Abramson RD, Watson R, et al. 1991. Detection of specific polymerase chain reaction product by utilizing the 5'-3' exonuclease activity of *Thermus aquaticus* DNA polymerase. Proc Natl Acad Sci USA 88, 7276–7280.

Mehdizadeh Gohari I, Parreira VR, Nowell VJ, et al. 2015. A novel pore-forming toxin in type A Clostridium perfringens is associated with both fatal canine hemorrhagic gastroenteritis and fatal foal necrotizing enterocolitis. PLoS One 10, e0122684.

Powell DG. 2000. The significance of surveillance and reporting on the prevention and control of equine diseases. Vet Clin North Am Equine Pract, 16: 389–403.

Pusterla N, Madigan JE, and Leutenegger CM. 2006. Real-time polymerase chain reaction: a novel molecular diagnostic tool for equine infectious diseases. J Vet Intern Med, 20: 3–12.

Wilhelm J and Pingoud A. 2003. Real-time polymerase chain reaction. Chembiochem, 7(4): 1120–1128.

Wolk D, Mitchell S, and Patel R. 2001. Principles of molecular microbiology testing methods. Infect Dis Clin North Am, 15: 1157–1204.

52

Equine Genetic Testing

Carrie J. Finno

Department of Population Health and Reproduction, School of Veterinary Medicine, University of California, California, USA

52.1 Introduction

Genetic testing typically involves the analysis of an animal's DNA to determine the individual's genotype for an inherited disorder or trait. Genetic testing may be used for permanent individual identification and parentage determination; many breed registries now require such verification to ensure the accuracy of their pedigrees. Genetic testing is also used to test for specific diseases or traits. In order to interpret genetic testing results for future breeding, an understanding of the mode of inheritance is required. At this time, many of the genetic tests available for horses are for an autosomal recessive disorder to determine if an animal is a carrier. Carriers are phenotypically normal but have the potential to produced diseased progeny. Dominant disorders also exist in the horse and genetic tests may be used to definitively diagnose affected horses (Table 52.1).

Horses have 31 pairs of autosomes, or non-sex chromosomes. Genetic mutations associated with diseases or traits can occur anywhere along the 31 autosomes, X or Y chromosomes. Mutations are often classified by their effect and can be due to point mutations, insertions, deletions, or chromosomal rearrangements. A point mutation can change an amino acid (*missense* mutation), shorten the amino acid chain (*nonsense* mutation) or alter expression or proper splicing. For example, a *missense* mutation has been shown to cause Type 1 polysaccharide storage myopathy (McCue et al., 2008). Insertions or deletions cause mutations by altering the translational frame, which ultimately causes protein truncation. In the horse, a 5-bp deletion in the DNA-protein kinase catalytic subunit gene (*DNA-PKcs*) leads to severe combined immunodeficiency of Arabian foals (Shin et al., 1997).

Initial genetic mutations in the horse were discovered through the use of comparative genomics. Genes involved in a specific disease were targeted because of equivalent disease in other species, namely humans. In the horse, the mutations for hyperkalemic periodic paralysis (HYPP) (Rudolph et al., 1992) and severe combined immunodeficiency (SCID) (Shin et al., 1997), were uncovered by evaluating candidate genes that had been associated with similar diseases in humans. Following the sequencing and annotation of whole genome maps, other disease were discovered through whole genome linkage mapping (hereditary regional dermal asthenia [HERDA]: Tryon et al., 2007), genome-wide association studies using both microsatellites (Type I polysaccharide storage myopathy [PSSM]: McCue et al., 2008) and single nucleotide polymorphisms (SNPs) (Lavender Foal syndrome: Brooks et al., 2010). The majority of genetic tests currently available are for diseases or traits that are inherited as autosomal recessive traits. This chapter focuses on the genetic diseases in the horse for which a mutation is currently known. Genetic tests for performance traits (gaitedness, best racing distance, etc.) will not be discussed in this chapter and readers are directed to a recent review for more information (Finno and Bannasch, 2014).

52.2 Hyperkalemic Periodic Paralysis (HYPP)

Breeds Affected
- Quarter horse (QH)
- American Paint Horse
- Appaloosa
- QH-cross

Mode of Inheritanc
- Autosomal semi-dominant

Clinical Signs
- May be asymptomatic
- Episodic weakness and paralysis; typically last between 15–60 min and horses may appear completely normal between episodes (Naylor, 1994, Spier et al., 1990, Rudolph et al., 1992)

Interpretation of Equine Laboratory Diagnostics, First Edition. Edited by Nicola Pusterla and Jill Higgins.

Table 52.1 Definitions of genetic terms.

Definitions of Genetic Terms	
Allele	One of the alternative forms of a gene or genetic locus
Base pairs	A DNA nucleotide is made of a molecule of sugar, a molecule of phosphoric acid and a molecule called a "base." The bases are the "letters" that spell out the genetic code. In DNA, the code letters are A (adenine), T (thymine), G (guanine), and C (cytosine)
Coding DNA (exons)	A sequence of a gene's DNA that transcribes into protein structures
Congenital	Conditions present at birth that may or may not be inherited. Some congenital conditions have a genetic origin while others may be due to metabolic derangements or toxic insults
Deletion	Loss of one or more nucleotide bases in a DNA sequence
Genotype	Genetic makeup, either at a single locus or at all loci
Genome-wide association study	A study that uses genome-wide markers, typically microsatellites or single nucleotide polymorphisms (SNPs) to determine an association between a phenotype and a region of a particular chromosome
Insertion	Addition of one or more nucleotide bases into a DNA sequence
Linked	Association of genes and markers that lie near each other on a chromosome; linked genes and markers tend to be inherited together
Locus	Place on a chromosome where a specific gene, DNA sequence or marker is located
Marker	Segment of DNA with a known location on a chromosome, the inheritance of which can be followed. A marker can be a gene or some section of DNA with no known function.
Microsatellite	Repetitive stretches of short sequences of DNA used as genetic markers to track inheritance within families
Point Mutation	Simple change in one base of the gene sequence
Non-coding DNA	Sequences of an organism's DNA that do not encode protein sequences. Some noncoding DNA is transcribed into functional non-coding RNA molecules
Phenotype	Observable traits or characteristics of an animal (e.g., coat color, weight, presence or absence of a disease)
Recombination	Genetic transmission process by which the combinations of alleles observed at different loci between two parental individuals become shuffled in offspring
Single nucleotide polymorphism (SNP)	Differences in single base pair of DNA (A,C,T,G) often used as genetic markers for linkage and association studies

- Muscle fasciculation and sweating in flanks, necks and shoulders
- During severe attacks, horses may dog-sit or become recumbent
- Homozygous horses may demonstrate respiratory stridor, dysphagia, or respiratory distress (Carr et al., 1996)

Genetic Etiology

- Missense mutation in the voltage-dependent skeletal muscle sodium channel alpha-subunit (*SCN4A*) (Rudolph et al., 1992)
- Mutation results in failure of a subpopulation of sodium channels to inactivate when serum potassium concentrations are increased. The excessive influx of sodium and efflux potassium results in persistent depolarization of muscle cells followed by temporary weakness.

Treatment

- Feeding grain or corn syrup to stimulate insulin-mediated movement of potassium across cell membranes may be of benefit.
- Acetazolamide (3 mg/kg every 8–12 h orally)

- Severe cases: calcium gluconate, IV dextrose, or sodium bicarbonate may be used
- With severe dyspenea, a tracheostomy may be required
- Prevent with regular exercise and frequent turnout
- Feed a balanced diet containing between 0.6 and 1.5% total potassium concentrations and meals containing <33 g of potassium (Reynolds et al., 1998)

Breeding

- Breeding a heterozygous affected horse (N/H) to a normal horse (N/N) results in a 50% chance of producing heterozygous affected (N/H) foal
- Breeding a homozygous affected horse (H/H) to a normal horse (N/N) results in a 100% chance of producing a heterozygous affected horse (N/H)

Breed Registry Regulations

- American Quarter Horse Association (AQHA)
  - Foals tracing to Impressive born in 1998 and later have a statement placed on their Certificate of Registration: "This horse has an ancestor known to carry HYPP, designated under AQHA rules as a

genetic defect, AQHA recommends testing to confirm presence or absence of this gene."
- Effective January 1, 2007, any foal testing homozygous positive for HYPP (H/H) is not eligible for registration with the AQHA.
- The American Paint Horse Association recommends testing for HYPP; however, it is not mandatory at this time.

52.3 Severe Combined Immunodeficiency (SCID)

Breeds Affected
- Arabian horses

Mode of Inheritance
- Autosomal recessive

Clinical Signs
- Normal at birth
- Develop infections by 6–10 weeks post-partum when colostral antibodies decline (McGuire et al., 1974, Perryman et al., 1978)
  - Adenovirus
  - *Pneumocystis carinii*
  - Secondary bacterial infections
  - Intermittent diarrhea
  - Other conditions include hepatic necrosis, ulcerative enteritis, focal myocardial necrosis, peritonitis, pleuritic and pericarditis (Perryman et al., 1978)

Genetic Etiology
- 5-bp deletion resulting in a frameshift mutation and a 967 amino acid deletion in DNA-protein kinase catalytic subunit (*DNA-PKcs*) (Shin et al., 1997)
- The mutation results in the ability to recombine particular gene segments in order to form coding sequences of immunoglobulin and T-cell antigen receptor variable regions (i.e., V(D)J recombination). SCID-affected foals lack both B and T lymphocytes

Treatment
- None; SCID-affected foals typically die by 5 months of age

Breeding
- Breeding a SCID-carrier to another SCID-carrier results in a 25% chance of producing a SCID-affected foal and a 50% chance of producing another carrier
- Breeding a carrier to a normal horse results in 50% chance of producing a SCID-carrier

Breed Registry Regulations
- The Arabian Horse Association requires disclosure of a horse's SCID status. According to their policy, "The AHA Code of Ethics requires members to disclose SCID, CA, LFS and HYPP status, if known, for any horse capable of reproducing that is being offered for breeding, sale, or lease. In addition, an owner of a mare that produces

affected SCID, LFS, CA, or HYPP offspring should immediately notify the stallion owner."

52.4 Ileocolonic Aganglionosis (Lethal White Foal Syndrome)

Breeds Affected
- American Paint Horse
- QH
- Thoroughbred (rare)
- Miniature Horse

Mode of Inheritance
- Autosomal semi-dominant; one copy of the mutation may result in a frame overo, highly white calico overo, and frame blend overo (Santschi et al., 2001) or solid coat color (Metallinos et al., 1998) while two copies of the mutation lead to the ileocolonic aganglionosis phenotype.

Clinical Signs
- All white or nearly all-white coat
- Colic with associated abdominal distension and failure to pass feces shortly after birth

Genetic Etiology
- Missense mutation in the endothelin receptor B gene (*EDNRB*) (Metallinos et al., 1998, Santschi et al., 1998)
- The mutation results in abnormal development of enteric ganglia and melanocytes within the neural crest

Treatment
- None

Breeding
- Breeding a heterozygote (N/O) to another heterozygote (N/O) results in a 25% chance of producing a foal affected with ileocolonic aganglionosis (O/O) and a 50% chance of producing another heterozygote (N/O)
- Breeding a heterozygote (N/O) to a normal horse (N/N) results in 50% chance of producing a heterozygote (N/O)

Breed Registry Regulations
- The American Paint Horse Association recommends testing for Lethal White Foal Syndrome; however, it is not mandatory at this time.

52.5 Junctional Epidermolysis Bullosa (JEB)

Breeds Affected
- Belgian draft
- European draft breeds: Breton, Comtois, Vlaams Paard, Italian draft
- American Saddlebred horses

Mode of Inheritance
- Autosomal recessive

Clinical Signs

- Irregular erosions and ulcerations develop in the skin and mouth over pressure points or after mild trauma (Shapiro and McEewen, 1995)
- Erosions may be present at mucocutaneous junctions of mouth, rectum, vulva, and along the coronary bands
- Granulation tissue along the coronary bands may result in sloughing of the hooves (Kohn et al., 1989)
- Dystrophic teeth and corneal ulcers (Shapiro and McEewen, 1995)

Genetic Etiology
- Belgian and European draft breeds
  - 1-bp insertion leading to a premature stop codon in the laminin γ2 subunit chain gene (*LAMC2*) (Spirito et al., 2002)
- American Saddlebred
  - 6589-bp deletion in the laminin α3 subunit chain (*LAMA3*) (Graves et al., 2009)
- These two genes (*LAMC2* and *LAMA3*), along with *LAMB3*, encode the polypeptide subunits that comprise the laminin 5 molecule. Laminin 5 is secreted by keratinocytes and is involved in cell adhesion, particularly at the dermal-epidermal junction (Rousselle et al., 1997). Mutations in these two subunits lead to ineffectual laminin 5.

Treatment
- None

Breeding
- Breeding a JEB-carrier (N/J) to another JEB-carrier (N/J) results in a 25% chance of producing a foal affected with JEB (J/J) and a 50% chance of producing another carrier (N/J).
- Breeding a carrier (N/J) to a normal horse (N/N) results in 50% chance of producing a carrier (N/J).

Breed Registry Regulations
- Belgian Draft Horse Corporation of America: JEB testing is mandatory for new breeding stallions upon DNA-typing for registration of his offspring. All mares are strictly a voluntary program. All results are placed on the registration certificate.
- American Saddlebred Association: DNA testing is mandatory for verification of parentage but there are no mandatory requirements for JEB-testing within this association at the time of writing.

52.6 Glycogen Branching Enzyme Deficiency (GBED)

Breeds Affected
- Quarter Horse (QH)
- American Paint Horse
- QH-related breeds

Mode of Inheritance
- Autosomal recessive

Clinical Signs (Valberg et al., 2001, Wagner et al., 2006)
- Stillbirth
- Transient flexural limb deformities
- Seizures
- Respiratory or cardiac failure

Genetic Etiology
- Nonsense mutation in the glycogen branching enzyme gene (*GBE1*) (Ward et al., 2004)
- Mutation results in the inability to create a branched structure of glycogen. As a result, cardiac and skeletal muscle, liver and brain cannot store or mobilize glycogen to maintain normal glucose homeostasis.

Treatment
- None

Breeding
- Breeding a GBED-carrier (G/g) to another GBED-carrier (G/g) results in a 25% chance of producing a foal affected with GBED (g/g) and a 50% chance of producing another carrier (G/g).
- Breeding a carrier (G/g) to a normal horse (G/G) results in 50% chance of producing a carrier (G/g).

Breed Registry Regulations
- AQHA, APHA: Genetic testing for GBED is recommended but not mandatory at this time.

52.7 Malignant Hyperthermia (MH)

Breeds Affected
- Quarter Horse

Mode of Inheritance
- Autosomal dominant

Clinical Signs (Aleman et al., 2005)
- Episodes initiated by exposure to halogenated anesthetics or upon stress/excitement
- Lactic acidosis, hyperthermia, muscle rigidity
- May lead to death

Genetic Etiology
- Missense mutation in the ryanodine receptor type 1 gene (*RYR1*) (Aleman et al., 2004)
- Mutation results in excessive release of calcium into the myoplasm and a hypermetabolic state

Treatment
- To prevent an episode: pre-treatment with dantrolene (4 mg/kg) 30–60 min prior to anesthesia (Valverde et al., 1990)
- During an episode: address hyperthermia and acidemia with alcohol, chilled intravenous fluids with sodium bicarbonate and mechanical ventilation

Breeding
- Breeding a heterozygous affected horse (N/MH) to a normal horse (N/MH) results in a 50% chance of producing heterozygous (N/MH) affected foal.

- To the author's knowledge, there have been no reported cases of horses homozygous (MH/MH) for the MH mutation (Dr. Monica Aleman, personal communication 2015).

Breed Registry Regulations
- AQHA: Genetic testing for MH is recommended but not mandatory at this time.

52.8 Hereditary Equine Regional Dermal Asthenia (HERDA)

Breeds Affected
- Quarter Horse (QH)
- QH-related breeds

Mode of Inheritance
- Autosomal recessive

Clinical Signs (White et al., 2007)
- Typically not evident until about 1.5 years of age (often associated with initial saddling or trauma)
- Seroma, hematoma, open wound or sloughing skin apparent
- Loose, easily tented skin primarily along the dorsum

Genetic Etiology
- Missense mutation in the cyclophilin B gene (*PPIB*) (Tryon et al., 2007)
- Mutation is hypothesized to effect protein folding of collagens

Treatment
- Maintain horses indoors and away from other horses to prevent development of progression of lesions
- No effective therapy

Breeding
- Breeding a HERDA-carrier (N/HRD) to another HERDA-carrier (N/HRD) results in a 25% chance of producing a foal affected with HERDA (HRD/HRD) and a 50% chance of producing another carrier (N/HRD).
- Breeding a carrier (N/HRD) to a normal horse (N/N) results in 50% chance of producing a carrier (N/HRD).

Breed Registry Regulations
- AQHA: Genetic testing for HERDA is recommended but not mandatory at this time.

52.9 Glanzmann Thrombasthenia (GT)

Breeds Affected
- Multiple

Mode of Inheritance
- Autosomal recessive

Clinical Signs
- Epistaxis and prolonged bleeding
- Coagulopathy characterized by

- Normal thrombocyte count
- Normal concentration of von Willebrand factor antigen
- Prolonged cutaneous bleeding time
- Abnormal clot retraction test
- Failure of platelet aggregation in response to agonists

Genetic Etiology
- Two identified mutations in platelet glycoprotein IIb of IIb/IIIa complex (*ITGA2B*)
  - Missense mutation in exon 2 (Christopherson et al., 2006)
  - 10-bp deletion spanning exon 11 and intron 11, resulting in the potential lack of splicing of intron 11 and nonsense-mediated decay of mRNA from this gene (Christopherson et al., 2007)

Treatment
- Cauterization of bleeding sites
- Anti-fibrinolytic drugs if needed

Breeding
- Breeding a GT-carrier to another GT-carrier results in a 25% chance of producing a foal affected with GT and a 50% chance of producing another carrier.
- Breeding a carrier to a normal horse results in 50% chance of producing a carrier.
- Compound heterozygote cases can occur (two heterogeneous recessive alleles at the *ITGA2B* locus that can cause disease in a heterozygous state; i.e., one allele has the exon 2 missense mutation + and the second allele has the 10 bp deletion) (Christopherson et al., 2007)

Breed Registry Regulations
- Genetic testing for GT is not mandatory for any breed association at this time.

52.10 Type 1 Polysaccharide Storage Myopathy (Type 1 PSSM)

Breeds Affected
- Quarter Horse
- American Paint Horses
- Appaloosas
- Draft breeds
- Ricky Mountain Horse
- Tennessee Walking Horse
- Morgan
- Haflinger

Mode of Inheritance
- Autosomal dominant

Clinical Signs
- May be asymptomatic
- Signs of exertional rhabdomyolysis (Firshman et al., 2003)

- Typically following <20 min of exercise at a walk and trot, particularly if the horse has rested for several days before exercise
- Muscle pain
- Stiffness and sweating
- Exercise intolerance and reluctance to move
- Muscle fasciculation and gait abnormalities (draft breeds)

Genetic Etiology
- Missense mutation in the glycogen synthase 1 gene (*GYS1*) (McCue et al., 2008)
- Mutation results in unregulated glyocogen synthesis and potentially impaired aerobic glycogen metabolism

Treatment
- Acute episodes: stall confinement may be indicated for <48 h
- Address hydration status and provide sedatives and anti-inflammatories to well-hydrated horses to relieve anxiety and pain
- Prevention of future episodes: gradual to exercise using incremental training along with dietary management aimed at providing adequate, but not excessive calories, by decreasing glucose load (dietary starch <10% daily digestible energy) and providing fat as an alternate energy source (up to 13% of daily digestible energy) (Ribeiro et al., 2004)

Breeding
- Breeding a heterozygous affected horse (P/N) to a normal horse (N/N) results in a 50% chance of producing heterozygous affected (P/N) foal.
- Breeding a homozygous affected horse (P/P) to a normal horse (N/N) results in a 100% chance of producing a heterozygous affected horse (P/N).

Breed Registry Regulations
- AQHA and APHA: Genetic testing for Type 1 PSSM is recommended but not mandatory at this time.

52.11 Lavender Foal Syndrome (LFS) or Coat Color Dilution Lethal

Breeds Affected
- Arabians

Mode of Inheritance
- Autosomal recessive

Clinical Signs (Page et al., 2006)
- Dilute silver or lavender hair coat
- Tetanic episodes from birth including opisthotonos, extensor rigidity, and paddling

Genetic Etiology
- 1-bp deletion in myosin 5a (*MYO5A*), leading to a frameshift mutation and premature stop codon (Brooks et al., 2010)
- Based on comparative data, it is hypothesized that the mutation leads to abnormal trafficking of melanosomes to the periphery of the cell in addition to abnormal trafficking of dendritic cargo in neurons.

Treatment
- None

Breeding
- Breeding a carrier (N/LFS) to another carrier (N/LFS) results in a 25% chance of producing an affected foal (LFS/LFS) and a 50% chance of producing another carrier (N/LFS).
- Breeding a carrier (N/LFS) to a normal horse (N/N) results in 50% chance of producing a carrier (N/LFS).

Breed Registry Regulations
- The Arabian Horse Association requires disclosure of a horses' SCID status. According to their policy, "The AHA Code of Ethics requires members to disclose SCID, CA, LFS, and HYPP status, if known, for any horse capable of reproducing that is being offered for breeding, sale, or lease. In addition, an owner of a mare that produces affected SCID, LFS, CA, or HYPP offspring should immediately notify the stallion owner."

52.12 Cerebellar Abiotrophy (CA)

Breeds Affected
- Primarily Arabians
- Carriers identified in Bashkir Curly Horses, Trakehners, and Welsh ponies (most likely due to Arabian ancestry) (Brault and Penedo, 2011)

Mode of Inheritance
- Autosomal recessive

Clinical Signs (DeBowes et al., 1987)
- Cerebellar ataxia (dysmetria, spasticity, wide-based stance, intention tremors, and a lack of menace response) with an age of onset around 2.5–6 months of age

Genetic Etiology (Brault et al., 2011)
- Missense mutation in *Target of EGR1* (*TOE1*)
- This mutation, although residing in *TOE1*, resides approximately 1200 base pairs upstream of *MUTYH*, a gene that encodes a DNA glycosylase involved in oxidative DNA damage repair. It is hypothesized that

the SNP may either have an effect on *TOE1* or a regulatory effect on *MUTYH* by affecting the binding affinity of the transcription factor *GATA2*

Treatment
- None

Breeding
- Breeding a carrier (N/CA) to another carrier (N/CA) results in a 25% chance of producing an affected foal (CA/CA) and a 50% chance of producing another carrier (N/CA).
- Breeding a carrier (N/CA) to a normal horse (N/N) results in 50% chance of producing a carrier (N/CA).

Breed Registry Regulations
- The Arabian Horse Association requires disclosure of a horses' SCID status. According to their policy, "The AHA Code of Ethics requires members to disclose SCID, CA, LFS and HYPP status, if known, for any horse capable of reproducing that is being offered for breeding, sale, or lease. In addition, an owner of a mare that produces affected SCID, LFS, CA or HYPP offspring should immediately notify the stallion owner."

52.13   Foal Immunodeficiency Syndrome (Immunodeficiency of Fell Ponies)

Breeds Affected
- Fell and Dales ponies

Mode of Inheritance
- Autosomal recessive

Clinical Signs (Scholes et al., 1998)
- 2–4 weeks age of onset
- Weakness, dyspnea, poor growth, diarrhea
- Anemia
- Immunodeficiency (depleted B lymphocytes and low immunoglobulin concentrations) (Thomas et al., 2005)
- Peripheral ganglionopathy

Genetic Etiology (Fox-Clipsham et al., 2011)
- Missense mutation in the sodium/myo-inositol cotransporter gene (*SLC5A3*)
- It is hypothesized that this mutation alters the function of *SCL5A3*, leading to erythropoiesis failure and compromise of the immune system.

Treatment
- None

Breeding
- Breeding a carrier (n/FIS) to another carrier (n/FIS) results in a 25% chance of producing a foal affected with foal immunodeficiency syndrome (FIS/FIS) and a 50% chance of producing another carrier (n/FIS).
- Breeding a carrier (n/FIS) to a normal pony (n/n) results in 50% chance of producing a carrier (n/FIS).

Breed Registry Regulations
- Currently, there are no mandatory testing requirements within the Fell pony society.

52.14   Congenital Myotonia

Breeds Affected
- New Forest pony

Mode of Inheritance
- Autosomal recessive

Clinical Signs
- Typically well-muscled due to bilateral dimpling of the thigh and rump muscles
- Recurrent episodes of muscle stiffness and weakness
- Hyperreactive when stimulated; third eyelid protrusion may occur
- Severe muscle rigidity resulting in decreased flexion of distal limbs

Genetic Etiology
- Missense mutation in the chloride channel, voltage sensitive 1 gene (*CLCN1*) (Wijnberg et al., 2012)
- A missense mutation in *CLCN1* also cause the severe acute muscle stiffness demonstrated in "fainting" goats (Beck et al., 1996)

Treatment
- In humans and dogs, quinidine, procainamide and phenytoin are used
- Efficacy of these drugs is currently unknown in equine congenital myotonia

Breeding
- Breeding a carrier to another carrier results in a 25% chance of producing a foal affected with congenital myoptonia and a 50% chance of producing another carrier
- Breeding a carrier to a normal pony results in 50% chance of producing a carrier

Breed Registry Regulations
- Currently, there are no mandatory testing requirements within the New Forest pony Association and Registry

52.15 Multiple Ocular Defects (Anterior Segment Dysgenesis or Congenital Aniridia)

Breeds Affected
- American Miniature Horse
- Icelandic
- Rocky Mountain Horse
- Kentucky Mountain Saddle Horse
- Shetland ponies
- Morgans

Mode of Inheritance
- Autosomal semi-dominant

Clinical Signs
- Silver coat color
- Wide range of eye anomalies (Andersson et al., 2013)
  - Uveal cysts
  - Cornea globose
  - Iris stromal hypoplasia
  - Abnormal pectinate ligaments
  - Cataracts
  - Iris hypoplasia
  - Heterozygotes may have the less severe cyst phenotype with cysts originating from the temporal ciliary body, iris, or retina

Genetic Etiology (Andersson et al., 2013)
- Missense mutation in the melanocyte protein 17 precursor gene, *PMEL17*
- Causes both the silver coat color and the multiple ocular defect syndrome

Treatment
- Treatment is specific to anomalies present

Breeding
- Breeding a heterozygous affected horse (N/Z) to a normal horse (N/N) results in a 50% chance of producing heterozygous affected foal (N/Z).
- Breeding a homozygous affected horse (Z/Z) to a normal horse (N/N) results in a 100% chance of producing a heterozygous affected horse (N/Z).

Breed Registry Regulations
- Currently, there are no mandatory testing requirements within the Rocky Mountain Horse Association

52.16 Congenital Stationary Night Blindness (CSNB)

Breeds Affected
- Multiple; occurs in homozygotes for the incompletely dominant allele that confers Leopard complex spotting

Mode of Inheritance
- Autosomal semi-dominant; one copy of the mutation results in leopard complex spotting while two copies of the mutation lead to the CSNB phenotype

Clinical Signs
- Non-progressive impaired vision in dark conditions
- Electroretinogram abnormalities include an absent b-wave and increased amplitude of the a-wave (Witzel et al., 1978)

Genetic Etiology (Bellone et al., 2013)
- Retroviral insertion in the transient receptor potential cation channel, subfamily M, member 1 (*TRPM1*)
- Insertion leads to premature poly-adenylation, leading to decreased *TRPM1* expression 3' of the insertion

Treatment
- Detect CSNB-affected horses and advise owners to use caution when handling or riding in dark conditions.

Breeding
- Breeding a heterozygote (LP/lp) to another heterozygote (LP/lp) results in a 25% chance of producing a foal that may become affected with CSNB (LP/LP) and a 50% chance of producing another carrier (LP/lp).
- Breeding a heterozygote (LP/lp) to a normal horse (lp/lp) results in 50% chance of producing a heterozygote (LP/lp).

Breed Registry Regulations
- Currently, there are no mandatory testing requirements for CSNB within the Appaloosa Horse Club

52.17 Incontinentia Pigmenti

Breeds Affected
- Breed was not reported in the single publication

Mode of Inheritance
- X-linked dominant

Clinical Signs (Towers et al., 2013)
- Pruritic, exudative skin lesions that develop soon after birth and progress to areas of alopecia
- Streaks of darker and lighter coat coloration that followed the lines of Blaschko
- Defects in tooth, hoof, and ocular development reported

Genetic Etiology (Towers et al., 2013)
- Nonsense mutation in Inhibitor of *Kappa Light Polypeptide Gene Enhancer in B cells, Kinase (IKBKG)*

- Leads to truncation of more than 85% of IKBKG protein

Treatment
- None

Breeding
- In the one reported family, all affected animals were females descended from one affected founded mare
- Males die *in utero*

Breed Registry Regulations
- None at this time

52.18 Dwarfism

Breeds Affected
- American Miniature Horse

Mode of Inheritance
- Autosomal recessive

Clinical Signs (Eberth, 2013)
- Disproportionate dwarfism characterized by several of the following:
  - Severely shortened stature
  - Shortened limbs relative to overall body size
  - Bowed forelegs
  - Shortened neck
  - Disproportionally large cranium
  - Flat faces with prominent eyes, low nasal bridge, severe underbite
  - Cleft palate
  - Large abdominal hernia

Genetic Etiology (Eberth, 2013)
- Four variants in *aggrecan (ACAN)*; labeled as D1 through D4
  - 1-bp deletion in exon 2, leading to a frameshift mutation and premature stop codon (D1)
    - Associated with fetal lethality
  - Missense mutation in exon 6 (D2)
  - 1-bp deletion in exon 11, leading to a frameshift mutation and premature stop codon (D3)
  - 21-bp deletion in exon 15 (D4)

Treatment
- None

Breeding (Eberth, 2013)
- Genetic testing for all variants (D1 through D4) is recommended
- Breeding of a carrier (N/D*, where * represents variants 1–4) to another carrier (N/D*) will result in a 25% chance of an affected foal (D*/D*) and a 50% chance of a carrier (N/D*)
- The dwarf phenotype has been reported with the following genotypes:
  - D2/D2
  - D2/D3

- D2/D4
- D3/D4
- A lethal (aborted or resorbed phenotype) is reported with the following genotypes:
  - D1/D1
  - D1/D2
  - D1/D3
  - D1/D4

Breed Registry Regulations
- None at this time

52.19 Disorders of Sexual Development

52.19.1 Androgen Insensitivity Syndrome (AIS)

Breeds Affected
- Multiple; the mutation was identified in the Quarter Horse

Mode of Inheritance
- X-linked recessive

Clinical Signs
- Affected individuals are XY with undescended testicles and female secondary sex characteristics, including female external genitalia

Genetic Etiology (Revay et al., 2012)
- Missense mutation (GTG mutation in the start codon) of the *androgen receptor (AR)*
- Leads to a reduced amount of functional androgen receptor expressed during critical periods of development in the XY male embryo

Treatment
- None

Breeding
- Breeding of a carrier mare to a normal stallion results in a 25% chance of producing an carrier female, a 25% chance of producing a normal female, a 25% chance of producing an affected male and a 25% chance of producing a normal male

Breed Registry Regulations
- None at this time

52.19.2 Ovotesticular Disorder of Sexual Development (Sex Reversal: XY Female)

Breeds Affected
- Multiple

Mode of Inheritance
- Y-linked

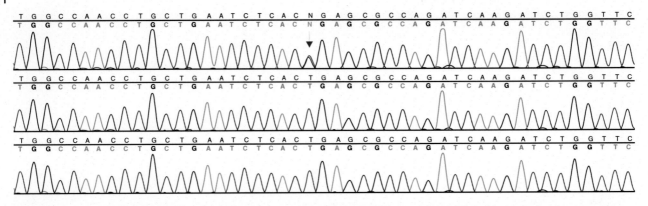

Figure 52.1 Sequencing chromatogram generated from an automated Sanger DNA sequencer of three horses. Each color represents a nucleotide. The pink arrow points to a single nucleotide variant where the first horse (top panel with arrow) is heterozygous (T/C) while the second (middle panel) and third (bottom panel) horses are homozygous T/T. The letter "N" may appear over these sites to denote that the sequencer was unable to determine only one base pair at this location.

Clinical Signs
- Small uterus and ovaries
- Male-like behavior

Genetic Etiology (Pailhoux et al., 1995, Raudsepp et al., 2010)
- DNA-binding domain of the sex determining region of Y gene, *SRY*, is deleted from the Y chromosome in the XY mare

Treatment
- None

Breeding
- Affected XY-individuals obtained the defective Y chromosome from their sire

Breed Registry Regulations
- None at this time

52.20 DNA Testing through Licensed Laboratories

DNA can be prepared from any type of tissue, hair follicle or heparinized blood sample. When performing DNA testing for a known mutation, only a small amount of DNA is required. Therefore, DNA testing is currently performed on hair follicles (20 mane or tail hairs with roots intact). The hair bulbs are the source of the DNA so hair that has been cut cannot be used for testing. Alternatively, 3–7 mL of blood collected in a purple top EDTA tube can be used to extract DNA from the buffy coat cell layer.

The basis for DNA testing is PCR. Primers can be designed specifically to amplify either the disease-causing allele or the normal allele. Alternatively, the PCR product can be digested with a restriction enzyme that cleaves the DNA at a particular sequence of bases. A restriction enzyme is chosen that shows a different cleavage pattern between the mutant and the normal version of the PCR product. Direct sequencing of a section of DNA can also be used to determine the animal's genotype (Figure 52.1). Many different methods are available to assay changes in DNA that lead to disease. Each company that offers a test may choose a different type of assay for the same mutation. Additionally, there are limits to all genetic testing. In mutation tests for the diseases described previously, the specific mutation being assayed is the only factor being evaluated. An animal may have a different mutation in that gene or a mutation in a different gene that causes the same phenotype (phenocopy). It is therefore correct to state that an animal has been "DNA tested negative" for this specific mutation rather than "DNA tested clear" of the disease.

It is important to realize that no association or committee evaluates quality control of DNA tests that are available in animals. Most tests are published in the scientific literature not as tests, but as articles describing the discovery of the mutation. Because some cases involve patent issues, some tests are offered before publication. Much of the research done to identify the mutations involved in the tests is performed at universities and funded by granting agencies that have both financial and intellectual interest in patenting the tests. Companies then license the rights to offer the tests. A list of *licensed* testing labs in the United States is included in Table 52.2. Veterinarians should contact the laboratories to inquire about available genetic tests for large animal species because laboratories are licensed to only run particular tests. The author strongly recommends against having genetic testing performed at laboratories that do not hold testing licenses. *For the 5-panel AQHA test, only UC Davis Veterinary Genetics Laboratory is licensed to perform this testing for the purposes of registration in any animal after October 1, 2013.* This testing standard has been established in order to ensure that testing procedures are consistent and performed within licensed laboratories.

Table 52.2 US laboratories offering *licensed* genetic testing for horses.

Testing facility	Licensed genetic tests offered as of January 1, 2015
Animal Genetic Testing and Research Laboratory Department of Veterinary Science Gluck Equine Research Center University of Kentucky Lexington, KY 40546 (859) 218-1212 www.ca.uky.edu/gluck	Saddlebred JEB LWFS Congenital myotonia ACAN Dwarfism in Miniature Horses
Animal Health Diagnostic Center Cornell University College of Veterinary Medicine P.O. Box 5786 Ithaca, NY 14852-5786 (607) 253-3935 http://ahdc.vet.cornell.edu/test/	LFS
Maxxam Analytics 335 Laird Road, Unit 2 Guelph, Ontario N1H 6J3 Canada (519) 836-2400 http://maxxam.ca/services/dna-testing/animal-dna-testing/animal-dna-diagnostic-testing	HYPP LWFS
Progressive Molecular Diagnostics 6455 US Highway 377 Tioga, TX 76271 (888)-837-8362 www.progressivemoleculardiagnostics.com/~shop/main.html	GBED HERDA HYPP LWFS MH PSSM1
Veterinary Diagnostic Laboratory University of Minnesota 1333 Gortner Avenue St. Paul, MN 55108-1098 (612) 625-8787 www.vdl.umn.edu/	MH PSSM1
Veterinary Genetics Laboratory University of California, Davis PO Box 1102 Davis, CA 95617-1102 (530) 752-2211 www.vgl.ucdavis.edu/	CA LFS Silver coat color (multiple ocular anomalies) GBED HERDA HYPP Leopard complex mutation (CSNB) AQHA 5 panel test: GBED, HERDA, HYPP, MH, PSSM1 2-panel test (Arabians): CA and LFS
VetGen 3728 Plaza Drive, Suite 1 Ann Arbor, Michigan, 48108 USA (734) 669-8440 www.vetgen.com	GBED SCID LFS CA 3-panel test (Arabian) SCID, LFS, CA

CA = cerebellar abiotrophy, CSNB = congenital stationary night blindness, GBED = glycogen branching enzyme deficiency, JEB = junctional epidermolysis bullosa, LFS = lavender foal syndrome, LWFS = lethal white foal syndrome, HERDA = hereditary equine regional dermal asthenia, HYPP = hyperkalemic periodic paralysis, MH = malignant hyperthermia, PSSM1 = polysaccharide storage myopathy, type 1, SCID = severe combined immunodeficiency

References

Aleman M, Brosnan RJ, Williams DC, Lecouteur RA, Imai A, Tharp BR, and Steffey EP. 2005. Malignant hyperthermia in a horse anesthetized with halothane. J Vet Intern Med, 19: 363–366.

Aleman M, Riehl J, Aldridge BM, Lecouteur RA, Stott JL, and Pessah IN. 2004. Association of a mutation in the ryanodine receptor 1 gene with equine malignant hyperthermia. Muscle Nerve, 30: 356–365.

Andersson LS, Wilbe M, Viluma A, Cothran G, Eksesten B, Ewart S, and Lindgren G. 2013. Equine multiple congenital ocular anomalies and silver coat colour result from the pleiotropic effects of mutant PMEL. PLoS One, 8: e75639.

Beck CL, Fahlke C, and George AL, Jr. 1996. Molecular basis for decreased muscle chloride conductance in the myotonic goat. Proc Natl Acad Sci U S A, 93: 11248–11252.

Bellon RR, Holl H, Setaluri V, Devi S, Maddodi N, Archer S, et al. 2013. Evidence for a retroviral insertion in TRPM1 as the cause of congenital stationary night blindness and leopard complex spotting in the horse. PLoS One, 8: e78280.

Brault LS, Cooper CA, Famula TR, Murray JD, and Penedo MC. 2011. Mapping of equine cerebellar abiotrophy to ECA2 and identification of a potential causative mutation affecting expression of MUTYH. Genomics, 97: 121–129.

Brault LS and Penedo MC. 2011. The frequency of the equine cerebellar abiotrophy mutation in non-Arabian horse breeds. Equine Vet J, 43: 727–731.

Brooks SA, Gabreski N, Miller D, Brisbin A, Brown HE, Streeter C, et al. 2010. Whole-genome SNP association in the horse: identification of a deletion in myosin Va responsible for Lavender Foal Syndrome. PLoS Genet, 6: e1000909.

Carr EA, Spier SJ, Kortz GD, and Hoffman EP. 1996. Laryngeal and pharyngeal dysfunction in horses homozygous for hyperkalemic periodic paralysis. J Am Vet Med Assoc, 209: 798–803.

Christopherson PW, Insalaco TA, Van Santen VL, Livesey L, Bourne C, and Boudreaux MK. 2006. Characterization of the cDNA Encoding alphaIIb and beta3 in normal horses and two horses with Glanzmann thrombasthenia. Vet Pathol, 43: 78–82.

Christopherson PW, Van Santen VL, Livesey L, and Boudreaux MK. 2007. A 10-base-pair deletion in the gene encoding platelet glycoprotein IIb associated with Glanzmann thrombasthenia in a horse. J Vet Intern Med, 21: 196–198.

Debowes RM, Leipold HW, and Turner-Beatty M. 1987. Cerebellar abiotrophy. Vet Clin North Am Equine Pract, 3: 345–3452.

Eberth JE. 2013. Chondrodysplasia-Like Dwarfism in the Miniature Horse. M.S., University of Gluck.

Finno CJ and Bannasch DL. 2014. Applied equine genetics. Equine Vet J, 46: 538–544.

Firshman AM, Valberg SJ, Bender JB, and Finno CJ. 2003. Epidemiologic characteristics and management of polysaccharide storage myopathy in Quarter Horses. Am J Vet Res, 64: 1319–1327.

Fox-Clipsham LY, Carter SD, Goodhead I, Hall N, Knottenbelt DC, May PD, et al. 2011. Identification of a mutation associated with fatal Foal Immunodeficiency Syndrome in the Fell and Dales pony. PLoS Genet, 7: e1002133.

Graves KT, Henney PJ, and Ennis RB. 2009. Partial deletion of the LAMA3 gene is responsible for hereditary junctional epidermolysis bullosa in the American Saddlebred Horse. Anim Genet, 40: 35–41.

Kohn CW, Johnson GC, Garry F, Johnson CW, Martin S, and Scott DW. 1989. Mechanobullous disease in two Belgian foals. Equine Vet J, 21: 297–301.

Mccue ME, Valberg SJ, Miller MB, Wade C, Dimauro S, Akman HO, and Mickelson JR 2008. Glycogen synthase (GYS1) mutation causes a novel skeletal muscle glycogenosis. Genomics, 91: 458–466.

McGuire TC, Poppie MJ, and Banks KL. 1974. Combined (B- and T-lymphocyte) immunodeficiency: a fatal genetic disease in Arabian foals. J Am Vet Med Assoc, 164: 70–76.

Metallinos DL, Bowling AT, and Rine J. 1998. A missense mutation in the endothelin-B receptor gene is associated with Lethal White Foal Syndrome: an equine version of Hirschsprung disease. Mamm Genome, 9: 426–431.

Naylor JM. 1994. Equine hyperkalemic periodic paralysis: review and implications. Can Vet J, 35, 279–285.

Page P, Parker R, Harper C, Guthrie A, and Neser J. 2006. Clinical, clinicopathologic, postmortem examination findings and familial history of 3 Arabians with lavender foal syndrome. J Vet Intern Med, 20: 1491–1494.

Pailhoux E, Cribiu EP, Parma P, and Cotinot C. 1995. Molecular analysis of an XY mare with gonadal dysgenesis. Hereditas, 122: 109–112.

Perryman LE, McGuire TC, and Crawford TB. 1978. Maintenance of foals with combined immunodeficiency: causes and control of secondary infections. Am J Vet Res, 39: 1043–1047.

Raudsepp T, Durkin K, Lear TL, Das PJ, Avila F, Kachroo P, and Chowdhary BP. 2010. Molecular heterogeneity of XY sex reversal in horses. Anim Genet, 41 Suppl 2: 41–52.

Revay T, Villagomez DA, Brewer D, Chenier T, and King WA. 2012. GTG mutation in the start codon of the androgen receptor gene in a family of horses with 64,XY disorder of sex development. Sex Dev, 6: 108–116.

Reynolds JA, Potter GD, Green LW, Wu G, Carter GK, Martin MT, et al. 1998. Genetic-diet interactions in the hyperkalemic periodic paralysis syndrome in Quarter horses fed varying amounts of potassium: III. The relationship between plasma potassium concentration and HYPP Symptoms. J Equine Vet Science, 18: 731–735.

Ribeiro WP, Valberg SJ, Pagan JD, and Gustavsson BE. 2004. The effect of varying dietary starch and fat content on serum creatine kinase activity and substrate availability in equine polysaccharide storage myopathy. J Vet Intern Med, 18: 887–894.

Rousselle P, Keene DR, Ruggiero F, Champliaud MF, Rest M, and Burgeson RE. 1997. Laminin 5 binds the NC-1 domain of type VII collagen. J Cell Biol, 138: 719–728.

Rudolph JA, Spier SJ, Byrns G, Rojas CV, Bernoco D, and Hoffman EP. 1992. Periodic paralysis in quarter horses: a sodium channel mutation disseminated by selective breeding. Nat Genet, 2: 144–147.

Santschi EM, Purdy AK, Valberg SJ, Vrotsos PD, Kaese H, and Mickelson JR. 1998. Endothelin receptor B polymorphism associated with lethal white foal syndrome in horses. Mamm Genome, 9: 306–309.

Santschi EM, Vrotsos PD, Purdy AK, and Mickelson JR. 2001. Incidence of the endothelin receptor B mutation that causes lethal white foal syndrome in white-patterned horses. Am J Vet Res, 62: 97–103.

Scholes SF, Holliman A, May PD, and Holmes MA. 1998. A syndrome of anaemia, immunodeficiency and peripheral ganglionopathy in Fell pony foals. Vet Rec, 142: 128–134.

Shapiro J. and McEewen B. 1995. Mechanobullous disease in a Belgian foal in eastern Ontario. Can Vet J, 36: 572.

Shin EK, Perryman LE, and Meek K. 1997. A kinase-negative mutation of DNA-PK(CS) in equine SCID results in defective coding and signal joint formation. J Immunol, 158: 3565–3569.

Spier SJ, Carlson GP, Holliday TA, Cardinet GH, 3rd and Pickar JG. 1990. Hyperkalemic periodic paralysis in horses. J Am Vet Med Assoc, 197: 1009–1017.

Spirito F, Charlesworth A, Linder K, Ortonne JP, Baird J, and Meneguzzi G. 2002. Animal models for skin blistering conditions: absence of laminin 5 causes hereditary junctional mechanobullous disease in the Belgian horse. J Invest Dermatol, 119: 684–691.

Thomas GW, Bell SC, and Carter SD. 2005. Immunoglobulin and peripheral B-lymphocyte concentrations in Fell pony foal syndrome. Equine Vet J, 37: 48–52.

Towers RE, Murgiano L, Millar DS, Glen E, Topf A, Jagannathan V, et al. 2013. A nonsense mutation in the IKBKG gene in mares with incontinentia pigmenti. PLoS One, 8: e81625.

Tryon RC, White SD, and Bannasch DL. 2007. Homozygosity mapping approach identifies a missense mutation in equine cyclophilin B (PPIB) associated with HERDA in the American Quarter Horse. Genomics, 90: 93–102.

Valberg SJ, Ward TL, Rush B, Kinde H, Hiraragi H, Nahey D, et al. 2001. Glycogen branching enzyme deficiency in quarter horse foals. J Vet Intern Med, 15: 572–580.

Valverde A, Boyd CJ, Dyson DH, and Pascoe PJ. 1990. Prophylactic use of dantrolene associated with prolonged postanesthetic recumbency in a horse. J Am Vet Med Assoc, 197: 1051–1053.

Wagner ML, Valberg SJ, Ames EG, Bauer MM, Wiseman JA, Penedo MC, et al. 2006. Allele frequency and likely impact of the glycogen branching enzyme deficiency gene in Quarter Horse and Paint Horse populations. J Vet Intern Med, 20: 1207–1211.

Ward TL, Valberg SJ, Adelson DL, Abbey CA, Binns MM, and Mickelson JR. 2004. Glycogen branching enzyme (GBE1) mutation causing equine glycogen storage disease IV. Mamm Genome, 15: 570–577.

White SD, Affolter VK, Schultheiss PC, Ball BA, Wessel MT, Kass P, et al. 2007. Clinical and pathological findings in a HERDA-affected foal for 1.5 years of life. Vet Dermatol, 18: 36–40.

Wijnberg ID, Owczarek-Lipska M, Sacchetto R, Mascarello F, Pascoli F, Grunberg W, et al. 2012. A missense mutation in the skeletal muscle chloride channel 1 (CLCN1) as candidate causal mutation for congenital myotonia in a New Forest pony. Neuromuscul Disord, 22: 361–367.

Witzel DA, Springer MD, and Mollenhauer HH. 1978. Cone and rod photoreceptors in the white-tailed deer Odocoileus virginianus. Am J Vet Res, 39: 699–701.

53

Genetic Tests for Equine Coat Color

M. Cecilia T. Penedo

Veterinary Genetics Laboratory, School of Veterinary Medicine, University of California, California, USA

53.1 Clinical Background

Genetic testing for horse coat color and white patterns has become increasingly popular as owners apply information from such tests to breeding programs for more consistent production of colors that enhance the esthetic and economic value of animals. Owners also rely on these diagnostic tests to clarify the genetic makeup and better define color of horses whose phenotypes are ambiguous. Common reasons for requests of molecular tests for coat color are:

- Testing of breeding stock to identify homozygotes (two copies) for color variants in genes such as Extension (black pigment), Champagne, Dun, Gray, Roan, or Tobiano. All offspring of such homozygotes will possess the trait of interest.
- Dilutions genes such as Cream and Champagne can produce similar phenotypes. Coat color tests determine which dilution variant is present. Description of color gains accuracy when genetic content is known.
- Screening breeding stock for Lethal White Overo.
- Testing for multiple genes to establish genetic makeup and expected outcomes of foal color.

Variations in color and pattern phenotypes are under genetic control and result from mutations in genes involved with different aspects of melanogenesis, pigment trafficking, and packaging, melanocyte differentiation, migration, and proliferation during embryonic development. In general, most or all known mutations are present in many breeds. Exceptions to this are, for example, absence of Roan in Thoroughbreds, absence of white spotting mutations in breeds that exclude spotting from standards or breeds with restricted color standards, such as Norwegian Fjords that are all Dun. Coat color mutations generally do not impact the health of animals but known exceptions are Silver dilution and the white patterns known as Appaloosa (also known as Leopard Complex), Lethal White Overo (LWO), Gray (Progressive Graying with Age), and homozygous lethal White (Dominant White).

The mutations responsible for the major coat color and white patterns have been determined (Table 53.1). DNA diagnostic tests are available to establish the genetic makeup of horses for selected genes. Dun and Roan have been mapped to genes but the specific mutations have yet to be identified. DNA tests via linked markers that co-segregate with Dun or Roan are available through some laboratories. Classification of coat color phenotypes is not always straightforward and thus the availability of genetic tests has greatly improved phenotypic description.

Horse owners are generally knowledgeable about basic genetics of coat color but often veterinarians are consulted to explain test results, or to assess breeding potential of horses for foal color production. Knowledge of health problems associated with specific colors helps to facilitate diagnosis and considerations for treatment and management. This chapter provides a brief overview of inheritance of coat color in horses and genetic testing applications. Detailed description of specific colors and white patterns can be found in Sponenberg (2009).

The base colors of horses – bay, black, brown, or chestnut – are determined by the interaction of two genes, Extension (Melanocortin 1 Receptor or MC1R) and Agouti (Agouti Signaling Protein or ASIP). Signaling through MC1R with the agonist alpha-melanocyte stimulating hormone (α-MSH) leads to synthesis of black pigment (eumelanin), while binding of MC1R with the antagonist ASIP results in synthesis of red pigment (phaeomelanin). The wild-type, normal Extension and Agouti genes code for dominant alleles symbolized by *E* and *A*, respectively, which are present in at least one copy in all bay horses and whose typical phenotype is

Table 53.1 Genes, allelic variants, and molecular nature of coat color mutations. DNA changes are described in reference to location on the horse genome reference sequence assembly EquCab2.0.

Effect/Locus name	Gene	Alleles	Mutation description	Reference
Base Color				
Extension	*MC1R*	*E* (black), *e* (red)	ECA3g.36259552C > T	Marklund et al., 1996
		e[a] (red)	ECA3g.36259552 T, g.36259555G > A	Wagner and Reissmann, 2000
Agouti	*ASIP*	*A* (bay), *a* (black)	a: ECA22g.25168579–25168589del	Rieder et al., 2001
Color Dilution				
Cream	*SLC45A2*	*N,Cr*	ECA21g.30666626G > A	Mariat et al., 2003
Pearl	*SLC45A2*	*N, Prl*	ECA21: unpublished	MCT Penedo (unpublished)
Dun	*TBX3*	*N, D*	ECA8:linked SNP[*]	MCT Penedo (unpublished)
Champagne	*SLC36A1*	*N, Ch*	ECAg.14:26701114C > G	Cook et al., 2008
Silver	*PMEL17*	*N, Z*	ECA6g.73665315C > T	Brunberg et al., 2006, Andersson et al., 2013
White pattern				
Gray[+]	*STX17*	*N, G*	ECA15: intron 6, 4.6 Kb duplication	Rosengren Pielberg et al., 2008
Roan	*KIT*	*N, Rn*	ECA3, linked markers	MCT Penedo (unpublished)
Appaloosa (Leopard)	*TRPM1*	*N, Lp*	ECA1: 1378 base pairs insertion	Bellone et al., 2013
Overo (LWO)[+]	*EDNRB3*	*N, O*	ECA17g.50624681–50624682TC > AG	Metallinos et al., 1998
Sabino-1	*KIT*	*N, SB1*	ECA3g.77735542 T > A	Brooks and Bailey, 2005
Splashed White	*MITF*	*N, SW1, SW3*	SW1: ECA16g. 20117302Tdelins11 SW3: ECA16:g.20105348_52del5	Hauswirth et al., 2013
	PAX3	*N, SW2*	SW2: ECA6g.11429753C > T	Hauswirth et al., 2013
Tobiano[+]	*KIT*	*N, TO*	ECA3, large inversion (47 Mb)	Brooks et al., 2007
White	*KIT*	*N, W1-W20*	Many variants (see refs)	Haase et al., 2007, 2009

+ Intellectual property rights apply for commercial testing.

* SNP: single nucleotide polymorphism.

reddish body hair with black points. Black color results from the recessive Agouti allele named *a* which leads to black pigment synthesis only and uniform pigment distribution throughout body. Chestnut color results from recessive Extension alleles *e* and the rare *e*[a] that preclude eumelanin synthesis (Marklund et al., 1996, Wagner and Reissmann, 2000). Brown, also known as seal brown, is thought to be caused by another Agouti mutation (A[t]) yet to be described (Sponenberg 2009). For purposes of simplification, brown is grouped here with bay. All horses can be classified into one of the three base colors, either phenotypically or with aid of molecular tests.

Base colors can be modified by mutations in other genes involved with pigmentation which result in lightening of color (dilution). Color dilutions produced distinct phenotypes defined by the color name: Cream, Pearl, Champagne, Dun and Silver. Except for Dun, the specific mutations that produce these dilutions are known. In terms of mode of inheritance, Cream (*Cr*) is an incomplete-dominant allele over its wild-type

(*N*) allele and exhibits dosage-dependent phenotype such that buckskins, smoky blacks and palominos have one copy of Cream (*N/Cr*) and mostly dilution of red pigment only; perlinos, smoky creams, and cremellos have two copies (*Cr/Cr*) and dilution of both black and red pigments in hair, and also pink skin and blue eyes. Pearl (*Prl*), another allele in the Cream gene, is recessive and dilutes both black and red pigments in hair. Champagne (*Ch*), Dun (*D*), and Silver (*Z*) are dominant alleles over the corresponding wild-type *N* alleles with little or no dosage effect.

The Silver allele causes multiple congenital ocular anomalies (MCOA) syndrome (Andersson et al., 2013) regardless of base color. Homozygotes for Silver (*Z/Z*) have the MCOA phenotype with impaired vision resulting from a host of anomalies that include uveal cysts, cornea globosa, iris stromal hypoplasia, abnormal pectinate ligaments, cataracts, and iris hypoplasia. Heterozygotes (*N/Z*) have less severe ocular problems (Cyst-phenotype), often displaying peripheral cysts of the iris, cilliary body, or retina. Silver color is present in several breeds including American Miniature Horse, Exmoor Pony, Icelandic Horse, Shetland Pony, Belgian Draft, Morgan Horse, Rocky Mountain Horse, and its related breeds Kentucky Mountain Saddle Horse, and Mountain Pleasure Horse. Breeding between Silver horses should be avoided in order to reduce incidence of MCOA. Breeding of Silver to Not-Silver are preferred but chance is 50% for a Silver-colored foal.

Depigmentation (Gray and Roan) and white spotting patterns can overlay any base color and dilution phenotype. Gray is associated with increased susceptibility to dermal melanoma in older horses, with prevalence rates as high as 80% in horses 15 years of age and older (Phillips and Lembcke, 2013). Melanomas are usually benign but some can metastasize to internal organs if left untreated. They typically appear as firm, black nodules in the dermis of glabrous skin under the tail base, anal, perianal and genital regions, perineum, lips, and eyelids. Vitiligo is also common in gray horses. Homozygous Gray (*G/G*) horses have higher incidence of melanomas and turn white faster than heterozygotes (*N/G*). The Gray allele produces the progressive graying with age phenotype via up-regulation of *STX17* gene with hyperproliferation and depletion of melanocyte stem cells in hair follicles, but not the skin (Rosengren Pielberg et al., 2008). Breeding schemes that reduce incidence of homozygous Gray horses can be beneficial.

Appaloosa spotting in homozygous condition (*Lp/Lp*) is associated with congenital stationary night blindness (CSNB) (Bellone et al., 2013), a condition thought to be caused by defective neural transmission through the rod pathway involving the inner nuclear layer of the retina (Sandmeyer et al., 2007). The defect is present at birth and is characterized by impaired vision in dark conditions. Elimination of CSNB through selective breeding is not necessary as most affected horses function very well and often the condition is not diagnosed. Diagnosis of CSNB enables adjustments to handling and training routines to improve safety for horse and human contacts. One modifier of the Appaloosa pattern, named Pattern-1 or PATN1, has recently been identified (Holl et al., 2016) in the RING finger and WD repeat domain 3 gene (RFWD3), which increases the extent of white spotting in horses that possess at least one copy of the Appaloosa gene. The PATN1 mutation is relevant for breeders who seek to produce Appaloosa horses and ponies with increased amount of white spotting.

Dominant white is a complex white-spotting pattern associated with mutations in KIT (Haase et al., 2007, 2009, 2011) and with variable expression of phenotypes that range from minimum spotting to all white phenotypes. Typically, both skin and hair show depigmentation but the eyes remain darkly pigmented. Twenty different alleles, named W1 to W20, have been identified to date (Haase et al., 2007, 2009, Hauswirth et al., 2013). The majority of these mutations are considered to be homozygous lethals based on predicted effects on KIT protein function and most are family-specific and rare within breeds. There is very little demand for genetic testing of dominant white mutations. In contrast, there is more demand for LWO testing to determine if horses with overo or mixed-pattern phenotypes carry the mutation. Although prevalent in horses with frame pattern, LWO occurs with other patterns, and in horses with minimal to no visible spotting (Santschi et al., 1998). Breeders of white-spotted horses should test their breeding stock to avoid mattings between LWO-carriers that could result in lethal white foals.

Unilateral or bilateral deafness is often associated with extensive head and limb white spotting and tends to occur more often, but not always, in horses with Frame Overo, Splashed White, or combinations of these patterns. With appropriate training, deaf horses can be used successfully in performance events. Hearing test (BAER test) is recommended as part of pre-purchase examinations.

53.2 Tests Available

DNA tests for color and patterns genes shown in Table 53.1 are performed by laboratories that provide horse genotyping services. Not all laboratories offer comprehensive testing for all genes; information about test options is available on websites. A partial list of service providers in the USA and other countries is presented in Table 53.2. For most laboratories, tests can be ordered online and prices range between $25.00–40.00 per test, with discounts options for multiple testing of genes or samples. Tests for Dominant White have been limited to W3 (one Arabian family), W4 (Camarillo White), W5 (one Thoroughbred family), and W10 (one Quarter Horse family) and demand is very limited. Some breed registries, such as the American Quarter Horse Association and American Paint Horse Association, offer a discounted fee for coat color panel testing (all genes) to members, and incorporate test results in the registration record, but tests have to be ordered through the registry.

PCR-based DNA tests are designed to detect presence or absence of specific mutations but there is no uniform method used across laboratories. Different assay strategies such as allele-specific amplification in end-point or real-time PCR modalities, single-nucleotide extension, Taqman assays or restriction enzyme digestion, among others, are appropriate for testing. Detection systems are

Table 53.2 Partial list of service laboratories that provide horse coat color tests.

Laboratory name	Country	Website
Animal Genetics, Inc	USA, UK	www.animalgenetics.us www.animalgenetics.eu
Animal Genetics Laboratory	USA	http//:vetmed.tamu.edu/vibs/service-labs
Animal Genetic Testing and Research Laboratory (UKY)	USA	www.ca.uky.edu/gluck/AGTRL.asp
Animal Health Trust	UK	www.aht.org.uk
Australian Equine Genetics Research Centre	Australia	www.aegrc.uq.edu.au
Certagen Gmbh	Germany	www.certagen.de
dr. van Haeringen Laboratorium b.v.	Netherlands	www.vhlgenetics.com/vhl
GeneControl GmbH	Germany	www.genecontrol.de/main.html
Laboklin	Germany, UK	www.laboklin.de, www.laboklin.co.uk
VetGen	USA	www.vetgen.com
Veterinary Genetics Laboratory	USA	www.vgl.ucdavis.edu

commonly based on fluorescence dyes attached to PCR products. Key to any diagnostic test is sufficient validation with known reference samples to ensure that results are accurate and robust. Examples of assays based on fluorescence-tagged, allele-specific PCR amplification and detection by capillary electrophoresis with laser-assisted optics for image analysis are shown in Figure 53.1. The images show how each possible genotype for Extension, Agouti, and Cream can be clearly identified by this method and are representative of assays used for other coat color genes.

53.3 Sample Collection and Submission

Information about sample collection and submission is available online from service provider websites. About 20–30 hair roots pulled from mane or tail, or about 1–5 ml of whole blood in EDTA blood tubes (purple top), or blood spots in blood cards are common sample types processed by all laboratories. Hairs with attached roots are preferably placed in plain paper envelopes marked with animal identifiers or taped to test request forms. Hair root sampling is non-invasive and overall less expensive than blood alternatives. Refrigeration is not needed for shipping either hair or blood as DNA is very stable under most conditions. Alternative types of samples, for example, semen, tissue biopsy, postmortem bone or teeth, are also good sources of DNA but only used in special circumstances. It should be determined in advance if these are acceptable and additional processing costs as DNA extractions require use of more labor-intensive procedures.

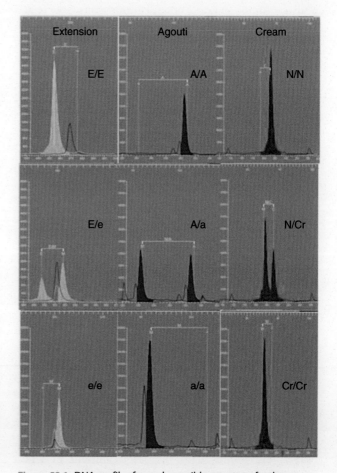

Figure 53.1 DNA profiles for each possible genotype for the Extension, Agouti, and Cream genes. Colored peaks in yellow, blue, and red are fluorescence-labeled PCR products separated by laser-assisted capillary electrophoresis followed by fragment size analysis of imaging data. For each gene, alleles are identified by the length in base pairs of PCR product (*x*-axis). Signal intensity (*y*-axis) only reflects yield of product in the PCR reaction.

53.4   Interpretation of Test Results

Coat color results are reported as genotypes (genetic makeup) determined for each test requested. There is no standardized nomenclature to represent allelic variants but genotype designations are similar among laboratories. The allele designations shown in Table 53.3 are those used by the Veterinary Genetics Laboratory, University of California, Davis, CA, USA. Extension and Agouti alleles are historically named E and e, A, and a, respectively. For remaining genes, wild-type alleles are represented by "N" (normal) and mutant alleles by abbreviations related to the specific gene/mutation. A brief explanation of results is typically included in test reports to facilitate understanding of genetic implications for color determination or breeding.

The phenotypic effects of coat color and pattern alleles depend on the mode of inheritance (dominant, incomplete-dominant, or recessive) and, if present, the combined action of mutant alleles present in different genes. Expectations of standard phenotypes for individual genes are described in Table 53.4. Because of its limited application, Dominant White was omitted from the table but expectations are that horses carrying one copy of a mutant allele will be white spotted. Except for W20/W20 genotypes, homozygotes for most dominant white alleles are not expected to be viable and have not been documented. Base color phenotypes of bay, black, and chestnut are modified by presence of mutant alleles in the other known genes, as well as by other unknown genes. Results of coat color tests define the genetic makeup and clarify coat color classification for the major genes but may not explain all displays color phenotypes. Testing for all known genes (panel testing) is needed in order to fully define a coat color phenotype but, frequently, requests are made for selected genes of interest to owners. For example, common requests are for tests of Extension and Agouti to determine whether breeding stock can consistently produce only bay- or only black-based foals. Breeders of Tobiano or Roan horses often seek to identify homozygotes (TO/TO or Rn/Rn) for use as breeding stock that will produce only Tobiano or Roan foals.

The following example of coat test for an American Miniature Horse mare (Figure 53.2) illustrates how genetic tests resolve the underlying genetic makeup of ambiguous phenotypes. The mare displays a pale-cream body color, flaxen mane and tail, white markings in four legs, thin dorsal list along the back. Eye color is described as amber or light-brown and skin color as light pink with freckles.

Coat color test results: Extension: **e/e**; Agouti: **a/a**; Cream/Pearl: **N/N**; Champagne: **N/Ch**; Dun: **N/D**; Silver: **N/Z**; Gray: **N/N**; Roan: **N/N**; Appaloosa: **N/N**; LWO: **N/N**; Sabino-1: **N/N**; Splashed White: **N/N**, Tobiano: **N/TO**. These define the color of the mare as Tobiano, Dun,

Table 53.3 Genotypes reported in coat color tests and mode of inheritance mutations.

Gene	Possible genotypes	Mode of inheritance
Extension	E/E, E/e, e/e	e: recessive
Agouti	A/A, A/a, a/a	a: recessive
Cream	N/N, N/Cr, Cr/Cr	Cr: incomplete dominant
Pearl	N/N, N/Prl, Prl/Prl	Prl: recessive
Dun	N/N, N/D, D/D	D: dominant
Champagne	N/N, N/Ch, Ch/Ch	Ch: dominant
Silver	N/N, N/Z, Z/Z	Z: dominant
Gray	N/N, N/G, G/G	G: dominant
Roan	N/N, N/Rn, Rn/Rn	Rn: dominant
Appaloosa (Leopard)	N/N, N/Lp, Lp/Lp	Lp: incomplete dominant
Lethal White Overo	N/N, N/O, O/O	O: dominant; homozygous lethal
Sabino-1	N/N, N/SB1, SB1/SB1	SB1: partial-dominant, not lethal
Splashed White	N/N, N/SW1, N/SW2, N/SW3, SW1/SW1, SW3/SW3	SW1: dominant; not homozygous lethal SW2: dominant; likely homozygous lethal SW3: dominant, likely deleterious in homozygous state (microphthalmia)
Tobiano	N/N, N/TO, TO/TO	TO: dominant
White	N/N, N/Wx, Wx/Wx	x = W1-W20: dominant, variable expression

Table 53.4 Coat color genotypes and genetic implications for color and breeding potential.

Locus/Genotype		Interpretation of genotype result
Extension		
	E/E	2 copies of black pigment allele. Base color is bay or black. All foals will be black-pigmented. Cannot have chestnut foals.
	E/e	1 copy of black pigment allele. Carries 1 copy of chestnut allele (e). Can produce bay, black or chestnut foals depending on the color of the mate. Base color is bay or black depending on genotype at Agouti locus.
	e/e	2 copies of red pigment allele. Base color is chestnut. Cannot produce black-pigmented foals when mated to another chestnut.
Agouti		
	A/A	2 copies of Agouti allele. Base color is bay in E/E or E/e background. All black-pigmented foals will be bay. No effect on red pigment (ee).
	A/a	1 copy of Agouti allele. Carries 1 copy of Non-Agouti (a). Base color is bay in E/E or E/e background. Can produce foals with bay, black or chestnut base color, depending on the color of the mate. No effect on red pigment (ee).
	a/a	2 copies of Non-Agouti allele. Base color is black in E/E or E/e background. Can produce foals with bay, black or chestnut base colors depending on color of mate.
Cream and Pearl		
	N/N	Cream or Pearl not present.
	N/Cr	1 copy of Cream allele. Diluted red pigment in body hair. Chestnut is diluted to palomino, bay to buckskin and black to smoky black. Horse can produce Cream-diluted and non-diluted foals.
	Cr/Cr	2 copies of Cream allele. Diluted black and red pigments in body, mane and tail hair; pink skin and blue eyes. Chestnut dilutes to cremello, bay to perlino and black to smoky cream. All offspring are Cream-diluted.
	Cr/Prl	1 copy each of Cream and Pearl. Diluted black and red pigments in body, mane and tail hair; pink skin and blue eyes. Horse color mimics Cr/Cr phenotypes but will not breed true for Cream. Can produce diluted and non-diluted foals.
	N/Prl	1 copy of Pearl allele. Color not diluted. Base colors are chestnut, bay or black.
	Prl/Prl	2 copies of Pearl allele. Diluted color for both red and black pigments. Dilution more intense in body hair than mane and tail; mimics Champagne phenotypes. Purplish skin color with some freckling. Eye color diluted.
Champagne		
	N/N	Champagne not present.
	N/Ch	1 copy of Champagne allele. Dilutes chestnut to gold, bay to tan with brown points (amber) and black to darker tan with brown points (classic). Skin is purplish with mottling.
	Ch/Ch	2 copies of Champagne allele. Dilutes chestnut to gold, bay to tan with brown points (amber) and black to darker tan with brown points (classic). Skin is purplish with mottling. All offspring will be Champagne diluted.
Dun		
	N/N	Dun not present.
	N/D	1 copy of Dun allele. Body hair diluted to pale red in chestnut, to tan in bay and to slate in black base colors. Primitive marks usually present.
	D/D	2 copies of Dun allele. Body hair diluted to pale red in chestnut, to tan in bay and to slate in black base colors. Primitive marks usually present. All offspring will be Dun diluted.
Silver		
	N/N	Silver not present.
	N/Z	1 copy of Silver allele. Bay-based horses have lightened black pigment on lower legs and flaxen mane and tail. Black-based horses have chocolate body color with flaxen mane and tail. No effect on chestnut. Horse is at risk for ocular cysts.
	Z/Z	2 copies of Silver allele. Bay-based horses have lightened black pigment on lower legs and flaxen mane and tail. Black-based horses have chocolate body color with flaxen mane and tail. No effect on chestnut. All bay and black offspring will be Silver diluted. Horse has or will develop MCOA and impaired vision.

Table 53.4 (Continued)

Locus/Genotype		Interpretation of genotype result
Gray		
	N/N	Gray not present.
	N/G	1 copy of Gray allele. Horse is or will turn Gray with age. Skin and eye are pigmented. Horse can produce Gray and Not-Gray offspring. Increased risk for melanomas at older age.
	G/G	2 copies of Gray allele. Horse is or will turn Gray with age. Skin and eye are pigmented. All offspring will be Gray. Increased risk for melanomas at older age.
Roan		
	N/N	Roan not present.
	N/Rn	1 copy of classic Roan allele. Horse is Roan with mixed colored and white hairs over body and darker head, lower legs, mane and tail. Horse will produce Roan and Not-Roan offspring.
	Rn/Rn	2 copies of classic Roan allele. Horse is Roan with mixed colored and white hairs over body and darker head, lower legs, mane and tail. All offspring will be Roan.
Appaloosa		
	N/N	Appaloosa spotting not present.
	N/Lp	1 copy of Appaloosa spotting. Variable amount of white; pigmented spots in white areas are common. Mottled skin, striped hooves and white sclera.
	Lp/Lp	2 copies of Appaloosa spotting. Variable amount of white; few pigmented spots in white areas. Mottled skin, striped hooves and white sclera. All foals will have Appaloosa spotting. Horse has congenital stationary night blindness (CSNB).
Lethal White Overo		
	N/N	LWO spotting not present.
	N/O	1 copy of LWO allele. Horse has white spotting of variable expression. If bred to another N/O, there is a 25% chance of producing a LWO foal.
	O/O	2 copies of LWO allele. Foal is all white. It has, or will present shortly after birth, intestinal tract abnormalities (ileocolonic aganglionosis) incompatible with life.
Sabino-1		
	N/N	Sabino-1 spotting not present.
	N/SB1	1 copy of Sabino-1 allele. Horse typically displays 2 or more white legs, blaze, spots or roaning in the midsection, jagged margins around white areas.
	SB1/SB1	2 copies of Sabino-1. All or nearly all white. Also called sabino-white. Not lethal.
Tobiano		
	N/N	Tobiano spotting not present.
	N/TO	1 copy of Tobiano allele. Horse has Tobiano spotting and will produce Tobiano and Not-Tobiano foals.
	TO/TO	2 copies of Tobiano allele. Horse has Tobiano spotting. All foals will be Tobiano.

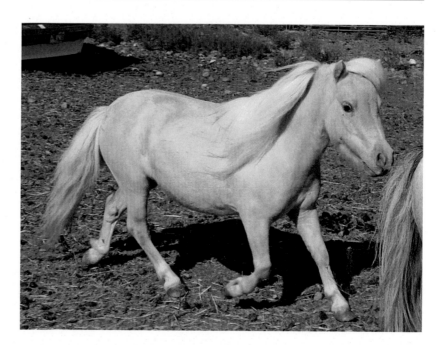

Figure 53.2 American Miniature Horse mare with diluted color phenotype. *Source:* Courtesy of Susan Oberg.

Gold, or Champagne. In addition, the mare carries Silver, not expressed on the chestnut background, and can produce Silver-colored foals if base colors are bay or black. The restricted Tobiano pattern of the mare (described as left front stocking, right front fetlock, left rear white to hock, right rear high fetlock) illustrates atypical display of white spotting commonly observed in Miniature horses. In normal-sized horses, Tobiano spotting extends over the top midline somewhere between the withers and top of the tail. Given the independent segregation of the coat color genes during meiosis, this mare has the potential to produce a plethora of different colors in offspring ranging from standard base colors to numerous possibilities of single or multiple dilutions, with or without Tobiano spotting. The genetic makeup of this mare could not have been fully predicted by inspection of her phenotype alone, even if parental colors were taken into consideration.

References

Andersson LS, Wilbe M, Viluma A, Cothran G, Ekesten B, Ewart S, and Lindgren G. 2013. Equine multiple congenital ocular anomalies and silver coat colour result from the pleiotropic effects of mutant PMEL. Plos One, 8: e75639.

Bellone RR, Holl H, Setaluri V, Devi S, Maddodi N, Archer S, et al. 2013. Evidence for a retroviral insertion in TRPM1 as the cause of congenital stationary night blindness and leopard complex spotting in the horse. Plos One, 8: e78280.

Brooks SA and Bailey E. 2005. Exon skipping in the KIT gene causes a Sabino spotting pattern in horses. Mamm Genome, 16: 893–902.

Brooks SA, Lear TL, Adelson DL, and Bailey E. 2007. A chromosome inversion near the KIT gene and the Tobiano spotting pattern in horses. Cytogenet Genome Res, 119: 225–230.

Brunberg E, Andersson L, Cothran G, Sandberg K, Mikko S, and Lindgren G. 2006. A missense mutation in PMEL17 is associated with the Silver coat color in the horse. BMC Genet, 7: 46.

Cook D, Brooks S, Bellone R, and Bailey E. 2008. Missense mutation in exon 2 of SLC36A1 responsible for champagne dilution in horses. PLoS Genet. 4: e1000195.

Haase B, Brooks SA, Schlumbaum A, Azor PJ, Bailey E, Alaeddine F, et al. 2007. Allelic heterogeneity at the equine KIT locus in dominant white (W) horses. PLoS Genet, 3: e195.

Haase B, Brooks SA, Tozaki T, Burger D, Poncet PA, Rieder S, et al. 2009. Seven novel KIT mutations in horses with white coat colour phenotypes. Anim Genet, 40: 623–629.

Haase B, Rieder S, Tozaki T, Hasegawa T, Penedo MC, Jude R, and Leeb T. 2011. Five novel KIT mutations in horses with white coat colour phenotypes. Anim Genet, 42: 337–339.

Hauswirth R, Jude R, Haase B, Bellone RR, Archer S, Holl H, et al. 2013. Novel variants in the KIT and PAX3 genes in horses with white-spotted coat colour phenotypes. Anim Genet, 44: 763–765.

Holl H, Brooks S, Archer S, Brown K, Malvick J, Penedo MC, and Bellone R. 2016. Variant in the RFWD3 gene associated with PATN1, a modifier of Leopard Complex spotting. Anim Genet, 47(1): 91–101.

Marklund L, Moller MJ, Sandberg K, and Andersson L. 1996. A missense mutation in the gene for melanocyte-stimulating hormone receptor (MC1R) is associated with the chestnut coat color in horses. Mamm Genome, 7: 895–899.

Metallinos DL, Bowling AT, and Rine J. 1998; A missense mutation in the endothelin-B receptor gene is associated with Lethal White Foal Syndrome: an equine version of Hirschsprung disease. Mamm Genome, 9: 426–431.

Phillips JC and Lembcke LM. 2013. Equine melanocytic tumors. Vet Clin North Am Equine Pract, 29: 673–687.

Rieder S, Taourit S, Mariat D, Langlois B, and Guérin G. 2001. Mutations in the agouti (ASIP), the extension (MC1R), and the brown (TYRP1) loci and their association to coat color phenotypes in horses (*Equus caballus*). Mamm Genome, 12: 450–455.

Rosengren Pielberg G, Golovko A, Sundstrom E, Curik I, Lennartsson J, Seltenhammer MH, et al. 2008. A cis-acting regulatory mutation causes premature hair graying and susceptibility to melanoma in the horse. Nat Genet, 40: 1004–1009.

Sandmeyer LS, Breaux CB, Archer S, and Grahn BH. 2007. Clinical and electroretinographic characteristics of congenital stationary night blindness in the Appaloosa and the association with the leopard complex. Vet Ophthalmol, 10: 368–375.

Santschi EM, Purdy AK, Valberg SJ, Vrotsos PD, Kaese H, and Mickelson JR. 1998. Endothelin receptor B polymorphism associated with lethal white foal syndrome in horses. Mamm Genome, 9: 306–309.

Sponenberg DP. 2009. *Equine Color Genetics*. Singapore: Wiley-Blackwell.

Wagner HJ and Reissmann M. 2000. New polymorphism detected in the horse MC1R gene. Anim Genet, 31: 289–290.

54

Peritoneal Fluid

Jorge Nieto

Department of Surgical and Radiological Sciences, School of Veterinary Medicine, University of California, California, USA

54.1 Introduction

Peritoneal fluid is a clear liquid that lubricates the serosal surfaces of abdominal organs. Normal peritoneal fluid is clear pale yellow, has low concentration of protein, and low cellularity. Abdominocentesis for collection of peritoneal fluid in horses was reported in 1964 to aid in the diagnosis and prognosis of colic, dystocia, and inflammatory and non-inflammatory conditions (Maksic, 1964). Collection of peritoneal fluid is performed in most horses referred with colic at referral centers and is considered a valuable diagnostic technique for evaluation of intra-abdominal disease in horses. If possible abdominocentesis should be performed after rectal and ultrasonographic evaluation of the abdomen to try to prevent enterocentesis or puncture of the spleen. Cases at risk of enterocentesis are horses with large colon impactions, especially sand impactions, and horses at risk of puncture of the spleen are horses with nephrosplenic entrapment, where the spleen is pushed to midline. If no ultrasound is available to select a pocket of fluid, usually the abdominocentesis is performed on the most dependent part of the abdomen to the right of midline. Collection of peritoneal fluid is performed after aseptic preparation with either an 18–19G 1.5-inch sharp needle, or a teat or bitch catheter. Collection of fluid using a sharp needle does not require the use of local anesthetic; however, the use of blunt catheters require the use of a small amount of local anesthetic and making a small incision with a #15 scalpel blade through the skin and subcutaneous tissue. To prevent blood contamination from the stab skin incision the catheter is pushed through a sterile gauze swab. If the abdominocentesis is performed with needles, the use of a second needle 1-inch from the first one is commonly used to eliminate the negative pressure in the abdominal cavity. Collection of peritoneal fluid with needles, in foals or

horses that may kick while having the procedure performed, may predispose to septic peritonitis by producing bowel perforation or lacerations. Although enterocentesis or spleen punctures rarely cause a clinical problem they affect the diagnostic evaluation of peritoneal fluid. The peritoneal fluid is usually collected by gravity flow into plain tubes for microbial culture, EDTA containing tubes for cytology or heparin containing tubes for biochemistry evaluation.

54.2 Visual Inspection

Visual evaluation of peritoneal fluid is usually performed at the time of collection. If serosanguineous fluid is obtained it is recommended to allow some fluid to drain out to remove blood contamination from a bleeding skin or muscle vessel. The normal appearance of peritoneal fluid is straw color. Changes in total protein concentration or increase number of nucleated cells or erythrocytes will change the appearance of the fluid to cloudy, dark yellow, orange, or red. Several studies have found a strong correlation between the presence of orange or serosanguineous peritoneal fluid with the presence of small intestinal strangulating obstructions (Latson et al., 2005, Nieto et al., 2005, Yamout et al., 2011). A recent study found a correlation between abnormal peritoneal fluid for strangulating obstructions involving the small intestine but not the large colon (colon volvulus). It is possible that cases of colon volvulus have severe signs of pain with rapid deterioration of the clinical condition and are referred earlier and thus have fewer changes on the abdominal fluid. In addition, due to the degree of pain those cases are immediately taken to surgery to increase the chances of survival and therefore evaluation of peritoneal fluid is not always performed. Horses with abnormal appearance of peritoneal fluid (orange or red)

(A)

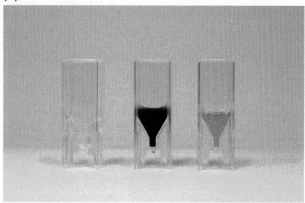

(B)

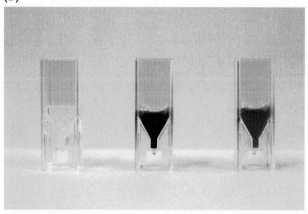

Figure 54.1 Peritoneal fluid of a horse with blood contamination at collection (A) and a horse with a strangulating obstruction (B). Left sample is distilled water for comparison, middle sample is non-centrifuged peritoneal fluid and right sample is centrifuged peritoneal fluid).

Box 54.1 Cytological and biochemical values of normal peritoneal fluid in adult horses.

Color	Pale Yellow
Total protein	<2.5 g/dL
Erythrocytes	Absent
Total nucleated cell count	<5000/μL
Neutrophils	20–90%
Mononuclear cells	5–60%
Lymphocytes	0–35%
Eosinophils	0–5%
Basophiles	0–1%
Glucose	90–115 mg/dL
Creatinine	1.8–2.7 mg/dL
Lactate	0.3–1 mmol/L
Amylase	0–14 IU/L
Lipase	0–36 IU/L

were more likely to have a small intestinal strangulating obstruction compared to horses with yellow appearance of peritoneal fluid (odds ratio (OR): 4) with a high positive predictive value of 86%, and a sensitivity and specificity of 67%. The presence of orange/red peritoneal fluid after centrifugation indicates lyses of erythrocytes due to a prolonged strangulating obstruction (Figure 54.1). The presence of a hematocrit higher than the peripheral blood hematocrit in a sample of hemorrhagic peritoneal fluid is indicative of a splenic puncture. Reddish brown-green peritoneal fluid with or without visible plant material indicates bowel rupture.

54.3 Cytological Evaluation

Cytological evaluation of peritoneal fluid is commonly used for the diagnosis of horses with colic (Box 54.1). Although normal peritoneal fluid of adult horses should have no erythrocytes, blood contamination is common during collection. A study found that >20,000 erythrocytes/μL were considered a sensitive indication for the need of surgical intervention in horses with colic. However, detection of red coloration of peritoneal fluid by laboratory technicians using visual inspection is not accurate up to 40,000 erythrocytes/μL (Weimann et al., 2002). To determine subtle changes in the color of peritoneal fluid a spectrophotometer can be used to detect hemoglobin concentrations in centrifuged fluid that has a higher sensitivity and specificity than visual evaluation. In cases of abdominal hemorrhage erythrophagocytosis by mononuclear cells and the absence of platelets indicates the presence of previous bleeding.

Protein content of peritoneal fluid is estimated biochemically using automated analyzers or by refractometry, which depends on the physical properties of protein in solution. Although there are variations on the total protein concentration depending on the method used, studies have shown that results for protein estimates from hand-held refractometers correlate well with biochemical methods (biuret method). The refractometer measures the refractive index of a sample relative to the refractive index of water. The reading is actually a measurement of total solids and is only an estimation of protein concentration. Therefore, other solids in the sample besides protein, or the presence of turbid, hemolyzed, or lipemic samples may affect the results. Peritoneal fluid in adult horses and foals has a low protein concentration (1.1 g/dL) and an elevation is consistent with inflammation. Horses with peritoneal fluid concentrations >2.6 g/dL were more likely to have a small intestinal strangulating obstruction (OR: 20; with high sensitivity 76% and specificity 86%).

Although normal peritoneal fluid has been reported to have 5000–10,000 nucleated cells/µL, most normal horses have less than 3000 cells/µL. The leukocyte differential in normal peritoneal fluid is 2:1 neutrophils to mononuclear cells, with sporadic mesothelial cells. Since blood contamination is common during collection a study evaluating the effects of blood contamination concluded that up to 17% blood contamination of peritoneal fluid did not significantly alter interpretation of nucleated cell count or protein concentration (Malark et al., 1992). Intraperitoneal extravasation of erythrocytes and protein occurs during strangulating obstructions of bowel due to an increase in capillary hydrostatic pressure, follow by passive congestion of the strangulated bowel. The entrance of toxins and/or bacteria into the abdominal cavity as consequence of devitalization of bowel causes massive influx of granulocytes from the blood (Morris and Johnston, 1986). There is a positive correlation between the duration of infarction and the elevation of peritoneal fluid nucleated cells. Changes in peritoneal fluid can be evident 1–2 h after unset of a strangulating obstruction. Common numbers of leukocytes in horses with strangulating obstructions are 5000–30,000 cells/µL with 90–95% neutrophils and they can increase up to 150,000 cells/µL as the intestine deteriorates. In addition of the increase in cell numbers, degeneration changes also occur included nuclear pyknosis, karyorrhexis, karyolysis, and cytoplasmic vacuolization (Rowe and White, 2008). Horses with septic peritonitis or non-strangulated infarctions also can have elevated total protein and leucocytes count (300,000–400,000 cells/µL), however, on these cases the number of red cells often is low (Figure 54.2).

Evaluation of peritoneal fluid after abdominal surgery has been studied in healthy horses and ponies after exploratory celiotomy alone, or after resection and anastomosis (Santschi et al., 1988, Hanson et al., 1992). Increases in erythrocyte count (212,000 cells/µL), leukocyte count (199,800 cells/µL), percentage of neutrophils (91%), and concentration of total protein (6 g/dL) were observed and remain higher than baseline values for more than 7 days post surgery. In addition, changes in nucleated cell count in peritoneal fluid are detected as early as 4 h after entero or cecocentesis. Horses with septic peritonitis due to leakage of devitalized bowel, gastrointestinal rupture or primary peritonitis will have elevated numbers of total nucleated cells in the peritoneal fluid. Bacteria can be identified by a Gram stain and the presence of a mixed population of bacteria is indicative of bowel rupture while a single type of bacteria may indicate primary peritonitis. The presence of pleomorphic Gram-negative rods may be

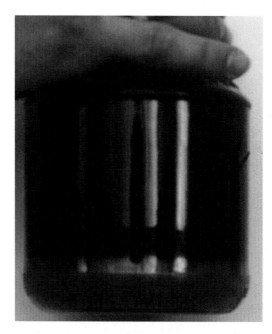

Figure 54.2 Peritoneal fluid from a horse with septic peritonitis due to a cecocentesis. Fluid was serosanguineous, had a high protein, and elevated number of nucleated cells.

suggested of *Actinobacillus equili* peritonitis. However, gram staining of peritoneal fluid samples only reveals bacteria in 27–33% of cases. If septic peritonitis is suspected aerobic and anaerobic culture and sensitivity is critical to assist in the selection of the most appropriate antimicrobial. The use of commercially available blood culture media may increase the likelihood of obtaining a positive culture. The presence of greenish brown and turbid peritoneal fluid indicates bowel rupture. In cases where rupture is suspected based on the color of the abdominal fluid, it is recommended to repeat the abdominocentesis using the ultrasound to select a pocket of fluid and avoid an enterocentesis. Cytological evaluation usually confirmed the diagnosis of bowel rupture by observing plant debris, large number of toxic and degenerated neutrophils, and free and intracellular bacteria. However, in some occasions of rupture bowel nucleated cell may be low due to dilution form the intraluminal fluid (Figure 54.3).

Peritoneal fluid nucleated cells, protein and fibrinogen concentrations and specific gravity in mares that have recently foaled should be normal. Therefore abnormalities detected in peritoneal fluid of mares within a week of foaling should be attributed to a systemic or gastrointestinal problem and not to the foaling process (Van Hoogmoed et al., 1996). In contrast castration increased the nucleated cell count >10,000 cells/µL in 63% of clinically normal horses castrated by routine methods. The same study also found that 88% of the horses had blood-tinged peritoneal fluid (Schumacher et al., 1988).

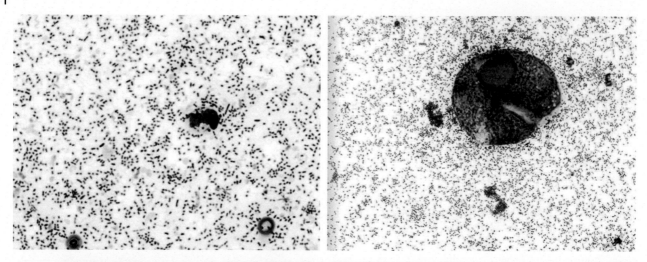

Figure 54.3 Peritoneal fluid of a horse with rupture bowel. The fluid had a total of 0.1 g/dL protein, 420 nucleated cells/μL, and lactate total of 7.9 mmol/L (peripheral lactate was 13.7 mmol/L). There is heterogeneous population of bacteria and protozoa and the presence of intracellular bacteria within karyolitic neutrophils indicating rupture bowel.

54.4 Biochemical Evaluation

Biochemical evaluation of peritoneal fluid is commonly used in the diagnosis and prognosis of horses with colic, and in horses with a suspicion of septic peritonitis or uroperitoneum. Recently several studies have shown that peritoneal fluid lactate can be used in the diagnosis of horses with colic. Lactate is the end product of glycolysis and is most commonly elevated due to poor tissue perfusion an anaerobic glycolysis. Intestinal ischemia has a negative effect on cell membrane permeability with intracellular byproducts such as lactate being release into the systemic circulation and peritoneal cavity. Lactate in the peritoneal fluid of normal horses is low (<1 mmol/L) and it is increased in horses with colic. Horses with colic (strangulating or non-strangulating obstructions) have higher concentrations of lactate in the peritoneal fluid compared with blood lactate concentrations. However, lactate is a small diffusible molecule and in cases of severe hypovolemia or reduction in oxygen delivery, blood lactate can diffuse into the abdomen producing similar concentrations in blood and peritoneal fluid. Horses with strangulating obstructions have higher concentrations of peritoneal lactate (8.45 mmol/L) compared to horses with non-strangulating obstructions (2.09 mmol/) (Latson et al., 2005). A cut-off concentration of peritoneal lactate of 2.8 mmol/L had a sensitivity of 88% and a specificity of 67% to differentiate between non-strangulating and strangulating obstructions (Yamout et al., 2011). A study evaluating peritoneal fluid variables in horses with colic found that changes in gross appearance, pH, and concentrations of chloride and lactate have the strongest correlation with the presence of strangulating obstructions. By using those variables, a model to estimate the probability of a horse having a strangulating obstruction was created. The model is routinely used at our clinic in most horses with colic:

$$p = 1/1 + e^{-[10.908 + 146.527\log 10\,Ab.Lact - 0.288\,Ab.Cl + 2.043\,Ab.pH + 1.823\,Abcolor - 19.081\log 10\,AbLact^*AbdpH]}$$

Where p = probability of finding necrotic intestine, Ab.Lact = abdominal lactate, Ab.Cl = abdominal chloride, Ab.pH = abdominal pH, Ab.color = presence of clear abdominal fluid (1) or presence of cloudy or serosanguineous abdominal fluid (2), and Ab.Lact = value of abdominal lactate.

Some horses with early strangulating obstructions may have low values of peritoneal fluid lactate on presentation. However, an increase in peritoneal fluid lactate concentration after 1–6 h of medical treatment (intravenous fluid) is a strong predictor for selection of horses with strangulating obstructions (sensitivity 95%, specificity 77%) (Peloso and Cohen, 2012).

Bench top lactate analyzers are expensive and time consuming to maintain, and therefore are limited to use in hospital settings. Because the increased use of lactate in human athletes to monitor training and performance in field situations, several affordable, portable, and easy to use hand-held blood lactate analyzers are commercially available. However, those machines are validated only for the measurement of lactate concentrations in the blood of humans. The hand-held portable analyzers are relatively affordable (~$300–500), run on disposable strips with a life of 1 year from manufacture, and the cost per strip/sample is from $2–$3 dollars. A recent study compared the three handheld portable analyzers available in the United States (Lactate Scout[+], Lactate Plus, and Lactate Pro) and measured levels of agreement for peritoneal fluid compared to a bench top

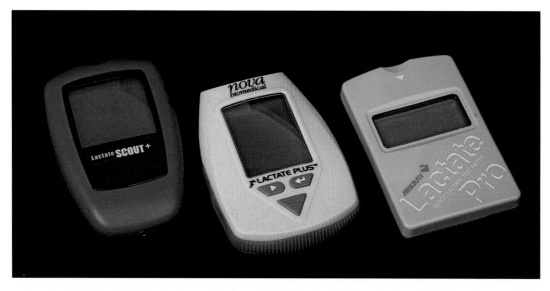

Figure 54.4 Hand-held lactate portable analyzers available in the United States. Peritoneal fluid was analyzed by the portable analyzers and compared to a bench top analyzer and to a chromogenic assay. The Lactate Pro analyzer has the highest level of agreement in peritoneal fluid of horses.

analyzer and a chromogenic assay (Nieto et al., 2015) (Figure 54.4). Portable lactate analyzers had good agreement with the bench top analyzer at low concentration of lactate in both blood and peritoneal fluid; however, as concentration of lactate increases, the difference between the bench top and the portable analyzers also increases.

Peritoneal fluid pH and glucose concentrations can be used to assist in the identification of horses with septic peritonitis. Peritoneal fluid pH <7.3, serum-to-peritoneal fluid glucose concentration differences >50 mg/dL, glucose concentrations < 30 mg/dL, and fibrinogen peritoneal fluid concentrations > 200 mg/dL are highly indicative of septic peritonitis (Van Hoogmoed et al., 1999). Peritoneal fluid is usually collected by gravity flow into an open vacutainer tube, exposing the collected fluid to air. Exposure of peritoneal fluid to room air has a significant effect increasing pH values (Romero et al., 2011). Therefore, if peritoneal pH is used for diagnostic purposes the time from collection to analysis needs to be minimized to provide the best clinical interpretation.

Uroperitoneum is a sporadic cause of abdominal distension and obtundation in the neonatal foal, and is a rare condition in adult horses. The diagnosis can be performed by ultrasonographic observation of large volumes of free, nonechogenic fluid within the abdomen and a small, irregular shape collapse bladder. Abdominocentesis usually produces a free flow of peritoneal fluid with a low cell count, low specific gravity, and at least twice the creatinine concentration of peripherally blood. In most uncomplicated cases of uroperitoneum the total nucleated cell count and total protein may be normal or have low values due to dilution. However, in some cases evaluation of peritoneal fluid may show increase total nucleated cells count, high concentrations of total protein, and the presence of bacteria suggesting peritonitis. If laboratory facilities are not available, new methylene blue can be infused into the bladder by a urinary catheter and the collection blue tinged peritoneal fluid by abdominocentesis will indicate a rupture bladder. However, this technique may not allow detection of other causes of uroperitoneum such as a ruptured ureter or the distal urachus.

References

Hanson RR, Wright JC, Schumacher J, Baird AN, Humburg J, and Pugh DG. 1992. Evaluation of peritoneal fluid following intestinal resection and anastomosis in horses. Am J Vet Res, 53: 216–221.

Latson KM, Nieto JE, Beldomenico PM, and Snyder JR. 2005. Evaluation of peritoneal fluid lactate as a marker of intestinal ischaemia in equine colic. Equine Vet J, 37: 342–346.

Maksic D. 1964. Abdominal paracentesis and its use in diagnosis in the horse. 20th Ann Con Am Assoc Equine Prctnr, pp. 319–321.

Malark JA, Peyton LC, and Galvin MJ. 1992 Effects of blood contamination on equine peritoneal fluid analysis. J Am Vet Med Assoc, 201: 1545–1548.

Morris DD and Johnston JK (1986) Peritoneal fluid constituents in horses with colic due to small intestinal disease. Equine Colic Symposium, pp. 134–142.

Nieto JE, Aldridge BM, Beldomenico PM, Aleman M, and Snyder JR. 2005. Characterization of equine intestinal fatty acid binding protein and its use in managing horses with colic. Am J Vet Res, 66: 223–232.

Nieto JE, Dechant JE, le Jeune SS, and Snyder JR. 2015. Evaluation of 3 handheld portable analyzers for measurement of l-lactate concentrations in blood and peritoneal fluid of horses with colic. Vet Surg, 44: 366–372.

Peloso JG and Cohen ND. 2012. Use of serial measurements of peritoneal fluid lactate concentration to identify strangulating intestinal lesions in referred horses with signs of colic. J Am Vet Med Assoc, 240: 1208–1217.

Romero AE, Nieto JE, Dechant JE, Hopper K, and Aleman M. 2011. Effects of aerobic and anaerobic fluid collection on biochemical analysis of peritoneal fluid in healthy horses and horses with colic. Vet Surg, 40: 40–45.

Rowe EL and White NA. 2008. Diagnosis of gastrointestinal disease. In NA White, JN Moore and TS Mair (eds), *The Equine Acute Abdomen7*. USA: Teton NewMedia, pp. 235–28.

Santschi EM, Grindem CB, Tate LP Jr, and Corbett WT. 1988. Peritoneal fluid analysis in ponies after abdominal surgery. Vet Surg, 17: 6–9.

Schumacher J, Schumacher J, Spano JS, McGuire J, Scrutchfield WL, and Feldman RG. 1988. Effects of castration on peritoneal fluid in the horse. J Vet Intern Med, 2: 22–25.

Van Hoogmoed L, Rodger LD, Spier SJ, Gardner IA, Yarbrough TB, and Snyder JR. 1999. Evaluation of peritoneal fluid pH, glucose concentration, and lactate dehydrogenase activity for detection of septic peritonitis in horses. J Am Vet Med Assoc, 214: 1032–1036.

Van Hoogmoed L, Snyder JR, Christopher M, and Vatistas N. 1996. Peritoneal fluid analysis in peripartum mares. J Am Vet Med Assoc, 209: 1280–1282.

Weimann CD, Thoefner MB, and Jensen AL. 2002. Spectrophotometric assessment of peritoneal fluid haemoglobin in colic horses: an aid to selecting medical vs. surgical treatment. Equine Vet J, 34: 523–527.

Yamout SZ, Nieto JE, Beldomenico PM, Dechant JE, leJeune S, and Snyder JR. 2011. Peritoneal and plasma D-lactate concentrations in horses with colic. Vet Surg, 40: 817–824.

55

Respiratory Secretions
Melissa Mazan

Cummings School of Veterinary Medicine, Tufts University, Massachusetts, USA

55.1   Introduction

Respiratory fluid was first examined microscopically at about the time of the American Civil War (Johnston and Frable, 1979), but it was not until the 1980s that the tracheal wash (Seals 1980) and the BAL were described in veterinary medical literature (Derksen et al., 1985). In the ensuing time, it has become commonplace for the equine practitioner to sample the secretions of the lower respiratory tract, usually in order to rule out infectious and non-infectious inflammatory disease, and, less commonly to detect neoplastic disease. Specific indications may include coughing, nasal discharge, or poor performance in the case of non-septic diseases; with septic diseases, we may also note apparent dyspnea, fever, and weight loss. In this chapter, we will discuss what can be done with aspirates of the lower airways – namely, tracheal aspirates and bronchoalveolar lavage.

55.2   How to Decide Which Sample to Take

When we sample these respiratory spaces, we have a choice of doing cytology, biochemical analysis (e.g., glucose, lactose, pH, protein), bacterial culture or viral isolation, or PCR, depending on the question being asked. In order to choose the right sample – and to do the right test on that sample – it is important to have a reasonable idea of what the disease process is and to have some idea of the pathophysiology of that disease. In general, if the practitioner suspects that the problem is infection of the parenchyma or airways, then it is important to take a sample that is representative of the lesion and which is uncontaminated by the normal flora of the upper airways. If the practitioner suspects a diffuse non-septic disease such as inflammatory airway disease (IAD) or heaves (recurrent airway

obstruction, or RAO) then a BAL is more appropriate. Although a tracheal aspirate is often touted as being easier to obtain in the field, with practice a BAL becomes quite easy and quick to perform. Moreover, the cells obtained by tracheal aspirate are not representative of the cells obtained by BAL (Derksen et al., 1985); rather, they likely represent a combination of backflow from nasal discharge and secretions from the trachea itself, in addition to the forward flow of secretions from the lower airways and lung. If pleural effusion is suspected, then pleurocentesis may be indicated, but it is important to remember that the majority of pleural effusions in the horse are an extension of initial pneumonia, and in the early stages, these parapeumonic effusions are often sterile. Thus, the practitioner is more likely to find the offending microorganisms using a tracheal aspirate for culture rather than a pleural fluid sample. Moreover, because the disease may be localized within the lung, BAL may also yield a sterile sample (Rossier et al., 1991). In the less common case of fungal disease such as pneumocystis, a BAL is more likely to yield an answer. Regardless of the test being done, there are a few practicalities that are important in order to ensure that the optimum sample for cytology, culture, or biochemical analysis can be obtained.

In this chapter, we will first discuss samples that arise from lung (TA and BAL). We will briefly discuss pertinent aspects of the acquisition of the pulmonary fluids, and then processing fluid to provide samples for cytological diagnosis as well as appropriate sampling and interpretation of microbiology.

55.3   Performing the Tracheal Aspirate

Tracheal aspirates can be acquired by either a transtracheal approach or through an endoscope. Although a transtracheal aspirate is usually considered an appropriate

Interpretation of Equine Laboratory Diagnostics, First Edition. Edited by Nicola Pusterla and Jill Higgins.
© 2018 John Wiley & Sons, Inc. Published 2018 by John Wiley & Sons, Inc.

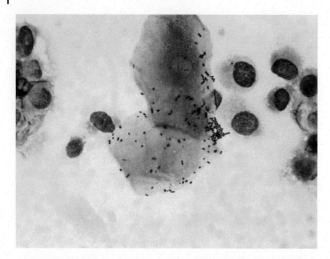

Figure 55.1 Squamous cell with attached bacteria but no accompanying inflammatory cells indicates nasopharyngeal contamination.

sample for culture, if the horse coughs sufficiently to retroflex the catheter into the oropharynx, the culture will be irretrievably contaminated. If you suspect this to be the case, assess the cytology before submitting for microbiology, as you will be able to see squamous cells with their attendant bacteria (Figure 55.1). As a caveat, the horse with dysphagia may develop aspiration pneumonia, in which case, the squamous cells do not indicate a tracheal aspirate gone awry, rather, they reflect the pathogenesis of the disease. When the tracheal aspirate is acquired by use of endoscopy, the catheter must be doubly guarded in order to ensure that bacteria from the nasopharynx are not dragged into the sampling area (Hoffman et al., 1991). It is useful to deposit lidocaine on the larynx before approaching the trachea in order to decrease coughing. When using a guarded catheter, make sure not to advance the endoscope itself distal to the sampling site. Visualize the tracheal puddle and, taking care to stay several centimeters proximal, advance the catheter into the puddle, and aspirate.

In horses with mild disease, or when sampling blindly, as with a transtracheal aspirate, it is often necessary to wash the trachea with 10–20 ml of preservative-free saline. In horses with plentiful mucus, it will not be necessary unless the mucus is very thick and tenacious. When performing a blind sample of the tracheal fluid, it helps to pre-measure to the spot at which you expect you will find fluid, that is, the tracheal puddle. The tracheal puddle is not at the carina, it is 5–15 cm proximal to the carina. Use the smallest amount of saline possible (usually about 10 ml) and flush the fluid into the trachea rapidly. Then, using constant suction, slowly withdraw the catheter until negative pressure is felt and fluid can be seen coming into the syringe. If you do not act quickly, the fluid may be lost into the rest of the lung.

If you decide that you would like to sample both the tracheal fluid and perform a BAL, the tracheal fluid should always be sampled first.

55.3.1 Other Factors Affecting the Results of the Tracheal Aspirate

Tracheal aspirates done approximately one hour after exercise are more likely to yield evidence of inflammation and less likely to have pharyngeal contamination (Malikides et al., 2003, Martinet et al., 1999). High speed exercise is likely to elicit at least microscopically evident pulmonary hemorrhage in most horses. Horses that have had their heads elevated (for instance, when being transported) for even 4–6 h may have an elevated percentage of neutrophils and intracellular bacteria in the tracheal aspirate, because normal drainage of the airways has been prevented by the enforced head carriage (Raidal et al., 1997).

55.4 Performing the Bronchoalveolar Lavage

The BAL can be performed blindly, using a specially made tube by Bivona or can be done endoscopically. In order to do an endoscopic BAL on an average sized horse, you will need an endoscope that is 200–250 cm long. The diameter of the scope may vary, but a general principle is that the smaller the diameter, the smaller the area that is sampled and consequently the less representative is the sample of the entire lung. The Bivona tube usually has a diameter of 11 mm, which allows for a sample of subsegmental bronchioles without being so narrow as to give a non-representative sample.

In order to perform a good BAL, equipment and supplies should be carefully set up ahead of time (Figure 55.2): including 500 ml of saline warmed to body temperature. It is always prudent to warn the owner that the horse will do some impressive coughing, but in order to decrease coughing, it helps to give the horse 4–5 puffs of albuterol (360–450 µg) via a metered dose inhaler. It has also been demonstrated that dilute lidocaine solution (0.66% – 20 ml of 2% lidocaine with 40 ml of sterile saline added) and sedation with butorphanol tartar (0.01 mg/kg) reduce coughing (Westermann et al., 2005), although dilute lidocaine is the most effective. Next, the horse must be properly sedated – poor sedation results in a poor BAL. The level of sedation should be such that the horse easily drops its nose to the ground and does not resist insertion of the Bivona tube or endoscope past the larynx. A twitch helps to stabilize the head. If you are doing a blind BAL, it is helpful to pre-measure the

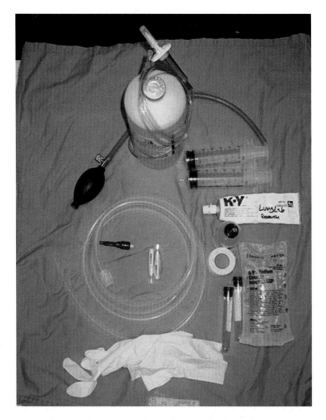

Figure 55.2 Material routinely used to collect BAL fluid includes a Bivona Tube, a puffer, an infusion set, 60-ml syringes, dilute lidocaine (0.66%), lubricant, and red top tubes.

distance from the nose to the larynx so that you can deposit dilute lidocaine before proceeding further. If you are doing an endoscopic BAL, then you will be able to directly visualize the larynx. Continue to dribble dilute lidocaine throughout the trachea and bronchi each time the horse coughs. When a blind BAL is performed, the tube almost always ends up in the right dorsal bronchus. Bronchoscopically guided BAL sampling allows targeting specific lung areas. Make sure that the BAL tube or endoscope is well wedged, or you will fail to retrieve fluid representative of the small airways and alveoli. Use gentle suction when retrieving fluid. In the field, the practitioner will often use manual suction, but recently a study in dogs showed that a suction pump using 5 kPa pressure resulted in better retrieval than manual efforts (Woods et al., 2014).

The amount of saline used will influence the results of the BAL. Smaller volumes result in a sample with a higher percentage of neutrophils. In our clinic, we routinely use two aliquots of 250 ml of saline. Either the return from the second aliquot or a pooled sample should be used for analysis, as the first sample will often have an increased number of neutrophils and possibly epithelial cells (Jean et al., 2011). Check your fluid grossly before making slides – it should have a nice head of froth representing surfactant and signaling that you have obtained a true bronchoalveolar sample. You will always see at least scant flocculent material, which is mucus, but in the severely affected horse with inflammatory airway disease or heaves you will see Curschmann's spirals that are visible to the naked eye. The recent bleeder will often have pink to overtly red tinged fluid.

55.4.1 Other Factors Affecting the Outcome of the BAL

It is useful to standardize the conditions under which a BAL is performed, or at the least to have a complete history so that the BAL can be interpreted accordingly. Long transport can increase the neutrophil percentage, so it is better not to sample by BAL for at least 12 h after shipping long distances. Exercise, including exercise in cold air can increase the neutrophil percentage (Davis et al., 2007), A recent study in a large number of clinically normal horses has shown that when the right lung is sampled, there is a higher percentage of both neutrophils and hemosiderophages as well as hemosiderophage to macrophage ratio, but not mast cells (Depecker et al., 2014). The authors posit that this may be for the same reason the aspiration pneumonia tends to be more severe on the right side; namely, that the right bronchus has a straighter ventral approach.

When performing BAL blindly, the BAL tube usually ends up in the right dorsal lung (McKane and Rose, 1993) but when doing the BAL with an endoscope, it is wise to ensure that the practitioner either samples both sides or always samples the same side for consistency's sake.

55.5 Processing Fluid from the BAL or Tracheal Aspirate

It is rare that a practitioner will be able to rely on a lab being so close that slides will be made within a few hours of the sample being taken. The quality of the slides that are made or the culture that is submitted will have a direct impact on the resultant diagnostic reliability. It is always disappointing when a sample that has taken time, effort, expenses, and a certain amount of invasiveness to obtain is left to languish in a truck and the receiving laboratory is left with a fluid that contains variable numbers of fragmented cells and bacterial overgrowth. Bacterial overgrowth is a problem for two reasons – first, it would be unfortunate to have a sample read out as septic when the problem is one of contamination, and second, bacterial overgrowth tends to lead to death and destruction of the cells of interest. Diagnoses can be compromised for

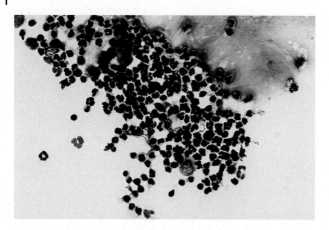

Figure 55.3 These neutrophils appear degenerate, however, even very segmented neutrophils, when left in saline without the benefit of being in a pocket of mucus or adding protein to the sample in the form of serum, will become degenerate in appearance after several hours.

other reasons when slide preparation is delayed; for instance, if there are red cells in the BAL fluid due to iatrogenic trauma, over the course of several hours, macrophages may engulf the red blood cells, leading to an erroneous diagnosis of chronic pulmonary hemorrhage. Neutrophils, if left for several hours in the collected fluid before being processed, will take on a degenerate appearance, with swollen nuclei (Figure 55.3). We often observe that the cells that are in large clumps of mucus retain a more normal appearance, whereas cells that have been unprotected in saline appear more degenerate (Dr. Tracy Sokol, personal communication).

55.5.1   How to Make Good Cytology Slides

First, it is important to remember that most respiratory secretions have a low concentration of cells. Along with this low cell count, most respiratory secretions also have low protein concentrations; this renders the cells quite fragile, especially lymphocytes that will be quickly destroyed. Adding serum helps the cells to survive, but will not prevent bacterial overgrowth. Because most samples have a relatively low cell count, most samples must be centrifuged in some way. In the case that there is a highly cellular sample, for instance in a tracheal aspirate from a horse with pneumonia or a sample from a highly cellular pleural effusion, it may be possible to do a "pick-and-smear" technique, in which a toothpick is used to pick out bits of material that can then be smeared onto the glass. For low-cell samples, cytocentrifuge preparations tend to be very uniform and easy to read, but most practitioners do not have access to a cytocentrifuge. In this case, the practitioner can centrifuge the sample, discard the supernatant, and make a smear of the sediment.

Although one study showed that samples should survive in a purple top tube at room temperature for 8–24h (Pickles et al., 2002a), the best cytological results are achieved by processing the samples immediately or placing the collected fluids on ice. If the sample is to be processed immediately, it is better not to use preservatives, but to keep it in several 10-ml red top tubes. If it is going to be several hours or longer before the sample is processed, and ice is not available, it can be preserved with formalin or alcohol, but the cytology will be inferior. EDTA is not a particularly good preservative. Its primary purpose is to prevent clotting. If you use formalin, remember that you will no longer be able to use Romanowsky stains (e.g., Dif Quik, Wright's, and Giemsa).

Normal horses have, in general, fewer than 1000 cells/μl in the BALF, depending on the extent of airway inflammation. When collecting fluid from the pulmonary epithelial lining of the lung, it is inevitable that there will be considerable dilution of cells (Hewson and Viel, 2002). It is possible to correct for this dilution, but the process is fraught with error and not necessary for clinical diagnosis. Calculation of cell count using a reference such as albumin or urea is well-discussed by Hewson and Viel and is more suited for research purposes (Hewson and Viel, 2002).

When you are making a sediment preparation, use 10-ml red top tubes and spin at approximately 500g for 5–10min. If you spin at much higher speeds than that, you risk rupturing the cells. When the fluid has finished spinning, remove the tubes from the centrifuge; you will note a whitish spot on the bottom and slightly to the side of the tube where the centrifugal force has thrown the cells. Dump out the supernatant with impunity – the cells will stick nicely to the glass of the tube, and you will not lose them. Give the tube a second brisk shake to get rid of any excessive fluid. You may then re-suspend the cell pellet in the fluid that will inevitably be left by lightly flicking the tube until the fluid looks cloudy.

It is important to label your slides clearly. Slides with frosted ends are the easiest to use. A #2 pencil works well for writing important information, such as horse name, owner name, date and source of the biological sample (BAL, TA, etc.). Most "sharpie" type pens will wash off in alcohol – if you use one, it must be one that can withstand bathing in various solvents and stains. Multiple different techniques can be used to make the slide, but the goal for all should be the same – to have cells on the slide, and to make sure that those cells are only one layer thick. A blood smear type preparation works well in some peoples' hands. Never squash the sample – cells are fragile and they will rupture. The author prefers to dip a swab in the resuspended fluid, and then gently roll that swab across the slide. When done correctly, this will keep you from breaking apart the cells, and will result in a thin, readable smear. However, do not use a cotton swab if you are concerned about the possible presence of

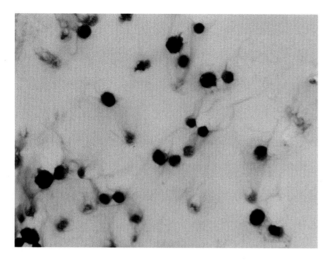

Figure 55.4 This BAL slide was not dried quickly and although there is an appropriate single cell layer, the cells have all shrunk and it is impossible to distinguish cell type. This is an example of "Blue Dot Disease."

plant material in the sample, as with, for instance, a broncho-esophageal fistula, as cotton is a plant material and can render the cytology confusing.

Thereafter it is critical to dry slides rapidly. You can keep a little fan for this purpose, or you can use a hairdryer. Make sure that the air or heat do not directly contact the cells, always apply to the back of the slide. If you do not dry cells rapidly, they will shrink and once they are stained, they will all look alike (Bue Dot Disease, Figure 55.4).

At this point, you may choose to send out your samples, or you may choose to assess them yourself. If money is an issue, then there is quite a bit of information that you can glean from assessing the cytology yourself. Ideally, you will look at the cytology yourself to have a quick

assessment and then send the slides to a laboratory. Send unstained slides – a cytology lab will almost always do a better job at staining slides than you can do yourself. If you are new at this, you may also wish to send fluid preserved in alcohol or formalin – make sure that the fixative is clearly identified on the tube. Regardless of which route you choose, before you discard your precious fluid and spend money sending out samples, it is a good idea to stain a few slides yourself to assess whether you have a good sample. Make enough slides so that you can stain them lighter or darker as you need. If a slide is too light, let the next one stay in the staining solution longer. If it is too dark, a dip or two in alcohol will usually destain the slide to the desired amount. As long as you do not use oil or mounting medium on your slides, you can always destain and re-stain. Regardless of the number of slides you stain, you should change out your stain regularly (of course cleaning the Coplin jars as you do), as the water and methanol will evaporate leaving you with uncertain concentrations of stain, and the solution will become dirty. The debris found in dirty stain may easily be mistaken for bacteria, as may granules from degranulated mast cells or eosinophils, as well as mucus globules.

The most commonly used stain is a modified Romanowsky, such as Dif-quik. This stain is, as the name implies, quick and effective, but, unfortunately, will not stain mast cells (Leclere et al., 2006). It will be necessary, in this case, to keep an extra slide for staining with Toluidine Blue. This is an easy stain to perform. Fix the slide in the first of the Dif-quik stains (methanol-based fixative), and then immerse in Toluidine Blue for at least 15 min. The metachromatic granules of the mast cells will stain a brilliant magenta color, whereas the other cells will be a dull, washed out blue (Figure 55.5).

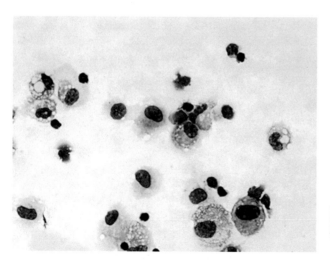 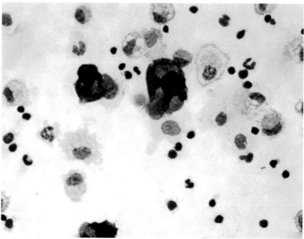

Figure 55.5 Dif-Quik and other Romanowsky stains do not stain mast cells. On the left, a seemingly innocuous BAL stained with Dif-Quik from a horse with pronounced airway hyper-responsiveness. On the right, the same slide stained with Toluidine Blue. Mast cells are easy to detect with their magenta granules.

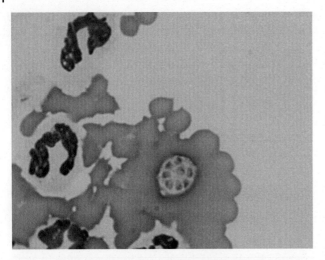

Figure 55.6 *Pneumocystis jirovecci* is considered an opportunistic infection which can be found in the lungs of even normal people and presumably normal horses. If the immune system is suppressed, the fungus can cause severe disease.

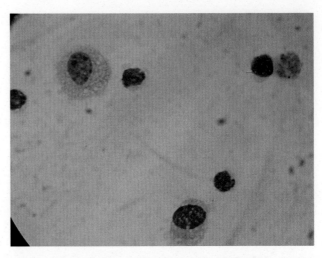

Figure 55.7 Typical BALF cytology from a normal horse. The predominant cells types are alveolar macrophages and lymphocytes.

If you suspect bacterial or fungal disease, almost all micro-organisms stain dark blue with Dif-Quik. For those of us who suffered the vagaries of Bunsen burners in microbiology lab in attempts to make Gram stains, there are now kits on the market that render Gram staining surprisingly easy without application of flame. An initial microscopic examination of the fluid will often help you to initiate treatment. For instance, you will be able to see if you have Gram positive or Gram-negative bacteria, clusters suggesting *Staphylococcus* spp. versus chains suggesting *Streptococcus* spp., or small rods versus large rods that might suggest anaerobes. In the rather rare case of *Pneumocystis*, staining with Toluidine Blue may reveal the 4–8 intracytoplasmic bodies (trophozoites: Figure 55.6) and PAS (which is, again, rather easy to perform if you buy the kit) may help you in detecting fungal organisms. This is, of course, no substitute for culture and analysis by a clinical pathologist.

55.6 Cells and Cellular Products Seen on BAL or TA

First, make sure that your microscope is well-maintained and clean. Then, assess the cytology on low magnification (4× or 10×) to see if it generally looks uniform or if there are areas with large clumps of mucus or rafts of cells. If you have a polarizing lens, this is a good time to take a quick look to see if there are refractile particles present. It is useful now to look with the 40× (high dry), but it will be necessary to do your final cell count with oil-immersion at 63–100× to ensure that you have an adequate assessment

of cell morphology. In order to recognize the abnormal, you must first know what is normal.

On the normal BAL, it is possible to recover alveolar macrophages, lymphocytes, neutrophils, mast cells, eosinophils, erythrocytes, plasma cells, epithelial cells, megakaryocytes, erythrocytes, alveolar type I and type II epithelial cells, and endothelial cells, however, the vast majority of cells should comprise alveolar macrophages with a smaller percentage of lymphocytes and even fewer neutrophils and epithelial cells (Figure 55.7). Many reference ranges have been published. To a certain extent, the method of making slides influences the cell differential, as there will be a greater percentage of macrophages, mast cells, and eosinophils on cytocentrifuge preparations (Pickles et al., 2002b). In our laboratory, we count at least 400 cells with an oil objective (63–100×). A recent study showed that with low-percentage cells such as mast cells or eosinophils it may be more reliable to evaluate five microscopic fields at at least 50×, regardless of the total number of cells counted. Regardless of method, best results were achieved when there were at least 100 cells per hpf (Fernandez et al., 2013). We consider a normal BAL to have 50–70% alveolar macrophages, 30–50% lymphocytes, less than 2% mast cells, less than 0.1% eosinophils, and occasional non-ciliated epithelial cells including goblet cells. On the normal tracheal aspirate, far more epithelial cells and neutrophils are seen, and the cytology has much greater variability than that of the BAL, with up to 15% neutrophils found in the normal horse (Derksen et al., 1989). The remainder of the cells should be alveolar macrophages with a scattering of lymphocytes. It is of interest to note that neutrophils may migrate to the respiratory system within 5 h of insult

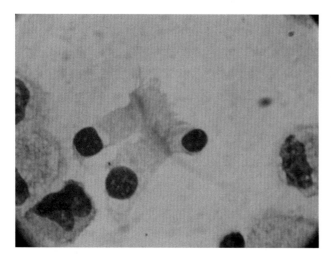

Figure 55.8 Epithelial cells have a basally located nucleus and a columnar shape. These epithelial cells are easy to recognize because they are ciliated.

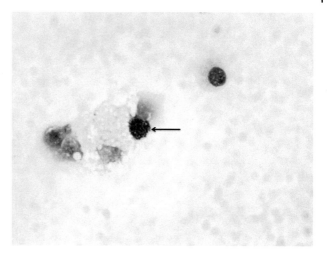

Figure 55.9 Goblet cells (arrow) may look unexpectedly round for an epithelial cell and would possibly be mistaken for a mast cell, but the granules are very large and stain dark blue.

(Brazil et al., 2005) If the practitioner is interested in doing sequential evaluations of the lower lung, both tracheal aspirate and BAL can be performed at 24-h intervals without changing the cytological picture (Jean et al., 2011).

Epithelial cells can be recognized by their somewhat columnar shape and because their nucleus is at the basal aspect of the cell; the presence of cilia on some epithelial cells renders them even more clearly recognizable (Figure 55.8). The more distal you travel in the lung, the fewer ciliated epithelial cells there will be, and the less columnar they will be. The nucleus of *goblet cells* (epithelial) is also at the basal aspect, but they often contain mucus granules and do not have cilia (Figure 55.9). On a BAL, especially a cytospin preparation, the goblet cell may look rather rounder than expected, but it can be distinguished from mast cells or eosinophils because the mucus granules stain a dark blue and are significantly larger than the granules in mast cells or eosinophils. Proliferation of type II alveolar epithelial cells (AEC) may be seen after acute lung injury, and it is possible to mistake these cells for macrophages (Linssen et al., 2004). However, although they are approximately the size of alveolar macrophages and stain similarly, the cytoplasm is usually scant. It is normal to have epithelial cells on a tracheal aspirate, but the presence of more than an occasional epithelial cell on a BAL indicates that you have achieved a bronchial lavage, and not a lavage of the alveolar spaces. Large numbers of ciliated epithelial cells or detached cilia plates may be seen in horses with severe coughing or after viral disease (Figure 55.10). Clumps of reactive epithelial cells (creola) (Najafi et al., 2003) can also be seen with chronic inflammation such as IAD or RAO. (Figure 55.11)

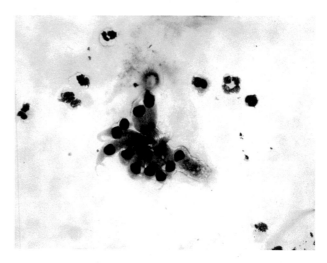

Figure 55.10 Large numbers of cliated epithelial cells can be seen in horses with severe coughing, after viral disease, when the BAL is traumatic, or if a bronchial lavage has been performed rather than a bronchoalveolar lavage.

Alveolar macrophages should be the predominant population in any tracheal wash or BAL. They are the biggest of the cells, and are recognized by a large, somewhat foamy or lacy cytoplasm and a round or often oval nucleus. They may be multinucleate, and it is not unusual even in a clinically normal horse for see engulfed debris in some of the macrophages (Figure 55.12).

Lymphocytes are the next most prevalent cell type. The majority of the cell is taken up by the dense blue nucleus. The respiratory secretions of horses contain both large and small lymphocytes, with the large lymphocytes having somewhat less densely staining nuclei than the small lymphocytes (Hewson and Viel, 2002, Figure 55.13).

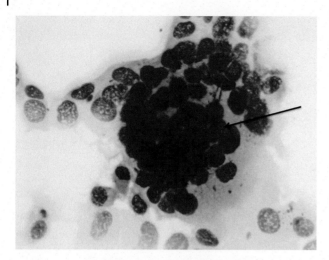

Figure 55.11 Clumps of reactive epithelial cells (arrow), also called *creola*, can be seen in horses with chronic airway inflammation.

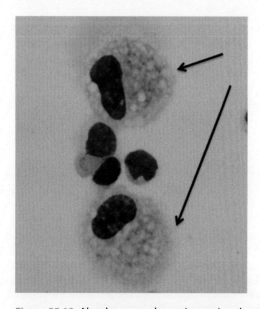

Figure 55.12 Alveolar macrophages (arrows) are large cells with lacy cytoplasm. They should be the predominant cell in the normal BAL cytology.

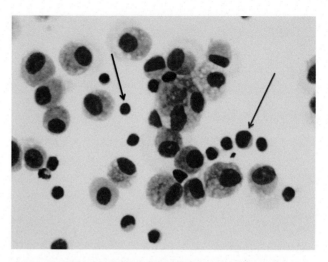

Figure 55.13 The normal BAL cytology in the horse should have approximately 40% lymphocytes, and these will be a mixture of small lymphocytes with scant cytoplasm (black arrow) and larger lymphocytes with a lighter and more obvious cytoplasm (red arrow).

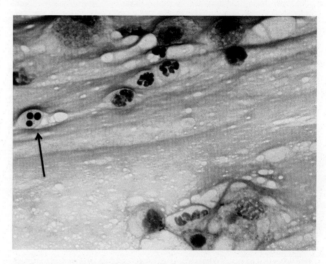

Figure 55.14 Neutrophil with pyknotic nucleus (black arrow) in a pool of mucus.

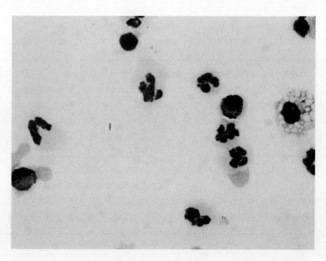

Figure 55.15 Mixed neutrophilic and eosinophilic inflammation.

Neutrophils are scarce in normal respiratory secretions, although, as stated previously, higher percentages are normal in the TA. In the normal BAL, neutrophils should have a tightly segmented morphology, and horses with heaves often have pyknotic neutrophils (Figure 55.14). Degenerate neutrophils develop a more swollen appearing nucleus, there is a loss of detail, and the cytoplasm may appear more bluish (Figure 55.15). It is important to remember that neutrophils can obtain a degenerate appearance if the BAL is left sitting for more than one hour or so, whereas regardless of etiology, neutrophils from tracheal aspirates may look degenerate.

Mast cells are approximately the same size as alveolar macrophages, and although their cytoplasm tends to be more finely stippled than that of alveolar macrophages, it is not possible to be certain in identifying them without Toluidine Blue staining or by using a stain such as May-Grunewald-Giemsa (Figure 55.5).

Eosinophils are usually easily detected by noting their mulberry shaped granules (Figure 55.15). Charcot-Leyden crystals are orange-ish bits of degenerating eosinophils that may be seen in the less common case of eosinophilic IAD or other eosinophilic respiratory diseases (Cibas and Ducatman, 2009).

Mucus is often ignored, but is a very important component of especially the BAL. It stains pinkish to bluish, and can range from a filmy amorphous appearance to a well-organized, more fibrillar or striated appearance (Figure 55.16). It often contains clumps of cells or non-cellular elements, to the extent that if only the non-mucus portion is assessed, a neutrophilic BAL could easily be underestimated (Figure 55.17).

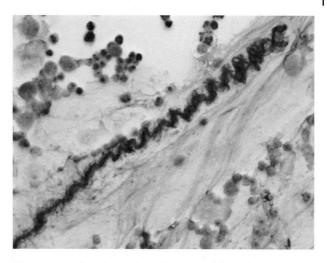

Figure 55.18 Curschmann's spirals are spiral-shaped mucus plugs that reflect the shape of mucus gland ducts or bronchioles. They can be seen in cases with long-standing mucus accumulation, and are not specific to any one disease.

A recognizable element of mucus is the Curschmann's spiral, which is more commonly seen in horses with long-standing inflammatory diseases such as IAD or RAO (Figure 55.18).

55.7 Non-Cellular Elements Seen on BAL or TA

Pollen can often be seen in BAL or TA samples, both extracellularly and engulfed by macrophages. Pollen may be round, with a spiky appearing coat, or may be more egg-shaped, with apparent creases, depending on the species and whether it is moist or has dried out (Figure 55.19).

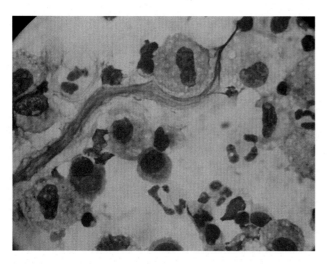

Figure 55.16 When airway inflammation becomes chronic, mucus will become more fibrillar, forming long, tightly compacted strands.

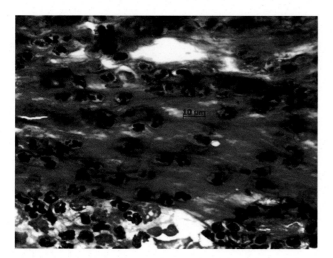

Figure 55.17 Hypercellular mucus often contains large numbers of degenerate-appearing neutrophils. This trapping of neutrophils can falsely decrease the reported neutrophil percentage.

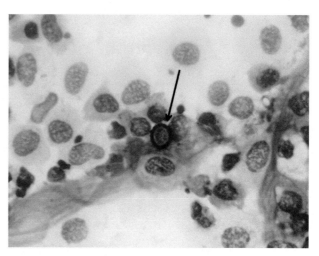

Figure 55.19 Mucus and pollen (arrow) in a horse with a recent onset cough. Alveolar macrophages dominate the cell population but occasional neutrophils are also seen.

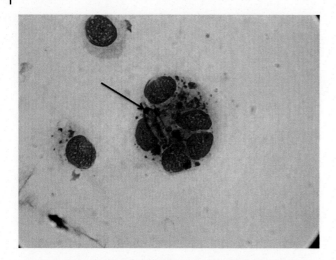

Figure 55.20 Giant cell containing many particulates (dark blue staining within cytoplasm) and a hay spore (arrow).

Mold spores are also often seen in BAL samples, again, both intracellulary and extracellularly. *Alternaria* spp., with one wider end and one thin-tailed end can look somewhat like a mite, and *Cladosporium* spp., which is small and ovoid, are the most common molds seen (Figure 55.20). It is important to remember that their presence does not denote infection, rather, they represent the environment from which the horse inhales from.

Silicates usually appear as dark blue staining particulates within macrophages; with polarizing microscopy, they will be refractile (Figure 55.21).

Glove powder will be extracellular; it also will be refractile with polarizing microscopy. On light microscopy, it will appear round-to oval and will have a dot in the center. On polarized microscopy, it will have a characteristic birefringent Maltese cross appearance (Jadhav et al., 2010).

55.8 Submitting Samples for Bacterial or Viral Culture

If you are lucky enough to be in close proximity to a laboratory, you can collect the fluid into a sterile container and submit it promptly at room temperature. If you use a red top tube for submission of samples, clean the top with alcohol and allow it to dry for at least 1 min before injecting the fluid through the cap. If you use a sterile container, be careful to adhere to aseptic technique. If you suspect a bacterial origin for the disease, at the minimum, a culture for aerobic organisms should be done, as well as antibiotic sensitivity testing. If the sample cannot be submitted immediately (within an hour), then the fluid should be refrigerated or a minimum of 10 ml should be injected into a blood culture vial. Culture swabs are convenient but do not provide as good a yield as a decent volume of fluid submitted in a sterile container or a blood culture bottle (strive for at least 1.0 ml, 10 ml is better). If you are submitting a sample for viral culture alone, then viral culture media is best. If you wish to submit for both bacterial and viral cultures, then a sterile container is best. Be cognizant of maintaining the sterility of the container when opening it and depositing the sample.

The question of how to interpret culture of tracheal fluid can be troublesome. Thirty years ago, Sweeney and coworkers (1985) noted that potentially pathogenic bacteria can be isolated from the trachea of clinically normal horses, and only 28% of tracheal aspirates from clinically healthy, pastured horses failed to grow any bacteria. This highlights the difficulty to assess whether culture of bacteria from the trachea reveals a true infection, a defect in clearance, or merely reflects the presence of a normal microbiome. Indeed, it has been

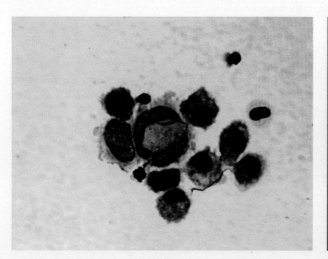
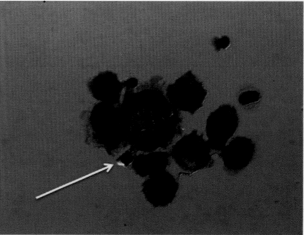

Figure 55.21 Birefringent particulates (arrow) can only be seen with a polarizing lens.

suggested logically that a low level of nonpathogenic bacteria likely guard against colonization from pathogenic bacteria (Cardwell et al., 2013). If bacteria which are possible commensals (including *Streptococcus equi* ss. *zooepidemicus*) are found, then quantitative bacteriology is most appropriate. It has been suggested (Christley and Rush, 2007) that it is necessary to have at least 100 CFU/μl with concurrent neutrophilic inflammation to call the pulmonary fluid infectious. It is suggested that a true infection is more likely if a heavy growth of one type of bacteria is present, rather than the more normal sparse population of three or more bacterial microorganisms (Wood et al., 2005). Interestingly, the lower airways of clinically normal foals contain both extra- and intra-cellular bacteria (Hoffman et al., 1991) and on post-mortem examination, cultures of the lower respiratory tract of adult horses without clinically evident respiratory disease or signs of inflammation grew bacteria in almost a third of them (Blunden and Mackintosh, 1991).

The take-home message for the practitioner is that light bacterial growth is not unexpected from the trachea of the clinically normal horse and may even be found in the BAL of normal horses. Positive culture results should always be viewed in light of cytologic and clinical findings. If you have a febrile horse whose respiratory secretions contain degenerate neutrophils with intracellular bacteria, then it is most reasonable to accept the results of bacteriology as a true infection. The converse is also true; a failure to grow bacteria in the face of a clinically ill horse and a supportive cytology argues that there was an issue with the bacteriological culture. For instance, perhaps the sample was accidentally placed in an EDTA tube, or formalin was added, or the horse was being treated with antimicrobials that suppressed bacterial growth. Another reason may be that the sample sat in inappropriate conditions leading to decreased bacterial viability. When the response to treatment does not match the culture findings it is possible that more than one bacterial species is causing disease, but only one was successfully cultured. It is therefore important to assess all laboratory findings with respect to the horse's clinical progress.

It is generally not recommended to look for microorganisms in BALF. However, interstitial pulmonary diseases such as *Pneumocystis* spp. infection may be more easily found on BALF, and a positive PCR result for EHV-5 is more clinically significant when on BAL than on nasal swab or tracheal aspirate to support a diagnosis of equine multinodular pulmonary fibrosis.

Common pathogens in equine pulmonary infections include *Streptococcus equi* ss. *zooepidemicus*, *Actinobacillus equuli equuli*, *Actinobacillus equuli haemolyticus*, *Pasteurella* spp., *Mycoplasma* spp., *Escherichia coli*, and *Klebsiella pneumonia*. Likely contaminants, on the other hand, include coagulase negative *Staphylococcus* spp., alpha-hemolytic *Streptococcus* spp., *Pseudomonas* spp. (very often a contaminant from improperly cleaned endoscopes), *Bacillus* spp., and *Proteus* spp. (Richard et al., 2010). Although *Nicotella semolina* has been implicated as a potential pulmonary pathogen, it was equally likely to be found in respiratory secretions of both control and affected horses (Hansson et al., 2013). On the other hand, *Stenotrophomonas maltophilia* was associated with chronic lower airway disease without clinical signs of sepsis, questioning the role of this bacteria as a true respiratory pathogen (Winther et al., 2010).

55.9 Secretions of the Lower Respiratory System and Diagnosis of Disease

55.9.1 Inflammatory Airway Disease and Recurrent Airway Obstruction

The diagnosis of inflammatory airway disease (IAD) has elicited much discussion and some resulting disagreement. The North American consensus, as developed at a Havemeyer conference and solidified in a 2007 consensus statement by the American College of Veterinary Internal Medicine recommends, at a minimum, the findings of:

> exercise intolerance, poor performance, or coughing with or without excess tracheal mucus; nonseptic inflammation detected by cytologic examination of BALF or pulmonary dysfunction based on evidence of lower airway obstruction, airway hyper-responsiveness, or impaired blood gas exchange at rest or during exercise; and the absence of evidence of systemic signs of infection (fever, hematologic abnormalities compatible with infection, increased respiratory efforts at rest). (Couetil et al., 2007)

Tracheal wash is considered inappropriate for the diagnosis of IAD, both because of the lack of correspondence between BAL and TA (Derksen et al., 1989) and because of the lack of evidence linking TA cytology to poor performance (Holcombe et al., 2006). The statement goes on to describe BAL cytology as having mild neutrophilia, lymphocytosis, or monocytosis, or eosinophilia or mastocytosis.

Despite the ACVIM consensus statement, many practitioners, especially those in Great Britain, continue to use TA as a measure of IAD, as they find it easier to collect in the field. A cut-off of 20% neutrophils on the

TA is commonly held to be within normal limits, but a recent study in clinically normal Quarter horses suggests that the number may be as high as 25% or more after exercise (Azevedo et al., 2014). Moreover, it is important to note that although tracheal mucus is associated with poor performance, neutrophils are not. This argues that the syndrome of tracheal inflammation in young race-horses that may or may not be associated with bacterial infection is best diagnosed by endoscopic visualization of mucus, and not by enumeration of neutrophils.

With this in mind, the respiratory fluid of choice for the diagnosis of IAD and of RAO is that obtained by BAL. Although horses with IAD generally have mild neutrophilia and horses with RAO generally have more pronounced neutrophilia, there is a large percentage of cases that cannot be distinguished on the basis of BAL cytology alone. In horses with RAO, it has been noted that as clinical signs worsen, the neutrophil percentage increases (Vrins et al., 1991). Increases in many different cell types have been reported in horses with IAD; the important finding to remember is that inflammation does not, in this case, equal infection.

Unlike with tracheal aspirate, there is a functional correlation between abnormal BAL cytology and performance and clinical signs. Specific findings include a clear relationship between BAL mast cell percentage and airway hyper-responsiveness (Hoffman et al., 1998), and neutrophil percentage and cough (Bedenice et al., 2008). Horses with IAD were also shown to have greater derangements of arterial blood gases during exercise (Sanchez et al., 2005).

Although horses with RAO have increased tissue mast cells, they rarely have mastocytosis on BAL (Kaup et al., 1990) whereas in our laboratory we find that at least 50% of horses with IAD have increased mast cells. It is far rarer to find horses with increased numbers of eosino-phils, and our clinical impression is that BAL eosino-philia may have a seasonal nature (Riihimaki et al., 2008). Certainly, if there are persistent increases in eosinophils one would look for parasitism, eosinophilic pneumonia or eosinophilic epitheliotrophic disease.

It is difficult to know if BAL from stabled horses can be determined to be normal. Multiple studies have shown that neutrophils increase in a dramatic fashion in horses with heaves when they are removed from pasture and placed in a stable, but what is often overlooked is that clinically normal horses also have an increase in BAL neutrophils when they are stabled (Holcombe et al., 2001, Pirie et al., 2003, Tremblay et al., 1993). This brings up the question whether the 5% neutrophil cut-off is too stringent. Depecker et al. (2014) found that when they classified clinically normal horses in active race training based on this cutoff, 93.5% would be classified as having IAD with only 6% being classified as definitively normal. If they used the less stringent cutoff of 10% PMNs (Hare

and Viel, 1998), 56.5% of horses would be classified as having IAD. It is of course possible that almost 100% of horses in race training had IAD; however, it is unlikely that IAD posed a performance-limiting problem for all of them. Our lab would certainly argue that lung-function testing with histamine bronchoprovocation would be necessary to determine the functional significance of this cytological finding. A second question posed by this group was whether it mattered if the right versus the left lung was sampled. Surprisingly, between 12 and 17% of horses with IAD would have been misclassified as controls if only the right or left lung would have been sampled and cytology would have focused only on the neutrophil count rather than the number of mast cells.

55.9.2 Exercise Induced Pulmonary Hemorrhage (EIPH)

Until recently, we commonly held that only horses, greyhounds, and racing camels experience pulmonary hemorrhage during exercise but more recently EIPH has been occasionally recognized in elite human athletes and even in non-athletic humans (Diwakar and Schmidt, 2014). It is far more common in horses that work at a sufficiently high speed (Birks et al., 2003). The best explanation remains the high hydrostatic pulmonary capillary pressure combined with very negative pleural pressures that horses experience during intense exercise, resulting in even greater transmural pressures across the pulmonary capillaries (West et al., 1993).

Considering that all horses working at high intensity probably experience some degree of EIPH resulting in higher RBC percentages in the BAL (Meyer et al., 1998) it is necessary to decide what the laboratory definition of EIPH will be. The fact that the BAL itself may elicit hemorrhage if pressures are too high may complicate the diagnosis, thus more than RBCs must be seen to have confidence in the findings (Langsetmo, 2000). Moreover, the exact link between pulmonary hemorrhage and performance is not well-understood.

Hemosiderophages are found in horses with no history or signs of EIPH (Doucet and Viel, 2002a,b) including healthy polo ponies that worked at high intensities (Donaldson, 1991). Unfortunately, there is no definitive gold standard in diagnosing EIPH, however, the following suggestions should be followed. It takes approximately 1 week after intense exercise to see hemosiderophages, and it takes approximately 1 week for red cells to be completely phagocytosed (Doucet and Viel, 2002a,b). After hemosiderophages appear, they will remain detectable for about 3 weeks. These time points can help to stage when bleeding must have occurred in the horse. The BALF hemosiderophage to macrophage ratio (H/M) is often used to determine if a significant bleeding episode has occurred, with a ratio of hemosiderophages to macrophages greater than 20% being considered pertinent (Richard et al., 2010). Others have suggested that more than 50% of the macrophages in tracheal aspirate must be hemosiderophages to give a diagnosis of EIPH, and a hemosiderin score has been shown to reflect a history of clinical EIPH (Doucet and Viel, 2002a,b). However, none of these methods is entirely satisfactory, as none has been correlated to performance. Similar to the findings for IAD, both lungs are not equivalent when looking for EIPH on BAL examination (Depecker et al., 2014).

Although it is commonly stated that Prussian Blue stain is necessary to detect hemosiderophages, most are clearly visible on Dif Quik or similar staining. The hemosiderin may be light golden brown and diffuse to dark blue-black and may be so dense that it is difficult to see the nucleus of the cell. Frequently, hemosiderophages form giant cells. In rare cases, pigment-laden macrophages may contain melanin or carbon. Prussian Blue staining will distinguish the iron content in hemosiderin. If a hemosiderin score is to be used Prussian Blue staining is more diagnostic than Dif Quik. (Doucet and Viel, 2002a,b, Figure 55.22).

55.9.3 Silicosis

The earth's crust is composed primarily of silica, yet most horses do not have silicosis. The history most frequently reported is not unlike that in advanced heaves, with chronic weight loss, respiratory distress, and tachypnea. Reported cases have all come from California (Berry et al., 1991) but in our laboratory, we have seen cases with corresponding clinical signs that come from other areas of the West or that live next to cement factories or quarries. The BAL may appear to be innocuous with primarily macrophages, but polarizing microscopy will reveal birefringent intra- and extra-cellular particles that are consistent with silica (Figure 55.21). Use of loose fiberglass in the ceilings of barns can also result in the horse inhaling the fine silica particles that make up fiberglass with ensuing acute pulmonary hemorrhage or chronic disease (Figure 55.23).

55.9.4 Smoke Inhalation

Horses that survive barn fires will often have thermal damage to the respiratory system. Because of the long half-life of alveolar macrophages, carbon particles, similar to those in smokers' lungs, may persist for years in macrophages (Murphy et al., 2008, Figure 55.24).

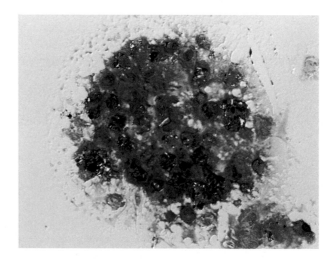

Figure 55.23 Within this giant cell are multiple scintillating refractile particles. This can only be seen with polarizing microscopy (Picture courtesy of Dr. Andrew Hoffman).

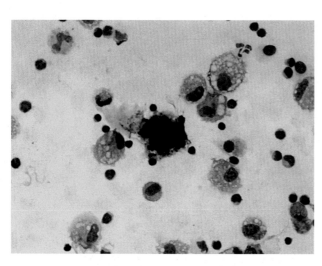

Figure 55.22 BAL cytology from a horse with EIPH that raced 10 days before sample collection. Note the dark black pigment within the hemosiderophage, and the lack of free red cells.

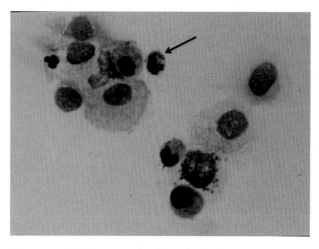

Figure 55.24 This BAL was taken from a horse that had been in a barn fire several months previously. Carbon particles (arrows) are still evident engulfed in alveolar macrophages. Alveolar macrophages are extremely long-lived, and these particles will be evident on BAL for years.

References

Azevedo N, Vasconcelos M, DeLima P, and Filho H. 2014. Analysis of tracheal secretion in healthy horses undergoing a vaquejada simulation test. Open J Vet Med 4(10).

Bedenice D, Mazan MR, and Hoffman AM. 2008. Association between cough and cytology of bronchoalveolar lavage fluid and pulmonary function in horses diagnosed with inflammatory airway disease. J Vet Intern Med/Am College Vet Intern Med, 22(4): 1022–1028.

Berry CR, O'Brien TR, Madigan JE, and Hager DA. 1991. Thoracic radiographic features of silicosis in 19 horses. J Vet Intern Med/Am College Vet Intern Med, 5(4): 248–256.

Birks EK, Durando MM, and McBride S. 2003. Exercise-induced pulmonary hemorrhage. Vet Clin N Am-Equine, 19(1): 87–100.

Blunden AS and Mackintosh ME. 1991. The microflora of the lower respiratory tract of the horse: An autopsy study. Brit Vet J 147(3): 238–250.

Brazil TJ, Dagleish MP, McGorum BC, Dixon PM, Haslett C, and Chilvers ER. 2005. Kinetics of pulmonary neutrophil recruitment and clearance in a natural and spontaneously resolving model of airway inflammation. Clin Exp Allergy, 35(7): 854–865.

Cardwell JM, Smith KC, Wood JL, and Newton JR. 2013. A longitudinal study of respiratory infections in British national hunt racehorses. Vet Rec, 172(24): 637.

Christley R and Rush BR. 2007. Inflammatory airway disease. In BC McGorum (ed.), *Equine Respiratory Medicine and Surgery*. Philadelphia: Saunders Elsevier, pp. 591–595.

Cibas E and Ducatman B. 2009. *Cytology: Diagnostic Principles and Clinical Correlates*. Philadelphia: Saunders Elsevier.

Couetil LL, Hoffman AM, Hodgson J, Buechner-Maxwell V, Viel L, Wood JL, and Lavoie JP. 2007. Inflammatory airway disease of horses. J Vet Intern Med/Am College Vet Intern Med, 21(2): 356–361.

Davis MS, Williams CC, Meinkoth JH, Malayer RJ, Royer CM, Williamson KK, and McKenzie EC. 2007. Influx of neutrophils and persistence of cytokine expression in airways of horses after performing exercise while breathing cold air. Am J Vet Res, 68(2): 185–189.

Depecker M, Richard EA, Pitel PH, Fortier G, Leleu C, and Courouce-Malblanc A. 2014. "Bronchoalveolar lavage fluid in standardbred racehorses: Influence of unilateral/bilateral profiles and cut-off values on lower airway disease diagnosis. Vet J, 199(1): 150–156.

Derksen FJ, Brown CM, Sonea I, Darien BJ, and Robinson NE. 1989. Comparison of transtracheal aspirate and bronchoalveolar lavage cytology in 50 horses with chronic lung disease. Equine Vet J, 21(1): 23–26.

Derksen FJ, Scott JS, Miller C, Slocombe RF, and Robinson NE. 1985. Bronchoalveolar lavage in ponies with recurrent airway obstruction (heaves). Am Rev Resp Disease, 132(5): 1066–1070.

Diwakar A and Schmidt GA. 2014. Exercise-induced pulmonary hemorrhage in a nonathlete: case report and review of physiology. Lung, 192(2): 329–331.

Donaldson LL. 1991. A review of the pathophysiology of exercise-induced pulmonary haemorrhage in the equine athlete. Vet Res Comm, 15(3): 211–226.

Doucet MY and Viel L. 2002. Alveolar macrophage graded hemosiderin score from bronchoalveolar lavage in horses with exercise-induced pulmonary hemorrhage and controls. J Vet Intern Med/Am College Vet Intern Med, 16(3): 281–286.

Doucet MY and Viel L. 2002. Clinical, radiographic, endoscopic, bronchoalveolar lavage and lung biopsy findings in horses with exercise-induced pulmonary hemorrhage. Can Vet J, 43(3): 195–202.

Fernandez NJ, Hecker KG, Gilroy CV, Warren AL, and Leguillette R. 2013. Reliability of 400-cell and 5-field leukocyte differential counts for equine bronchoalveolar lavage fluid. Vet Clin Pathol, 42(1): 92–98.

Hansson I, Johansson KE, Persson M, and Riihimaki M. 2013. The clinical significance of *Nicotella semolina* in horses with respiratory disorders and a screening of the bacterial flora in the airways of horses. Vet Microbiol, 162(2–4): 695–699.

Hare JE and Viel L. 1998. Pulmonary eosinophilia associated with increased airway responsiveness in young racing horses. J Vet Intern Med/Am College Vet Intern Med, 12(3): 163–170.

Hewson J and Viel L. 2002. Sampling, microbiology, and cytology of the respiratory tract. In PM Lekeux (ed.), *Equine Respiratory Diseases*, Ithaca, NY: International Veterinary Information Service.

Hoffman AM, Mazan MR, and Ellenberg S. 1998. association between bronchoalveolar lavage cytologic features and airway reactivity in horses with a history of exercise intolerance. Am J Vet Res, 59(2): 176–181.

Hoffman AM, Viel L, Muckle CA, and Tesarowski DB. 1991. Evaluation of a guarded bronchoscopic method for microbial sampling of the lower airways in foals. Can J Vet Res, 55(4): 325–331.

Holcombe SJ, Jackson C, Gerber V, Jefcoat A, Berney C, Eberhardt S, and Robinson NE. 2001. Stabling is associated with airway inflammation in young Arabian horses. Equine Vet J, 33(3): 244–249.

Holcombe SJ, Robinson NE, Derksen FJ, Bertold B, Genovese R, Miller R, de Feiter Rupp H, et al. 2006. Effect of tracheal mucus and tracheal cytology on racing performance in Thoroughbred racehorses. Equine Vet J, 38(4): 300–304.

Jadhav KB, Gupta N, and Ahmed MB. 2010. Maltese Cross: Starch artifact in oral cytology, divulged through polarized microscopy. J Cytol, 27(1): 40–41.

Jean D. Vrins A, Beauchamp G, and Lavoie JP. 2011. Evaluation of variations in bronchoalveolar lavage fluid in horses with recurrent airway obstruction. Am J Vet Res, 72(6): 838–842.

Johnston WW and Frable WJ. 1979. *Diagnostic Respiratory Cytopathology*. Masson Publications.

Kaup FJ, Drommer W, Damsch S, and Deegen E. 1990. Ultrastructural findings in horses with chronic obstructive pulmonary disease (COPD). II: Pathomorphological changes of the terminal airways and the alveolar region. Equine Vet J, 22(5): 349–355.

Langsetmo I, Meyer MR, and Erickson HH. 2000. Relationship of pulmonary arterial pressure to pulmonary haemorrhage in exercising horses. Equine Vet J, 32: 379–384.

Leclere M, Desnoyers M, Beauchamp G, and Lavoie JP. 2006. Comparison of four staining methods for detection of mast cells in equine bronchoalveolar lavage fluid. J Vet Intern Med/Am College Vet Intern Med, 20(2): 377–381.

Linssen KC, Jacobs JA, Poletti VE, van Mook W, Cornelissen EI, and Drent M. 2004. Reactive type II pneumocytes in bronchoalveolar lavage fluid. Acta Cytol, 48(4): 497–504.

Malikides N, Hughes KJ, Hodgson DR, and Hodgson JL. 2003. Comparison of tracheal aspirates and bronchoalveolar lavage in racehorses. 2. Evaluation of the diagnostic significance of neutrophil percentage. Aust Vet J, 81(11): 685–687.

Martin BB, Jr, Beech J, and Parente EJ. 1999. Cytologic examination of specimens obtained by means of tracheal washes performed before and after high-speed treadmill exercise in horses with a history of poor performance. J Am Vet Med Assoc, 214(5): 673–677.

McKane SA and Rose RJ. 1993. Radiographic determination of the location of a blindly passed bronchoalveolar lavage catheter. Equine Vet Educ, 5(6): 329–332.

Meyer TS, Fedde MR, Gaughan EM, Langsetmo I, and Erickson HH. 1998. Quantification of exercise-induced pulmonary haemorrhage with bronchoalveolar lavage. Equine Vet J, 30(4): 284–288.

Murphy J, Summer R, Wilson AA, Kotton DN, and Fine A. 2008. The prolonged life-span of alveolar macrophages. Am J Resp Cell Mol Biol, 38(4): 380–385.

Najafi N, Demanet C, Dab I, De Waele M, and Malfroot A. 2003. Differential cytology of bronchoalveolar lavage fluid in asthmatic children. Ped Pulmonol, 35(4): 302–308.

Pickles K, Pirie RS, Rhind S, Dixon PM, and McGorum BC. 2002. Cytological analysis of equine bronchoalveolar lavage fluid. Part 2: Comparison of smear and cytocentrifuged preparations. Equine Vet J, 34(3): 292–296.

Pickles K, Pirie RS, Rhind S, Dixon PM, and McGorum BC. 2002. Cytological analysis of equine bronchoalveolar lavage fluid. Part 3: The effect of time, temperature and fixatives. Equine Vet J, 34(3): 297–301.

Pirie RS, Collie DD, Dixon PM, and McGorum BC. 2003. Inhaled endotoxin and organic dust particulates have synergistic proinflammatory effects in equine heaves (organic dust-induced asthma). Clin Exp Allergy, 33(5): 676–683.

Raidal SL, Taplin RH, Bailey GD, and Love DN. 1997. antibiotic prophylaxis of lower respiratory tract contamination in horses confined with head elevation for 24 or 48 hours. Aust Vet J, 75(2): 126–131.

Richard EA, Fortier GD, Lekeux PM, and Van Erck E. 2010. Laboratory findings in respiratory fluids of the poorly-performing horse. Vet J, 185 (2): 115–122.

Riihimaki M, Lilliehook I, Raine A, Berg M, and Pringle J. 2008. Clinical alterations and mRNA levels of IL-4 and IL-5 in bronchoalveolar cells of horses with transient pulmonary eosinophilia. Res Vete Sci, 85(1): 52–55.

Rossier Y, Sweeney CR, and Ziemer EL. 1991. Bronchoalveolar lavage fluid cytologic findings in horses with pneumonia or pleuropneumonia. J Am Vet Med Assoc, 198(6): 1001–1004.

Sanchez A, Couetil LL, Ward MP, and Clark SP. 2005. Effect of airway disease on blood gas exchange in racehorses. J Vet Intern Med/Am College Vet Intern Med, 19(1): 87–92.

Seals W. 1980. Tracheal wash as a way to diagnose equine respiratory infection. Vet Med, Small Animal 75 (12): 1893–1894.

Sweeney CR, Beech J, and Roby KA. 1985. Bacterial isolates from tracheobronchial aspirates of healthy horses. Am J Vet Res, 46(12): 2562–2565.

Tremblay GM, Ferland C, Lapointe JM, Vrins A, Lavoie JP, and Cormier Y. 1993. Effect of stabling on bronchoalveolar cells obtained from normal and COPD horses. Equine Vet J, 25(3): 194–197.

Vrins A, Doucet M, and Nunez-Ochoa L. 1991. A retrospective study of bronchoalveolar lavage cytology in horses with clinical findings of small airway disease. Zentralblatt Fur Veterinarmedizin Reihe A 38(6): 472–479.

West JB, Mathieu-Costello O, Jones JH, Birks EK, Logemann RB, Pascoe JR, and Tyler WS. 1993. Stress failure of pulmonary capillaries in racehorses with exercise-induced pulmonary hemorrhage. J Appl Physiol (Bethesda, MD: 1985), 75(3): 1097–1109.

Westermann CM, Laan TT, van Nieuwstadt RA, Bull S, and Fink-Gremmels J. 2005. Effects of antitussive agents administered before bronchoalveolar lavage in horses. Am J Vet Res, 66(8): 1420–1424.

Winther L, Andersen RM, Baptiste KE, Aalbæk B, and Guardabassi L. 2010. Association of *Stenotrophomonas maltophilia* infection with lower airway disease in the horse: a retrospective case series. Vet J, 186(3): 358–363.

Wood JL, Newton JR, Chanter N, and Mumford JA. 2005. Inflammatory airway disease, nasal discharge and respiratory infections in young British racehorses. Equine Vet J, 37(3): 236–242.

Woods KS, Defarges AM, Abrams-Ogg AC, Viel L, Brisson BA, and Bienzle D. 2014. Comparison of manual and suction pump aspiration techniques for performing bronchoalveolar lavage in 18 dogs with respiratory tract disease. J Vet Intern Med/Am College Vet Intern Med, 28(5): 1398–1404.

56

Pleural Fluid

Melissa Mazan

Cummings School of Veterinary Medicine, Tufts University, Massachusetts, USA

56.1   Introduction

There are a few points about the normal anatomy of the pleural space that are important to keep in mind. First, although the horse's mediastinum is considered to be fenestrated, those fenestrations often become plugged with fibrin when there is an inflammatory condition of the pleurae. This can be useful, as it makes bilateral pneumothorax less likely, but it also means that it is difficult and sometimes impossible to predict the cytologic or bacteriologic condition of one side of the chest by sampling the other side. Second, although the parietal pleura is supplied by the systemic vasculature as in most mammals, in animals with thick pleurae, such as the horse, pig, sheep, and perhaps human, the visceral pleura is supplied by the bronchial circulation, rather than the pulmonary circulation (Bouros, 2009). The functional significance of this is that thin-pleura species, such as dogs and cats, can rely on the lower-pressure visceral pleura absorbing increased fluid, whereas in horses, the lymph system must pick up the slack. This may explain the readiness with which horses develop parapneumonic effusions. Regardless of the vascular supply and drainage, pleural effusion develops when more fluid is produced than is absorbed, applying the Starling principles. The pleural vessels are normally somewhat "leakier" than other vessels, and with inflammation, they become even leakier, allowing protein to escape into the pleural space. The higher protein level causes a higher oncotic pressure in the pleural space, drawing yet more fluid into the pleural space.

56.2   Causes of Pleural Effusion

The pleural fluid is sampled when there is suspicion of a pleural effusion. Pleural effusion may be due to primary disease of the lungs, including pneumonia, abscess, or neoplasia, which secondarily affects the pleura, termed a parapneumonic effusion; or it may, rarely, be due to a primary pleural disease, such as hematogenous pleuritis or mesothelioma. By far the most common type of pleural effusion is infectious, that is parapneumonic effusion secondary to aspiration pneumonia (Mair, 1991). Rarely, an adult horse may have a chylous effusion. Other causes, which are uncommon, include hypoproteinemia, heart failure, or mediastinal mass. In the latter conditions, the pleural fluid should be sterile. Unlike fluid from the trachea, there is no commensal population of bacteria within the pleural fluid.

A parapneumonic effusion is most commonly suspected when a horse has an appropriate history (travel, general anesthesia, recent racing, recent viral infection) along with fever, cough, and apparent dyspnea. The diagnosis is made more solid when on auscultation the horse has normal or harsh lung sounds over the dorsal lung fields, and dull to absent lung sounds ventrally. Confirmation of pleural effusion is made easily with ultrasound.

56.3   Pleurocentesis

Although there are published references for blind centesis of the pleural space (7th to 8th rib spaces, approximately 4 cm above the costochondral junction, and avoiding the lateral thoracic vein), by far the best approach is under ultrasound guidance, looking for the most ventral fluid and avoiding the heart. If, on ultrasound, the fluid is loculated, it may be necessary to tap more than one area. The area to be tapped should be clipped and aseptically prepared. Local anesthesia is used to facilitate the tap. It helps to remember that the pleura itself is quite sensitive. A 14-gauge catheter can be used to obtain a sample without first placing a stab incision; if a teat cannula or chest tube is to be placed,

Interpretation of Equine Laboratory Diagnostics, First Edition. Edited by Nicola Pusterla and Jill Higgins.
© 2018 John Wiley & Sons, Inc. Published 2018 by John Wiley & Sons, Inc.

then a stab incision will be necessary. If there is a large amount of fluid in the chest, then there is little danger of stabbing the lung itself as long as a modicum of caution is used. It takes a bit of effort to get through the skin, subcutaneous tissue and intercostal muscle. The mediastinum of the horse is fenestrated but in most inflammatory effusions, the openings are plugged with fibrin, making it essentially non-fenestrated. Thus, both sides of the chest should be tapped if an inflammatory condition is suspected. An aliquot of the fluid should be placed in an EDTA (purple top) tube for cytology – failure to use an anti-coagulant will make it difficult to read the cytology if there is inflammation – and a further aliquot should be placed in a sterile container for culture. It would be reasonable to submit the pleural fluid for both anaerobic and aerobic culture, the former especially if there is a putrid smell. However, culture of the pleural fluid is no substitute for culture from a tracheal aspirate if a parapneumonic effusion is suspected.

56.4 Assessment of Pleural Fluid

56.4.1 Gross Appearance

Normal pleural fluid is light yellow, thin, and clear. If there is an infectious pleuritis the fluid may be a dark yellow or reddish brown in the case of vascular compromise, or rarely it may look like frank pus. Pleural fluid is often reddish with neoplastic lesions (rare) as well as with infection, but neoplastic lesions rarely have a putrid smell; the latter being associated with anaerobic infection. Hemorrhagic taps usually are red throughout the tap, whereas traumatic taps usually clear as the fluid continues to flow. Rarely, the fluid is greenish; in this case, if you are sure that you are in the pleural space, the most likely cause is intra-thoracic esophageal rupture or diaphragmatic hernia with inadvertent penetration of the entrapped gut. Even more rarely, the fluid may be thin and white, in which case a chylous effusion may be suspected; chylous effusions may also appear serous or sanguinous; the best distinguishing test is usually triglyceride levels (see below).

56.4.2 Cytology of the Pleural Fluid

The same principles that are used in making slides for BAL or TA apply for pleurocentesis, although with the usual higher cell count, it may not be necessary to centrifuge the sample. Pleural taps, even in the normal horse, are reported to have higher red cell counts than peritoneal fluid. If the cause of the effusion is hemorrhage, then there should be hemosiderophages in the fluid. Note, however, that if the fluid is left to stand, macrophages in the fluid may ingest red cells; however, there should not have been enough time for macrophages to process the hemoglobin and produce hemosiderin. It may be useful in this case to distinguish between erythrophagia and hemosiderophages. In contrast to humans, wherein >1000 cells/µl is abnormal (Karkhanis and Joshi 2012), horses may have up to 5000 cells/µl (Piviani, 2014). The cell population mostly comprises mature neutrophils (50–80%), thus unlike with joint fluid the mere predominance of neutrophils does not predict sepsis (Piviani, 2014). However, neutrophils in the normal pleural space should have tightly organized and sometimes pyknotic nuclei. Degenerate neutrophils raise the suspicion of infection and toxic neutrophils raise the suspicion of severe systemic disease (Piviani, 2014). As a caveat, however, as with BAL or TA samples, if the sample was left to languish too long before being submitted to the laboratory, the neutrophils may acquire a degenerate appearance. Acute inflammation usually results in a primarily neutrophilic cell population, whereas chronic inflammation may result in increased numbers of lymphocytes or macrophages. Increased numbers of lymphocytes may also be seen with chylous effusion. Mesothelial cells may also be seen, albeit rarely, in pleural fluid. It can be difficult to distinguish activated mesothelial cells from rare neoplastic cells; the diagnosis may require biopsy or immunohistochemical testing (Piviani, 2014). Large, immature lymphocytes may indicate lymphoma. If plant material or protozoa are seen, one should suspect intra-thoracic esophageal rupture (which may be spontaneous or more rarely, traumatic secondary to intubation with a nasogastric tube), accidental centesis of a viscus, or presence of gut in the thoracic cavity secondary to diaphragmatic hernia.

56.4.3 Biochemical Evaluation

Biochemical evaluation can be very useful in evaluating a pleural effusion. Protein measured by refractometer should be less than 2.5 g/dl. EDTA can raise protein levels when total solids are measured with a refractometer, especially when the EDTA tube is partially full. Since water soluble molecules easily diffuse into the pleural space, a horse that has high peripheral lactate will generally have a high lactate in the pleural space as well. In the face of an infection, the pleural space will have a high lactate (>2 mmol/l) regardless of the blood level due to lactate production by white cells and bacteria. Conversely, white cells and bacteria consume glucose, therefore a low glucose (<60 mg/dl) is generally associated with a septic pleuritis (Brumbaugh and Benson, 1990). In humans, effusions with a triglyceride level greater than 113 mg/dl are usually diagnostic for chylous (Maldonado et al., 2009).

56.4.4 Microbiology

As for BAL and TA, most microorganisms will stain dark blue with Dif Quik and a Gram stain will help even further with initial antimicrobial choice while awaiting culture results. Because pleuropneumonia is usually due to aspiration, in a positive sample you may find a mixed population of Gram-negative, Gram-positive, and anaerobic bacteria. (Figure 56.1).

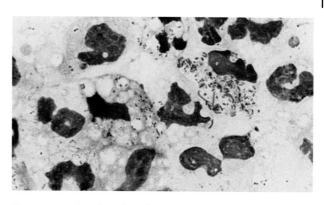

Figure 56.1 Pleural cytology from a horse with pleuropneumonia secondary to esophageal obstruction. Note the degenerate appearance of the neutrophils as well as a mixed population of intracellular bacteria.

References

Bouros D. 2009. *Pleural Disease*. Boca Raton, FL: CRC Press.

Brumbaugh GW and Benson PA. 1990. Partial pressures of oxygen and carbon dioxide, pH, and concentrations of bicarbonate, lactate, and glucose in pleural fluid from horses. Am J Vet Res, 51(7): 1032–1037.

Karkhanis VS and Joshi IM. 2012. Pleural effusion: diagnosis, treatment, and management. Open Access Emerg Med, 4: 31–52.

Mair T. 1991. Treatment and complications of pleuropneumonia. Equine Vet J, 23(1): 5.

Maldonado F, Hawkins FJ, Daniels CE, Doerr CH, Decker PA, and Ryu JH. 2009. Pleural fluid characteristics of chylothorax. Mayo Clinic Proc, 84(2): 129–133.

Piviani M. 2014. Cytology of the lower respiratory tract. In R Walton (ed.), *Equine Clinical Pathology*, Ames, Iowa: Wiley Blackwell, pp. 233–251.

57

Urine Analysis
Leslie Sharkey

Department of Veterinary Clinical Sciences, College of Veterinary Medicine, University of Minnesota, Minnesota, USA

57.1 Introduction

Urinalysis is considered part of the minimum laboratory database and ideally should be performed simultaneously with the CBC and serum biochemical profile prior to any treatment for the initial diagnostic evaluation. The method of collection, usually free catch or via urinary catheter in horses, should be noted because it can be relevant to interpretation. Interpretation of urinalysis data should be in the context of the history, presenting clinical signs and physical examination findings, and should be integrated with the other laboratory data. In particular, historical information should include any changes in fluid intake or in the volume of urine produced, and any observations about changes in behavior related to urination such as straining or increased/decreased frequency. A complete treatment history is critical, including any fluid therapy, treatment with diuretics, and any potentially nephrotoxic medications such as nonsteroidal anti-inflammatories or antibiotics. Particularly pertinent physical examination findings include hydration and perfusion status (tacky mucous membranes, capillary refill time, mucous membrane color, sunken eyes, pulse quality), the presence of dental tartar that can be associated with chronic renal insufficiency, body condition, and any abnormalities of the upper or lower urinary tract identified on physical examination or imaging studies. Urine samples should be submitted and analyzed as rapidly as possible after collection because of the potential for degradation of cellular elements and overgrowth of bacteria. Microscopy in particular should be performed within a few hours if feasible.

57.2 Gross Evaluation

Color and clarity are the two most notable features of the gross evaluation. Normal fresh equine urine is light to dark yellow and clear to cloudy. The cloudiness is due to the presence of mucus and calcium carbonate crystals. *In vitro* oxidation of some plant compounds eliminated in urine can lead to orange or red discoloration, illustrating the importance of examination of fresh specimens (Savage, 2008). Red or brown freshly voided urine indicates the presence of hematuria or pigmenturia. Urine should be examined for the presence of blood clots, and blood in the urine usually results in increased turbidity, except for cases in which erythrocytes have lysed in the urine. Hematuria can be distinguished from pigmenturia because centrifugation should clear the red blood cells in urine and result in formation of cell pellets, however, if hemolysis has occurred in the urine, microscopic evaluation for the presence of red cell ghosts (lysed cellular membrane remnants) may be required. Hematuria can originate in any segment of the urogenital tract due to a variety of underlying inflammatory, infectious, and neoplastic conditions, urolithiasis, or occasionally because of idiopathic renal hematuria best documented in Arabians (Schumacher, 2007, Vits, 2008). Hematuria can be severe enough to cause clinically significant anemia.

Pathologic pigmenturia is most often associated with hemoglobinuria, myoglobinuria or bilirubinemia. Hemoglobinuria is associated with hemolysis, so evaluation of a complete blood count including examination of the plasma for hemolysis and careful microscopic evaluation of red cell morphology for suggestive abnormalities (ghost cells, eccentrocytes, Heinz bodies, schistocytes) is required for confirmation; ghost cells are not expected to be present in the urine with hemoglobinuria. Clinical signs and physical examination findings supportive of anemia are likely to be present. Myoglobinuria also leads to discoloration of urine. Clinical signs of myopathy as well as moderate to marked increases in serum creatine kinase and AST activity are expected. The degree of pigmenturia will diminish as myoglobin is cleared after an acute episode (Figure 57.1). Pigmenturia can interfere with dipstick analysis when sufficiently severe.

Interpretation of Equine Laboratory Diagnostics, First Edition. Edited by Nicola Pusterla and Jill Higgins.
© 2018 John Wiley & Sons, Inc. Published 2018 by John Wiley & Sons, Inc.

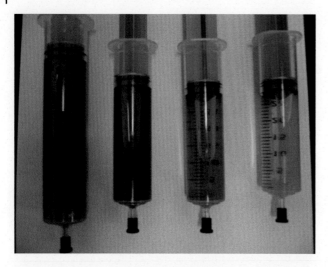

Figure 57.1 Urine with clearing myoglobin after an acute episode of myopathy. The urine was collected on the day of presentation and the subsequent 3 days of hospitalization (left to right).

Pigmenturia can also be associated with non-pathologic conditions including the administration of drugs (rifampin, phenothiazine, nitazoxanide, doxycycline) and ingestion of certain plants.

57.3 Chemical Evaluation

57.3.1 Urine Specific Gravity

Urine specific gravity measurement should be performed using a well maintained and calibrated refractometer; dipstick values can be unreliable. Depending on recent activity, water intake, and hydration status, healthy horses can have a wide range of urine specific gravity values. Values between 1.008 and 1.014 are considered isosthenuric with plasma. Values below that range can be normal or associated with disease processes that increase water intake or interfere with the action of anti-diuretic hormone on renal tubules. Normal horses should be able to concentrate their urine to a specific gravity of >1.030 in response to physiologic need, so values between isosthenuria and 1.030 can be interpreted as "inappropriate" and concerning for decreased renal tubular function in dehydrated or azotemic horses. Fluid therapy and diuretics can reduce renal concentrating ability, and glucosuria and ketonuria can result in osmotic diuresis. The presence of large amounts of protein and glucose can increase the urine specific gravity, occasionally misrepresenting renal concentrating ability.

57.3.2 Dipstick Evaluation

While useful, dipstick evaluation can be negatively impacted by several factors. The use of inappropriately stored or out of date strips predispose to erroneous results. Testing should be performed only on fresh urine that is at room temperature, and strips must be read within the specified time frames after application of urine. The use of discolored urine can bias results as well. Results are usually reported semiquantitatively as negative through 3 or 4 +.

- *Bilirubin* dipsticks preferentially measure conjugated bilirubin because of increased water solubility and renal excretion; increases are most often seen in horses with post-hepatic cholestasis.
- *Blood* is best evaluated by microscopic evaluation of the urine, so dipstick results should be verified with a complete urinalysis.
- *Glucose* in urine can be attributed to hyperglycemia exceeding the ability of the renal tubular reabsorption, in which case osmotic diuresis may reduce the urine specific gravity. Alternatively, if glucosuria is observed with relatively normal blood glucose concentrations, renal tubular dysfunction, typically acute tubular necrosis, should be considered.
- *Ketones* are rarely positive in equine urine, but could indicate metabolic stress.
- *pH* measured by dipstick should be considered a rough estimate, and a pH meter should be used if more accuracy is required. Normal equine urine is alkaline based on a forage diet; however, high grain diets can result in slightly acid to neutral urine. Aciduria can also reflect metabolic disorders.
- *Protein* is only estimated by the dipstick method, and a more quantitative protein:creatinine ratio should be performed if glomerular pathology is the suspected cause. Proteinuria is often classified in a similar manner to azotemia, using a pre-renal, renal, and post-renal scheme in which more than one source is possible in a patient. Proteinuria is classified as pre-renal if it is attributable to unusual amounts of protein in the plasma spilling over into the urine. This is most commonly observed with myopathy or gammopathies, although it can be transiently observed after colostrum ingestion in foals. Renal proteinuria is due to glomerular or tubular pathology. Glomerular pathology results in mild to severe proteinuria, and when sufficiently advanced, is often associated with hypoalbuminemia. In the early stages of glomerular disease, renal concentrating ability may be preserved and azotemia may be absent, while tubular disease is typically associated with inappropriately concentrated urine and azotemia. In contrast, tubular proteinuria is typically milder and does not often directly cause decreased serum albumin concentration. Post-renal proteinuria originates from disease distal to the kidney. Post-renal proteinuria due to hemorrhagic and inflammatory lesions should be excluded before a more extensive evaluation for glomerulopathies is undertaken. Clinicians should

keep in mind that the presence of one source of proteinuria does not exclude others, and serial evaluation after correction of pre-renal or post-renal sources may be required to exclude renal proteinuria in some cases.

57.3.3 Urine Protein: Creatinine Ratio

The urine protein:creatinine ratio can be used as a more quantitative assessment of proteinuria, although like dipstick protein analysis of urine, it does not localize the source of the protein. To normalize the protein excretion for the glomerular filtration rate, the concentration of protein is expressed proportionally to the urine creatinine concentration because creatinine is neither secreted nor reabosorbed. Because the high urinary concentration of creatinine and the low concentration of urine protein are often outside the linearity of assays developed for evaluation of serum, samples are sent to reference laboratories and should not be performed on in-clinic point of care analyzers. One relatively small study of horses and ponies observed minimal day to day variation and suggests that a value of <1 is likely normal (Uberti, 2009).

57.3.4 Urinary GGT

GGT is among a number of enzymes expressed by renal tubular epithelial cells that can be released into the urine with cell damage and thus measured diagnostically and is the most commonly utilized. Like protein, it is usually expressed as a ratio to creatinine, with values in healthy horses being less than 25 (Savage, 2008). Ratios of between 25 and 60 are equivocal, whereas values over 60 are interpreted to be indicative of renal tubular cell damage. Beyond 100, the degree of increase is not necessarily proportional to the extent or severity of cell damage, however, trends have prognostic value. See Box 6.3, Chapter 6 for a clinical case example.

57.3.5 Urinary Fractional Excretion of Electrolytes

The kidney is responsible for electrolyte and fluid balance, typically reabsorbing most of the filtered sodium and chloride, excreting excess potassium, and eliminating or retaining calcium and phosphorus depending on dietary intake and physiologic requirements. Fractional excretion is calculated in proportion to creatinine elimination, calculated using the following formula

$$FE_{electrolyte}(\%) = [electrolyte]_{urine} / [electrolyte]_{plasma} \times [Cr]_{plasma} / [Cr]_{urine} \times 100$$

As with most renal parameters, urinary fractional excretions should be performed using pre-treatment samples with special attention paid to a history of fluid or diuretic administration. Reference values are <1% for sodium, <1.7% for chloride, >25% for potassium, >2.5% for calcium, and <4% for phosphorus (Savage, 2008). Abnormal fractional excretions can suggest renal tubular dysfunction or dietary issues. However, one needs to keep in mind that fractional excretion should not be used in horses receiving polyionic fluids or sedated prior to urine collection.

57.4 Sediment Evaluation

It is important for clinicians to recognize that significant pathology can be identified in the urine sediment even when biochemical evaluation of the serum and urine is unremarkable, so a sediment examination is warranted for most or all initial diagnostic evaluations. Urine samples are typically concentrated for microscopic evaluation centrifuging a few milliliters of fresh mixed urine at 1500–2000 rpm for approximately 5 min. The supernatant is decanted, and then the cell pellet is re-suspended in the remaining urine by gentle agitation of the tube. A small volume of the concentrated sample is placed on a glass slide and a coverslip is used to spread the sample to an even thickness. The light is reduced to increase the refractivity for better viewing. Staining is not always necessary. For more detailed evaluation of the cellular elements of the sediment, cytology samples can be prepared from the concentrated samples using the same technique used for body cavity fluid samples. Smears are then dried and a Diff-Quik or Gram stain can be applied.

57.4.1 Cells

Erythrocytes, leukocytes, and epithelial cells are the most common cells identified in the sediment examination. These can be identified in wet preps without staining, however as noted above, better cell detail can be visualized using standard cytologic techniques in selected cases for evaluation of morphology. Cells do have a tendency to be poorly preserved in urine. Erythrocytes can be present due to hemorrhage or inflammation in any part of the urinary tract, normal urine typically has fewer than 5–10 red blood cells/high power field. The same is true of leukocytes, although with hemorrhage the ratio of erythrocytes to leukocytes is high, while with inflammation it is low. Epithelial cells should be observed for signs of atypia, which is most commonly associated with reactive changes secondary to inflammation, but neoplasia may be a consideration in some cases. Bacteria can also be visualized on wet preparations; however, Gram staining can improve identification and subclassification by morphology and staining characteristics that can be useful in preliminary antibiotic selection prior to the availability of urine culture results. Rarely, parasites or eggs can be identified in equine urine.

57.4.2 Casts

Casts are small cylindrical structures reflecting the aggregation of substances within the renal tubule, and thus reflect renal pathology. They can be comprised of protein, erythrocytes, leukocytes, and or sloughed renal tubular cells. Casts are unstable in urine, and are most likely to be identified in samples evaluated shortly after collection, especially since they have a particular tendency to dissolve in alkaline equine urine. They can also be shed in "showers" rather than at a constant rate, so evaluation of multiple samples may be required to identify casts.

57.4.3 Crystals

Horses frequently have variable numbers of calcium carbonate crystals in their urine, however calcium phosphate and calcium oxalate crystals may also be observed in healthy animals (Figure 57.2). Acidification

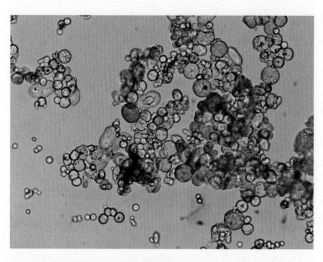

Figure 57.2 Calcium oxalate crystals in the urine of a healthy horse. Unstained direct wet preparation, 200×.

of the urine (2–10% acetic acid) can clear crystals to facilitate microscopic evaluation of other elements of the sediment. Pathologic equine urolithiasis is uncommon (Duesterdieck-Zellmer, 2007).

References

Duesterdieck-Zellmer KF. 2007. Equine urolithiasis. Vet Clin Equine, 23: 613–629.

Savage CJ. (2008) Urinary clinical pathologic findings and glomerular filtration rate in the horse. Vet Clin Equine, 24: 387–404.

Schumacher J. 2007. Hematuria and pigmenturia of horses. Vet Clin Equine, 23: 655–675.

Uberti B, Eberle B, Pressler BM, Moore GE, and Sojka JE. 2009. Determination of and correlation between urine protein excretion and urine protein-to-creatinine ratio values during a 24-hour period in healthy horses and ponies. Am J Vet Res, 70: 1551–1556.

Vits L, Araya O, Bustamante, Mohr F, and Galecio S. 2008. Idiopathic renal haematuria in a 15 year old Arabian mare. Vet Rec, 162: 251–252.

58

Synovial Fluid

Jorge Nieto and Jan Trela

Department of Surgical and Radiological Sciences, School of Veterinary Medicine, University of California, California, USA

58.1 Introduction

Synovial fluid (SF) is produced in tendon sheaths, bursas, and joints. Functions of synovial fluid include lubrication to reduce friction, as well as source of nutritional and regulatory factors for the articular cartilage. Synovial fluid is a filtrate of plasma through the synovial membrane where several macromolecules are secreted. The SF is normally a clear to pale yellow viscous fluid composed primarily of plasma filtrate, which is similar to blood plasma, except that it contains fewer proteins. The synovial membrane is a thin lining composed of tissue macrophage A cells, fibroblast-like B cells, and fenestrated capillaries (Steel, 2008). Underneath the synovial membrane lies the subsynovium (subintima), a thicker layer of loose connective tissue that contains an extensive system of lymphatics for clearance of transported molecules. The extracellular matrix of the synovium contains collagen and other molecules like hyaluronan (HA), glycosaminoglycans, and proteoglycans. The SF total protein concentration is approximately 25–35% of the plasma protein concentration of the horse.

Alterations in synoviocyte metabolism reflected by changes in joint fluid parameters may occur as a response to a variety of disease conditions. Evaluation of the SF can provide the clinician with valuable information that in conjunction with history, physical examination findings, ultrasonography, and radiography may assist in the diagnosis of those conditions.

The most common reason for analyzing synovial fluid in the horse is for suspected synovial contamination and infection. Analysis provides an indication of the degree of synovitis within the joint. Although differentiation in many cases is straightforward, it can be challenging in some patients because of the large variation in clinical sings and fluid alterations, including the high rate of false negative bacterial cultures results in clinically confirmed septic synovitis.

58.2 Sample Collection

Synovial fluid collection is performed by synoviocentesis and must be performed under strict aseptic conditions. Introduction of a needle through contaminated or infected skin may lead to infection in a sterile synovial cavity or contamination of septic structure with additional organisms. Although the reported risk of sepsis is low, that is, 0.08% after intraarticular injections (Steel et al., 2013) and 0.07% after elective arthroscopy (Borg and Carmalt, 2013), the consequences can be disastrous.

Synovial fluid sample without iatrogenic hemorrhage or contamination is necessary for accurate interpretation. The patient should be appropriately restrained. Proper help as well as sedation and in some cases local analgesia can be used to minimize patient movement. The site for aspiration should always be as far as possible from skin injuries (wounds) and areas of soft tissue swelling. This not only reduces the risk of blood contamination of the sample but also the risk of introducing bacteria to the synovial cavity from periarticular sites of infection.

Knowledge of all approaches for joint injection, including both dorsal and palmar/plantar pouches is essential. The use of ultrasound can assist to detect cellulitis, identify fluid (quantity and quality), and to collect synovial fluid under ultrasound guidance. After needle insertion, if fluid flows out through the needle it should be caught into the tube before any attempt is made to aspirate the fluid with a syringe. If suction is required it should be applied very gently using a small syringe (i.e., 3 mL). Aspirated fluid can be collected into an ethylenediamine tetraacetic acid (EDTA) blood collection tube for cytology and total protein analysis, red top tube or enrichment medium for culture and sensitivity, and a heparinized tube for chemical analysis.

In some cases, if there is not enough fluid for testing, a sample obtained following injection of sterile physiological fluid into the synovial cavity may provide some

Interpretation of Equine Laboratory Diagnostics, First Edition. Edited by Nicola Pusterla and Jill Higgins.

information (nucleated cell differential). Sterile 0.9% saline or lactated Ringer's solution can be injected into the synovial structure and then the fluid can be aspirated. This technique will dilute the synovial fluid and affect the clinicopathologic parameters however, because the urea concentration in synovial fluid normally mimics that in serum, the urea concentrations in synovial fluid and serum collected simultaneously can be compared to determine the degree of dilution (Gough et al., 2002); however, this is infrequently performed in practice.

After sample collection, the fluid often becomes gelatinous but doesn't clot. Gentle mixing of the sample returns it to its fluid state. This phenomenon is called thixotropy (Hlavacek, 2001). If there is blood contamination of the sample from hemarthrosis or iatrogenic causes, or a marked elevation of total protein concentration, the sample may actually clot. It is very important to immediately transfer the sample to a sterile tube containing anticoagulants.

58.3 Fluid Analysis

Complete analysis consists of a description of the gross appearance of the fluid, cytology (including total cell count and differential), total protein concentration, and biochemistry evaluation. In addition, Gram stain and aerobic and anaerobic cultures can also be performed if indicated.

The most accurate clinically important parameter for the diagnosis of septic synovial structures is cytology including total nucleated cell count and differential. When the volume of fluid obtained is limited, cytologic examination is the single most useful test.

Visual assessment of synovial fluid is useful and frequently accurate (Wright et al., 2003). Normal synovial fluid is transparent, clear to pale yellow, and highly viscous. It lacks fibrinogen and other clotting factors, which prevents it from clotting. Sanguineous fluid is not unusual and must be distinguished between iatrogenic hemorrhage at the time of collection and hemarthrosis where fluid is uniformly bloody. Chronic hemorrhage is characterized by dark yellow or yellow-orange discoloration that is called xanthochromia. It occurs due to the presence of hemoglobin breakdown pigments and is often associated with chronic traumatic arthritis.

Septic synovial fluid is usually turbid, cloudy and with decreased viscosity (Figure 58.1). Infection is strongly considered if the degree of turbidity prevents newspaper print to be read through the sample and the cell count is greater than 30,000/μL (Bertone, 1999). The color of septic synovial fluid varies from pale yellow to orange or red with bloody fluid being not unusual. The color of synovial

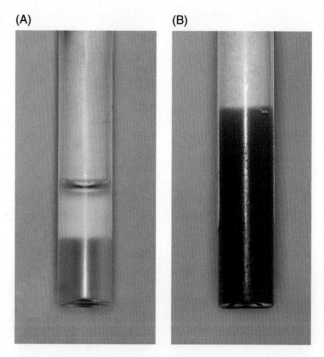

(A)   **(B)**

Figure 58.1 Synovial fluid collected from a horse with a dorsal carpal laceration. Fluid from the midcarpal joint (A) is cloudy yellow, with a total protein of 2.1 g/dL, good mucin clot, 2400 total nucleated cells/μL, and 60% neutrophils. Fluid from the radiocalrpal joint (B) is cloudy and pink, with a total protein of 5.3 g/dL, poor mucin clot, 86,800 total nucleated cells/μL, and 99% neutrophils. Samples were collected before antimicrobials were administered and bacterial cultures yielded no growth.

fluid by itself should not be used to diagnose sepsis by itself, since trauma around synovial structures can produce the presence of serosanguinous fluid.

If clinical signs are combined with risk factors such as history of recent joint injection or presence of a wound over a synovial structure immediate initiation of treatment is important. In these cases, if the gross appearance of the SF is consistent with sepsis, appropriate treatment including intravenous broad-spectrum antimicrobials and lavage, should be initiated before the diagnosis is confirmed with laboratory analysis (Steel, 2008). Viscosity is usually reduced with synovitis and is directly related to the quantity and degree of polymerization of HA (Persson, 1971). This implies inflammation but not necessarily infection. The lower viscosity of septic SF is attributable to a lower HA concentration and may also be the result of decreased HA synthesis (Hardy et al., 1998) and can be evaluated qualitatively during cytologic examination or subjectively by observing the length of the strand formed between the thumb and the index finger, with separation of the thumb and finger normally producing a string 4–5 cm long before breaking. Decreased stringing occurs with decreased viscosity.

Total protein concentration can easily be measured on a hand-held refractometer or by biochemical assays. Levels become elevated early (<24 h) in the pathogenesis and frequently exceed 4.0 g/dL in septic joints (Tulamo et al., 1989). However, in some cases levels may vary with ranges reported from 2.2–9.8 g/dL (Frees et al., 2002, Schneider et al., 1992, Wright et al., 2003). The reference total protein value for normal horses has been reported as 1.8 +/– 0.3 g/dL (RW 1974) and in general, a value less than 2.0 g/dL is considered normal (McIlwraith, 1980).

Total nucleated cell count rises early following microbial contamination and typically exceeds 30,000 cells/μL (Wright et al., 2003). Marked variation, however, has been reported from 1100–380,000 cells/μL (Frees et al., 2002, Lapointe et al., 1992, Schneider et al., 1992, Wright et al., 2003). Nucleated cell count can be measured manually using a microscope and hemocytometer, or by automated analyzer that dilutes the specimen in isotonic buffer. Fluid from a tendon sheath is similar to joint fluid with reference values reported as 200–3500 cells/μL (Malark et al., 1991). If there is a small number or low virulent bacteria in the sample the increase of the WBC count may be delayed. Therefore, if early infection is suspected, fluid evaluation can be repeated after 12–24 h. It must be recognized that repeat sampling may also cause increase in the nucleated cell count (Dykgraaf et al., 2007).

Cytologic examination is often the part of the analysis of synovial fluid that defines between septic and non-septic structure (Box 58.1). Fluid smears are prepared for differential cell counts in a similar way to peripheral blood smears. Initial examination of the smear should include subjective evaluation of cellularity and the number of erythrocytes follows by a thorough microscopic examination. Normal SF consists of synoviocytes, macrophages, and large mononuclear cells in addition to fewer small mononuclear cells or lymphocytes. Neutrophils usually constitute less than 10% and eosinophils 1% of the nucleated cells (McIlwraith, 1980). In contaminated or septic

synovial structures (Figure 58.2A and 58.2B) neutrophil count typically exceeds 80% (Schneider et al., 1992, Wright et al., 2003). Identification of microorganisms is uncommon, although positive identification on a gram stain provides an early guide to antimicrobial selection. However, identification of bacteria by Gram stains only occurs in approximately 25% of the cases with septic infection.

Biochemical evaluation of synovial fluid can be useful in the clinical diagnosis of synovial sepsis. Biochemical analysis of septic synovial fluid is supported by a pH < 6.9, lactate concentration > 4.9 mmol/L, and serum-synovial glucose differences > 39.6 mg/dL (2.2 mmol/L) (Dechant et al., 2011, Lloyd et al., 1990, Schneider et al., 1992, Tulamo et al., 1989).

(A)

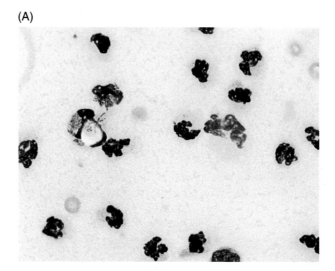

(B)

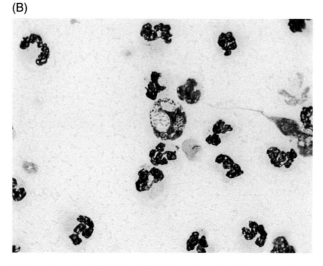

Figure 58.2 A and B. Synovial fluid sample (100×) from a tendon sheath showing increased cellularity with a pale pink finely stippled background and scattered erythrocytes. Neutrophils show moderate degeneration. Scattered neutrophils contain intracellular cocci and short rods. Rarely bacteria of similar morphology were also noted extracellularly. Source: Courtesy of Dr. Diana Schwartz.

Box 58.1 Cytological and biochemical values of normal and septic synovial fluid in adult horses.

	Normal	Septic Synovitis
Total leukocytes (/uL)	<300	>30,000
Neutrophils (%)	<10	>80
Total Protein (g/dL)	<2	>4
pH	7.39–7.53	<6.9
Lactate (mmol/L)	0.42–3.9	>4.9
Glucose	80–97	54
Serum/synovial glucose difference (mg/dL)	<39.6	>39.6

58.4   Diagnostic Imaging

Diagnostic imaging techniques are important in the diagnosis of synovial sepsis. Radiographs should be taken in all horses suspected to have synovial sepsis. Although bony lesions caused by sepsis may not be evident in the early stages, radiographs may show the presence of metallic foreign bodies or air in the synovial structure. Since synoviocentesis may allow the entrance of air, radiographs should be taken before fluid collection. Bone scintigraphy is highly specific and visualizes bony lesions earlier that radiographic methods; however, it is not a very specific method. In an effort to get an earlier diagnosis of septic bone in humans other scintigraphic methods are used, including 99mTc-labeled antibodies or antibody fragments, and leukocytes labeled *in vitro* with 99mTc-HMPAO (hexamethyl-propylene amine oxime) or 111In Oxine (8-hydroxyquinoline) (Sudol-Szopinska and Cwikla, 2013).

Ultrasonography allows evaluation of periarticular wounds, joint effusion, the quality of the synovial fluid, synovial inflammation, presence of foreign bodies, involvement of soft tissues and may assist with fluid collection (Figure 58.3). A recent retrospective study, reporting ultrasonographic findings in horses with confirmed septic synovial structures, found that 81% had marked effusion, 69% had moderate to severe synovial thickening, and in 55% the synovial fluid was echogenic (Beccati et al., 2015).

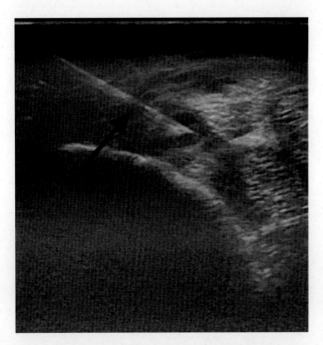

Figure 58.3 Ultrasonographic image of a septic proximal interphalangeal joint. The image shows slightly echogenic effusion within the dorsal recess of the joint with moderate synovial thickening. A 19G needle was inserted under ultrasound guidance and was used to collect synovial fluid. Source: Courtesy of Dr. Pablo Espinosa.

In humans, magnetic resonance imaging (MRI) is an important tool for evaluation of musculoskeletal infections and has been considered the gold standard for the diagnosis of human septic arthritis, osteomyelitis, and soft tissue infection (Graif et al., 1999). A recent study evaluating horses with septic arthritis by MRI found diffuse hyperintensity within bone and extracapsular tissue in 100% of the cases, joint effusion, synovial proliferation, and capsular thickening in 93%, bone sclerosis in 78%, and evidence of cartilage and subchondral bone damage in 57% (Easley et al., 2011). The authors have found standing MRI a very useful tool in the diagnosis of septic synovial structures in horses with nail penetrations in the hoof.

58.5   Polymerase Chain Reaction (PCR)

Since the reported success rate for a positive culture from synovial fluid is highly variable, detection of bacteria by PCR has been evaluated in vitro and in clinical cases (Crabill et al., 1996, Elmas et al., 2013, Pille et al., 2004, 2007). Synovial fluid was inoculated with different bacteria ranging in quantity from 1 to 1,000 colony forming units per milliliter (Crabill et al., 1996). In that study, PCR was able to detect bacteria by PCR in all inoculated samples but was unable to detect bacteria in bacteria-free control synovial fluid samples. A recent study in clinical cases compared a universal bacterial real-time PCR assay with bacterial culture (Elmas et al., 2013). The study found a higher sensitivity (87 vs 72%) but lower specificity (56 vs 86%) of a universal bacterial real-time PCR assay compared to bacterial culture. Due to the quick turn-around-time (approximately 4 h) and the high analytical sensitivity, PCR may assist in the early diagnosis and improve outcome in horses with septic synovitis.

58.6   Bacterial Culture and Sensitivity

The most common microorganisms cultured from septic synovial structures are aerobic or facultative anaerobes; and the most common genus of bacteria is *Enterobacteriacea* followed by *Streptococcus* and *Staphylococcus* (Moore et al., 1992). Although the gold standard for the diagnosis of septic synovitis is a positive bacterial culture from the synovial fluid, absence of bacterial growth is a common finding. Therefore, a negative culture does not preclude a diagnosis of septic synovitis. The range of successful bacterial cultures has been reported to range from 22 to 74% (Honnas et al., 1992, Lavoie et al., 1991, Madison et al., 1991, Schneider et al., 1992). Factors that may influence the outcome of a positive culture include the number of bacteria, phagocytized microorganisms, sequestration of bacteria in the synovial membranes, bactericidal qualities of the synovial fluid, and previous administration of antimicrobials. Culture of synovial membranes in addition to synovial fluid increases the likelihood of a positive bacterial culture. However, culturing of synovial fluid yielded bacterial growth more often than did culturing of synovial membrane (Madison et al., 1991). It has been shown in horses with septic synovitis that the use of blood culture enrichment medium is superior for isolation of bacteria to direct agar culture or agar culture after conventional enrichment (Dumoulin et al., 2010). The addition of resins and/or sodium polyanethole sulfonate to blood culture media may increase the bacterial growth by absorbing antimicrobials and inactivating growth inhibitors (Rohner et al., 1997).

58.7   Osteoarthritis Biomarkers

Diseases affecting joints are a major cause of chronic disability in horses. Researchers have attempted to find a biomarker of osteoarthritis in blood and synovial fluid by using in vitro and *in vivo* models. However, osteoarthritis is a progressive disease and the ideal single marker has not been identified. More recently researchers have investigated degradative and inflammatory events in both naturally occurring and experimental models of osteoarthritis (De Grauw 2011). Although there are exciting prospects relating to biomarkers for equine musculoskeletal diseases there is still considerable work to do before a clinical useful biomarker panel is available.

References

Beccati F, Gialletti R, Passamonti F, Nannarone S, Di Meo A. and Pepe M. 2015. Ultrasonographic findings in 38 horses with septic arthritis/tenosynovitis. Vet Radiol Ultrasound, 56: 68–76.

Bertone AL. 1999. Update on infectious arthritis in horses. Equine Vet Edu, 11: 143–152.

Borg H and Carmalt JL. 2013. Postoperative septic arthritis after elective equine arthroscopy without antimicrobial prophylaxis. Vet Surg, 42: 262–266.

Crabill MR, Cohen ND, Martin LJ, Simpson RB, and Burney N. 1996. Detection of bacteria in equine synovial fluid by use of the polymerase chain reaction. Vet Surg, 25: 195–198.

De Grauw JC. 2011. Molecular monitoring of equine joint homeostasis. Vet Q, 31: 77–86.

Dechant JE, Symm WA, and Nieto JE. 2011. Comparison of pH, lactate, and glucose analysis of equine synovial fluid using a portable clinical analyzer with a bench-top blood gas analyzer. Vet Surg, 40: 811–816.

Dumoulin M, Pille F, Van Den Abeele AM, Boyen F, Boussauw B, Oosterlinck M, et al. 2010. Use of blood culture medium enrichment for synovial fluid culture in horses: a comparison of different culture methods. Equine Vet J, 42: 541–546.

Dykgraaf S, Dechant J.E, Johns JL, Christopher MM, Bolt DM, and Snyder JR. 2007. Effect of intrathecal amikacin administration and repeated centesis on digital flexor tendon sheath synovial fluid in horses. Vet Surg, 36: 57–63.

Easley JT, Brokken MT, Zubrod CJ, Morton AJ, Garrett KS, and Holmes, SP. 2011. Magnetic resonance imaging findings in horses with septic arthritis. Vet Radiol Ultrasound, 52: 402–408.

Elmas CR, Koenig JB, Bienzle D, Cribb NC, Cernicchiaro N, Cote NM, and Weese JS. 2013. Evaluation of a broad range real-time polymerase chain reaction (RT-PCR) assay for the diagnosis of septic synovitis in horses. Can J Vet Res, 77: 211–217.

Frees KE, Lillich JD, Gaughan EM, and Debowes RM. 2002. Tenoscopic-assisted treatment of open digital flexor tendon sheath injuries in horses: 20 cases (1992–2001). J Am Vet Med Assoc, 220: 1823–1827.

Gough MR, Munroe GA, and Mayhew G. 2002. Urea as a measure of dilution of equine synovial fluid. Equine Vet J, 34: 76–79.

Graif M, Schweitzer ME, Deely D, and Matteucci T. 1999. The septic versus nonseptic inflamed joint: MRI characteristics. Skeletal Radiol, 28: 616–620.

Hardy J, Bertone AL, and Malemud, CJ. 1998. Effect of synovial membrane infection in vitro on equine synoviocytes and chondrocytes. Am J Vet Res, 59: 293–299.

Hlavacek M. 2001. The thixotropic effect of the synovial fluid in squeeze-film lubrication of the human hip joint. Biorheology, 38: 319–334.

Honnas CM, Welch RD, Ford TS, Vacek JR, and Watkins JP. 1992. Septic arthritis of the distal interphalangeal joint in 12 horses. Vet Surg, 21: 261–268.

Lapointe JM, Laverty S, and Lavoie JP. 1992. Septic arthritis in 15 standardbred racehorses after intra-articular injection. Equine Vet J, 24: 430–434.

Lavoie JP, Couture L, Higgins R, and Laverty S. 1991. Aerobic bacterial isolates in horses in a university hospital, 1986–1988. Can Vet J, 32: 292–294.

Lloyd KC, Stover SM, Pascoe JR, and Adams P. 1990. Synovial fluid pH, cytologic characteristics, and gentamicin concentration after intra-articular administration of the drug in an experimental model of infectious arthritis in horses. Am J Vet Res, 51: 1363–1369.

Madison JB, Sommer M, and Spencer PA. 1991. Relations among synovial membrane histopathologic findings, synovial fluid cytologic findings, and bacterial culture results in horses with suspected infectious arthritis: 64 cases (1979–1987). J Am Vet Med Assoc, 198: 1655–1661.

Malark JA, Nixon AJ, Skinner KL, and Mohammed H. 1991. Characteristics of digital flexor tendon sheath fluid from clinically normal horses. Am J Vet Res, 52: 1292–1294.

McIlwraith CW. 1980. Synovial fluid analysis in the diagnosis of equine joint disease. Equine Practice, 2: 44–48.

Moore RM, Schneider RK, Kowalski J, Bramlage LR, Mecklenburg LM, and Kohn CW. 1992. Antimicrobial susceptibility of bacterial isolates from 233 horses with musculoskeletal infection during 1979–1989. Equine Vet J, 24: 450–456.

Persson L. 1971. On the synovia in horses. A clinical and experimental study. Acta Vet Scand Suppl, Suppl 35: 3–77.

Pille F, Martens A, Schouls LM, Dewulf J, Decostere A, Vogelaers D, and Gasthuys F. 2007. Broad range 16S rRNA gene PCR compared to bacterial culture to confirm presumed synovial infection in horses. Vet J, 173: 73–78.

Pille F, Martens A, Schouls LM, Peelman L, Gasthuys F, Schot CS, et al. 2004. Detection of bacterial DNA in synovial fluid from horses with infectious synovitis. Res Vet Sci, 77: 189–195.

Rohner P, Pepey B, and Auckenthaler R. 1997. Advantage of combining resin with lytic BACTEC blood culture media. J Clin Microbiol, 35: 2634–2638.

Van Pelt RW. 1974. Interpretation of synovial fluid findings in the horse. J Am Vet Med Assoc, 165: 91–95.

Schneider RK, Bramlage LR, Moore RM, Mecklenburg LM, Kohn CW, and Gabel AA. 1992. A retrospective study of 192 horses affected with septic arthritis/tenosynovitis. Equine Vet J, 24: 436–442.

Steel CM. 2008. Equine synovial fluid analysis. Vet Clin North Am Equine Pract, 24: 437–454, viii.

Steel CM, Pannirselvam RR, and Anderson GA. 2013. Risk of septic arthritis after intra-articular medication: a study of 16,624 injections in Thoroughbred racehorses. Aust Vet J, 91: 268–273.

Sudol-Szopinska I and Cwikla JB. 2013. Current imaging techniques in rheumatology: MRI, scintigraphy and PET. Pol J Radiol, 78: 48–56.

Tulamo RM, Bramlage LR, and Gabel AA. 1989. Sequential clinical and synovial fluid changes associated with acute infectious arthritis in the horse. Equine Vet J, 21: 325–331.

Wright IM, Smith MR, Humphrey DJ, Eaton-Evans TC, and Hillyer MH. 2003. Endoscopic surgery in the treatment of contaminated and infected synovial cavities. Equine Vet J, 35: 613–619.

59

Cerebrospinal Fluid

Monica Aleman

Department of Medicine and Epidemiology, School of Veterinary Medicine, University of California, California, USA

59.1 Introduction

Cerebrospinal fluid (CSF) is a transparent colorless and odorless ultrafiltrate from plasma. The major functions of CSF include providing physical support to neural structures, excretory actions, transport, and control of neurochemical environment of the central nervous system (Vernau et al., 2008). Cerebrospinal fluid is produced at the following sites:

- Choroidal by capillaries (filtration) and epithelium (secretion) of the choroid plexus in the lateral, third, and fourth ventricles of the brain
  - 60–70% production
  - Most produced at lateral and third ventricles
- Extrachoroidal by ependymal lining, pia mater, and leptomeningeal capillaries
  - 30–40% production

The rate of formation of CSF is continuous and varies among species but it has been estimated at 0.02–0.5 mL/min. Cerebrospinal fluid formation rate directly parallels the rate of sodium exchange. Therefore, formation is influenced by osmotic pressure in blood (e.g., altered CSF formation in cases of hyponatremia or hypernatremia). Certain drugs have been associated with increased (e.g., phenylephrine) or decreased (e.g., acetazolamide, furosemide, diazepam analogues, dopamine D_1 agonists, noradrenaline, omeprazole, serotonin agonists, vasopressin) CSF formation in other species but it is unknown if these drugs would have a similar effect in horses.

Before discussing the circulation of CSF, it is important to review the meninges. The meninges consists of three layers of connective tissue that line the entire CNS. The pachymeninx (thick fibrous layer) consists of the dura mater, and the leptomeninges (thin layers) consist of the arachnoid and pia mater. The dura mater is the most external layer attached to the skull and adjacent to the vertebral canal. The arachnoid and pia mater are the inner layers. The pia mater is lining the brain and spinal cord. Cerebrospinal fluid occupies and circulates the ventricular system of the brain, central canal of the spinal cord, and subarachnoid space (the space between the leptomeninges [arachnoid and pia mater]) of both, brain, and spinal cord.

Cerebrospinal circulation is mainly unidirectional from site of production to site of absorption. Circulation is promoted by continuous production of CSF, ciliary action of ventricular ependymal, respiratory, and vascular pulsations, and pressure gradient across the arachnoid villi. Its absorption occurs mainly at the arachnoid villi in the venous sinuses. CSF also gets absorbed in veins and lymphatics found around nerve roots and nerves at intervertebral foramina; and olfactory, optic, and vestibulocochlear nerves as they pass through the skull. Absorption of CSF is the primary mechanism of homeostasis to maintain intracranial cerebral pressure (ICP). The total volume of CSF is produced and absorbed about 3–5 times a day.

59.2 Cerebrospinal Fluid Collection

The collection of CSF from the subarachnoid space can be done at various sites. However, routine collection comprises the atlanto-occipital (AO or cerebellomedullary cisterna, or cisterna magna) and lumbosacral (LS) spaces (Mayhew, 1975). For a full description of the landmarks, the reader is referred to Mayhew's study listed here (1975). More recently, CSF centesis has been described at the space between C1 and C2 vertebrae through a dorso-ventro-lateral approach (Pease et al., 2012). All three approaches can be performed under general anesthesia, while C1-C2 and LS approaches can

Interpretation of Equine Laboratory Diagnostics, First Edition. Edited by Nicola Pusterla and Jill Higgins.
© 2018 John Wiley & Sons, Inc. Published 2018 by John Wiley & Sons, Inc.

also be done under sedation. It is beyond the scope of this text to discuss protocols for anesthesia and/or sedation for CSF collection. Ultrasound-guided standing AO centesis under sedation has been reported but there is a risk of injuring the spinal cord and even caudal brainstem if the horse moves as centesis is being performed. Caution must be practiced while performing CSF centesis regardless of anatomical site. Ultrasound-guided or assisted techniques have been described for all three sites of CSF collection. Ultrasound can be particularly helpful in horses with abnormal anatomy or variable conformation.

Site of collection is going to depend on several factors; such as neuroanatomical localization (AO centesis preferred for suspected brain disease versus LS centesis for disease of the cauda equina), patient's temperament, safety, and financial concerns. Whenever possible, it is recommended to collect CSF as close to lesion location. Volume of CSF collected can depend on various factors and site of collection from a few to several milliliters. Collection of CSF can be done in a syringe or vacutainer tube with no anticoagulant because this will dilute the CSF, and in most cases CSF will not clot unless there is hemorrhage or high protein concentration. In hospitals with no laboratory or in the field situation, 1–2 mL could be collected in a vacutainer with EDTA for cytologic analysis if there is a suspected risk of CSF clotting (grossly abnormal and opaque). Save CSF with no anticoagulant for other tests (such as microbial culture, see next sections). Cytologic analysis must be performed as soon as possible shortly after collection to avoid cell degeneration, activation of monocytes in the collection device, clotting, and alteration of biochemical parameters (e.g., glucose, potassium). In the field situation, transportation of CSF on ice to the closest laboratory is acceptable. Alternatively, a small volume of CSF can be spin down and the pellet resuspended in 1–2 drops of plasma and do smears for cytologic evaluation. It is important to mention that CSF must not be frozen for cytologic evaluation. For all other tests, CSF can be frozen until further processing.

59.3 Cerebrospinal Fluid Constitution

Certain CSF parameters might vary depending on the site of collection. For example, the content of protein will be slightly higher if CSF is collected from the lumbosacral space compared to the atlanto-occipital space in normal individuals due to cranial to caudal flow of CSF (Andrews et al., 1990). Age can have an effect in CSF protein concentration (Andrews et al., 1994, Furr and

Bender, 1994). Neonatal foals tend to have a higher concentration of protein in CSF than non-neonatal foals and older animals due to a more permeable blood brain barrier and blood-CSF barrier (Furr and Bender, 1994). Neonatal foals also have higher creatine kinase concentrations than non-neonatal and adult horses but values fall towards adult values by 40 h after birth (Furr and Bender, 1994). The biochemical constitution of CSF is addressed in following sections.

59.4 Cerebrospinal Fluid Analysis/Interpretation

Analysis of CSF often provides evidence of presence of disease; however, cytological alterations might not be specific for particular disorders. Occasionally, CSF analysis can provide a definitive diagnosis (e.g., bacterial meningitis, *Cryptococcus neoformans*, rarely parasites, some cases of lymphoma and melanoma). This should not be a reason for not performing CSF analysis. Identifying abnormalities in CSF can be associated to type, location, severity, and duration of disease. Meningeal and paraventricular diseases (e.g., meningitis) can produce greater abnormalities in CSF than parenchymal disease. Previous or concurrent therapy might also affect cytological findings. It is important to mention that a normal CSF does not rule out abnormality of the CNS.

59.4.1 Color

Normal CSF is transparent, colorless, and has a viscosity similar to water (Figure 59.1A). The CSF specific gravity is 1.004–1.008, and refractive index is 1.3343–1.3349. Discolored CSF could be due to presence of increased number of cells (e.g., meningitis), cellular breakdown products (e.g., hemoglobin, bilirubin), or presence of blood (Figure 59.1). Discolored CSF, often red/pink, orange, or yellow, is called xanthochromic (Greek: xanthos = yellow). If red, a distinction between pathologic (e.g., trauma, vasculitis, CNS hemorrhage) versus iatrogenic (e.g., centesis) hemorrhage must be made. Centrifugation of an aliquot of CSF could aid in the distinction. A xanthochromic supernatant supports pathologic hemorrhage versus a colorless supernatant suggests blood contamination.

Presence of bilirubin gives a marked yellow color. Presence of bilirubin could be due to erythrocyte breakdown from previous hemorrhage or by the crossing of unconjugated bilirubin of the blood brain barrier (BBB) in cases of markedly elevated serum bilirubin. In damaged BBB, both conjugated and unconjugated bilirubin can cross this barrier.

(A)

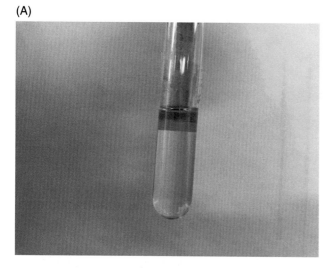

(B)

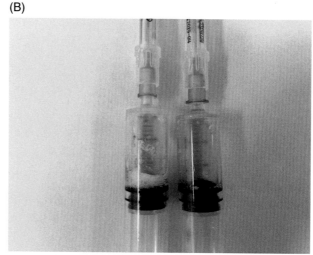

Figure 59.1 Cerebrospinal fluid. Xanthochromic transparent CSF from a horse with herpesvirus myeloencephalopathy (A); Xanthochromic cloudy opaque CSF from a horse with bacterial meningitis (B).

Cloudy yellow to green discoloration can be seen in cases of bacterial meningitis on which the total nucleated cell count is high due to increased neutrophils. Black CSF supports presence of melanin (e.g., melanoma). Cloudy CSF is seen when the number of total nucleated cells are elevated at approximately above 500 cells/µL. Turbid fluid can also be observed with the presence of fat. It is important to make the distinction (cytology: lipid).

59.4.2 Protein Concentration

Protein concentration in CSF is substantially less than in any other body fluid. Therefore, it cannot be measured by refractometry (measurement in g/dL). Several methods of protein quantification in mg/dL have been reported such as turbidimetry, biuret procedures, Lowry's method, Coomassie brilliant blue, Ponceau S red, and Pyrogallol red (Vernau et al., 2008). Reference ranges must be determined by the diagnostic laboratory. Total protein (TP) concentration in healthy adult horses has been reported to have a wide range from 29 mg/dL to 170 mg/dL. Most references support that TP concentration should not exceed 100 mg/dL (Mayhew et al., 1997). It is the experience of the author that healthy adult horses usually do not have TP exceeding 80 mg/dL regardless of site of collection. Protein concentrations in healthy neonatal foals usually do not exceed 100–120 mg/dL (Furr and Bender, 1994, Rossdale et al., 1982) but higher concentrations have also been reported (up to 210 mg/dL).

Almost all proteins in CSF are derived from serum. Exceptions include transthyretin (prealbumin), transferrin, beta and gamma trace proteins, tau protein, glial fibrillary acidic protein, and myelin basic protein (Vernau et al., 2008). Serum proteins with a high molecular weight (160,000 daltons or more) are usually not present in CSF, unless the BBB is not intact. A number of techniques have been used for fractionation of CSF proteins. Two methods used for the determination of albumin and immunoglobulins include high resolution protein electrophoresis and nephelometry (fast and requires < 1 mL of CSF). The major protein in CSF is albumin which is only synthesized by the liver. Immunoelectrophoresis can determine alpha, beta, and gamma globulin fractions in CSF. The gamma globulin fraction contains immunoglobulins IgG, IgM, IgA, and others. The major immunoglobulin in CSF is IgG which originates from serum. In inflammatory disease processes, the gamma globulin fraction is increased due to disrupted BBB or intrathecal production. During early stages of disease, IgM is the first immunoglobulin to be detected and the first to return to baseline values once the antigenic stimulation disappears. This is the basis for the diagnosis of some serologic and CSF tests (e.g., West Nile virus infection and other encephalitis). In cases of increased total protein concentration, electrophoresis and immunoelectrophoresis might aid in the diagnosis of an infectious or inflammatory (polyclonal gammopathy) versus a neoplastic (usually monoclonal gammopathy) process. It is important to emphasize that reference values must be determined for individual diagnostic laboratories (different methods used, Table 59.1).

Increased protein concentration with normal total nucleated cell count is known as albuminocytological dissociation and can occur with various diseases including extradural compressive lesions, spinal cord disease, ischemic events, trauma, vasculitis, and any CNS disease resulting in intrathecal globulin production.

Table 59.1 Protein content in CSF for atlanto-occipital (AO) and lumbosacral (LS) spaces for adults and neonatal foals reported by several authors (Andrews et al., 1990, 1994, Kirk et al., 1974, Kristensen et al., 1977).

Parameter	Adults				Neonatal foals		
	Kirk et al. 1974	Kristensen, Firth 1977	Andrews et al. 1990	Andrews et al. 1990	Andrews et al. 1994	Andrews et al. 1994	Unit
	AO	AO	AO	LS	AO	LS	
Total Protein	40.1 ± 3.1		87 ± 17	93 ± 16	82.8 ± 19.2	83.6 ± 16.1	mg/dL
Albumin	15.3 ± 1.2	43.4 ± 6.8	35.8 ± 9.7	37.8 ± 11.2	52 ± 8.6	53.8 ± 15.7	mg/dL
Albumin quotient			1.4 ± 0.4	1.5 ± 0.4	1.86 ± 0.29	1.85 ± 0.51	
Globulins							mg/dL
Alpha1	5.2 ± 0.9	5.3 ± 1.3					mg/dL
Alpha2	6.7 ± 0.4						mg/dL
Alpha2a		3.3 ± 0.8					mg/dL
Alpha2bc		6.4 ± 1.8					mg/dL
Beta	5.8 ± 0.6						mg/dL
Beta1		17 ± 3.2					mg/dL
Beta2		7.8 ± 2.3					mg/dL
Gamma	5.7 ± 0.8	14.8 ± 3.3					mg/dL
IgG			5.6 ± 1.4	6 ± 2.1	10.2 ± 5.5	9.9 ± 5.7	mg/dL
IgG index			0.19 ± 0.046	0.194 ± 0.05	$0.519 + 0.284$	$0.482 + 0.27$	

59.4.3 Albumin Quotient

Albumin quotient (AQ, Table 59.1), also known as albumin index, is a ratio of CSF to serum albumin used as an indicator of barrier dysfunction (blood brain/CSF barrier) in the absence of pathologic or iatrogenic hemorrhage (Andrews et al., 1994). Values above reference range (see Table 59.1) support increased permeability. The formula to calculate albumin quotient is as follows:

$$\text{Albumin quotient} = \frac{\text{CSFAlbumin (mg/dL)}}{\text{SerumAlbumin (mg/dL)}} \times 100$$

59.4.4 IgG Index

IgG index is a ratio of CSF to serum IgG (Table 59.1). However, since IgG can originate intrathecally or from serum; calculation of this ratio to determine blood brain/CSF barrier dysfunction solely based on IgG might not be accurate. Since albumin is solely produced extrathecally (liver), adding albumin (serum, CSF) into the calculation of IgG index improves demonstration of intrathecal IgG synthesis (Andrews et al., 1994). Hemorrhage will affect accurate determination of intrathecal IgG. An IgG index > 1 might support intrathecal IgG production. For diagnostic uses of albumin quotient and IgG index in the

interpretation of antibody titers for equine protozoal myelitis (EPM), the reader is referred to appropriate section in this book.

$$\text{IgGindex} = \frac{\text{CSF}_{\text{IgG}} \text{ (mg/dL)}}{\text{Serum}_{\text{IgG}} \text{ (mg/dL)}} \times \frac{\text{Serum}_{\text{Albumin}} \text{ (mg/dL)}}{\text{CSF}_{\text{Albumin}} \text{ (mg/dL)}}$$

59.4.5 Cytology

Erythrocytes (RBC). Normal CSF does not contain erythrocytes. Blood contamination, either from disrupted BBB or iatrogenia, can affect CSF cytological findings and interpretation particularly antibody testing. For example, as few as 8 RBC/μL are enough to alter Western blot interpretation for *Sarcocystis neurona* (Miller et al., 1999). This is in contrast to no detectable effect on immunofluorescent antibody test at any serologic titer for *S. neurona* and *Neospora hughesi* when RBC are lower than 10,000/μL (Finno et al., 2007). However, RBC of > 10,000/μL had an effect on CSF for both pathogens when the corresponding titers were > 160 and > 80 for *S. neurona and N. hughesi*, respectively (Finno et al., 2007). If blood contamination is encountered, when possible (safety, patient cooperation, and "do no harm" principle) sequential aspirates are collected gently to reduce the amount of RBC in the CSF before submission

Figure 59.2 Blood contamination of LS CSF. Note sequential aspirates until CSF became as clear as possible.

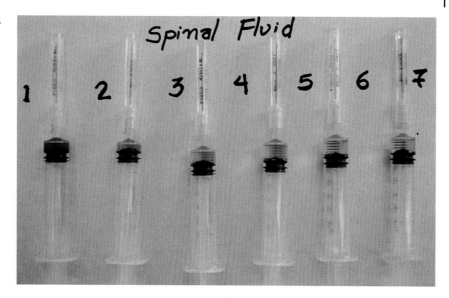

(Figure 59.2). The presence of erythrophagia, hemosiderophages (Prussian blue stains for iron [iron is derived from metabolized hemoglobin]), or hematoidin crystals (bilirubin products) supports hemorrhage not associated with CSF centesis. The presence of platelets and/or absence of erythrophagia or erythrocyte breakdown products supports iatrogenic blood contamination. If the CSF is pink in color, presence of blood should be suspected but a specific number of RBCs to give a pink coloration to CSF in horses is unknown and could be inaccurate.

Correction formulas for the estimation of leukocytes count and protein concentration for the effect of blood contamination in CSF have been used. It has been estimated in other species, that about 500–700 RBC/μL would contribute to 1 leukocyte/μL, and approximately 1000 RBC/μL would increase TP by 1 mg/dL. These guidelines should be interpreted with caution. Correction formula for leukocytes:

$$\text{White cells} = \text{WBC}_{\text{CSF}} - \frac{\text{WBC}_{\text{Blood}} \times \text{RBC}_{\text{CSF}}}{\text{RBC}_{\text{Blood}}}$$

Total nucleated cell count (TNCC). Total nucleated cell count has been reported to be < 5/μL for healthy foals and adults with one report of up to 6 cells/μL (Furr and Bender, 1994, Mayhew et al., 1977). It is the author's experience that TNCC is usually <3/μL for healthy foals and adults. An increased in TNCC is called pleocytosis and considered abnormal. There are no or rare neutrophils in normal CSF. Normal CSF TNCC consist of varying proportions of lymphocytes and monocytes. The proportion of lymphocytes has been reported to vary from 70–90% and monocytes from 10–30%. Eosinophils and plasma cells are not present in normal CSF. Pleocytosis could be neutrophilic, lymphocytic, eosinophilic, or mixed (2 or more cell types increased) according to increased cell type. Examples of neutrophilic pleocytosis include bacterial and fungal meningitis (e.g., *Cryptococcus*), but could also be observed in acute phases of other neurologic diseases. Absence of pleocytosis in early stages of meningitis can occur and a second CSF centesis might be necessary. Repeat CSF can aid in the diagnosis and follow up of cases. Lymphocytic pleocytosis is also a non-specific finding since it could be present in active or resolving infection, immunemediated, or neoplastic disorders. However, lymphocytic pleocytosis is a common finding in viral diseases (e.g., herpesvirus myeloencephalitis). Eosinophilic pleocytosis could be seen in parasitic and rare immunemediated (e.g., idiopathic) diseases. Mixed pleocytosis could be observed in cases of polyneuritis equi but it could be observed with other granulomatous inflammation. Presence of large foamy activated macrophages and reactive lymphocytes are not seen in normal CSF; and if seen support abnormality despite a TNCC within reference range.

Other cell types in CSF might be observed as the result of incidental aspiration (e.g., leptomeninges, ependymal cells, melanocytes from the skin). Occasionally, malignant cells can be seen (e.g., lymphoma, melanoma) in CSF.

59.4.6 Biochemical Constitution

Biochemical parameters reference values might vary with site of centesis, age, and different methodology used by individual diagnostic laboratories. The biochemical constitution of CSF compared to plasma is as follows (for more specific details, see Table 59.2):

- Similar or slightly higher sodium, chloride and magnesium
- Similar or slightly lower potassium and calcium
- Lower glucose and substantially lower protein concentration

Table 59.2 Biochemical parameters of normal CSF. Values presented here are derived from various publications and should only be used as a guideline (Furr and Bender, 1994, Jackson et al., 1996, Rossdale et al., 1982, Toth et al., 2012).* = Values from neonatal foals during anesthesia with isoflurane in 100% oxygen (Geiser et al., 1996).

Parameter	Reference range	Unit
Electrolytes		
Sodium	139–150	mmol/L
Potassium	1.3–3.9	mmol/L
Chloride	92–116	mmol/L
Magnesium	1.06–2.95	mg/dL
Calcium	2.5–6.98	mg/dL
Phosphorus	0.5–2.2	mg/dL
Enzymes		
Creatine kinase (adult)	0–8	IU/L
Creatine kinase (neonate)	4–33	IU/L
Aspartate transferase	0–50	IU/L
Alkaline phosphatase	0–8	IU/L
Lactate dehydrogenase	10–40	IU/L
Gamma glutamyl transferase	0.8–4.2	IU/L
Others		
Glucose	40–80	mg/dL
	40–70% of blood glucose	
Ammonia	Lower than blood (plasma: 5-59)	ug/dL
Blood Gases		
pH	7.35-7.4	
PO_2*	141.8 ± 6.79	mm/Hg
PCO_2*	37.8 ± 0.97	mm/Hg
HCO_3*	23.1 ± 0.19	mmol/L
TCO_2*	24.3 ± 0.2	mmol/L
L-lactate	<2	mmol/L
D-lactate	0	μmol/L

Glucose is derived from plasma by facilitated diffusion. This dependence on blood glucose concentration explains the detrimental effects of hypoglycemia in the brain especially in neonatal foals. Seizures and altered mentation are the most common manifestations of profound hypoglycemia. In addition, CSF glucose depends on the rate of glucose transport and metabolism in the central nervous system, and its concentration in the CSF of healthy horses has been reported to range from 40–80% of blood glucose concentration. However, in a recent study of infectious meningitis in horses showed that most affected horses had CSF glucose much lower than 50% of blood glucose

concentrations and in some cases CSF glucose was profoundly low (11 mg/dL) (Toth et al., 2012).

59.4.7 Other CSF Parameters

Other constituents and neurotransmitters have been measured in CSF. Ubiquitin C-terminal hydrolase 1 (UCHL1) in CSF was found to be a potential marker of brain injury in foals with neonatal hypoxic encephalopathy. However, this marker was not studied in neonatal foals with other neurologic disorders to determine if elevations in UCHL1 are exclusively seen in cases of hypoxic injury. Hypocretin, also known as orexin, is a neurotransmitter produced in the hypothalamus that regulates arousal, wakefulness, and appetite. Hypocretin has been found in low concentrations in CSF from horses with pituitary pars intermedia dysfunction and in a single Icelandic foal diagnosed with narcolepsy. Cytokine profiles in CSF from horses with various neurologic disorders have been studied but overlap of values occurs. Lymphocyte phenotype subsets in CSF have been reported for healthy horses and few horses with presumed EPM but no significant differences were noted. A larger number of horses with confirmed disease are necessary to fully investigate if differences in lymphocyte profile exist.

59.5 Other Diagnostic Tests in CSF

Other diagnostic tests that can be done in CSF include microbial culture (bacterial [aerobic, anaerobic], fungal), PCR for the detection of infectious pathogens (viral, bacterial, rickettsial, fungal, parasitic), and antibody/antigen testing (viral, bacterial, spirochetes [Multiplex assay for *Borrelia burgdorferi*], fungal, protozoae; e.g., immunofluorescent antibody test and ELISA for surface antigens for the detection of *S. neurona* and *N. hughesi*). For more specific information of diagnosis through PCR and antibody/antigen testing, the reader is referred to other sections in this book.

59.5.1 Microbial Culture

Microbial isolation of bacteria in CSF has been reportedly of low yield. However, this should not discourage the clinician from attempting microbial culture. Bacterial growth was seen in 17% (n = 4/23 horses) and 57% (n = 13/23) of CSF samples collected antemortem and postmortem, respectively in a retrospective study of bacterial meningitis by Toth et al. (2012) Combining antemortem and postmortem CSF samples, bacterial growth was observed in 65% of the cases (n = 15/23 horses). It is worthy attempting bacterial culture in suspected cases of bacterial meningitis. Microbial culture combined with PCR testing might increase the

Table 59.3 Bacterial pathogens reported to cause meningitis/meningoencephalomyelitis in horses. F = facultative, all other anaerobic organisms are obligate anaerobes (Toth et al., 2012). Two other organisms reported in horses with sinusitis and meningitis but not isolated in CSF include *Acinetobacter* spp. and *Prevotella* spp.

Adults

Aerobic

Gram Positive	*Gram Negative*	**Anaerobic**	
		Gram Positive	*Gram Negative*
Corynebacterium pseudotuberculosis	*Actinobacillus equuli*	*Listeria monocytogenes* (F)	*Bacteroides* sp.
Listeria monocytogenes	*Capnocytophaga canimorsus*	*Peptostreptococcus* sp.	*Fusobacterium* sp.
Meticillin resistant Staphylococcus aureus	*Klebsiella pneumoniae*		
Staphylococcus aureus	*Pasteurella caballi*		
Staphylococcus spp.	*Proteus* sp.		
Streptococcus acidominimus	*Sphingobacterium multivorum*		
Streptococcus equi equi			
S. equi zooepidemicus			
Streptococcus suis			

Foals

Pathogens causing sepsis

Aerobic

Gram Positive	*Gram Negative*	**Anaerobic**	
		Gram Positive	*Gram Negative*
Corynebacterium pseudotuberculosis	*Escherichia coli*	*Listeria monocytogenes* (F)	
Listeria monocytogenes	*Klebsiella pneumoniae*		
Rhodococcus equi	*Klebsiella oxytoca*		
Staphylococcus aureus	*Salmonella agona*		
Streptococcus equi equi			
S. equi zooepidemicus			

diagnostic value of CSF in such cases. Table 59.3 presents reported bacterial pathogens causing meningitis or meningoencephalomyelitis in horses. Infectious meningitis and meningoencephalomyelitis can also be caused by other pathogens such as *Cryptococcus* sp., *Borrelia burgdorferi*, parasites, and viruses.

59.5.2 CSF Antigen-Specific Antibodies

Specific antibodies to antigens in the CNS should be in greater proportion of total immunoglobulin than that found in serum. Two indices have been used to evaluate this proportion: the Goldman-Witmer coefficient or C-value, and the antibody index (AI) (Furr et al., 2011). These two tests require the determination of specific antigen-specific antibody titer; therefore these tests are not applicable for non-quantitative methods such as Western blot. The upper limit of normal for both tests is

<1. Blood contamination of CSF with up to 10^5 RBC/μL does not alter the C-value and AI.

Titer = specific antibody titer (e.g., *S. neurona* ELISA), QAb = Specific antibody quotient. For more detailed information of the use and interpretation of these CSF indices as a diagnostic aid for EPM and Lyme's disease, refer to other sections in this book.

$$\text{C-value} = \frac{\text{CSF Titer} \times \text{Total serum IgG (mg/dL)}}{\text{Total CSF IgG (mg/dL)} \times \text{Serum Titer}}$$

$$\text{AI} = \frac{\text{QAb}}{(\text{CSF Albumin/Serum Albumin}) \times 1000}$$

$$\text{QAb} = \frac{\text{CSF Titer} \times 1000}{\text{Serum Titer}}$$

References

Andrews FM, Geiser DR, Sommardahl CS, et al. 1994. Albumin quotient, IgG concentration, and IgG index determinations in cerebrospinal fluid of neonatal foals. Am J Vet Res, 55: 741–745.

Andrews FM, Maddux JM, and Faulk D. 1990. Total protein, albumin quotient, IgG and IgG index determinations for horse cerebrospinal fluid. Prog Vet Neurol, 1: 197–204.

Finno CJ, Packham AE, Wilson WD, et al. 2007. Effects of blood contamination of cerebrospinal fluid on results of indirect fluorescent antibody tests for detection of antibodies against Sarcocystis neurona and Neospora hughesi. J Vet Diagn Invest, 19: 286–289.

Furr M and Bender H. 1994. Cerebrospinal fluid variables in clinically normal foals from birth to 42 days of age. Am J Vet Res, 55: 781–784.

Furr M, Howe D, Reed S, et al. 2011. Antibody coefficients for the diagnosis of equine protozoal myeloencephalitis. J Vet Intern Med, 25: 138–142.

Geiser DR, Andrews FM, Rohrbach BW, et al. 1996. Cerebrospinal fluid acid-base status during normocapnia and acute hypercapnia in equine neonates. Am J Vet Res, 57: 1483–1487.

Jackson C, de Lahunta A, Divers T, et al. 1996. The diagnostic utility of cerebrospinal fluid creatine kinase activity in the horse. J Vet Intern Med, 10: 246–251.

Kirk GR, Neate S, McClure RC, et al. 1974. Electrophoretic pattern of equine cerebrospinal fluid. Am J Vet Res, 35: 1263–1264.

Kristensen F and Firth EC. 1977. Analysis of serum proteins and cerebrospinal fluid in clinically normal horses, using agarose electrophoresis. Am J Vet Res, 38: 1089–1092.

Mayhew IG, Whitlock RH, Tasker JB. 1977. Equine cerebrospinal fluid: reference values of normal horses. Am J Vet Res, 38: 1271–1274.

Mayhew IG. 1975. Collection of cerebrospinal fluid from the horse. Cornell Vet, 500–511.

Miller MM, Sweeney CR, Russell GE, et al. 1999. Effects of blood contamination of cerebrospinal fluid on western blot analysis for detection of antibodies against Sarcocystis neurona and on albumin quotient and immunoglobulin G index in horses. J Am Vet Med Assoc, 215: 67–71.

Pease A, Behan A, and Bohart G. 2012. Ultrasound-guided cervical centesis to obtain cerebrospinal fluid in the standing horse. Vet Radiol Ultrasound, 53: 92–95.

Rossdale PD, Cash RSG, and Leadon DP. 1982. Biochemical constituents of cerebrospinal fluid in premature and full term foals. Equine Vet J, 14: 134–138.

Toth B, Aleman M, Nogradi N, et al. 2012. Meningitis and meningoencephalomyelitis in horses: 28 cases (1985–2010). J Am Vet Med Assoc, 240: 580–587.

Vernau W, Vernau KA, and Bailey CS. 2008. Cerebrospinal fluid. In JJ Kaneko, JW Harvey, ML Bruss (eds), *Clinical Biochemistry of Domestic Animals*. 6th Edn. San Diego, CA: Elsevier, pp. 769–819.

60

Laboratory Testing for Endocrine and Metabolic Disorders
Nicholas Frank

Department of Clinical Sciences, Cummings School of Veterinary Medicine, Tufts University, Massachusetts, USA

60.1 Introduction

Laboratory tests are often used to confirm the diagnosis of endocrine and metabolic disorders in horses and results are easily interpreted when advanced/severe disease is encountered. Diagnosis is much more challenging, however, at earlier time points in the development of endocrine and metabolic disorders when clinical signs are subtle and results fall closer to reference intervals. Endocrine and metabolic disorders often have an insidious onset and the disorder may be present before clinical signs are recognized. These cases are more difficult to evaluate and the practitioner must interpret laboratory results within the context of the patient's signalment, history, and clinical signs and diagnostic decisions should be based upon all of the available information. It is often necessary to repeat testing to evaluate responses to management recommendations and assess disease progression.

A general shift is occurring in the measurement of hormone concentrations as laboratories discontinue use of radioimmunoassays because of reduced availability of reagents and the additional burden of working with radioisotopes. Hormones are being measured by enzyme-linked immunosorbent (ELISA) or chemilumnescent assays instead and this brings into question the applicability of previously established reference intervals. If reference intervals were established using a radioimmunoassay, it cannot be assumed that the same cut-off values are appropriate for ELISA or chemilumnescent assays.

As more information becomes available, it is also likely that breed-specific reference intervals will be established for hormone and metabolite measurements. Differences between pony and horse breeds have already been identified for plasma triglyceride concentrations and breed-specific reference intervals are being developed for insulin. Sample collection conditions are also important for many hormone measurements. Insulin and glucose serve as good examples because higher concentrations are detected after feeding and some feed increase glucose and insulin concentrations more than others. A final point is that *reference interval* is preferred over *reference range* and cut-off values represent the upper value of a 95% confidence interval or 97.5th percentile value.

60.2 Pituitary Pars Intermedia Dysfunction

Laboratory tests for pituitary pars intermedia dysfunction (PPID) include measurement of adrenocorticotropin hormone (ACTH) and cortisol hormones. High cortisol concentrations might be expected with PPID, but this hormone follows an ultradian rhythm and fluctuations make it difficult to differentiate horses with PPID from healthy animals. Cortisol also follows a diurnal rhythm with approximately 30% higher concentrations detected in the morning. A diurnal cortisol rhythm test has been suggested for the diagnosis of PPID, but is not recommended because blunting of the diurnal cortisol rhythm can also occur in healthy aged horses (Cordero et al., 2012). Age is therefore a significant confounding factor and this is of particular concern because PPID is an age-associated endocrine disorder.

Two diagnostic tests are recommended for detecting PPID and one additional test is acceptable, but not recommended. The currently recommended tests for PPID are measurement of resting ACTH concentrations and the thyrotropin-releasing hormone (TRH) stimulation test for early PPID (Table 60.1). An overnight dexamethasone suppression test is an acceptable substitute for measuring the resting ACTH concentration, but is no longer recommended because of the inconvenience of collecting blood on 2 days and small risk of laminitis

Interpretation of Equine Laboratory Diagnostics, First Edition. Edited by Nicola Pusterla and Jill Higgins.
© 2018 John Wiley & Sons, Inc. Published 2018 by John Wiley & Sons, Inc.

Table 60.1 Recommended diagnostic tests for pituitary pars intermedia dysfunction.

Test	Procedure	Interpretation
Plasma adrenocorticotropic hormone (ACTH) concentration	Fasting is not required unless also assessing insulin status. Collect blood in glass or plastic tubes containing EDTA. Tubes should be placed in a cooler with ice packs or refrigerated. Centrifuge the same day. Submit for measurement of ACTH.	*December to June* Positive if ACTH > 35 pg/mL* and clinical signs present. *Mid-July to mid-November* Positive if ACTH > 100 pg/mL and clinical signs present. If no clinical signs of PPID, monitor and recheck in 3–6 months.
Thyrotropin-releasing hormone (TRH) stimulation test	No cut-off values for mid-July to mid-November. Fasting is not required unless also evaluating insulin status. Collect baseline blood sample and then inject 1.0 mg (total dose) TRH intravenously as a bolus. Collect a second blood sample 10 or 30 min later.	Baseline ACTH concentration interpreted as above. Positive if ACTH > 110 pg/mL at 10 minutes (December–June) Positive if ACTH > 75 pg/mL at 30 minutes (December–June)
Insulin status	Measure fasting glucose and insulin concentrations as a screening test. Further assess by performing an oral sugar test.	

* Cut-off values for ACTH concentrations measured using a chemiluminescent assay by the Animal Health Diagnostic Laboratory at Cornell Veterinary, Ithaca, NY.
Information adapted from tables provided by the Equine Endocrinology Group (http://sites.tufts.edu/equineendogroup).
Source: Adapted from Equine Endocrinology Group, 2016, http://sites.tufts.edu/equineendogroup/.

secondary to dexamethasone administration in horses with insulin dysregulation.

When clinical signs of PPID are readily apparent and the condition is more advanced, a diagnostic testing is straightforward because affected horses have high resting ACTH concentrations. An EDTA plasma sample is collected and a higher than normal ACTH concentration is detected. Plasma ACTH concentrations normally increase in the late summer as day length starts to decrease, reach their highest point in September and October, and then return to lower concentrations by December (Copas and Durham, 2012). It is important to account for these seasonal changes when interpreting ACTH results and some referral laboratories have established season-specific reference intervals. Monthly reference intervals can be expected in the future.

A TRH stimulation test is recommended when early PPID is suspected and a dynamic test is required to confirm the diagnosis (Beech et al., 2007). Melanotropes of the pars intermedia express TRH receptors and stimulation of these cells by TRH induces secretion of hormones, including ACTH (McFarlane et al., 2006). Higher ACTH concentrations are detected in horses with PPID when measured 10 and/or 30 min following intravenous injection of 1 mg TRH solution. Thyrotropin-releasing hormone solution is not available as a labeled drug, but can be purchased from reliable compounding pharmacies (Goodale et al., 2015). Cut-off values have not been established for ACTH concentrations measured between mid-July to mid-November, so use of the TRH stimulation test is limited to December to June at present.

Monitoring of horses with PPID is accomplished by measuring resting ACTH concentrations and the first recheck is recommended 30 days after initiating pergolide treatment. A follow-up TRH stimulation test can be performed for horses with early PPID, but is rarely necessary because most horses respond well to pergolide treatment at this stage of the disorder. Since both recommended diagnostic tests rely upon ACTH measurements, it should be mentioned that results from a recent study indicate that equine ACTH is more resistant to degradation than previously assumed (Rendle et al., 2014). Blood samples should ideally be transported on ice packs and centrifuged the same day, but it is not necessary to centrifuge samples immediately and this makes testing easier to perform in the field. Physiological stress can raise plasma ACTH concentrations in horses that are transported, hospitalized, painful, or suffering from systemic illness, but these increases are usually modest (<75 pg/mL) (Ayala et al., 2012, Fazio, 2013).

60.3 Adrenal Disorders

60.3.1 Critical Illness-Related Corticosteroid Insufficiency

Critical illness-related corticosteroid insufficiency (CIRCI) should be considered in premature foals and neonates with sepsis that do not respond well to treatment. This condition is also referred to as relative adrenal insufficiency and foals with this endocrine disorder are less capable of withstanding neonatal disease because of inadequate corticosteroid secretion from the adrenal glands. The adrenal glands of the horse do not fully develop until after birth, and foals born prematurely can have reduced adrenal function (Fowden et al., 2012). Relative adrenal insufficiency is important when the body is challenged by systemic disease such as sepsis and manifestations of this condition include hypoglycemia, hypotension, weakness, and poor response to treatment of the primary disease.

An ACTH stimulation test is recommended to confirm the diagnosis of CIRCI and is performed by administering 100 μg synthetic ACTH (cosyntropin) intravenously and collecting blood at times of 0 and 90 min to measure plasma cortisol concentrations (Hart et al., 2009). A two- to four-fold increase in cortisol concentration is expected in healthy foals <7 days of age and a diminished response supports the diagnosis of CIRCI. A paired low dose (10 μg)/high dose (100 μg) ACTH stimulation test has also been described (Hart et al., 2009). Low-dose hydrocortisone therapy is recommended for foals with CIRCI and new treatment protocols are being developed.

60.4 Adrenal Exhaustion (Steroid Withdrawal)

Relative adrenal insufficiency is occasionally detected in adult horses and is most often associated with prolonged stress or use of performance-enhancing drugs and hormones in competition horses, or following withdrawal of corticosteroids administered for the management of diseases such as recurrent airway obstruction, purpura hemorrhagica, or immune-mediated hemolytic anemia. Secretion of corticosteroids, and sometimes also mineralocorticoids, from the adrenal glands is inadequate in these situations and affected horses are lethargic and perform poorly. Resting or exercise-induced hypoglycemia may be detected and electrolyte imbalances consistent with hypoaldosteronism can be present, including hyponatremia, hypochloremia, and hyperkalemia. An ACTH stimulation test can be performed to confirm the diagnosis using the procedure described before. Horses are managed by administering prednisolone orally according to a slowly tapering treatment regimen.

60.5 Insulin Dysregulation and Equine Metabolic Syndrome .

Fasting hyperinsulinemia, excessive insulin responses to ingested sugars, and tissue insulin resistance are collectively referred to as insulin dysregulation (ID), and these abnormalities are components of equine metabolic syndrome (EMS), a collection of risk factors for predicting the development of laminitis in horses, ponies, and donkeys (Frank and Tadros, 2014, Frank et al., 2010). Hyperinsulinemia has been associated with laminitis in horses and it is hypothesized that laminar tissues sustain damage when insulin concentrations remain high for several days (Asplin et al., 2007, de Laat et al., 2010). Grazing on pasture grass raises insulin concentrations and genetically susceptible horses with EMS have higher blood insulin concentrations in response to oral sugars than other horses. This can be referred to as postprandial hyperinsulinemia and horses affected by EMS are at risk for developing laminitis when permitted to graze on pasture grass with high sugar content.

Laboratory testing is required to measure glucose and insulin concentrations and identify animals with hyperglycemia and/or hyperinsulinemia (Table 60.2). Diabetes mellitus is occasionally diagnosed in horses, often in association with PPID, but glucose concentrations usually fall within reference interval. Hyperinsulinemia is more commonly detected. More severely affected animals have fasting hyperinsulinemia whereas mildly affected horses are only identified when postprandial insulin responses to sugars are assessed.

There are two approaches to diagnosing ID. Resting insulin concentrations are measured under fed or fasted conditions, or an oral sugar test (OST) is performed to assess postprandial insulin responses to ingested sugars. Fasting hyperinsulinemia is defined by an insulin concentration > 20 μU/mL, if insulin is measured using a radioimmunoassay. Insulin concentrations > 30 μU/mL are suggestive of ID when measured under fed conditions, if only hay with low non-structural carbohydrate content is consumed. If testing is to be performed under fasting conditions, the horse should be given one flake of hay before 10 pm the night before and then feed is withheld until after a blood sample is collected the next morning. An endocrine and metabolic panel that includes triglyceride and leptin concentrations can be recommended to evaluate lipid metabolism and adipokine release. Hypertriglyceridemia is a predictor of laminitis risk in ponies, with cut-off values of 57 and 94 mg/dL established from two studies (Treiber et al., 2006, Carter et al., 2009). Hyperleptinemia (>4 ng/mL) indicates that leptin secretion from adipocytes is excessive, which suggests that adipose tissues are adversely affecting the health of the animal. Blood leptin concentrations are positively correlated with adiposity, so hyperleptinemia is expected in the obese horse (Kearns et al., 2006). When leptin measurements are used in clinical practice, they are more useful for assessing horses with a leaner body type because detection of hyperleptinemia in these animals suggests that internal adipose deposits are contributing to metabolic

Table 60.2 Recommended diagnostic tests for equine metabolic syndrome.

Test	Procedure	Interpretation[a]
Endocrine and metabolic panel Glucose Insulin Triglycerides Leptin ACTH	Fasting required. Leave only one flake of hay in the stall after 10 PM the night before and collect blood in the morning. Collect blood into one EDTA and one serum tube (leptin).	Persistent hyperglycemia indicates diabetes mellitus (insulin is normal or increased) Hyperinsulinemia if fasting insulin concentration > 20 µU/mL (mU/L) Fed insulin concentration > 30 µU/mL is a concern if only fed low non-structural carbohydrate hay. Hypertriglyceridemia if > 50 mg/dL; concern if > 27 mg/dL Hyperleptinemia if serum leptin concentration > 4 ng/mL Refer to Table 60.1 for ACTH interpretation
Oral sugar test (OST) This test is recommended to assess the combined effects of incretin hormones, pancreatic beta cell insulin secretion, and insulin resistance on insulin concentrations. If the owner has concerns about inducing laminitis, a two-step approach is recommended. First, measure fasting insulin concentrations. If within reference range, proceed to the OST.	Fasting required (see above) Owner administers 0.15 mL per kg (approximately 75 mL) Karo Light[b] corn syrup orally using 60-mL catheter-tip syringes. Collect blood 60 and 90 minutes after administration of corn syrup. Measure glucose and insulin concentrations.	Normal if insulin concentration < 45 µU/mL at 60 and 90 min. Strong evidence if insulin concentration > 60 µU/mL at 60 or 90 min. Weak evidence if insulin concentration 45 to 60 µU/mL at 60 or 90 min. Excessive glucose response if glucose concentration > 125 mg/dL at 60 or 90 min

a) Cut-off values for assays performed by the Animal Health Diagnostic Laboratory at Cornell University, Ithaca, NY. Insulin and leptin measured by radioimmunoassay and ACTH by chemiluminescent assay.
b) Karo Light®; ACH Food Companies, Inc, Cordova, TN.
ACTH = Adrenocorticotropic hormone. PPID = Pituitary pars intermedia dysfunction.

dysregulation. Lower blood concentrations of high-molecular weight adiponectin have also been detected in obese horses and this adipokine may be included on panels in the future (Wooldridge et al., 2010).

The OST is performed under fasting conditions and 15 mL per 100 kg (75 mL for a 500-kg horse) Karo® Light corn syrup is administered by mouth using 60-mL catheter-tip syringes (Schuver et al., 2014). Blood is collected into tubes containing EDTA at 60 and 90 min and plasma glucose and insulin concentrations are measured. Results are normal if plasma insulin concentrations remain < 45 µU/mL at 60 and 90 min and positive if insulin concentrations are above 45 µU/mL at either time point. Detection of insulin concentrations above 60 µU/mL at 60 or 90 min is a strong indication of ID whereas concentrations between 45 and 60 µU/mL provide weaker evidence. Glucose concentrations > 125 mg/dL at 60 or 90 min indicate loss of glycemic control during the OST. If horse owners express concern about performing the OST, a two-step approach is recommended where the fasting insulin concentration is measured first. If the insulin concentration falls within reference interval, an OST is performed as a second step to confirm that the horse is healthy.

Stress and exogenous corticosteroids are potential confounding factors when assessing insulin status because cortisol antagonizes the action of insulin. Horses in the acute stages of laminitis that are very painful have increased endogenous cortisol and catecholamine concentrations, so testing should be delayed until pain subsides. However, it is important to test horses for ID as close to the laminitis episode as possible, before management changes lower insulin concentrations. Testing is therefore recommended as soon as pain levels decrease and the horse walks freely around the stall or enclosure and consumes feed with normal appetite. It is not necessary to wait until non-steroidal anti-inflammatory drugs such as phenylbutazone are discontinued before testing for ID.

60.6 Equine Hyperlipemia

Plasma triglyceride (TG) concentrations increase beyond reference interval (<65 mg/dL) when anorexia develops in horses and fat stores are mobilized to meet energy demands. *Hyperlipidemia* refers to increased TG and/or cholesterol concentrations within the blood, whereas e*quine hyperlipemia* (EH) is a metabolic disorder accompanied by clinical signs that develops as hyperlipidemia progresses. All equids mobilize lipids in response to negative energy balance, but ponies, donkeys, and pregnant and lactating mares are at higher risk for EH. Clinical signs of EH include anorexia and depression, and plasma biochemical analysis results include hypertriglyceridemia, along with azotemia and increased liver enzyme activities in severely affected animals with organ failure resulting from fat infiltration. Plasma TG concentrations often exceed 500 mg/dL in clinically affected patients and severe hyperlipidemia can be detected in the field by observing milky opaque serum in a tube of clotted blood. Blood TG concentrations are likely to be high if it is not possible to read newsprint through the serum.

Equine hyperlipemia usually develops as a secondary medical problem when horses become stressed and enter negative energy balance as a result of colic, dental disease, or systemic illness (Dunkel et al., 2014). A vicious cycle develops when high blood lipid concentrations further suppress appetite. Type 2 diabetes mellitus can contribute to EH and is a concern in some horses with PPID (Durham et al., 2009) when they encounter stress associated with illness or hospitalization. Blood glucose concentrations should be measured in all horses with PPID, and insulin therapy considered if hyperglycemia and hypertriglyceridemia develop.

Hypertriglyceridemia is detected in advance of clinical signs of EH, and indicates that the animal has entered a negative energy balance and is mobilizing lipids. Clinicians should anticipate the development of EH in at-risk patients and provide nutritional support to restore positive energy balance. At-risk horses deprived of feed for 24 h will develop hyperlipidemia that progresses to EH when left untreated. Risk factors for EH include genetic predisposition (pony, miniature horse, or donkey), obesity, pregnancy, lactation, and endocrine disorders including PPID and EMS. Obesity is a key risk factor for EH because affected animals release more fatty acids from their adipose tissues in response to negative energy balance. Insulin resistance is also a contributing factor because insulin normally inhibits the activity of hormone-sensitive lipase. This enzyme catalyzes the conversion of TG to free fatty acids and glycerol, and is stimulated when fats are required for energy. Equine hyperlipemia is a disorder of increased hormone-sensitive lipase activity and excessive fatty acid mobilization from adipose tissues. Fatty acids are reassembled into triglyceride in the liver and secreted into the blood within very-low density lipoproteins. As EH progresses, lipid also accumulates in the liver and other tissues, leading to hepatic lipidosis, steatorrhea, and renal failure. Clinical signs progress as organs fail and the animal develops azotemia and hepatic encephalopathy.

60.7 Parathyroid Hormone Disorders

Hypocalcemia is the most common and clinically important calcium disorder of horses and is associated with clinical signs of weakness, muscle fasciculations, and synchronous diaphragmatic flutter. Rapid contraction of the diaphragm against the liver creates a sound referred to as *thumps* and movement of the diaphragm can be observed externally, occurring at the same rate as heart contractions. In these situations, hypocalcemia has lowered threshold potential within the phrenic nerve, and depolarization of the nerve occurs as electric impulses move through the myocardium of the heart. This phenomenon is seen in the horse because of the close proximity of the phrenic nerve to the heart and synchronous diaphragmatic flutter is an important indicator of hypocalcemia. Decreased dietary calcium intake, systemic inflammation, and sweating are common causes of hypocalcemia and the risk of this problem increases in late pregnancy and lactation. Calcium-containing intravenous fluids (e.g., 23% calcium borogluconate solution) should be administered to address hypocalcemia.

Hypercalcemia is also detected in horses and neoplastic disease and renal failure are the most common causes of this problem. Primary hyperparathyroidism also causes hypercalcemia and is discussed below, but very rarely occurs. Hyperphosphatemia can also be detected with renal failure as glomerular filtration rate decreases, although calcium and phosphorous concentrations vary considerably in horses with renal disease and are affected by diet. It is important to note that the upper limit of reference interval for phosphorous is much higher in the growing horse. Hypophosphatemia is associated with refeeding syndrome in horses and can develop when a starved animal is fed grain after being deprived of energy for many weeks or months. Calcium and phosphorous abnormalities are discussed in greater detail in Chapter 10.

Parathyroid hormone is secreted by chief cells in response to decreasing calcium concentrations and acts on the bone, kidney, and intestine to raise calcium concentrations. Hypoparathyroidism and hyperparathyroidism are rare endocrine disorders in the horse. Primary hypoparathyroidism should be considered if hypocalcemia and synchronous diaphragmatic flutter develop in the absence of common predisposing factors. Very few cases of hypoparathyroidism have been reported and affected horses are managed by increasing dietary calcium intake (Couetil et al., 1998). Hyperparathyroidism can occur as primary disease, as a result of a parathyroid tumor or develop as a secondary problem to dietary calcium/phosphorous imbalance and/or reduced calcium absorption by the intestine. Hypercalcemia and hypophosphatemia accompany primary hyperparathyroidism, whereas hyperphosphatemia (with normocalcemia or hypocalcemia) is a feature of nutritional secondary hyperparathyroidism. Hypercalcemia of malignancy results from increased release of parathyroid hormone-related peptide (PTHrp) from neoplastic tissue and this condition has the same electrolyte profile as primary hyperparathyroidism.

Primary hyperparathyroidism develops when a parathyroid tumor is present and secreting intact parathyroid hormone (iPTH). Parathyroid tumors are very difficult to locate because horses do not have discrete parathyroid glands, as seen in dogs, but instead have nests of chief cells within the thyroid gland, adjacent to the thyroid gland, or along the neck down to the mediastinum. Surgical removal of parathyroid gland tumors has been reported, for tumors that are located within or adjacent to the thyroid gland. Hyperparathyroidism can be first detected when routine blood tests are performed or a chronically affected animal might present with bilateral facial enlargement, which is commonly referred to as *Big Head Disease* (Frank et al., 1998). Facial structures enlarge over the thin bones of the sinuses as bone is replaced by fibrous connective tissue (fibrous osteodystrophy). A third manifestation of hyperparathyroidism is radiolucency of bones detected on radiographs of the limbs. Primary hyperparathyroidism is distinguished from nutritional secondary hyperparathyroidism by the finding of hypophosphatemia (versus normophosphatemia or hyperphosphatemia with nutritional secondary hyperparathyroidism). Urinary fractional clearance of phosphorous is increased and higher iPTH concentrations are detected. Only a few referral laboratories offer measurement of iPTH and PTHrp concentrations, so additional research may be required to locate an appropriate laboratory.

Hypercalcemia of malignancy is associated with neoplastic disease in horses and ameloblastoma and multiple myeloma are two tumor types that have been associated with this problem (Rosol et al., 1994, Barton et al., 2004). Increased secretion of PTHrp raises plasma calcium concentrations and lowers phosphorous concentrations in the same manner as primary hyperparathyroidism. Urinary fractional clearance of phosphorous is also higher than normal. If PTHrp concentrations cannot be measured, a low iPTH concentration supports the diagnosis of hypercalcemia of malignancy.

Nutritional secondary hyperparathyroidism induces osteodystrophia fibrosa and bilateral enlargement of the facial bones, in the same manner as primary hyperparathyroidism, but is caused by dietary calcium/phosphorous imbalance. It is also referred to as *Bran Disease* or *Miller's Disease* and these names were applied in the nineteenth century when horses working in mills developed the disorder as a result of being fed grain husks or bran. Carriage horses working in cities during the same period were also at risk for this disorder because they were fed grain and had limited access to forages or pasture. Nutritional secondary hyperparathyroidism results from a relative deficiency of calcium and high phosphorous intake. Bran and grains are rich in phosphorous and horses on grain-only diets can have a dietary calcium to phosphorous ratio closer to 1:1 or 1:2, compared to the recommended ratio of 2:1. Relative calcium deficiency increases secretion of PTH from the parathyroid glands and induces the same clinical signs as primary hyperparathyroidism. Nutritional secondary hyperparathyroidism is distinguished from primary hyperparathyroidism by the horse's dietary history and detection of normophosphatemia or hyperphosphatemia (as a result of excess phosphorous in the diet) and normal or high calcium concentrations. Increased plasma iPTH concentrations are detected in both primary and nutritional secondary hyperparathyroidism.

Impaired calcium absorption within the intestine can also induce or contribute to nutritional secondary hyperparathyroidism and causes include hypovitaminosis D and ingestion of oxalates. Horses grazing on grasses containing large amounts of oxalates such as Buffel grass, green and blue Panic grasses, and Argentine or Dallis grass are at risk for developing dietary calcium/phosphorous imbalance because oxalates bind to calcium and reduce its absorption in the intestine.

60.8 Thyroid Disorders

Low serum total triiodothyronine (tT_3) and total thyroxine (tT_4) concentrations are detected in horses with EMS or PPID, and also occur with systemic disease. Measurement of free triiodothyronine (fT_3) and free thyroxine (fT_4) hormones by dialysis is recommended to more fully assess thyroid status (Breuhaus et al., 2006) and detection of low fT_3 and fT_4 concentrations warrants further investigation. It would be ideal to measure serum thyroid-stimulating hormone (TSH) concentrations in horses, but this test is not commercially available and assays for measuring canine or human TSH cannot be used. If an equine TSH assay were available from referral laboratories, low concentrations of this pituitary hormone would be suggestive of secondary hypothyroidism, whereas primary hypothyroidism raises TSH concentrations as the body attempts to increase thyroid gland function. A TSH stimulation test is not used in the horse because of the limited availability of synthetic TSH, but the TRH stimulation test can be performed to assess the hypothalamic-pituitary-thyroid axis.

When the TRH stimulation test is performed to assess thyroid status, a pre-injection blood sample is collected and 1.0 mg TRH solution (1 mg/mL) is injected intravenously. Blood samples are then collected 2 and 4 h post-injection and fT_3, tT_3, fT_4, and tT_4 concentrations measured. Most laboratories measure thyroid hormones in serum, so tubes without anticoagulant should be selected. Healthy horses are expected to show > 1.5-fold increases in fT_3 and tT_3 concentrations at 2 h and fT_4 and tT_4 concentrations increase by the same magnitude at 4 h. A diagnosis of hypothyroidism is supported when resting hormone concentrations are low and do not increase appropriately in response to TRH stimulation.

It is more difficult to interpret results when only one thyroid hormone concentration is low and this is a subject of debate among clinicians. One view is that these are clinically insignificant findings that are simply reflective of metabolic status, while the other view is that horses suffer from mild hypothyroidism that requires treatment with levothyroxine. The author favors the former view and only prescribes levothyroxine for horses with consistently low fT_3 and fT_4 concentrations or abnormal TRH stimulation test results. Metabolic status, systemic disease (nonthyroidal illness) and feed deprivation lower thyroid hormone concentrations in horses and are important factors to consider when interpreting results (Christensen et al., 1997). Serum tT4 concentrations also decrease with administration of phenylbutazone and other protein-bound drugs.

Congenital hypothyroidism is a rare endocrine disorder of foals and has been associated with dietary iodine deficiency or excess in mares. Goiter is evident in most, but not all cases, and a syndrome of thyroid gland hyperplasia and musculoskeletal deformities (TH-MSD) occurs with greater frequency in foals from the Pacific Northwest of the United States and Canada (Allen et al., 1994). Foals with this syndrome are often born after prolonged gestation (340–400 days) and show characteristic clinical signs of dysmaturity, including a short silky hair coat, pliable ears, muscle weakness, and incomplete skeletal development. Mandibular prognathism is often observed as well as incomplete ossification of cuboidal bones. Most affected foals have goiter. The diagnosis is confirmed by measuring resting thyroid hormone concentrations, using age appropriate reference intervals because thyroid hormone concentrations are normally higher in foals. A TRH stimulation test can also be performed, as described previously. Foals can be treated with levothyroxine or closely monitored to ensure that thyroid function is increasing over time.

Hyperthyroidism is rare endocrine disorder in horses and should be considered if a thyroid mass is detected and clinical signs of hyperthyroidism are evident, including emaciation, hyperexcitability, polyphagia, tachycardia, and polydipsia (Alberts et al., 2000, Ramirez et al., 1998). Increased thyroid hormone concentrations are sometimes, but not always detected. Active thyroid tumors should be surgically removed or propylthiouracil can be administered to inhibit thyroid hormone production (Tan et al., 2008). Although hyperthyroidism is a potential complication of thyroid tumors, it should be noted that most thyroid masses are benign nonfunctional thyroid adenomas.

References

Alberts MK, McCann JP, and Woods PR. 2000. Hemithyroidectomy in a horse with confirmed hyperthyroidism. J Am Vet Med Assoc, 217: 1051–1054.

Allen AL, Doige CE, Fretz PB, et al. 1994. Hyperplasia of the thyroid gland and concurrent musculoskeletal deformities in western Canadian foals: reexamination of a previously described syndrome. Can Vet J, 35: 31–38.

Asplin KE, Sillence MN, Pollitt CC, et al. 2007. Induction of laminitis by prolonged hyperinsulinaemia in clinically normal ponies. Vet J, 174: 530–535.

Ayala I, Martos NF, Silvan G, et al. 2012. Cortisol, adrenocorticotropic hormone, serotonin, adrenaline and noradrenaline serum concentrations in relation to disease and stress in the horse. Res Vet Sci, 93: 103–107.

Barton MH, Sharma P, LeRoy BE, et al. 2004. Hypercalcemia and high serum parathyroid hormone-related protein concentration in a horse with multiple myeloma. J Am Vet Med Assoc, 225: 409–413, 376.

Beech J, Boston R, Lindborg S, et al. 2007. Adrenocorticotropin concentration following administration of thyrotropin-releasing hormone in healthy horses and those with pituitary pars intermedia dysfunction and pituitary gland hyperplasia. J Am Vet Med Assoc, 231: 417–426.

Breuhaus BA, Refsal KR, and Beyerlein SL. 2006. Measurement of free thyroxine concentration in horses by equilibrium dialysis. J Vet Intern Med, 20: 371–376.

Carter RA, Treiber KH, Geor RJ, et al. 2009. Prediction of incipient pasture-associated laminitis from hyperinsulinaemia, hyperleptinaemia and generalised and localised obesity in a cohort of ponies. Equine Vet J, 41: 171–178.

Christensen RA, Malinowski K, Massenzio AM, et al. 1997. Acute effects of short-term feed deprivation and refeeding on circulating concentrations of metabolites, insulin-like growth factor I, insulin-like growth factor binding proteins, somatotropin, and thyroid hormones in adult geldings. J Anim Sci, 75: 1351–1358.

Copas VE and Durham AE. 2012. Circannual variation in plasma adrenocorticotropic hormone concentrations in the UK in normal horses and ponies, and those with pituitary pars intermedia dysfunction. Equine Vet J, 44: 440–443.

Cordero M, Brorsen BW, and McFarlane D. 2012. Circadian and circannual rhythms of cortisol, ACTH, and alpha-melanocyte-stimulating hormone in healthy horses. Domest Anim Endocrinol, 43: 317–324.

Couetil LL, Sojka JE, and Nachreiner RF. 1998. Primary hypoparathyroidism in a horse. J Vet Intern Med 12: 45–49.

de Laat MA, McGowan CM, Sillence MN, et al. 2010. Equine laminitis: induced by 48 h hyperinsulinaemia in Standardbred horses. Equine Vet J, 42: 129–135.

Dunkel B, Wilford SA, Parkinson NJ, et al. 2014. Severe hypertriglyceridaemia in horses and ponies with endocrine disorders. Equine Vet J, 46: 118–122.

Durham AE, Hughes KJ, Cottle HJ, et al. 2009. Type 2 diabetes mellitus with pancreatic beta cell dysfunction in 3 horses confirmed with minimal model analysis. Equine Vet J, 41: 924–929.

Fazio E, Medica P, Cravana C, et al. 2013. Comparative endocrinological responses to short transportation of Equidae (*Equus asinus* and *Equus caballus*). Anim Sci J 84: 258–263.

Fowden AL, Forhead AJ, and Ousey JC. 2012. *Endocrine adaptations in the foal over the perinatal period*. Equine Vet J, Suppl: 130–139.

Frank N and Tadros EM. 2014. Insulin dysregulation. Equine Vet J, 46: 103–112.

Frank N, Geor RJ, Bailey SR, et al. 2010. Equine Metabolic Syndrome. J Vet Intern Med, 24: 467–475.

Frank N, Hawkins JF, Couetil LL, et al. 1998. Primary hyperparathyroidism with osteodystrophia fibrosa of the facial bones in a pony. J Am Vet Med Assoc, 212: 84–86.

Goodale L, Frank N, Hermida P, et al. 2015. Evaluation of a thyrotropin-releasing hormone solution stored at room temperature for pituitary pars intermedia dysfunction testing in horses. Am J Vet Res, 76: 437–444.

Hart KA, Heusner GL, Norton NA, et al. 2009. Hypothalamic-pituitary-adrenal axis assessment in healthy term neonatal foals utilizing a paired low dose/high dose ACTH stimulation test. J Vet Intern Med, 23: 344–351.

Kearns CF, McKeever KH, Roegner V, et al. 2006. Adiponectin and leptin are related to fat mass in horses. Vet J, 172: 460–465.

McFarlane D, Beech J, and Cribb A. 2006. Alpha-melanocyte stimulating hormone release in response to thyrotropin releasing hormone in healthy horses, horses with pituitary pars intermedia dysfunction and equine pars intermedia explants. Domest Anim Endocrinol 30, 276–288.

Ramirez S, McClure JJ, Moore RM, et al. 1998. Hyperthyroidism associated with a thyroid adenocarcinoma in a 21-year-old gelding. J Vet Intern Med, 12: 475–477.

Rendle DI, Litchfield E, Gough S, et al. 2015. The effects of sample handling and N-phenylmaleimide on concentration of adrenocorticotrophic hormone in equine plasma. Equine Vet J, 47: 587–591.

Rosol TJ, Nagode LA, Robertson JT, et al. 1994. Humoral hypercalcemia of malignancy associated with ameloblastoma in a horse. J Am Vet Med Assoc, 204: 1930–1933.

Schuver A, Frank N, Chameroy KA, et al. 2014. Assessment of insulin and glucose dynamics by using an oral sugar test in horses. J Equine Vet Sci, 34: 465–470.

Tan RH, Davies SE, Crisman MV, et al. 2008. Propylthiouracil for treatment of hyperthyroidism in a horse. J Vet Intern Med, 22: 1253–1258.

Treiber KH, Kronfeld DS, Hess TM, et al. 2006. Evaluation of genetic and metabolic predispositions and nutritional risk factors for pasture-associated laminitis in ponies. J Am Vet Med Assoc, 228: 1538–1545.

Wooldridge AA, Taylor DR, Zhong Q, et al. 2010. High molecular weight adiponectin is reduced in horses with obesity and inflammatory disease. J Vet Intern Med, (abstract); 24: 781.

61

Endocrine Testing for Reproductive Conditions in Horses

Alan Conley[1] and Barry Ball[2]

[1] Department of Population Health and Reproduction, School of Veterinary Medicine, University of California, California, USA
[2] Gluck Equine Research Center, Department of Veterinary Science, University of Kentucky, Kentucky, USA

61.1 Introduction and Overview

There are two major types of hormones that can be analyzed commercially and can be of value in supporting a diagnosis of reproductive conditions in horses (see Box 61.1). The sex steroid hormones (such as testosterone, estradiol, estrone sulfate, and progesterone) are the easiest and most reliably measured across species because, for the most part, these same steroids exist in all mammals (if at different concentrations) so assays are more generally available. The second type of hormones is of the protein type (such as inhibin and anti-Müllerian hormone). These differ among species in their chemical form (amino acid sequence and glycosylation), and immunoassays that rely on recognition with a primary antisera or antibody do not always recognize the same hormone in different species adequately enough to detect concentrations in physiological ranges. However, different laboratories utilize different primary antisera that have different cross-reactivity profiles with other, non-target analytes, and, therefore, reference ranges will differ among them and results from any laboratory should be evaluated based only on the reference ranges established by that laboratory.

61.2 Diagnostic Reproductive Hormone Analytes

61.2.1 Anti-Müllerian Hormone (AMH)

General properties:

- Homo-dimeric (two identical subunits), heavily glycosylated, protein hormone with a long, ≈36-hour half-life in serum so concentrations are more stable hour to hour and day to day because secretion is not gonadotropin-regulated (neither LH nor FSH-stimulated) or pulsatile in either males or females (reference range Table 61.1).
- In colts, secreted by the Sertoli cells of the testis at highest concentrations during fetal development, decreasing steadily with age after birth, continuing to decline through puberty.
- In fillies, also secreted by the granulosa cells of growing and small antral ovarian follicles as follicles develop after birth, reflecting follicle numbers in the ovaries (ovarian follicular reserve), decreasing with age as follicle reserve decline.
- Seasonal changes occur in stallions, such that concentrations are less in the non-breeding but increase during breeding season in stallions (range, ≈15–25 ng/ml; Claes et al., 2013a) but seasonal fluctuations are less than those seen for testosterone (≈0.60–1.3 ng/ml), which also varies seasonally in cryptorchids (Claes et al., 2013b).

61.2.2 Inhibin

General properties:

- Heterodimeric (α and β), glycosylated protein hormone with a half-life of several hours in sheep (Miller et al., 1997), though not determined for horses (Roser, personal communication), so concentrations are relatively stable but are gonadotropin-regulated and can change depending on physiological state.
- In colts, like AMH, secreted by the Sertoli cells of the testis; in contrast to AMH, however, concentrations of inhibin from birth increase through puberty and do not decrease with age in normal stallions (Roser et al., 1994).
- In fillies, like AMH, secreted by the granulosa cells of ovarian follicles but regulated by FSH and fluctuates during the cycle; highest at ovulation and lowest a week after ovulation.

Interpretation of Equine Laboratory Diagnostics, First Edition. Edited by Nicola Pusterla and Jill Higgins.
© 2018 John Wiley & Sons, Inc. Published 2018 by John Wiley & Sons, Inc.

Table 61.1 Reference range from common hormones established at the Clinical Endocrinology Laboratory, School of Veterinary Medicine, University of California at Davis.

Endocrine Hormone	Horse gender	Reference range
Anti-Müllerian Hormone	Gelding	<0.15 ng/ml
	Stallion	15–25 ng/ml
Testosterone	Mare (non-pregnant and pregnant)	0.1–4 ng/ml
Estrone sulfate		<50 pg/ml
Progesterone	Gelding	100–500 pg/ml
	Cryptorchid	500–2000 pg/ml
	Stallion	25–45 pg/ml
	Mare non-pregnant	up to 300 pg/ml
	Mare pregnant (dependents on stage)	<0.1 ng/ml
	Gelding	35–60 ng/ml
	Cryptorchid	140–200 ng/ml
	Stallion	0.6–6 ng/ml
	Non-pregnant mare (most breed)	0.1–60 ng/ml
	Non-pregnant miniature horse mare	>6 ng/ml
	Mare >45 days pregnancy (most breeds)	>60 ng/ml
	Miniature horse mare >80 days pregnancy	>1 ng/ml
	Functional luteal tissue Minimum considered safe for pregnancy maintenance	>4 ng/ml

61.2.3 Testosterone

General properties:

- Unconjugated, free steroid, short half-life of 1 h or less (reference range Table 61.1).
- Very low until puberty is initiated, and is virtually undetectable in newborn colts and fillies.
- Secreted by testicular Leydig (interstitial) cells (as is estrone sulfate) under trophic stimulation by LH and by the theca cells surrounding antral follicles in mares (Neto et al., 2010).
- Concentrations can be so variable hour to hour and month to month that diagnostic value is improved in

stallions by conducting a stimulation test acutely using either LH to measure response (usually at 1–2 h, though response at 24 or 48 h is more reliable) above baseline, when baseline concentrations are not in the stallion range (response to GnRH is more variable in cryptorchids, Arighi and Bosu, 1989).

- Low in mares, and secreted by a little less than half of diagnosed granulosa-cell tumors, but concentrations detected by immuno-assay increase dramatically during pregnancy.
- The adrenal gland may contribute to concentrations detected by immuno-assay.

61.2.4 Estrone Sulfate

General properties:

- Conjugated steroid hormone; the conjugated state is generally believed to extend the short half-life though it may still be less than an hour in horses (reference range Table 61.1).
- Secreted by testicular Leydig cells, but the increase at puberty is delayed relative to testosterone and there is no reliable acute stimulation after gonadotropic stimulation (Arighi and Bosu, 1989, Cox et al., 1986, Roser, 1995, Silberzahn et al., 1989).
- Detectable by immuno-assay in cyclic mares and concentrations increase with establishment of pregnancy at a point dependent on breed (diagnosis is delayed until much later and concentrations are higher in miniature breeds).

61.2.5 Progesterone

General properties:

- Unconjugated, free steroid, secreted by the corpus luteum in cyclic mares (but not present in prepubertal fillies) and in more limited amounts by the placenta of pregnant mares depending on stage of gestation, but not normally secreted in detectable amounts in stallions.
- Short half-life, 2–20 min (Ganjam et al., 1975)

61.2.6 Limitations of Interpreting Hormone Concentrations

- The interpretation of the results of endocrine testing for reproductive conditions can be more challenging than those for other endocrine diseases because reproductive hormones are particularly variable, sometimes hour by the hour, day by day, week by week, and season by season (Ganjam and Kenney, 1975). This is especially true of steroid hormones, but it is normal for reproductive hormones of all kinds to fluctuate with development and reproductive state to a degree not seen in other endocrine systems. The concentrations of steroid hormones secreted by the gonads and placenta are variable in systemic blood for a variety of reasons, and it has a significant effect on how concentrations are interpreted physiologically and clinically.

- Age and reproductive state are major factors in determining what constitutes a normal androgen (and estrogen) concentration in colts and stallions, or in cyclic and pregnant mares. For the diagnosis of cryptorchidism (see next), therefore, basal testosterone is fairly reliable but only when it is elevated (>100 pg/ml), and because of variations with age, the younger the colt at the time of testing, the less diagnostic a low basal concentration (<50 pg/ml) becomes for the presence of testicular tissue. Pregnancy markedly elevates measured testosterone in mares and becomes an unreliable indicator of granulosa cell tumors (GCTs, see later)
- Steroid secretion and testosterone concentrations for instance, are also pulsatile in stallions, responding to each pulse of LH released by the pituitary on an hourly basis.
- Steroid secretion in both stallions (Ganjam and Kenney, 1975) and mares is diurnal. For instance, testosterone concentrations are slightly elevated in stallions at midday (Kirkpatrick et al., 1976), the opposite diurnal pattern is true of progesterone concentrations in mares (Ginther et al., 2007).
- Steroid hormone secretion and circulating concentrations are lower in November and December in the northern hemisphere than in the breeding season, so using testosterone to test for cryptorchidism is less reliable in these months especially (Claes et al., 2013b).
- Testosterone in mature stallions can even vary with how the animal is housed (lower basal testosterone in stallions in bachelor herds than those running in a harem (McDonnell and Murray, 1995), or with sexual arousal (teasing) that can induce a rapid, reflex increase in testosterone secretion (Ganjam and Kenney, 1975, Villani et al., 2006) though perhaps not cryptorchids (Arighi and Bosu, 1989).
- Response tests, taking a baseline sample, introducing a stimulus (e.g., hCG; 2500–10,000 IU), and then taking a second sample later (typically 1–2 h, but with a secondary, higher peak at 24–48 h) that improves reliability and helps to mitigate the previously mentioned variation except perhaps that due to season.

61.2.7 Immuno-Assays

Almost all commercially available endocrine testing of horses seen in private veterinary practice at the present time are performed by immuno-assays, meaning that antisera raised against hormone analytes of interest are the basis for analyte recognition. These assays have many diagnostic advantages but also bear some disadvantages.

- Immuno-assays are generally sensitive, although, the diagnostic sensitivity of such assays depends on the volume of serum assayed and whether or not the sample is processed for extraction of steroids, usually with an ether solvent first. Analyses that use organic extraction of the serum sample allow for larger volumes (e.g., 0.5 ml) to be assayed, therefore improving the diagnostic sensitivity. Such methods allow detection of lower concentrations more reliably which is sometimes necessary for distinguishing some geldings from true cryptorchids. Cost is generally reasonable and assays are commercially accessible for practitioners, owners, and other clientele.
- Disadvantages of immuno-assays are that antisera cross-react with many different molecules (true for both steroids and protein hormonal analytes), so they necessarily lack specificity and values can be misleading if a cross-reacting analyte happens to be present in high concentrations. Further, the lower the concentration of a target analyte, the less specificity and the more confounding cross-reactants become.

61.2.8 Summary

In summary, natural variation in concentrations of reproductive hormones simply makes the interpretation of results more complex than hormones of almost any other body system and multiple samples are therefore always easier to interpret than single point-in-time determinations unless there is a very significant deviation from normal ranges. Reference ranges can be difficult to establish for reproductive conditions, in part because of these multiple sources of variation. Immuno-assays are sensitive and inexpensive but less specific than other assays, such as mass spectrometry, for instance, which is not readily available to veterinary practices or their clientele. Repeated analysis over time (days or weeks) does provide additional confidence in values obtained on any single day and therefore adds value diagnostically but with diminishing returns after the second or third sampling. Regardless of the method of analysis, values should only be interpreted in concert with the signalment, a complete history (reproductive and otherwise), a thorough clinical examination and all physical findings, and evaluated together for consistency.

61.3 Endocrine Diagnostic Aids for Cryptorchidism

Suspected cryptorchidism is common in horses presumed to have been gelded but showing stallion-like or aggressive behavior. Many times, the horse has changed owners multiple times and consequently, the castration history is vague or unreliable, no testes are palpable in the scrotum, but an inguinal or abdominal testis is suspected, most often because of behavior. The decision to anesthetize a horse in order to explore surgically is not a trivial one and endocrine testing is valuable for confirmation. The utility of testosterone, estrone sulfate, and testosterone after an hCG challenge (Arighi and Bosu, 1989, Cox et al., 1973, 2001, Roser, 1995, Silberzahn et al., 1989) in determining testicular function in normal, cryptorchid and gelded horses has been reviewed recently (Arighi, 2011). The use of AMH for the diagnosis of cryptorchidism is a recently developed, and likely a more efficient, test (Claes et al., 2013a).

61.3.1 Anti-Müllerian Hormone

Advantages when testing for cryptorchidism:

- Stability with time (hours, days, and weeks) and less seasonally variable than either testosterone or estrone sulfate.
- No need (or reason) for stimulation test.
- AMH is higher in prepubertal colts than stallions whereas testosterone is lower, so AMH is more reliable at younger ages when testosterone is least reliable.
- Cryptorchids may actually have higher AMH than intact stallions and may therefore be easier to distinguish.

Disadvantages when testing for cryptorchidism:

- As a single determination may be more expensive than a single steroid analysis (but still may be less expensive than the cost of collecting multiple blood samples and assaying testosterone in them after a stimulation test).
- Decreasing concentrations with age means that AMH may be less reliable in older cryptorchid animals (>10 y) and concentrations in very old cryptorchids with advanced testicular degeneration (from intra-abdominal temperatures) is unknown at present.

61.3.2 Testosterone and Estrone Sulfate

Advantages when testing for cryptorchidism:

- Testosterone and estrone sulfate are reliable and relatively inexpensive when baseline concentration is within the stallion range.

Disadvantages when testing for cryptorchidism:

- Less stable baseline affected more by variations hour to hour, seasonally, and by other environmental influences.
- More costly if baseline is equivocal and stimulation test is required.
- Estrone sulfate is particularly unreliable in younger horses

61.3.3 Test Interpretation

AMH is a more reliable indicator of cryptorchidism, especially in younger than older animals, it also is less variable seasonally and a single determination is reliable. The interpretation of AMH pertains only ever to basal secretion and, therefore, can and is made on a single sample, there is no need for a response test; there is none that could be done in fact (since there is nothing known that would stimulate AMH secretion acutely).

Testosterone and estrone sulfate concentrations are much more variable than AMH and therefore more prone to false negative interpretations in our experience. A testosterone concentration >100 pg/ml is reliably indicative of the presence of testicular tissue, and <50 pg ml is typical of geldings but less reliably so (false negatives more likely than false positives). Concentrations falling in the intermediate range of 50–100 pg/ml represent a diagnostic "gray zone" or equivocal result. Prior to the availability of AMH as an alternative analyte, such a result might trigger a hCG stimulation test, whereby testosterone is measured in two samples, one taken before hCG stimulation (2500–10,000 IU and a second taken afterwards (commonly 1–2 h but more reliably at 24 or 48 h). If testosterone concentrations double or more after stimulation, this is interpreted as an indicator of the existence of functional testicular tissue as long as stimulated concentrations exceed 100 pg/ml. If an hCG stimulation test is conducted in a suspect cryptorchid with a basal testosterone concentration <50 pg/ml, but even stimulated concentration remain <50 pg/ml, it is considered indicative that no residual testicular tissue exists. The decision to use a stimulation test incurs additional costs, which includes the hCG (or GnRH), the additional sample analysis, and the drawing of the second sample or more, but if neither basal testosterone nor AMH provide a clear interpretation, the extra expense may be justified. As noted before, testosterone secretion varies seasonally in stallions and we have shown similarly that there is seasonal variation in testosterone secretion by cryptorchid testes. Therefore, testing for cryptorchidism based on basal testosterone is more reliable during the breeding season whereas during November or December (in northern hemisphere) there is a greater chance that basal testosterone concentrations may give a low and false negative result. Like testosterone, estrone sulfate can be diagnostic for cryptorchidism if high concentrations are found, but estrogen secretion by the stallion testis is even more variable than testosterone, occurs at a later age and is therefore more difficult to interpret with confidence.

The measurement of two hormones is always better than only relying on the value of a single one, so running both testosterone and AMH will provide greatest confidence in interpretation. If cost is a concern, a rational compromise is to run a basal testosterone, and only if inconclusive, run an AMH subsequently (most endocrinology laboratories will save the sample if alerted to that possibility at the time the sample is submitted). A history is always useful, including the age of the horse, if an interpretation from the laboratory is of value, otherwise the endocrine results will be reported without diagnostic interpretation. An hCG stimulation test can be considered if neither basal testosterone nor AMH provides a clear result.

61.4 Endocrine Diagnostic Aids for Granulosa-Cell Tumors (GCT)

GCTs are by far the most common gonadal tumors in horses and one of the most common of all equine neoplasms (McCue et al., 2006). They can grow to impressive sizes, posing a surgical challenge when they do. When functional and in more advanced cases, they can disrupt cyclicity and therefore fertility unless removed. Altered or abnormal behavior is by far the most common presenting complaint and reason to seek hormone analysis for a possible GCT. However, actual signs associated with GCTs can vary from occasionally presenting as being uneasy under saddle, through exhibiting abnormal cyclicity, to erratic or abnormal reproductive behavior and dangerous aggression toward other horses and handlers. Whatever the presenting signs, until an ovary is palpably abnormal (loss of definition of the ovulation fossa as one subtle and early possible change) or clearly is abnormal otherwise any diagnosis of GCT must remain tentative, no matter what the endocrine findings. Even what might be considered convincing ultrasound evidence of a GCT can be misleading.

Endocrine tests that are an informative and valuable aid in the diagnosis of GCTs include anti-Müllerian hormone (AMH), inhibin, and testosterone. Progesterone or estrone sulfate may be added to provide information on the likelihood (or not) of pregnancy. It is important information because both inhibin and testosterone are elevated during pregnancy, greatly complicating diagnosis based on these analytes alone. AMH and inhibin are more often elevated together in functional GCTs (more positively correlated) than are inhibin and testosterone or AMH and testosterone, but no two tumors are alike. Analyzing all three hormones is better than any two, even if only marginally. If two analytes only are to be examined, AMH and inhibin are recommended. However, not all ovarian tumors are GCTs (dysgerminomas and teratomas among others), and not all GCTs are endocrinologically active. Multiple tumor types can co-exist on the same or different ovaries, however rare.

Endocrine testing is only an aid to clinical signs and findings are only ever consistent or not with the provisional diagnosis. GCTs do occur in pregnant mares, and foals can survive to term in the presence of a tumor. It is unlikely that tumor-derived hormones cross the placenta in significant amounts.

61.4.1 Anti-Müllerian Hormone

Advantages when testing for GCTs:

- Stability with time (hours, days, weeks, due to glycosylated state and thus long half-life).
- Concentrations do not change appreciably during pregnancy or during the normal estrous cycle.
- As a single analyte, more reliable than either inhibin or testosterone, >90% accuracy when >10 ng/ml.
- May be elevated earlier in the development of functional tumors.

Disadvantages when testing for GCTs:

- False negatives and false positives both still possible in a small percentage of cases.

61.4.2 Inhibin

Advantages when testing for GCTs:

- More stable than testosterone and therefore less variable.
- As a single analyte, more reliable than testosterone, perhaps >80% accuracy when >0.8 ng/ml.

Disadvantages when testing for GCTs:

- Less stable (more variable) than AMH.
- As a single analyte, not as predictive as AMH.
- Can be elevated during pregnancy and concentrations vary during the normal estrous cycle.

61.4.3 Testosterone

Advantages when testing for GCTs:

- Widely available through different laboratories.
- Relatively inexpensive.
- Reliable indicator of GCT when >100 pg/ml in nonpregnant mares.

Disadvantages when testing for GCTs:

- As a single analyte, not as accurate as either AMH or inhibin.
- More variable (shorter half-life) than either AMH or inhibin.
- Measured concentrations are greatly elevated during normal pregnancy.

61.4.4 Test Interpretation

Inhibin and testosterone have been the mainstay of GCT diagnosis for decades (McCue et al., 2006). Testosterone concentrations in mares are normally <45 pg/ml, and an increase above 45 pg/ml may indicate an early GCT. On its own, however, testosterone concentrations >45 pg/ml are seen in <50% of mares with confirmed GCTs at surgery, so many mares with GCTs do not develop an elevation of testosterone. However, the higher the testosterone concentration, the more confident is the interpretation. If testosterone concentrations exceed 100 pg/ml, a GCT is highly likely since alternative explanations of concentrations above this are essentially unknown in non-pregnant mares. Though it is often suspected that elevated testosterone might induce alterations in behavior, the correlation between testosterone concentrations and stallion-like or aggressive behavior is poor if testosterone is <100 pg/ml. It is believed that >100 pg/ml of testosterone is required to induce stallion-like behavior in mares with GCTs; these concentrations are reached in a minority of mares with GCT. Pregnancy is relevant in this regard also, because measured testosterone concentrations can exceed 250 pg/ml in pregnant mares without inducing behavioral problems. This lack of correlation between measured testosterone concentration and aggressive or stallion-like behavior may reflect more of a problem with immuno-assays than with the pathophysiology of the condition and new diagnostic approaches are being explored (see later). The possibility that testosterone concentrations in the range of 45–100 pg/ml in mares might be associated with adrenal secretion was explored. Testosterone concentrations in this range that were found in samples submitted to the Clinical Endocrinology Laboratory at Davis from mares in which confirmation of a GCT had not been made (mares did not go to surgery) were analyzed further to assess adreno-cortical function. In these samples measured testosterone concentrations were found to have a positive correlation with cortisol. This positive correlation suggests that the adrenal cortex might provide an alternative explanation for elevated immuno-reactive testosterone (45–100 pg/ml) in mares that do not have a GCT.

Elevated inhibin concentrations are a much better predictor of the presence of a GCT. Normally, inhibin concentrations in mares are <0.7 ng/ml (except during pregnancy), and concentrations >

0.7 ng/ml may indicate a developing GCT. Statistically, elevated inhibin concentrations are associated with about 80% confirmed GCT cases. In practice, when inhibin concentrations exceed 1 ng/ml, a GCT is likely because there are few other alternative explanations in a non-pregnant mare. Like testosterone, inhibins are elevated during normal pregnancy, so neither inhibins

nor testosterone are useful analytes as diagnostic aids for GCTs if a mare is pregnant, and a false positive could result if the lack of an existing pregnancy is not determined.

AMH is secreted by the granulosa cells of growing and small antral follicles in mares (Ball et al., 2008) but does not vary appreciably during the cycle or through pregnancy (Almeida et al., 2011, Ball et al., 2013). The lack of any associated increase in AMH during pregnancy adds additional value to this hormone as an indicator of a possible GCT in pregnant mares. An elevation of AMH >4 ng/ml in a mare with signs suggestive of a GCT is suspicious, but as for inhibins or testosterone, without palpable ovarian enlargement or very convincing ultrasound evidence of abnormal ovarian morphology, a diagnosis of GCT is entirely presumptive. Other ovarian tumors can cause abnormal enlargement or appear structurally abnormal on ultrasound examination, though none are functional from an endocrine perspective. Our experience has lead us to believe that an elevation of AMH concentration >10 ng/ml is almost certainly associated with a developing or existing GCT. In contrast, elevated AMH concentration in the range of 4–10 ng/ml (gray zone) is often not associated with ovarian enlargement, and the presence of a GCT can only be suspected until ovarian enlargement or morphological abnormality becomes obvious with repeated monitoring. We have examined ovaries from mares with AMH concentrations in the range of 4–10 ng/ml in which a GCT could not be found after surgical removal, so false positives are a reality.

Inhibins (Ellenberger et al., 2007) and AMH (Ball et al., 2008) are both secretory products of the granulosa cell or granulosa-derived cells in GCTs, whereas testosterone is secreted by the theca-derived cells of the GCT (Neto et al., 2010). It makes sense therefore that there is a more significant positive correlation between inhibin and AMH concentrations in mares with GCTs, but less correlation between testosterone and either AMH or inhibin (Ball et al., 2013). It is generally expected that as GCTs increase in size, so will concentrations of their secreted hormone products. Therefore, as a GCT grows, AMH, inhibin and testosterone concentrations in the grey zone are generally expected to continue to climb, and we have observed this in some cases. However, because tumors do what tumors do, and can differentiate in different ways, it is also possible for the secretory profile of a developing GCT to change in time from predominately one hormone (AMH or inhibin) to predominantly another (testosterone). We do not know but presume this might indicate differences in the rates of growth and differentiation of granulosa-derived versus theca-derived tissues with time. A post-surgical serum sample may be useful in order to confirm the complete removal of GCTs. The long (36 h) half-life of AMH means that this sample should be taken at least 1 week after surgical removal of the ovary.

AMH is a more reliable, early marker of developing GCTs because of its extended half-life, but because elevations may be seen before ovarian enlargement or other abnormalities develop, there is an associated increase in false positive, presumptive diagnoses. Repeated sampling certainly helps in cases where clinical signs persist. The lack of change in AMH during pregnancy makes it the only analyte of diagnostic value under those circumstances. Those cases seen with elevated AMH but no obvious GCT on dissection remain unexplained because no other tissue source (such as the adrenal gland) has been confirmed in horses. Until there is ovarian enlargement or demonstrable abnormalities in ovarian structure, any diagnosis is preliminary and presumptive, no matter what the hormonal results may be. Again, retesting 2–3-month intervals is useful in monitoring and assessing cases under these circumstances.

61.5 Pregnancy Diagnosis Aided by Estrone Sulfate and Progesterone Concentrations

Estrone sulfate and progesterone can be used as a diagnostic aid for pregnancy diagnosis in mares that are difficult to ultrasound or palpate. However, a breeding date and reproductive history is always informative in interpreting hormone concentrations and the likelihood of pregnancy. Confirmation of pregnancy a month or two later is advised to confirm that the expected increase in both estrone sulfate and progesterone (at least up through the seventh month of pregnancy) is occurring as it should with a viable pregnancy. Determination of progesterone concentration is also used as an indicator of the adequacy of progestogenic support of pregnancy. Based on a single publication (Shideler et al., 1982), 4 ng/ml is considered the minimal concentration compatible with the maintenance of pregnancy. Definitive evidence of luteal insufficiency remains lacking, however, as is the degree to which supplementation with a progestin can influence the rate of pregnancy loss (Allen, 2001). Recent studies have shown that a progesterone metabolite, dihydroprogesterone (DHP), which was long suspected of supporting pregnancy in the last third of equine gestation (Chavatte-Palmer et al., 2000, Holtan et al., 1991, Jewgenow and Meyer, 1998), is potently progestogenic, and can support pregnancy in the absence of the corpus luteum in early gestation (Scholtz et al., 2014). DHP can cross-react significantly with antisera used in commercially available assays, and those assays cannot discriminate progesterone

from DHP and possibly other metabolites as a result. Therefore, progesterone determinations by immuno-assays provide only an approximation of actual progesterone concentrations in mares. As noted previously, immuno-assays lack specificity for various circulating progesterone metabolites, but few commercially offered assays will likely detect altrenogest. Therefore, altrenogest is unlikely to interfere with progesterone determinations in those mares that are on treatment when sampled.

61.5.1 Estrone Sulfate

Advantages when testing for pregnancy:

- Reliable when elevated above 10 ng/ml after 45 days post-breeding (most breeds) or >60 ng/ml after 80 days post-breeding (mini-breeds).
- Additional elevation on a second test sample taken 3–4 weeks later is helpful for confirmation of pregnancy when concentrations are only marginally within the range considered consistent with pregnancy.
- Offered by multiple diagnostic laboratories and relatively inexpensive.

Disadvantages when testing for pregnancy:

- Immuno-reactive estrone sulfate can be elevated transiently in cyclic mares, so confirmation with a second sample taken a month or so later is advised.

61.5.2 Progesterone

Advantage when testing for pregnancy:

- Often used to assess adequacy of progesterone and perceived need for supplemental progestogens to sustain pregnancies.
- Low concentrations < 1 ng/ml are inconsistent with luteal function and viable pregnancy.

61.5.3 Test Interpretation

The normal range for cyclic mares is <6 ng/ml for estrone sulfate, and if it exceeds 6 ng/ml, 45 days or later after breeding, this is considered suspicious of pregnancy. However, rarely, cyclic mares can measure as much as 10 ng/ml of estrone sulfate, even in the presence of luteal phase concentrations of progesterone (>1 ng/ml), so interpretation is not foolproof based on these analytes alone, particularly without knowledge of the suspected stage of pregnancy (observed or known breeding date). Estrone sulfate concentrations <10 ng/ml should be treated as suspicious and the elevated concentrations confirmed in a second sample 3–4 weeks later if not confirmed by other means. If estrone sulfate concentrations have not increased during this interval, the possibility of pregnancy must remain in doubt. For reasons that are not understood, normal ranges are much higher for mares of miniature horse breeds, and estrone sulfate must exceed 60 ng/ml after 80 days post-breeding to be consistent with pregnancy in mares of miniature horse breeds.

There are several possible caveats to the diagnosis of pregnancy based on elevated estrone sulfate. Equine pregnancies have always been considered to rely on a minimum concentration of progesterone, which is generally accepted to be around 2–4 ng/ml (McKinnon et al., 1988, Shideler et al., 1982, Vanderwall et al., 2007). Therefore, based on the UC Davis assays and experience over the years, viable pregnancies in mares with progesterone concentrations that are <4 ng/ml (in mares that have elevated estrone sulfate) should also be confirmed by demonstrating an increase in estrone sulfate in a subsequent sample taken 3–4 weeks later. Estrone sulfate and progesterone concentrations are less reliable as mares near foaling (concentrations of both can decline at the end of pregnancy). Therefore, if breeding dates suggest that pregnancy could be at an advanced stage in mares with low estrone sulfate or progesterone, diagnosis is more problematic and results should be interpreted with caution.

A known breeding date is always helpful in interpreting estrone sulfate and progesterone concentrations for pregnancy diagnosis in mares in which a diagnosis by palpation is not possible or definitive. As with all endocrine tests, two samples a few weeks or months apart are also helpful because concentrations should increase as the pregnancy develops. This is particularly useful if the interpretation on the first sample is equivocal.

61.6 The Future of Endocrine Diagnostics for Reproductive Conditions in Horses

Endocrine diagnosis in all species has been based largely on immuno-assays for many decades. Immuno-assays are both relatively cheap and are potentially quite sensitive. However, since they rely on antibodies as the primary assay component, they lack specificity so that it is not always certain whether or not the desired analyte is actually being measured accurately; the measurement may be confounded by high concentrations of a cross-reacting analyte that yields a false positive result. This is

particularly important in steroid analysis where dozens, even hundreds, of related steroids can potentially confound an assay result. In fact, horses provide one of the best examples of this reality. While we use a progesterone immuno-assay to evaluate concentrations in pregnant mares in particular, these assays are not specific and measure a number of other related steroids with unknown physiological significance. It has been known for decades that if more specific assay methodology is used, progesterone is actually undetectable in the second half of pregnancy. We have shown recently that one particular 5alpha-reduced metabolite of progesterone, dihydroprogesterone (DHP), can substitute for progesterone in horses, stimulating endometrial growth, maintaining pregnancy after induced luteolysis in early pregnancy, and activating the equine progesterone receptor in an *in vitro* bioassay we developed recently. DHP is present in the luteal phase and in later pregnancy at concentrations that stimulate endometrial growth and maximally activate the equine progesterone receptor, but available immuno-assays cannot distinguish progesterone from DHP. This obviates the need to develop more specific assays for measuring progesterone and DHP, as well as other metabolites, and of determining their bioactivity and therefore physiological relevance. Work in our laboratory continues to this end, hoping to develop methods using mass spectrometry to establish more reliable and specific assays for pregnancy, cryptorchidism, and GCTs in the future. We have shown that progesterone circulates at higher concentrations than DHP in the luteal phase of cyclic mares and in early gestation. However, after 110 days of pregnancy, DHP concentrations overtake progesterone, the concentrations of which progressively disappear in most mares by 200 days of gestation. Therefore, a DHP concentration that exceeds the concentrations of progesterone is likely a very reliable indicator of pregnancy. Perhaps also measuring the bioactive steroids such as progesterone and DHP with greater specificity will allow us to predict the chances of embryonic loss in newly established pregnancies, or the health of pregnancies that are long established but at risk of abortion for whatever reason. This level of specificity and accuracy can be achieved with methods employing mass spectrometry, and we are pursuing the development of new assays for endocrine diagnostic testing using this more advanced technology.

References

Allen WR. 2001. Luteal deficiency and embryo mortality in the mare. Reprod. Domest. Anim, 36(3–4): 121–131 available from: PM:11555357.

Almeida J, Ball BA, Conley AJ, Place NJ, Liu IK, Scholtz EL, et al. 2011. Biological and clinical significance of anti-Mullerian hormone determination in blood serum of the mare. Theriogenology, 76(8): 1393–1403 available from: PM:21798581.

Arighi M. 2011, Testicular descent, In AO McKinnon (ed.), *Equine Reproduction*, 2nd Edn. Vol. 1. Oxford: Wiley-Blackwell, pp. 1099–1106.

Arighi M and Bosu WT. 1989. Comparison of hormonal methods for diagnosis of cryptorchidism in horses. Equine Vet Sci, 9(1): 20–26.

Ball BA, Almeida J, and Conley AJ. 2013. Determination of serum anti-Mullerian hormone concentrations for the diagnosis of granulosa-cell tumours in mares. Equine Vet J, 45 (2): 199–203 available from: PM:22779762.

Ball BA, Conley AJ, MacLaughlin DT, Grundy SA, Sabeur K, and Liu IK. 2008. Expression of anti-Mullerian hormone (AMH) in equine granulosa-cell tumors and in normal equine ovaries. Theriogenology, 70(6): 968–977 available from: PM:18599114.

Chavatte-Palmer P, Duchamp G, Palmer E, Ousey JC, Rossdale PD, and Lombes M. 2000. Progesterone, oestrogen and glucocorticoid receptors in the uterus and mammary glands of mares from mid- to late gestation. J Reprod Fertil Suppl, (56): 661–672 available from: PM:20681182.

Claes A, Ball BA, Almeida J, Corbin CJ, and Conley AJ. 2013a. Serum anti-Mullerian hormone concentrations in stallions: developmental changes, seasonal variation, and differences between intact stallions, cryptorchid stallions, and geldings. Theriogenology, 79(9): 1229–1235 available from: PM:23591325.

Claes A, Ball BA, Corbin CJ, and Conley AJ. 2013b. Age and season affect serum testosterone concentrations in cryptorchid stallions. Vet Rec, 173(7): 168 available from: PM:23812112.

Cox JE, Redhead PH, and Dawson FE. 1986. Comparison of the measurement of plasma testosterone and plasma oestrogens for the diagnosis of cryptorchidism in the horse. Equine Vet J, 18(3): 179–182 available from: PM:2874021.

Cox JE, Williams JH, Rowe PH, and Smith JA. 1973. Testosterone in normal, cryptorchid and castrated male horses. Equine Vet J, 5(2): 85–90 available from: PM:4151406.

Ellenberger C, Bartmann CP, Hoppen HO, Kratzsch J, Aupperle H, Klug E, et al. 2007. Histomorphological and immunohistochemical characterization of equine granulosa cell tumours. J Comp Pathol, 136(2–3): 167–176 available from: PM:17416235.

Ganjam VK and Kenney RM. 1975. Androgens and oestrogens in normal and cryptorchid stallions. J Reprod Fertil Suppl, (23): 67–73 available from: PM:1530.

Ganjam VK, Kenney RM, and Flickinger G. 1975. Effect of exogenous progesterone on its endogenous levels: biological half-life of progesterone and lack of progesterone binding in mares. J Reprod Fertil Suppl, (23): 183–188 available from: PM:1060775.

Ginther, OJ, Utt MD, and Beg MA. 2007. Follicle deviation and diurnal variation in circulating hormone concentrations in mares. Anim Reprod Sci, 100(1–2): 197–203 available from: PM:17000062.

Holtan DW, Houghton E, Silver M, Fowden AL, Ousey J, and Rossdale PD. 1991. Plasma progestagens in the mare, fetus and newborn foal. J Reprod Fertil Suppl, 44: 517–528 available from: PM:1795295.

Jewgenow K and Meyer HH. 1998. Comparative binding affinity study of progestins to the cytosol progestin receptor of endometrium in different mammals. Gen Comp Endocrinol, 110(2): 118–124 available from: PM:9570932.

McCue PM, Roser JF, Munro CJ, Liu IK, and Lasley BL. 2006. Granulosa cell tumors of the equine ovary. Vet Clin N Am-Equine Pract, 22(3): 799–817 available from: PM:17129804.

McDonnell SM and Murray SC. 1995. Bachelor and harem stallion behavior and endocrinology. Biol Rep Mon, 1: 577–590.

McKinnon AO, Squires EL, Carnevale EM, and Hermenet MJ. 1988. Ovariectomized steroid-treated mares as embryo transfer recipients and as a model to study the role of progestins in pregnancy maintenance. Theriogenology, 29(5): 1055–1063 available from: PM:16726427.

Miller S, Wongprasartsuk S, Young IR, Wlodek ME, McFarlane JR, De Kretser DM, and Jenkin G. 1997. Source of inhibin in ovine fetal plasma and amniotic fluid during late gestation: half-life of fetal inhibin. Biol Reprod, 57(2): 347–353 available from: PM:9241049.

Neto AC, Ball BA, Browne P, and Conley AJ. 2010. Cellular localization of androgen synthesis in equine granulosa-theca cell tumors: immunohistochemical expression of 17alpha-hydroxylase/17,20-lyase cytochrome P450. Theriogenology, 74(3): 393–401 available from: PM:20416939.

Parleviet JM, Bevers MM, van de Broek J, and Colenbrander B. 2001. Effect of GnRH and hCG administration in plasma LH and testosterone concentrations in normal stallions, aged stallions and stallions with lack of libido. Vet Quarter, 23(2): 84–87.

Roser JF. 1995. Endocrine profiles in fertile, subfertile and infertile stallions: testicular response to human chorionic gonadotropin in infertile stallions. Biol Repr Mon, 1: 661–669.

Roser JF, McCue PM, and Hoye E. 1994. Inhibin activity in the mare and stallion. Domest Anim Endocrinol, 11(1): 87–100 available from: PM:8124933.

Scholtz EL, Krishnan S, Ball BA, Corbin CJ, Moeller BC, Stanley SD, et al. 2014. Pregnancy without progesterone in horses defines a second endogenous biopotent progesterone receptor agonist, 5alpha-dihydroprogesterone. Proc Natl Acad Sci USA, available from: PM:24550466.

Shideler RK, Squires EL, Voss JL, Eikenberry DJ, and Pickett BW. 1982. Progestagen therapy of ovariectomized pregnant mares. J Reprod Fertil Suppl, 32: 459–464 available from: PM:6962883.

Silberzahn P, Pouret EJ, and Zwain I. 1989. Androgen and oestrogen response to a single injection of hCG in cryptorchid horses. Equine Vet J, 21(2): 126–129 available from: PM:2565228.

Vanderwall DK, Marquardt JL, and Woods GL. 2007. Use of a compounded long-acting progesterone formulation for equine pregnancy maintenance. J Eq Vet Sci, 27(2): 62–66.

Villani M, Cairoli F, Kindahl H, Galeati G, Faustini M, Carluccio A, and Veronesi MC. 2006. Effects of mating on plasma concentrations of testosterone, cortisol, oestrone sulfate and 15-ketodihydro-PGF2alpha in stallions. Reprod Domest Anim, 41(6): 544–548 available from: PM:17107515.

62

Foaling Predictor Tests

Ghislaine A. Dujovne[1] and Camilla. J. Scott[2]

[1] Department of Population Health Reproduction, School of Veterinary Medicine, University of California, California, USA
[2] William R. Pritchard Veterinary Medical Teaching Hospital, School of Veterinary Medicine, University of California, California, USA

62.1 Clinical Background

62.1.1 Key Points

No single foaling predictor test is 100% effective, but the use of these tests in conjunction with observation of physical signs and historical data gives us a good indication of the time of foaling. In the following are some key points that justify the use of specific tests as an aid to predict foaling in mares.

- Gestational length can vary greatly, ranging from 330–360 days (315–350 days for pony mares). Most mares will have similar gestational lengths from year to year so historical data in multiparous mares may help, but other factors such as day length can induce variation. For example, mares that are due to foal during short daylight hours are likely to have a longer gestation than mares due to foal during long daylight hours (McKinnon et al., 2011).
- Most mares foal at night (86% between 10 pm and 2 am), which makes it harder to have assistance at parturition (Rossdale and Short, 1967).
- Maiden mares may not show any of the typical signs of impending parturition and mares with placentitis or other causes of precocious mammary development often have early elevations in mammary calcium secretions.
- Foaling predictor tests are an aid in foaling management, no test claims to be 100% accurate.
- Foaling predictor tests enable evaluation of mares' readiness for spontaneous foaling and the extent of *in utero* fetal maturation.
- Individual variability between mares is great and predictability is unreliable.

62.1.2 Physical Signs of Impending Parturition

- Udder enlargement (typically in the last 2 weeks of gestation).
- Waxing on the teat ends (typically in the last 2 days of gestation).
- Changes in the quality of the mammary secretions from a watery straw-colored secretion to a thick honey-colored viscous secretion consistent with colostrum.
- Relaxation of the sacrosciatic ligaments of the tail head and gluteal muscle mass.
- Elongation of the vulvar lips.
- Changes in behavior such as restlessness, pacing, and intermittent rolling.

62.2 Tests Available

- Measurement of the components of mammary secretions pre-partum:
  - Most tests measure elevations in calcium carbonate in mammary secretions, numerous reports have shown calcium to rise rapidly in the mammary secretions of the prepartum mare (McKinnon et al., 2011).
  - Other changes seen in the mammary secretions include increased concentrations of potassium, calcium, citrate, and lactose and decreased concentrations of sodium (Douglas et al., 2002).
  - Inversion of the Na:K ratio in the secretions typically occurs 24–36 h prior to foaling with potassium concentrations becoming greater than sodium in the last few days of gestation (Peaker et al., 1979).
  - Precise measurement of electrolytes in mammary secretion requires a flame espectrophotometer or a laboratory chemistry analyzer. Using these systems, elevation of calcium above 40 mg/dL and potassium levels greater than sodium generally indicates fetal maturity in a normal equine pregnancy.

Interpretation of Equine Laboratory Diagnostics, First Edition. Edited by Nicola Pusterla and Jill Higgins.
© 2018 John Wiley & Sons, Inc. Published 2018 by John Wiley & Sons, Inc.

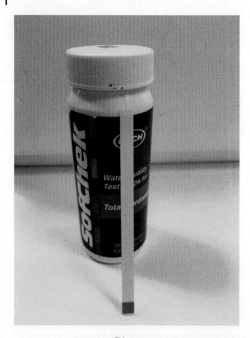

Figure 62.1 SofCheck™ test strips showing color change correlated to calcium levels from 0 ppm to 425 ppm.

This method is impractical for field veterinarians as most electrolyte changes happen late in the day and therefore sampling should be performed in the late afternoon or early evening (McKinnon et al., 2011, Ousey et al., 1984, Peaker et al., 1979, Leadon et al., 1984). An ionic score can also be calculated with greater than 35 points indicating a readiness for foaling (Ousey et al., 1984).

- Several stall-side tests are available; most of them are modified from water hardness tests (Figure 62.1). Some of these tests measure both divalent cations (Ca and Mg), which complicate their interpretation because the secretion of magnesium increases earlier than calcium and decreases before parturition (Table 62.1).

- It has been well established that 10 mmol/L (400 ppm) of calcium is a good indicator that the mare is ready to foal. (Ousey et al., 1984, Peaker et al., 1979, Leadon et al., 1984).

- Calcium in milk is not in the form of calcium carbonate; therefore, results from tests that measure calcium carbonate need to be converted to calcium for correct interpretation. To convert ppm of calcium carbonate to ppm of calcium (ppm = mmol × molecular weight), results should be divided by 2.5 because the molecular weight of calcium carbonate is 100 and the molecular weight of calcium is 40 (100/2.5 = 40).

- To prevent misinterpretation in water hardness tests for measuring calcium carbonate (i.e., Titrets; Chemetrics, Calvetron, VA) the dilution factor needs to be taken in consideration as well as the conversion from calcium carbonate to calcium. In the case of Foal Watch (CHEMetrics Inc., Calverton, VA) the dilution ratio used is 1:6, if we correct for dilution and convert 200 ppm calcium carbonate to calcium the real calcium value is 480 ppm, consistent with values described for foaling readiness. During routine use for foaling prediction these calculations are not necessary if you follow the packet insert for interpretation of each individual test, see next (McKinnon et al., 2011).

- The pH of the mammary secretion can also be determined using a portable pH device with a semi-micro electrode or pH paper (Figure 62.2). Canisso et al. (2013) suggests a 79% chance of foaling within 24 h when the pH drops below 7.0.

Table 62.1 Available stall-side tests.

Test kit	Type of test	Time of foaling	Advantages	Disadvantages
FoalWatch™ test kit (CHEMetrics Inc, Calverton, VA)	In house; Detects changes in Ca via titration	Ca <200 ppm = 99% probability that foaling will not occur in next 24 h Ca >200 ppm = 97% probability of foaling in 72 h *uncorrected values	Accurate Repeatable Quantitative Immediate results	More expensive and time consuming than other tests
Predict-A-Foal™ Test Mare Foaling predictor Kit (Animal Health Care Products, Vernon, CA)	Ca test, match strip to 5 squares, color bar changes	% Possibility of foaling in next 12 h No change/1 square = 1% 2 squares = 10% 3 squares = 40% 4/5 squares = 80%	Fast and easy Immediate results	More expensive than other semi-quantitative tests
SofCheck™ (Hatch Company, Loveland, CO) Company	PO Box 389, Loveland, CO	Water hardness test (ppm)	53% chance of foaling once levels of 250 ppm reached	Cheap Easy	Less reliable than other tests
pH paper	pH of mammary secretion	79% chance of foaling within 24 h once pH <7.0	Cheap Easy	Less reliable than other tests

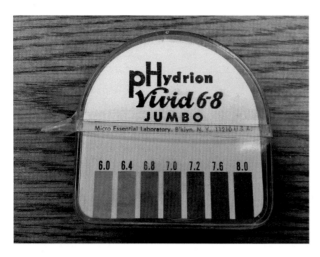

Figure 62.2 pH paper.

62.3 Sample Collection and Submission for FoalWatch™ Test Kit (CHEMetrics Inc., Calverton, VA)

- Start testing mammary secretions 10–14 d prior to the mare's due date or following signs of mammary development.
- Test in the late afternoon or early evening. Samples taken in the morning may be low and not reflect electrolyte changes, which are often seen in the evening or night.

- Follow the instructions provided with the kit carefully.
- Clean and dry the udder and teats prior to collecting a sample.
- Strip 2–5 ml total of mammary secretions from each teat into a clean sampling cup (provided with the kit).
- Draw up exactly 1.5 ml of mammary secretions using the syringe provided and place into the mixing vial.
- Add exactly 9 ml of distilled water to produce a 1:6 dilution and mix well.
- Add 1 drop of the indicator dye to the diluted sample and mix again.
- Attach the valve assembly over the glass titrettor and break the tip of the glass titret at the black line.
- Lift the control bar of the titrettor and insert the assembled titrettor into the body.
- Immerse the tip of the glass titret into the sample and press the control bar briefly to pull a small volume of sample into the titret.
- The fluid within the chamber will change color from orange to pink (Figure 62.3).
- Press the control bar briefly again to add more sample to the tube.
- After each addition of sample gently invert the entire titrettor and monitor for color change from orange to blue (Figure 62.3).
- Once the desired color change is achieved invert the glass titret chamber and read the titret scale.
- The units on the glass titret are calibrated to parts per million (ppm) of calcium carbonate.

Figure 62.3 FoalWatch™ Kit displaying color change from clear to orange to blue.

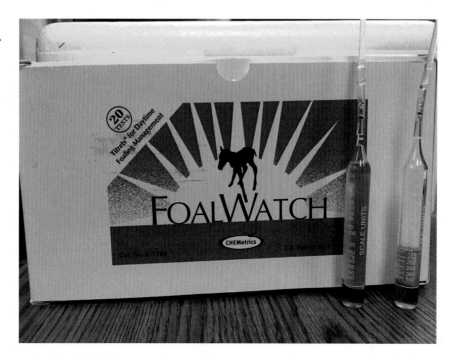

62.4 Interpretation of Test Results- Sensitivity, Specificity, and Positive Predictive Values of Measuring Calcium Carbonate in a Mare's Prepartum Mammary Secretions

- When prefoaling mammary secretions are less than 200 ppm (Ley at al., 1993):
  - 99% probability that foaling will not occur in the next 24 h
- When prefoaling mammary secretions exceed 200 ppm:
  - 51% probability of spontaneous foaling within the next 24 h
  - 84% probability of spontaneous foaling within the next 48 h
  - 97% probability of spontaneous foaling within the next 72 h
- Most mares foal within a short period of time once values of 300–500 ppm are obtained (see case example in Section 62.5).

62.5 Case Example

A 5-year-old maiden Warmblood mare presented at 320 days gestation for foal watch. Serial mammary gland secretions were testing using the FoalWatch™ test kit

Table 62.2 Case example calcium test results.

Gestation length (days)	Calcium level (ppm) *uncorrected values
320	175
321	200
322	225
323	200
324	225
325	240
326	260
327	340
328	Foaled

(CHEMetrics Inc., Calverton, VA) until foaling at 328 days gestation, the results in Table 62.2 were obtained.

Please note the fall from 225 ppm to 200 ppm from 322 days gestation to 323 days, in most cases this is just a normal biological variation but it is advisable to repeat the test to ensure accuracy in the testing method if unexpected values are obtained. Please also note the significant rise over the 24-h period from 326 to 327 days gestation that occurred 24-h prepartum. A rise such as this is often a good indicator of the mare approaching readiness for birth.

References

Canisso IF, Ball BA, Troedsson MH, et al. 2013. Decreasing pH of mammary gland secretions predict foaling and are correlated with electrolyte concentrations in prefoaling mares. Proceedings of the 59th Annual Convention of the American Association of Equine Practitioners- AAEP - December 7–11, Nashville, TN, USA.

Douglas CGB, Perkins NR, Stafford KJ, and Hedderley DI. 2002. Predicting of foaling using mammary secretion constituents. NZ Vet J, 50: 99–103.

Leadon DP, Jeffcott LB, and Rossdale PD. 1984. Mammary secretions in spontaneous and induced premature parturition in the mare Equine Vet J, 16: 256–259.

Ley WB, Bowen JM, Purswell BJ, et al. 1993. The sensitivity, specificity and predictive value of measuring calcium

carbonate in mares' prepartum mammary secretions. Theriogenology 40: 189–198.

McKinnon AO, Squires EL, Vaala WE, et al. 2011. Equine Reproduction, 2nd Edn, Chichester, UK: Wiley- Blackwell, Vol. 2.

Ousey JC, Dudan F, and Rossdale PD 1984. Preliminary studies of mammary secretions in the mare to assess foetal readiness for birth. Equine Vet J, 16: 259–263.

Peaker M, Rossdale PD, Forsyth IA, et al. 1979. Changes in mammary development and composition of secretion during late pregnancy in the mare. J Repro Fertil Suppl, (8): 555–561.

Rossdale PD, and Short RV. 1967. The time of foaling in thoroughbred mares. J Repro Fertil, 13: 341–343.

Index

Interpretation of Equine Laboratory Diagnostics, First Edition. Edited by Nicola Pusterla and Jill Higgins.
© 2018 John Wiley & Sons, Inc. Published 2018 by John Wiley & Sons, Inc.